SHELF-LIFE PEDIATRICS

SHELF-LIFE PEDIATRICS

Editors

Sonali Mehta Patel, MD, FAAP
Assistant Professor of Clinical Pediatrics
Rosalind Franklin University of Medicine
Associate Program Director
Pediatric Residency Program
Advocate Children's Hospital
Oak Lawn, Illinois

Kent Nelson, MD, FAAP
Lecturer of Clinical Pediatrics
Rosalind Franklin University of Medicine
Informatics Director
Pediatric Residency Program
Advocate Children's Hospital
Oak Lawn, Illinois

Stephanie R. Jennings, MD, FAAP
Associate Program Director
Pediatric Residency Program
Inpatient Director, Pediatrics
Advocate Children's Hospital
Oak Lawn, Illinois

Series Editors

Veeral Sudhakar Sheth, MD, FACS
Director, Scientific Affairs
University Retina and Macula Associates
Clinical Assistant Professor
University of Illinois at Chicago
Chicago, Illinois

Stanley Zaslau, MD, MBA, FACS
Professor and Chief
Urology Residency Program Director
Department of Surgery/Division of Urology
West Virginia University
Morgantown, West Virginia

Robert Casanova, MD
Assistant Dean of Clinical Sciences Curriculum
Associate Professor Obstetrics and Gynecology
Texas Tech University Health Sciences Center
Lubbock, Texas

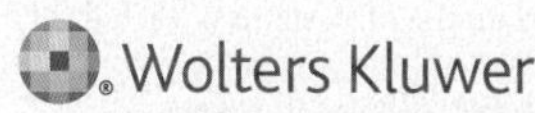

Health
Philadelphia • Baltimore • New York • London
Buenos Aires • Hong Kong • Sydney • Tokyo

Acquisitions Editor: Tari Broderick
Product Manager: Jenn Verbiar
Marketing Manager: Joy Fisher-Williams
Production Project Manager: Alicia Jackson
Designer: Stephen Druding
Compositor: Integra Software Services Pvt. Ltd.

351 West Camden Street
Baltimore, MD 21201

Two Commerce Square
2001 Market Street
Philadelphia, PA 19103

Printed in China

9 8 7 6 5 4 3 2 1

Library of Congress Cataloging-in-Publication Data
Shelf-life pediatrics/editors, Sonali Mehta Patel, Kent Nelson, Stephanie R. Jennings.
p. ; cm.
Includes index.
ISBN 978-1-4511-8957-5
I. Patel, Sonali Mehta, editor of compilation. II. Nelson, Kent, editor of compilation.
III. Jennings, Stephanie R., editor of compilation.
[DNLM: 1. Pediatrics—Problems and Exercises. WS 18.2]
RJ48.2
618.9200076—dc23
2013046934

To purchase additional copies of this book, call our customer service department at **(800) 638-3030** or fax orders to **(301) 223-2320**. International customers should call **(301) 223-2300.**

Visit Lippincott Williams & Wilkins on the Internet: http://www.lww.com. Lippincott Williams & Wilkins customer service representatives are available from 8:30 am to 6:00 pm, EST.

CCS0114

Contributors

Caitlin J. Agrawal, MD
Pediatric Hematology/Oncology Fellow
Department of Hematology/Oncology
Nationwide Children's Hospital
Columbus, Ohio

Tara Altepeter, MD
Pediatric Gastroenterology Fellow
Division of Pediatric Gastroenterology
Department of Pediatrics
Thomas Jefferson University
Philadelphia, Pennsylvania
Alfred I duPont Hospital for Children
Wilmington, Delaware

Joana Benayoun, MD
Attending Pediatrician
Atlanta, Georgia

Harit K. Bhatt, MD
University Retina and Macula Associates
Bedford Park, Illinois
Clinical Assistant Professor
Department of Ophthalmology & Visual Sciences
University of Illinois at Chicago
Chicago, Illinois

Diana C. Bottari, DO
Medical Director, Pediatric Pain and Sedation Services
Pediatric Pain Specialist
Pediatric Sedationist
Advocate Children's Hospital
Oak Lawn, Illinois

Mark M. Butterly, MD
Director Pediatric Residency Program
Department of Pediatrics
Advocate Children's Hospital
Oak Lawn, Illinois

Heather Dyer, MD
Instructor of Clinical Pediatrics
Rosalind Franklin University of Medicine & Science
North Chicago, Illinois
Director, Pediatric Hospitalist Program
Department of Pediatrics
Advocate Children's Hospital
Oak Lawn, Illinois

Corrie E. Fletcher, DO
Chief Resident, Pediatric Residency Program
Department of Pediatrics
Advocate Children's Hospital
Oak Lawn, Illinois

Rama D. Jager, MD, FACS
University Retina and Macula Associates
Oak Forest, Illinois
Clinical Professor
Department of Ophthalmology & Visual Sciences
University of Illinois at Chicago
Chicago, Illinois

Stephanie R. Jennings, MD, FAAP
Associate Program Director
Pediatric Residency Program
Inpatient Director, Pediatrics
Advocate Children's Hospital
Oak Lawn, Illinois

Nicole Keller, DO
Attending Physician
Department of Pediatrics
Advocate Children's Hospital
Oak Lawn, Illinois

Jason Mitchell, MD
Attending Physician
Division of Pediatric Cardiology
Department of Pediatric Subspecialties
Mid-Atlantic Permanente Medical Group
Washington, D.C.

Kent Nelson, MD
Assistant Professor of Clinical Pediatrics
Rosalind Franklin University of Medicine & Science
North Chicago, Illinois
Informatics Director, Pediatric Residency Program
Department of Pediatrics
Advocate Children's Hospital
Oak Lawn, Illinois

Patricia M. Notario, MD
Chief Resident, Pediatric Residency Program
Department of Pediatrics
Advocate Children's Hospital
Oak Lawn, Illinois

Rinku Patel, DO
Lecturer of Clinical Pediatrics
Rosalind Franklin University of Medicine and Science
North Chicago, Illinois
Academic Pediatric Hospitalist
Department of Pediatrics
Advocate Children's Hospital
Oak Lawn, Illinois

Sonali Mehta Patel, MD
Assistant Professor of Clinical Pediatrics
Rosalind Franklin University of Medicine and Science
North Chicago, Illinois
Associate Director, Pediatric Residency Program
Department of Pediatrics
Advocate Children's Hospital
Oak Lawn, Illinois

Nikita Williamson, MD
Academic Pediatric Hospitalist
Department of Pediatrics
Advocate Children's Hospital
Oak Lawn, Illinois

Introduction to the Shelf-Life Series

The Shelf-Life series is an entirely new concept. The books have been designed from the ground up with student input. With academic faculty helping guide the production of these books, the Shelf-Life series is meant to help supplement the student's educational experience while on clinical rotation as well as prepare the student for the end-of-rotation shelf-exam. We feel you will find these question books challenging but an irreplaceable part of the clinical rotation. With high-quality, up-to-date content and hundreds of images and tables, this resource will be something you will continue to refer to even after you have completed your rotation.

The series editors would like to thank Susan Rhyner for supporting this concept from its inception. We would like to express our appreciation to Catherine Noonan, Laura Blyton, Amanda Ingold, Ashley Fischer, Tari Broderick and Stacey Sebring, all of whom have been integral parts of the publishing team; their project management has been invaluable.

Veeral S. Sheth, MD, FACS
Stanley Zaslau, MD, MBA, FACS
Robert Casanova, MD

Acknowledgments

We would like to dedicate this book to all our medical students and the patients we serve. Without them the knowledge, guidance, and feedback to make this book would not have been possible. We would like to specifically thank, Dr. Savannah Ross, for her feedback as a medical student and future pediatrician on the construct, design, and information presented within this book. We are forever thankful to our many colleagues who helped author each chapter and each other for endless support along the way. Lastly, we would like to thank our families for their support and patience.

Stephanie R. Jennings, MD, FAAP
Kent Nelson, MD, FAAP
Sonali Mehta Patel, MD, FAAP

Contents

CHAPTER

1

General Pediatrics

NIKITA WILLIAMSON

1 A 6-month-old infant comes to clinic for her 6-month health maintenance visit. Her weight is at the 75th percentile and her height is at the 90th percentile. The child sits with assistance, rolls from prone to supine, and says "dada." The parents ask whether it is safe to place the baby in a front-facing car seat due to her size.

Of the following, what is the best advice to give these parents regarding car seat safety?

(A) Children should not be placed in a front-facing car seat until they are ≥24 months old
(B) Due to her size, she should be placed in a booster seat
(C) Car safety seat should face forward until the infant is 1 year old
(D) Car safety seat could be placed in the front seat as long as the vehicle is equipped with passenger-side airbags
(E) It is acceptable to use only the lap belt for restraint

The answer is A: Children should not be placed in a front-facing car seat until they are ≥24 months old. Car seat safety is a very important part of pediatric anticipatory guidance. Every infant should be secured in a rear-facing car seat whenever riding in a moving vehicle. **(C)** Children aged 0 to 24 months old should use rear-facing infant-only car seats or rear-facing convertible car seats. Children aged ≥24 months old can be placed in a convertible or forward-facing harness car seat. **(B)** Children aged 4 to 12 years, weighing ≥40 to 80 lb (18 to 36 kg), and shorter than 4' 9" (1.4 m) should be placed in a belt-positioning booster seat. **(D)** An infant car seat should never be placed in a seat equipped with airbags including front passenger-side and side-impact airbags. **(E)** The use of lap belts alone has been associated with a marked rise in seatbelt-related injuries.

2 At what ages is it recommended to routinely administer the DTaP (diphtheria, tetanus, and acellular pertussis) vaccine?

(A) 2, 4, 6, and 12 to 15 months
(B) 2, 4, 6, 15 to 18 months, and 4 to 6 years
(C) 12 months and 4 to 6 years
(D) Birth, 2, and 6 to 18 months
(E) 2, 4, and 6 months

The answer is B: 2, 4, 6, 15 to 18 months, and 4 to 6 years. The administration of the DTaP vaccine is routinely recommended at the following ages: 2 months, 4 months, 6 months, between 15 and 18 months, and between 4 and 6 years of age. The minimum age for administration of the first dose in this series is 6 weeks. The minimum interval between the second and third doses is 4 weeks and 6 months should pass between the third and fourth doses. The minimum age for the fifth dose is 4 years.

(A) Pneumococcal vaccine (13-valent) is recommended to be given at 2, 4, 6, and between 12 and 15 months. **(C)** The measles, mumps, and rubella and varicella vaccines are recommended at 12 months and between 4 and 6 years of age. **(D)** It is recommended to providers to give the hepatitis B vaccine prior to the infant's leaving the hospital (birth), at 2 months, and then between 6 and 18 months of age. The first and the last doses of the hepatitis B vaccine should be at least 6 months apart. **(E)** The rotavirus vaccine is a live oral vaccine commercially available in two different formulations. Both formulations are recommended to be given at 2 and 4 months of age. One of the formulations requires an additional dose at 6 months of age.

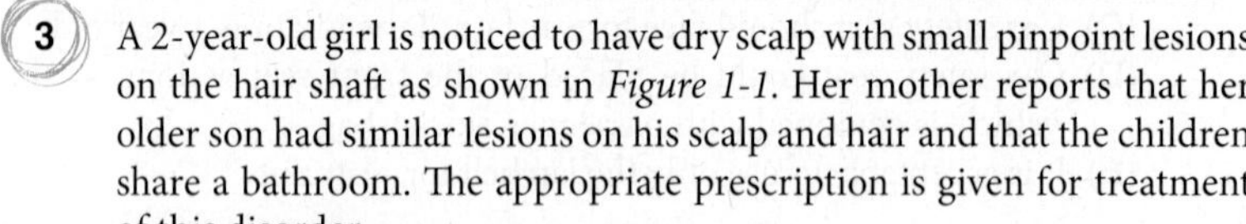

3 A 2-year-old girl is noticed to have dry scalp with small pinpoint lesions on the hair shaft as shown in *Figure 1-1*. Her mother reports that her older son had similar lesions on his scalp and hair and that the children share a bathroom. The appropriate prescription is given for treatment of this disorder.

Of the following, what is the most appropriate additional advice regarding this treatment?

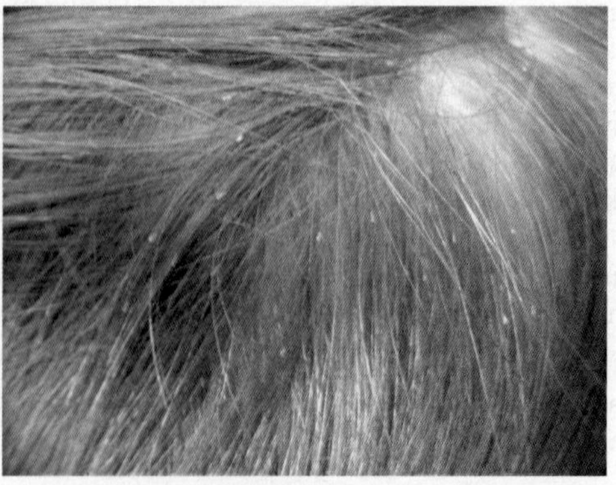

Figure 1-1

(A) Treatment should be applied only once
(B) Children cannot return to school for 2 weeks to ensure complete resolution of symptoms
(C) Apply the permethrin 5% cream from the neck to the toe
(D) Wash all clothing and linen in very hot water
(E) Apply lindane 1% cream to scalp

The answer is D: Wash all clothing and linen in very hot water. The child in the vignette has head lice infestation. There are three types of lice that affect humans: head louse (*Pediculosis capitis*), body louse (*Pediculosis corporis*), and pubic louse (*Pediculosis pubis*). Head lice can be transmitted from person to person by direct casual contact. Lice can easily be spread when children play together; share combs, headphones, towels, and bedding; and from articles of clothing. Symptoms usually include itchy, irritated, and dry scalp. The irritation is caused by a reaction from the lice saliva, which is injected into the skin while they feed. Diagnosis of lice is by examination of the scalp and hair. Whitish-gray insects are noticeable as well as eggs, or nits, that attach to the base of the hair shaft near the scalp. In children older than 2 years, topical, over-the-counter pediculicides can be used. The treatment of choice is permethrin 5% given its safety and improved efficacy as compared to lindane. **(E)** Lindane is not recommended because of resistance and its association with neurotoxicity. **(C)** Permethrin cream should be applied to dry hair only and left on for 12 hours. **(A)** A second application may be applied 7 to 9 days after the initial application. Neck to toe application is recommended if the child in the vignette had scabies. All household members should be treated at the same time regardless of symptoms. Nits should be removed with a fine-toothed comb after application of therapy. Brushes and combs should be discarded or cleaned in boiling water and advised to not share between family members. All clothing and bed linen should be dry cleaned or laundered in very hot water. **(B)** Children with head lice may return to school after the initial treatment has been completed.

4 An 18-month-old girl presents to the emergency department with complaints of irritability, inconsolable crying, fever, chills, and flushed skin. Her mother reports that the baby is teething and that she is giving acetaminophen and diphenhydramine every night for her fever and to help her sleep. She denies any previous illnesses or sick contacts but reports an older brother with attention-deficit hyperactivity disorder (ADHD). Her mother reports a dry diaper for the past 12 hours. Vital signs on presentation are temperature 39.7°C, pulse 150 beats per minute, respiratory rate 40 breaths per minute, and blood pressure 130/90 mmHg. On examination, she is inconsolable. Her skin is red and dry and her pupils are dilated but sluggish.

Of the following, which is the most likely cause of this infant's symptoms?

(A) Acetaminophen overdose
(B) Diphenhydramine overdose
(C) Meningitis
(D) Methylphenidate toxicity
(E) Dehydration

The answer is B: Diphenhydramine overdose. The patient in the vignette is experiencing symptoms consistent with anticholinergic toxicity secondary to antihistamine overdose. Classes of medications with anticholinergic properties include antihistamines (diphenhydramine), tricyclic antidepressants (amitriptyline), sleep aids (doxylamine), muscle relaxants (cyclobenzaprine), cold preparations (scopolamine), jimson weed, and belladonna alkaloids (glycopyrrolate). Anticholinergic medications block the action of acetylcholine by competitively binding to and blocking muscarinic receptors on the postganglionic cholinergic nerves. As a result, each organ system experiences a parasympathetic response. Clinical manifestations from anticholinergic toxicity include thirst, dry mucous membranes, warm and dry skin from inhibition of secretions from the salivary and sweat glands, flushed skin from dilatation of cutaneous blood vessels, fever from the inability to sweat, mydriasis (dilated pupils) with poor pupillary response, tachycardia, urinary retention, hypertension, decreased bowel sounds from inhibition of gastrointestinal motility, confusion and hallucinations, seizures, and coma. Tachycardia is the earliest and most reliable sign of anticholinergic toxicity. Treatment for anticholinergic toxicity includes supportive care, early decontamination, and antidotal therapy with physostigmine.

(A) Acetaminophen overdose is one of the most common poisonings worldwide. Children present with abdominal pain, diarrhea, irritability, nausea, vomiting, sweating, jaundice, and convulsions. Acetaminophen toxicity can cause serious liver damage requiring the need for a liver transplant. **(C)** In children with high fevers and history of recent illnesses or sick contacts, organic processes such as meningitis and sepsis should also be considered. **(D)** Sympathomimetic overdose (methylphenidate) can also mimic anticholinergic overdose with the presence of agitation, tachycardia, dilated pupils, and hyperthermia. Sweating and increased bowel sounds are hallmarks of sympathomimetic toxicity, whereas with anticholinergic toxicity there are decreased bowel sounds and lack of sweat. **(E)** Dehydration should be considered in a patient with dry mucous membranes, dry skin, and decreased urination; however, this is a less likely diagnosis given the history and physical findings of the patient in the vignette.

Of the following, which is a contraindication to giving the human papillomavirus (HPV) vaccine to adolescents?

(A) Breastfeeding mothers
(B) Positive HPV on Papanicolaou smear
(C) Immunocompetent patient
(D) Previous sexual exposure to genital warts
(E) Pregnant adolescents

The answer is E: **Pregnant adolescents.** HPV vaccine is a quadrivalent vaccine that protects individuals from HPV types 6, 11, 16, and 18. These types lead to various cancers including cervical, vulvar, vaginal, anal, and penile cancers. Immunizations are recommended for girls and boys aged 9 through 26 years old. The vaccine is administered as a three-injection series. The first and last doses must be given at least 6 months apart and the second dose is given at least 2 months after the initial dose. Individuals with life-threatening allergic reactions to any component of the HPV vaccine or to a previous dose of HPV vaccine should not receive the vaccine. **(A)** This vaccine is not recommended for pregnant women; however, breastfeeding mothers are able to safely receive it. **(B, C, D)** Previously positive HPV results on Papanicolaou smear, healthy individuals (immunocompetent), and recent exposure to genital warts are not contraindications to receiving the vaccine.

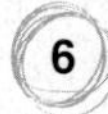

6 Of the following, which group of children should be identified and referred for early dental evaluation and preventative care?

(A) Premature infants
(B) Children with milk protein allergy
(C) Children who are thumb suckers
(D) Children with passive tobacco smoke exposure
(E) Children with a family history of dental caries

The answer is D: **Children with passive tobacco smoke exposure.** Because of the increased risk of development of dental caries and other oral health problems, children with the following risk factors should be referred for early dental evaluation, preventative care, and counseling:

- Prolonged breast or bottle feeding >12 months
- Exposure to maternal and passive tobacco smoke
- Frequent intake of sugary drinks and snacks
- Prolonged use of a training cup (sippy cup)
- Bottle use at bedtime
- Longer than 3-week use of liquid medication (teeth staining)
- Insufficient fluoride exposure
- Notable plaque on upper front teeth
- Enamel defects
- Children with special health-care needs

(A, B, C, E) The rest of the conditions should still have a formal dental evaluation at 1 year, but do not require earlier evaluation.

7 A sophomore in high school plans to participate in a Peace Corp project to Central Africa.

Of the following, which is the preferred chemoprophylactic therapy for malaria prior to her travel?

(A) Chloroquine
(B) Atovaquone–proguanil
(C) Primaquine phosphate
(D) Levofloxacin
(E) No prophylaxis indicated

The answer is B: Atovaquone–proguanil. Malaria is the most important preventable life-threatening, insect-borne illness that affects international travelers. Malaria is transmitted by the *Anopheles* mosquito and produces symptoms such as high fever, shaking chills, and flu-like illness. There are four species of *Plasmodium* that cause malaria: *P. falciparum*, *P. malariae*, *P. ovale*, and *P. vivax*. *P. falciparum* is the predominant species in Africa and Haiti, and it is the cause of the majority of fatalities in these regions. Although malaria can be fatal, morbidity and mortality can usually be prevented. Preventive measures include avoiding mosquito bites and maintaining antimalarial chemoprophylaxis when traveling. The Centers for Disease Control provides up-to-date listings of regions where malaria transmission occurs, the regions where antimalarial drug resistance is prevalent, and chemoprophylaxis recommendations for each specific region. Chemoprophylaxis should begin days to weeks prior to arrival to the endemic area depending on the recommended medication. Mefloquine should be initiated at least 2 weeks before arrival; chloroquine should be given 1 week prior; and both doxycycline and atovaquone–proguanil should be started 1 to 2 days prior to arrival. Therapy should be taken throughout the exposure time and continued 1 to 4 weeks after departure.

(E) The student in the vignette is traveling to Central Africa where malaria is highly prevalent and prophylaxis is highly recommended. *P. falciparum* accounts for a high majority of cases and this region has a high rate of chloroquine resistance, so the listed drug of choice for prophylaxis in this student is atovaquone–proguanil. **(A)** Chloroquine is not adequate therapy because of the high incidence of resistance. **(C)** Primaquine is recommended for prophylaxis in areas mostly exposed to *P. vivax*. Primaquine can cause hemolytic anemia in persons with glucose-6-phospate dehydrogenase deficiency; thus, patients must be screened prior to starting this medication. **(D)** Levofloxacin is a quinolone used to treat bacterial infections and has no role in malarial prophylaxis or treatment.

8 A 4-month-old infant is seen in the clinic because her mother reports that she is fussy and has a decreased appetite. She denies fevers. The child has tacky mucous membranes, mild erythema in the oropharynx, and white plaques inside her cheeks and on her hard palate.

Of the following, which is the best therapy for this condition?

(A) Acyclovir
(B) Viscous lidocaine
(C) Amoxicillin
(D) Nystatin suspension
(E) Acetaminophen

The answer is D: Nystatin suspension. The infant in the vignette has findings consistent with oral thrush. Oral thrush is a common infection of the mucus membranes affecting normal newborns. *Candida albicans* is the most common species found in thrush plaques. This infection is characterized by white, curd-like patches on the tongue, palate, and buccal mucosa. Oral thrush may be asymptomatic or can cause pain, fussiness, and decreased feeding leading to dehydration. Thrush is uncommon in immunocompetent children after 1 year of age although it can occur in children treated with antibiotics or inhaled corticosteroids without the use of a spacer. Persistent or recurrent thrush without explanation warrants further investigation for an underlying immunodeficiency. Oral nystatin is the first-line treatment of choice in children with uncomplicated thrush.

(A) Acyclovir is a treatment for herpes simplex virus. **(B)** Viscous lidocaine is not recommended for infants or young children due to the potential for swallowing and systemic absorption. **(C)** Amoxicillin is an antibiotic used to treat bacterial rather than fungal infections. **(E)** Acetaminophen is an analgesic and antipyretic and is used in many conditions as supportive care but is not the best therapy for thrush.

8 A previously healthy 8-year-old girl presents to the emergency department with complaints of nausea, vomiting, severe headache, dizziness, and lethargy. She noticed her symptoms today after traveling with her father and brother in a car from Chicago to Florida to visit her grandparents. Both her father and brother complain of moderate headaches at present. She denies fevers, chills, or nasal drainage. Of the following, what is the best initial management for this patient?

(A) 100% oxygen via a face mask
(B) Perform a lumbar puncture
(C) Obtain a magnetic resonance image of the head
(D) Administer intravenous morphine
(E) Consult neurosurgery for a possible intracranial process

The answer is A: 100% oxygen via a face mask. Carbon monoxide (CO) is an odorless, tasteless, colorless, nonirritating gas formed by incomplete hydrocarbon combustion. CO poisoning is responsible for many emergency department visits and carries a significant mortality risk. CO readily diffuses across the pulmonary capillary membrane and binds to the iron component of the heme molecule. Once CO binds to the heme molecule, it greatly diminishes the ability of the oxygen-binding sites to release oxygen to the peripheral tissues. CO poisoning may cause mild-to-severe symptoms, including nausea, slight dyspnea, headaches, dizziness, rapid fatigue, hypoxemia, hallucinations, confusion, and coma. Carboxyhemoglobin (HbCO) is not detected by pulse oximetry; thus, the PaO_2 value can be normal despite high HbCO concentrations. CO poisoning is treated with 100% oxygen, and in severe cases, patients may require hyperbaric oxygen therapy. Automobile exhaust contains high levels of CO and exposure during long car rides with inadequate or malfunctioning exhaust systems is a risk factor for CO poisoning. Old or malfunctioning home furnaces can also produce high levels of CO.

(B) The patient in the vignette is afebrile; and thus, less likely presenting with a central nervous system infection that would indicate a lumbar puncture. Even though this patient may eventually need further testing and therapies including **(C)** magnetic resonance imaging, **(D)** intravenous pain control, and **(E)** subspecialty consults, these steps would not be the best initial step in this patient's management.

10 A 5-year-old girl being treated for Kawasaki disease develops a cough, runny nose, sore throat, muscle aches, and a temperature of 40°C. Of the following illnesses, which is she at an increased risk of developing?

(A) Reye syndrome
(B) Osteomyelitis
(C) Pneumonia
(D) Septic arthritis
(E) Gastroenteritis

The answer is A: **Reye syndrome.** Patients with Kawasaki disease are treated with aspirin. The symptoms of the patient in the vignette are consistent with a viral illness, such as influenza. Reye syndrome is a rare but severe illness affecting children who use aspirin during a viral infection. The greatest risk is associated with influenza or varicella. The hallmark of this illness involves acute encephalopathy and fatty degeneration of the liver due to mitochondrial dysfunction. Patients with Reye syndrome present with vomiting and mental status changes. There is no definitive diagnostic testing; however, abnormal labs may include elevated liver enzymes, elevated ammonia, and low serum glucose levels. Treatment for Reye syndrome is supportive care. **(B, C, D, E)** Patients with Kawasaki disease are not at increased risk for osteomyelitis, pneumonia, septic arthritis, or gastroenteritis.

11 The back to sleep campaign has reduced the incidence of SIDS (sudden infant death syndrome) greatly. Of the following, which other preventative measure is important in reducing the incidence of SIDS?

(A) Use of bumper pads in cribs
(B) Cessation of maternal and secondhand cigarette smoking
(C) Cosleeping with parents
(D) Swaddling the infant
(E) Placing the infant on a propped pillow to avoid aspiration

The answer is B: **Cessation of maternal and secondhand cigarette smoking.** SIDS is the leading cause of infant mortality between 1 month and 1 year of age. A vast majority of SIDS cases are associated with one or more risk factors. Numerous risk factors for SIDS have been identified including young maternal age, maternal smoking during pregnancy, late or no prenatal care, preterm birth, low birth weight, prone sleeping position, **(A, E)** sleeping on a soft surface and/or with bedding accessories such as loose blankets and pillows, **(C)** bed sharing (cosleeping), and **(D)** overheating. Maternal smoking is a very important risk factor for SIDS. The rate of SIDS increases with the amount of smoke to which an infant is exposed. The strongest risk is from mothers who smoke during pregnancy; however, exposure to secondhand smoke is an additional independent risk factor for SIDS.

---

12 A 4-day-old, full-term newborn comes to clinic for her first newborn visit. During the examination, a small mobile mass is noted under the left breast with white drainage (see *Figure 1-2*). There is no redness or tenderness. The rest of her physical examination is unremarkable.

Of the following, what is the most appropriate next step in the diagnosis or treatment of this infant's breast mass?

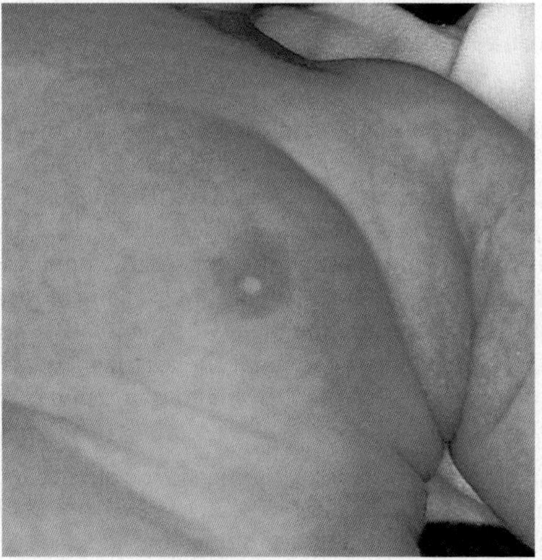

Figure 1-2

(A) Ultrasound of the breast
(B) Fine-needle aspiration of the breast mass
(C) Reassurance given to the parents
(D) Antibiotic therapy
(E) Excisional biopsy

The answer is C: Reassurance given to the parents. Breast enlargement in the newborn period is quite common and is called neonatal breast hypertrophy. This results from circulating maternal endogenous steroid hormones in the late gestational period. This condition is usually benign and no further management is necessary. **(A)** Ultrasound, **(B)** biopsies, and **(D)** antibiotics are not necessary for the resolution of this condition. On occasion, breast hypertrophy may be associated with mastitis, or inflammation of the breast tissue, which could be caused by staphylococcal or streptococcal infections. Mastitis is often accompanied by overlying skin inflammation with or without purulent discharge and is an indication for antibiotic administration. **(E)** Excision of the mass is contraindicated and results in abnormal development of the breast during adolescence.

13 Lactoferrin is a protein found in milk that assists with iron absorption. Of the following, which type of milk has the highest concentration of lactoferrin?

(A) Cow milk
(B) Goat milk
(C) Soy milk
(D) Human breast milk
(E) Human colostrum

The answer is E: Human colostrum. Human milk is recommended as the primary food source for feeding infants in the first 6 months of life with the addition of solids from 6 months to 12 months. Lactoferrin is a glycoprotein found in high concentrations in breast milk as well as mucosal secretions and has iron-binding properties. These properties have a bacteriostatic effect on microorganisms and contribute to the nonspecific immune system. The highest concentration of lactoferrin is found in human colostrum, followed by **(D)** breast milk, **(A)** cow milk, and then **(C)** soymilk. **(B)** Goat milk is not recommended for human infants because it contains inadequate quantities of iron, folate, lactoferrin, and several other vitamins and nutrients.

14 A 15-year-old boy presents to his primary care physician's office 1 week after returning from a class trip to South Africa. He complains of intermittent fevers, rigors, nausea, vomiting, and fatigue. He received his last set of immunizations upon entering high school last year. A complete blood count reveals a white blood count of 4.3×10^3 cells/μL, hemoglobin of 9.5 g/dL, hematocrit of 28%, and platelet count of 150×10^3 cells/μL. On examination, his sclerae are mildly icteric.

Of the following, which is his most likely diagnosis?

(A) Hepatitis A
(B) Yellow fever
(C) Dengue fever
(D) Malaria
(E) Acute lymphoblastic leukemia

The answer is D: Malaria. Malaria should be suspected in all patients with febrile illness after exposure to a region where malaria is endemic. Clinical manifestations are nonspecific and may include fever, chills, malaise, fatigue, tachycardia, tachypnea, headache, nausea, vomiting, abdominal pain, diarrhea, arthralgias, and myalgias. Physical findings may include mild anemia, jaundice, and splenomegaly. The patient in the vignette traveled to an endemic malaria location and has signs and symptoms consistent with this infection.

Like malaria, yellow fever and dengue fever are mostly found in endemic areas and transmitted via mosquito vector. **(B)** The clinical manifestations of yellow fever occur mostly in the liver and kidneys. Findings of yellow fever may also include hemorrhagic emesis, fever, epistaxis, jaundice, anuria, stupor, shock, and coma. **(C)** Dengue fever is endemic to the tropical and subtropic areas of the world. Mild dengue fever causes high fever, rash, muscle pain, and joint pain. The severe form of dengue fever can cause hemorrhage, shock, and death.

(A) Hepatitis A is a common infection in the United States, and because the virus is excreted in the stool, it is easily transmitted between children in daycare centers. Hepatitis A infection in children typically presents as an acute, self-limiting illness associated with fever, malaise, anorexia, vomiting, jaundice, diarrhea, and abdominal pain. Hepatitis A vaccine is recommended for children 1 year and older in a two-dose schedule based on the particular manufacturer of the vaccine. This vaccine must be given at least 2 weeks prior to foreign travel to an endemic area. **(E)** Leukemia is a cancer of the blood or bone marrow and patients suffer from an abnormal production of blood cells and can present with fever and pancytopenia; however, the history of travel to South Africa makes malaria the most likely diagnosis for the patient in the vignette.

15 A 12-month-old, previously healthy girl arrives in the emergency department with vomiting, poor appetite, lethargy, and a bulge on the right side of her head. Her father reports that the infant was napping on the couch and she rolled off onto a carpeted floor. Radiograph of the skull shows a small fracture of the parietal bone. Computed tomography (CT) of the head as shown in *Figure 1-3* reveals a small amount of acute bleeding in the subdural space.

Of the following, what is the most appropriate next step in the evaluation of this patient?

(A) Complete blood count (CBC)
(B) CT scan of the abdomen
(C) Radiographic skeletal survey
(D) Lumbar puncture
(E) Reassurance that this injury will heal without the need for intervention

The answer is C: Radiographic skeletal survey. Based on the history and physical examination findings of the child in the vignette, there is a high

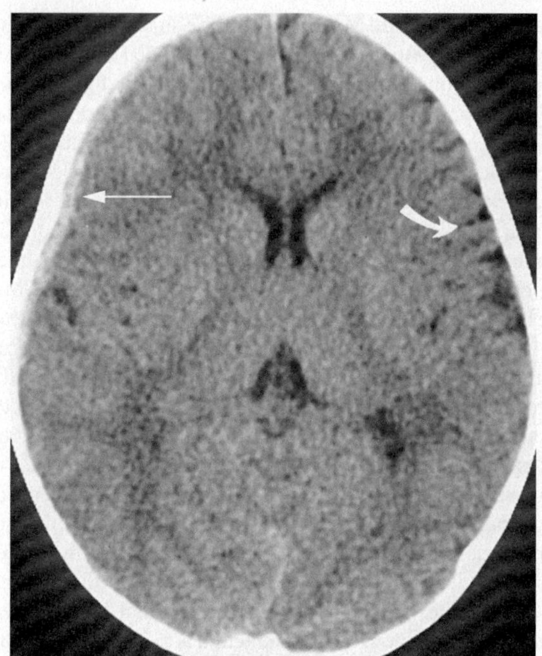

Figure 1-3

suspicion for nonaccidental head injury. Infants with nonaccidental injuries often present with nonspecific clinical features and may not have any admitted history of trauma. Shaken baby syndrome describes the development of cranial injury by the use of blunt force trauma, shaking, or more commonly, by a combination of forces. Violent shaking of an infant causes the brain to move within the skull yielding bruising of the brain parenchyma and shearing of the blood vessels often resulting in hemorrhage in the subdural and subarachnoid spaces, as well as retinal hemorrhages. These findings alone or in combination with other traumatic findings are consistent with nonaccidental injuries. When evaluating a child for suspicion of nonaccidental head injury, initial studies should include nonenhanced CT of the brain and a radiographic skeletal survey. In addition to making a diagnosis, these studies may provide a record of the level of extent and timing of the injuries.

(A) A CBC may be useful in children who present with bruising, pallor, fatigue, and fever to discover underlying infection, bleeding disorders, anemia, or oncologic illnesses. A CBC may be warranted in the patient in the vignette if there is concern for continued blood loss; however, a skeletal survey is more valuable in her evaluation. **(B)** Abdominal CT should be performed if the history and physical examinations suggest abdominal injury. Duodenal hematoma is concerning for abuse; however, the patient in the vignette does not have abdominal complaints. **(D)** Lumbar puncture should be obtained when considering meningitis, subarachnoid hemorrhage, or any central nervous system infections, which would be rare in a healthy, afebrile child. **(E)** Although the infant's injuries in the vignette may heal without intervention, she needs to be properly evaluated for abuse and a safe discharge plan established prior to sending her home.

16 A 13-year-old boy is brought to clinic for his high school sports physical examination. He denies any significant past medical history and his vaccines are up to date. On examination, he has a small amount of dark curly pubic hair, testicular enlargement, and gynecomastia. He denies any smoking, alcohol, or illicit drug use. His weight and height are at the 50th percentile. His mother is concerned about his breast enlargement and asks what she should do.

Of the following, what is the most appropriate next step in the management of this patient's gynecomastia?

(A) Refer him to a pediatric surgeon for a biopsy of the mass
(B) Refer to a pediatric endocrinologist for further evaluation
(C) Send for a urine toxicology screen
(D) Send for chromosome testing
(E) Reassure the mother and patient that this is a normal pubertal finding

The answer is E: **Reassure the mother and patient that this is a normal pubertal finding.** Puberty is a biological process in which a child experiences the anatomic and physiologic changes that lead to adulthood. These changes include the appearance of secondary sexual characteristics and development of reproductive capacity. Once the onset of puberty begins, the resulting sequence of somatic and physiologic changes gives rise to the sexual maturity rating (SMR) or Tanner stages. The first visible sign of puberty in a male is testicular enlargement (SMR 2). This characteristic can begin as early as age 9½ years. This is followed by development of small, curly pubic hair and penile lengthening (SMR 3). Growth acceleration begins in early adolescence and peak growth velocities are usually reached during SMR 3 to 4. Adolescent boys typically experience peak growth velocity approximately 2 to 3 years later than girls. Due to excess estrogenic stimulation, boys can display some degree of breast hypertrophy, typically bilateral, during SMR 2 to 3. See *Figure 1-4*.

(A) Since breast pathology is uncommon in this age group, sending for a surgical biopsy is not the next step in evaluation. **(C)** Marijuana use has been attributed to causing breast hypertrophy in adolescent boys, but if this were suspected, obtaining a thorough social history including a HEADSS examination (Home, Education, Activity, Drugs, Social, Suicidal ideation) would be recommended. **(D)** While gynecomastia in a phenotypic male could be the presentation of androgen insensitivity and diagnosed with karyotype testing,

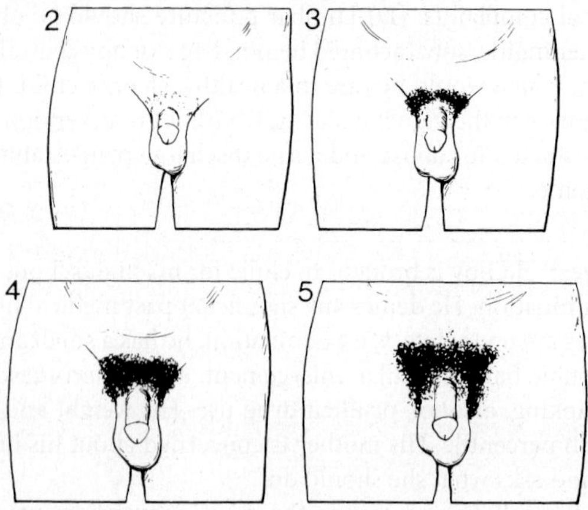

Figure 1-4

this is quite rare and would not be the most appropriate next step for the patient in the vignette. **(B)** A referral to an endocrinologist would be indicated for evaluation of abnormal or precocious puberty. Precocious puberty is the appearance of secondary sexual characteristics at an early age. Puberty is considered precocious if it occurs before the age of 8 years in girls and 9 years in boys. The patient in the vignette demonstrates normal somatic and physiologic changes of SMR stage 3.

17 The mother of a 4-year-old boy brings him to clinic for a well-child health maintenance visit. She reports that he spends 3 hours a day watching television; he likes looking up things on the computer, and drinks 24 ounces of chocolate milk per day. She describes mealtimes as chaotic and often spent in front of the television. His immunizations are up to date. His family history is significant for diabetes mellitus, hypertension, and hyperthyroidism. On examination, his height and weight are greater than the 97th percentile and his body mass index (BMI) is 22. Laboratory workup reveals his total cholesterol 210 mg/dL, low-density lipoprotein 115 mg/dL, and high-density lipoprotein 30 mg/L.

Of the following, what is the next best step in management?

(A) Initiate low-dose statin therapy
(B) Contact child protection services for nutritional neglect
(C) Draw growth hormone levels and thyroid function tests
(D) Work with mother to develop a nutritional plan and encourage daily exercise
(E) Reschedule for a follow-up appointment in 6 months for repeat cholesterol levels

The answer is D: Work with mother to develop a nutritional plan and encourage daily exercise. Obesity is an important public health problem affecting children and adolescents living in the United States and other developed countries. Obese children are more likely to be obese adults, thus increasing lifelong risk of serious health complications such as heart disease, diabetes, and stroke. BMI is a calculated value that takes both height and weight into account. It is calculated as follows: weight (kg)/height^2 (m^2). Interpretation of BMI varies for adults and children. In adults, a BMI value less than 25 is considered normal; 25 to 30 is considered overweight; >30, obese; and >35, morbidly obese. In children, BMI values are plotted on standardized chart, and percentiles are used to define overweight and obese categories. In children aged greater than 2 years, a BMI percentile of ≥95th percentile meets the criteria for obesity. The BMI percentile between the 85th and 95th percentiles defines the overweight range. A BMI of 22 in a 4-year-old boy is greater than the 97th percentile.

The laboratory workup for newly identified obese children includes fasting plasma glucose, triglycerides, low-density lipoprotein, high-density lipoprotein, total cholesterol, and liver function tests. Discussing obesity has been identified as a part of routine medical care for both children and adults. It is necessary to begin by helping the families to understand the importance of healthy living and healthy weights to maintain current and future health. Developing a good therapeutic relationship with families (including a food diary, nutritional plan, and scheduled daily activities) aids in successful management of obesity. The American Academy of Pediatrics recommends that screen time be restricted to no more than 2 hours per day for children >2 years old and that children <2 years old replace television by engaging in more physical activity.

The treatment of high cholesterol in children is a controversial issue. Most physicians believe that the best initial treatment for children with obesity and high cholesterol is diet and exercise. **(A)** Statin therapy is not routinely recommended for a 4-year-old child. **(C)** Growth hormone deficiency and hypothyroidism are unlikely causes for the patient in the vignette given his height and weight are concurrently elevated. **(B)** Contacting child protective services for neglect and **(E)** scheduling a follow-up appointment in 6 months are also not recommended as the next step in management in this patient.

---

18 A 2-year-old boy with no significant past medical history presents with acute intermittent episodes of nonproductive coughing, shortness of breath, and wheezing. He has scattered expiratory wheezing and his breath sounds are diminished on the right side. His parents deny any sick contacts and the boy is currently afebrile.

Of the following, which is this patient's most likely diagnosis?

(A) Asthma exacerbation
(B) Laryngotracheobronchitis
(C) Foreign body aspiration
(D) Vascular ring
(E) Bronchiolitis

The answer is C: **Foreign body aspiration.** Children younger than 3 years of age account for a high proportion cases involving foreign body aspiration. Signs and symptoms of foreign body aspiration can include unlabored breathing with intermittent, nonproductive cough, and expiratory wheezing that is best heard over the right lung field. Given the less acute angle of the right main stem bronchus from the trachea, aspirated foreign bodies are more likely to enter the right lung. Complications of foreign body aspirations may include, but are not limited to, fever, cough, atelectasis, hemoptysis, and pneumonia. The diagnostic workup for foreign body aspiration includes inspiratory and expiratory chest radiography showing differential air trapping on the affected side and definitive diagnosis and treatment by rigid bronchoscopy as indicated (see *Figure 1-5*).

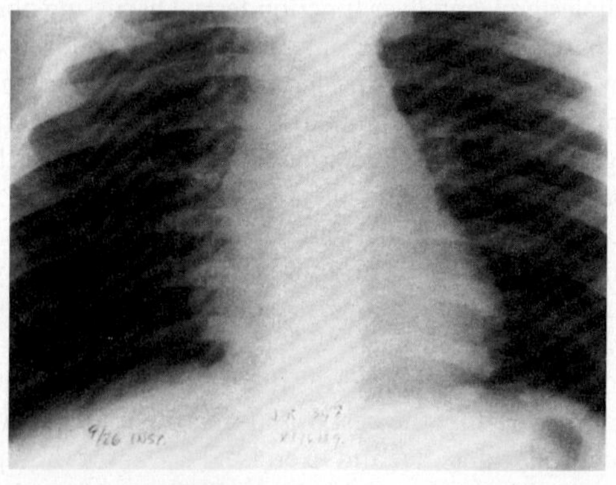

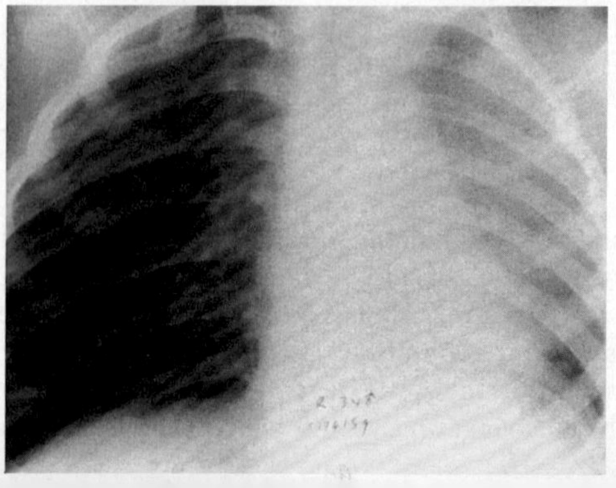

Wheezing represents an obstruction of small-to-medium pulmonary airways and is associated with many conditions such as asthma, vascular rings, and viral bronchiolitis. **(A)** Asthma is usually recurrent and responds to bronchodilators and inhaled steroid therapy. **(D)** A vascular ring is a congenital defect of the formation of the aorta and other large vessels around the esophagus and trachea that can lead to breathing and digestive difficulties. **(E)** Bronchiolitis involves inflammation of the bronchioles, or small airways, and is often secondary to a viral infection such as respiratory syncytial virus. **(B)** Children with viral croup, or laryngotracheobronchitis, present with a barky cough and inspiratory stridor secondary to inflammation of the upper airways.

---

19 A 10-year-old boy presents to the emergency department with fever, abdominal pain, headache, sore throat, and muffled speech that developed over the past 2 days. His pharyngeal examination is pictured in *Figure 1-6*.

Of the following, which organism is the most likely cause of his symptoms?

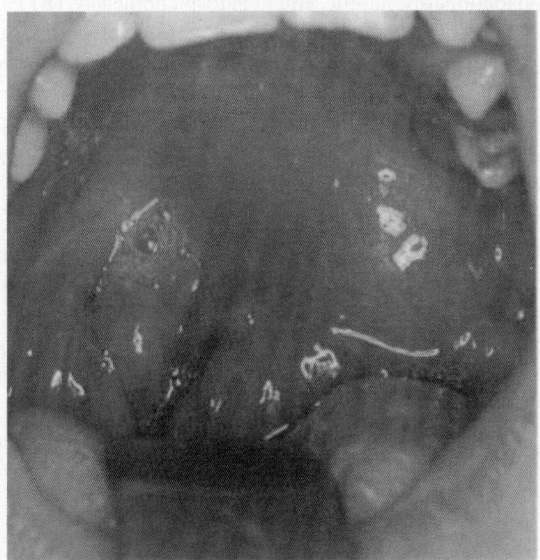

Figure 1-6

(A) Epstein-Barr virus (EBV)
(B) Parainfluenza virus
(C) *Corynebacterium diphtheriae*
(D) *Streptococcus pyogenes*
(E) *Streptococcus pneumoniae*

The answer is D: *Streptococcus pyogenes*. The image in the vignette demonstrates a peritonsillar abscess. A peritonsillar abscess develops between the superior pole of the tonsil and its capsule. The typical patient with a peritonsillar abscess is an adolescent with a recent history of acute pharyngotonsillitis. Physical examination often reveals an enlarged and erythematous tonsil with exudate and a deviated, edematous uvula. Group A streptococci or *S. pyogenes* is the most common pathogen isolated in a peritonsillar abscess and accounts for the majority of bacterial pharyngitis in children.

(C) *C. diphtheriae* is an uncommon cause of pharyngitis in developed countries since the initiation of the childhood vaccination program. It remains important to consider in patients from endemic areas or in suboptimally vaccinated individuals. Patients present with a gray, pseudomembranous appearance of the pharynx rather than as described in the vignette. Viruses are the most common cause of acute pharyngitis in children. Clinical features of pharyngitis secondary to a viral etiology may be accompanied by concurrent features such as conjunctivitis, coryza, cough, hoarseness, diarrhea, profound pharyngeal inflammation, and exanthematous rashes. **(A)** EBV is the cause of mononucleosis. It is characterized by severe exudative pharyngitis, fever, diffuse lymphadenopathy, fatigue, and hepatosplenomegaly. **(B)** Parainfluenza virus can cause both upper and lower respiratory tract infections, ranging from a mild cough to a severe pneumonia. Parainfluenza virus is the leading cause of croup or laryngotracheobronchitis in children. **(E)** *S. pneumoniae* is the leading cause of otitis media, pneumonia, and sinusitis. Of the above options, only the streptococci are associated with abscess formation, but *S. pyogenes* is the most likely of those listed.

---

20 A 2-year-old girl presents with crampy abdominal pain, malaise, and watery, foul-smelling stools over the past 2 weeks. Her mother denies blood or mucous in the stool, any recent medication use, or any sick contacts at home, but endorses that her daughter attends daycare 4 days per week. Rotavirus antigen testing and fecal occult blood assay are negative. Stool culture, fecal white blood cells, and ova/parasites testing are pending.

Of the following, what is the most likely etiologic agent of this patient's presentation?

(A) Rotavirus
(B) *Escherichia coli* O157:H7
(C) *Shigella sonnei*
(D) *Giardia intestinalis*
(E) *Clostridium difficile*

The answer is D: *Giardia intestinalis*. *G. intestinalis*, previously called *Giardia lamblia*, is a flagellated protozoan that affects the gastrointestinal tract. Groups at increased risk for giardiasis include children in daycare, international

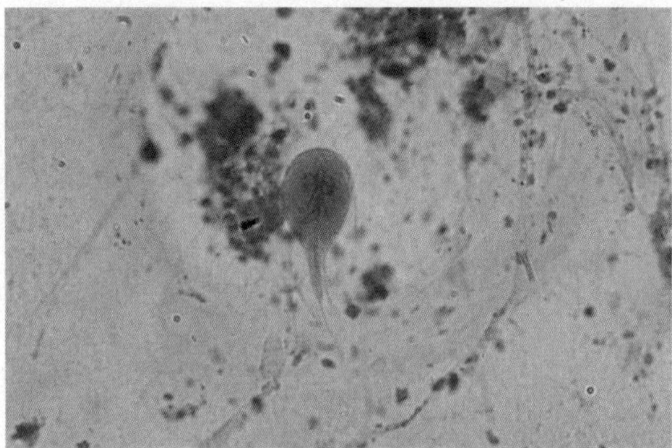

Figure 1-7

travelers, campers, immunocompromised individuals, and patients with cystic fibrosis. The cysts of *Giardia* are found in the feces of infected people and infection is spread by contamination of food with feces or direct fecal–oral contamination. The most common symptoms of giardiasis are foul-smelling diarrhea, crampy abdominal pain, bloating, nausea, vomiting, malaise, and fatigue. *Giardia* interferes with the absorption of fat from the intestines and may also cause weight loss. Fever is not usually present. Diagnosis of giardiasis is by antigen testing of the stool or direct examination of the stool under the microscope for cysts or flagellated trophozoites (see *Figure 1-7*). The drugs of choice for the treatment of giardiasis in the United States are tinidazole, metronidazole, or nitazoxanide.

(A) Rotavirus is the most common cause of diarrheal illnesses in children between 3 and 36 months of age. In the United States, infection occurs throughout the year, but the incidence peaks during the fall months in the southwest region and during the spring months in the northeast region. Incubation time is approximately 2 days and presenting symptoms include fever, vomiting, profuse watery diarrhea, and abdominal pain. Given the negative antigen testing for rotavirus, this diagnosis is less likely for the patient in the vignette. **(B)** *E. coli* O157:H7 is a gram-negative bacterium that infects the gastrointestinal tract and causes bloody diarrhea. It is an enteric pathogen and can be traced to contaminated and uncooked beef. This strain produces a shiga toxin that produces fever, vomiting, and abdominal cramping and also can lead to further complications such as hemolytic uremic syndrome. **(C)** *S. sonnei* also causes bloody diarrhea associated with fevers, bandemia, and seizure activity but is not the most likely cause for the patient in the vignette. **(E)** *C. difficile* is a bacterium that causes colonic infection leading to fever, abdominal pain, and bloody stools. History of antibiotic therapy in the previous several weeks is a risk factor for *C. difficile* infection.

CHAPTER

2

Newborn

KENT NELSON

1 A nurse in the special care nursery reports that a baby is moving strangely. The baby was delivered 12 hours ago by emergency cesarean section for nonreassuring heart tones to a G2P2 mother at 37 weeks' gestation. Apgar scores were 5 and 8 at 1 and 5 minutes, respectively. The 1-minute Apgar score was reduced secondary to respiratory depression among other findings. He was admitted to the special care nursery for observation and has had an uneventful course until now. On examination, the baby's eyes are deviated to the right and he continues to move his hands and arms despite attempts to hold them still. His fontanelle is flat and nonbulging. He has no heart murmur and the remainder of his examination is unremarkable. Blood glucose level is 87 mg/dL.

Of the following, what is the most likely cause of this baby's presentation?

(A) Hyponatremia
(B) Hypoglycemia
(C) Asphyxia
(D) Hypocalcemia
(E) Normal neonatal jitteriness

The answer is C: Asphyxia. Infants in the neonatal period are susceptible to seizure activity for a variety of reasons, including metabolic derangements, infectious causes, and anatomic abnormalities. Tonic–clonic seizures are not the norm in this age group due to immature brain myelination that hinders electrical propagation throughout the neonatal brain.

(C) The seizures described for the patient in the vignette are caused by the most common etiology of neonatal seizures, hypoxic–ischemic encephalopathy. This patient's hypoxic event likely occurred at birth and is reflected in the low 1-minute Apgar score. Long-term prognosis is good in children similar to the one in the vignette who only have a short period of hypoxia.

Metabolic issues may lead to seizures in the neonatal period, but the baby in the vignette does not show any signs supporting these possibilities. **(A)** Hyponatremia is a cause of neonatal seizures and is often seen secondary to incorrect formula mixing. Other causes of hyponatremia include the syndrome of inappropriate antidiuretic hormone or cerebral salt wasting; both can be seen following intracranial injury or hemorrhage. Diuretic use can also lead to hyponatremia.

(B) Hypoglycemia can cause jitteriness or exaggerated startle reflexes as well as seizures and is often seen in infants of diabetic mothers. **(D)** Hypocalcemia does not often cause seizures within the first 5 days of life. **(E)** Normal neonatal jitteriness would be easily stopped with attempts to hold the infant still and would not be associated with eye deviation.

2 A full-term baby girl is born to a mother who has received several intravenous medications during labor including magnesium sulfate. The baby is immediately brought to the warmer and the appropriate resuscitation protocol is begun. After 1 minute, the baby is lying awake in the crib with some crying and flexion of her extremities. Her body is mostly pink but her hands and feet are blue. Her heart rate is 132 beats per minute. She grimaces with nasal suctioning. At 5 minutes of life, the baby's activity has progressed and she is now more active and vigorous. She continues to have nasal discharge and sneezes with suctioning of her nares. Her cardiac, respiratory, and skin examinations are unchanged.

Of the following, which is the correct Apgar score at 1 and 5 minutes, respectively?

(A) 9 at 1 minute; 9 at 5 minutes
(B) 6 at 1 minute; 9 at 5 minutes
(C) 6 at 1 minute; 8 at 5 minutes
(D) 8 at 1 minute; 10 at 5 minutes
(E) 7 at 1 minute; 9 at 5 minutes

The answer is E: 7 at 1 minute; 9 at 5 minutes. The Apgar scoring system is a quick way to assess a newborn infant's transition from intrauterine to extrauterine life. The 1-minute Apgar score evaluates an infant's distress during the birthing procedure, while 5-, 10-, 15-, and 20-minute scores can act as indicators or predictors of the successful resuscitation. Apgar scores do not predict neurologic outcomes.

Sign	0	1	2
Heart rate	Absent	Below 100	Over 100
Respiratory effort	Absent	Slow, irregular	Good, crying
Muscle tone	Limp	Some flexion of extremities	Active motion
Response to catheter in nostril	No response	Grimace	Cough or sneeze
Color	Blue, pale	Body pink, extremities blue	Completely pink

3 A 27-year-old mother comes to the clinic to discuss her plans to have a second child. She is healthy and her first and only pregnancy 3 years ago was uneventful. Her blood type is A– and her son's blood type is O+. The son is healthy and developing normally.

Of the following, what is the best recommendation for this mother's upcoming prenatal course?

(A) A vitamin supplement including at least 400 mg of folate should be taken daily
(B) She should have an amniocentesis with her next pregnancy
(C) Anti-D antibody should be given to the new baby within 72 hours of delivery
(D) She should undergo first-trimester chorionic villus sampling
(E) There is no need for prenatal care since she and her first child are both healthy

The answer is A: **A vitamin supplement including at least 400 mg of folate should be taken daily.** Adequate prenatal care is very important for proper growth and development from embryo to fetus to infant. It is recommended that all women of childbearing age take a daily multivitamin with at least 400 mg of folate to decrease the risks of neural tube defects in the developing fetus.

In the case of maternal isoimmunization, specific care is recommended. A mother whose blood type is negative for the D antigen (Rh-factor negative) and gives birth to an Rh-positive baby is at risk for exposure to her neonate's D antigen during the birthing process. This can cause an antigen–antibody reaction in the mother that stimulates production of anti-D antibodies that can put future Rh-positive pregnancies at risk for a hemolytic anemia. **(C)** Administration of anti-D antibodies to the mother within 72 hours of the first birth, or miscarriage, can significantly decrease the risk to future pregnancies. A history of maternal isoimmunization is a relative contraindication to chorionic villus sampling. **(B, D)** Chorionic villus sampling and amniocentesis are tests done during pregnancy if there is concern for risk of genetic conditions such as trisomy 21. Chorionic villus sampling is done in the first trimester (10 to 12 weeks of gestation) and amniocentesis between weeks 15 and 17. The infant described in the vignette is not at an increased risk and therefore at this point amniocentesis would not be necessarily recommended. **(E)** Prenatal care is essential to every pregnancy no matter how many prior healthy pregnancies an individual has had.

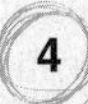

4 A 6-hour-old newborn boy, born at 38 weeks' gestation by elective cesarean section to a mother with gestational diabetes, is examined in the newborn nursery. His respiratory rate is 72 breaths per minute and therapy for suspected infectious causes are begun. His chest radiograph is pictured in *Figure 2-1*.

Based on the clinical presentation and radiographic findings, which of the following is the most likely diagnosis?

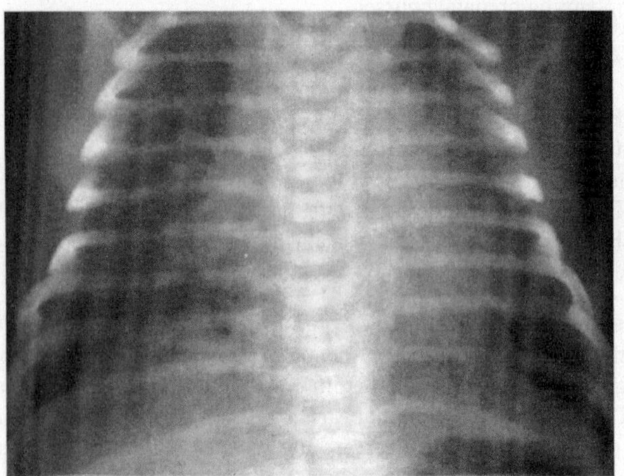

Figure 2-1

(A) Retained fetal lung fluid syndrome
(B) Meconium aspiration
(C) Respiratory distress syndrome
(D) Congenital diaphragmatic hernia
(E) Neonatal pneumonia

The answer is A: Retained fetal lung fluid syndrome. Respiratory distress in the newborn period is the most common cause of admission to the neonatal intensive care unit. Signs of respiratory distress include tachypnea, grunting, retractions, nasal flaring, hypoxia, cyanosis, decreased breath sounds with rales, and apnea. While infection and sepsis must be the first set of etiologies addressed, respiratory distress can arise because of several other noninfectious mechanisms, each with characteristic findings on chest radiograph. The patient in the vignette is full term and an infant of a diabetic mother. **(A)** He suffers from retained fetal lung fluid syndrome, also known as transient tachypnea of the newborn. It is thought to be caused by retained fluid in the neonatal lungs and is associated with cesarean section deliveries. It is usually short-lived and often resolves within 2 to 3 days. Chest radiographs show overaeration, prominent pulmonary markings, and retained fluid in the intralobar fissures.

(B) Meconium aspiration is characterized by patchy infiltrates, bilateral coarse streaking, with increased anteroposterior diameter and flattened diaphragm (see *Figure 2-2*). **(C)** Respiratory distress syndrome (RDS), also known as hyaline membrane disease, can affect premature infants with underdeveloped lungs and surfactant deficiency. These patients can present at birth with tachypnea, hypoxia, and cyanosis and chest radiographs show a characteristic diffuse ground-glass appearance with hypoaeration and air bronchograms (see *Figure 2-3*). **(E)** The radiographic findings of neonatal pneumonia are very similar to those of RDS but these infants are differentiated with clinical findings of infection. **(D)** Congenital diaphragmatic hernia results from a defect in the diaphragm and herniation of abdominal contents into the thorax. Severe hernias can retard normal pulmonary development and leave infants in distress secondary to inadequate pulmonary parenchyma. Chest radiographs show intestines and other abdominal contents within the thorax and occur most often on the left side (see *Figure 2-4*).

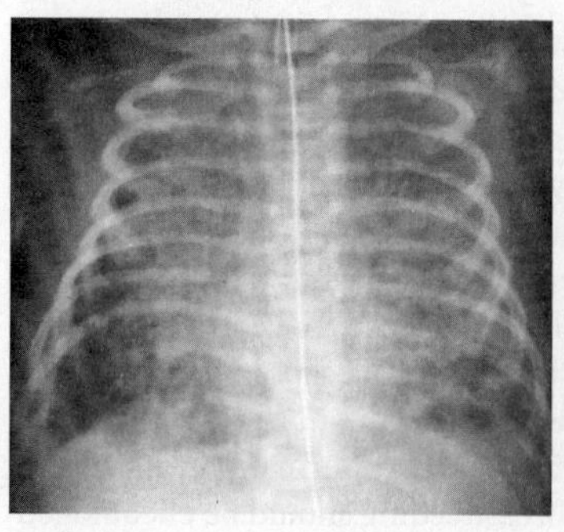

Figure 2-2

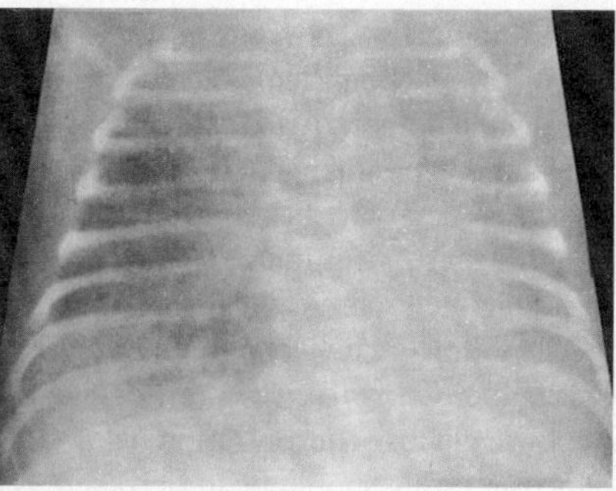

Figure 2-3

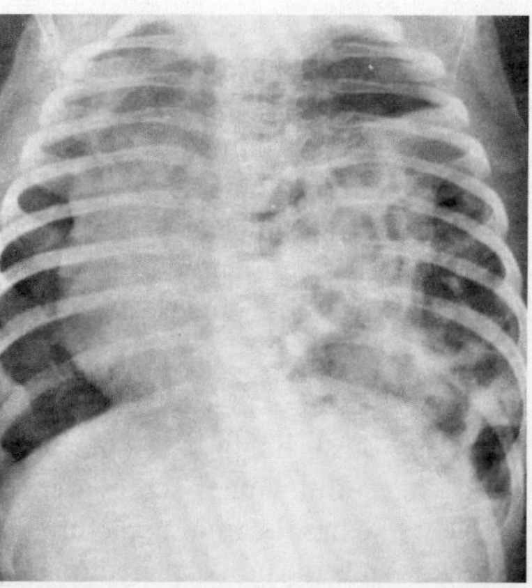

Figure 2-4

5 A full-term baby girl is born by cesarean section secondary to failure to progress to a G3P3 woman with poorly controlled type 1 diabetes mellitus. The baby's birth weight is 4.6 kg. Two hours following her delivery, the baby displays tremors and an exaggerated Moro reflex. Glucose oxidase strip analysis shows a glucose level of 30 mg/dL and serum glucose concentration is measured at 25 mg/dL.

Of the following, what is the most appropriate next step in the management of this baby?

(A) Observe closely and repeat serum glucose levels in 1 hour
(B) Wrap the baby tightly in a blanket and place her under the infrared warming lights
(C) Bring the baby to the mother for breastfeeding
(D) Give the baby 0.4 units of normal insulin intramuscularly
(E) Give an intravenous infusion of 8 mL of 10% glucose solution

The answer is E: Give an intravenous infusion of 8 mL of 10% glucose solution. Hypoglycemia is a common finding in infants of diabetic mothers, especially if maternal blood glucose concentrations were poorly controlled throughout pregnancy. The infant in the vignette is large for gestational age likely secondary to increased circulating insulin concentrations during development. At birth, this increased insulin concentration is abruptly stopped but the residual insulin increases the risk of falling blood glucose concentrations in the hours following delivery. Infants at risk for hypoglycemia should be monitored with glucose oxidase strip testing every few hours in the nursery. If the strips report a glucose concentration below 40 to 50 mg/dL, confirmation with serum glucose testing should be undertaken. **(C)** Breastfeeding should be encouraged once the acute symptomatic hypoglycemia is properly treated with glucose.

The infant in the vignette demonstrates clinical signs of hypoglycemia with increased tremors and an exaggerated Moro reflex. Symptomatic hypoglycemia needs to be addressed immediately with intravenous infusion of 10% dextrose solution. **(A)** Asymptomatic hypoglycemia can be monitored closely with repeat serum glucose levels and feeding.

(B) The tremors described in the vignette are secondary to hypoglycemia rather than cold stress so wrapping the baby in a blanket and placing under warming lights would not address the underlying cause. **(D)** Administration of normal insulin would cause lower serum glucose concentrations and therefore is contraindicated.

A full-term newborn girl is brought to the nursery. Her birth and prenatal course were uneventful. Apgar scores were 9 and 9 at 1 and 5 minutes, respectively. She has the finding pictured in *Figure 2-5*.

Of the following, what is the best explanation for this baby's physical examination findings?

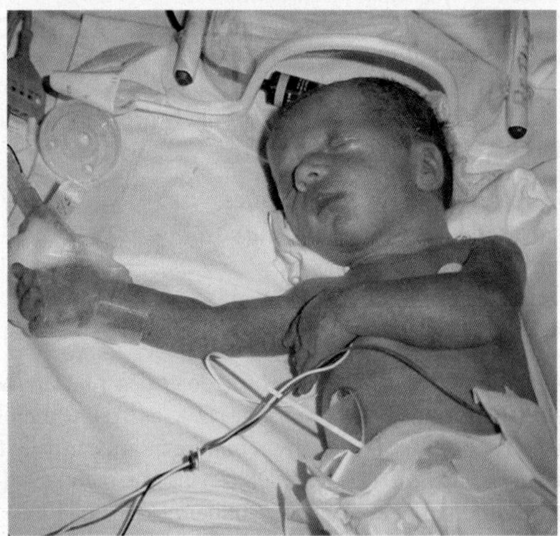

Figure 2-5

(A) Transposition of the great vessels
(B) Acrocyanosis
(C) Erythema toxicum
(D) Cutis marmorata
(E) Harlequin coloration

The answer is B: Acrocyanosis. Acrocyanosis, or bluish tint to the hands and feet, is a common and harmless condition in infants within the first several hours of life. This cyanosis is likely caused by vasomotor instability and sluggish peripheral blood flow. It can be exacerbated by cool temperatures but it rarely signifies any significant abnormalities in an otherwise healthy-appearing infant.

(E) Harlequin coloration, or harlequin color change, describes a stark division from forehead to pubis into pale and red halves. This harmless skin color change is also caused by vasomotor instability but is associated with pallor rather than cyanosis. **(A)** Central cyanosis is a bluish tint of the face, lips, and trunk. It is often secondary to hypoxemia and could be a sign of significant circulatory abnormalities like transposition of the great vessels. **(D)** Cutis marmorata can present as unilateral or bilateral mottled appearance of the skin on the extremities at birth. **(C)** Erythema toxicum is a blotchy, erythematous rash seen in about half of full-term infants secondary to a local immune response. It is not associated with any cyanosis and its course is self-limited.

7 A neonatal boy is born at 29 weeks' gestation by cesarean section secondary to chorioamnionitis. He has progressively worse respiratory distress and hypoxia on room air over the first several hours of life.

His mother did not receive antenatal steroids. An anteroposterior chest radiograph shows a uniform reticulogranular pattern and peripheral air bronchograms.

Of the following, what is the most likely primary mechanism of this disorder?

(A) Decreased chest wall compliance
(B) Increased intrathoracic pressure
(C) Pulmonary edema
(D) Bronchospasm
(E) Lack of surfactant

The answer is E: **Lack of surfactant.** The neonate described in the vignette has respiratory distress syndrome (RDS), also referred to as hyaline membrane disease of the newborn. This disorder is seen in premature infants, usually those born at gestational ages less than 32 weeks, but RDS can also be seen in full-term infants born to diabetic mothers. The etiology is secondary to lack of adequate surfactant production from immature alveolar lung cells. This results in a high surface tension and increased risk of alveolar collapse resulting in respiratory distress. Therapy includes antenatal steroids, postnatal respiratory support, and the administration of surfactant soon after birth. **(A, B, C, D)** Although neonates with RDS may have decreased chest wall compliance, increased intrathoracic pressure, pulmonary edema, and bronchospasm, the primary mechanism of RDS is lack of surfactant.

8 A 3-day-old newborn boy was born full term by normal, spontaneous vaginal delivery. His parents have no concerns since birth and are getting ready for discharge from the nursery. The results from his screening otoacoustic emissions test show that he did not pass.

Of the following, what is the most likely infectious cause for acquired sensorineural hearing loss?

(A) *Toxoplasma gondii*
(B) *Treponema pallidum*
(C) Rubella virus
(D) Cytomegalovirus (CMV)
(E) Herpes simplex virus

The answer is D: **Cytomegalovirus (CMV).** CMV is the most common infectious cause of acquired sensorineural hearing loss. A significant number of children are born in the United States with CMV infection; however, most have no obvious sequelae. Those with sequelae may present with microcephaly, intracerebral calcifications, intrauterine growth retardation, hepatosplenomegaly, chorioretinitis, or jaundice. **(A)** *Toxoplasma gondii* is a bacterial infection transmitted through cat feces. Symptomatic infants have microcephaly, hydrocephalus and intracranial calcifications, chorioretinitis, and seizures. **(B)** *Treponema palladium* is the causative agent of syphilis and transmission may occur at any time throughout pregnancy, but most often occurs during the first trimester. Infants have mucocutaneous lesions, eczema-like rash, snuffles, hepatosplenomegaly, osteochondritis, thrombocytopenia, and hemolytic anemia. **(C)** Congenitally transmitted rubella can result in congenital sensorineural hearing loss; however, CMV remains the most common infectious cause for acquired sensorineural hearing loss. Other symptoms of congenital rubella include cataracts, retinitis pigmentosa, glaucoma, microcephaly, and congenital heart disease such as persistent ductus arteriosus and pulmonary artery stenosis. **(E)** Herpes simplex virus is most often transmitted during vaginal delivery. Symptoms of infection include meningitis, involvement of lungs and liver, seizures, and vesicular skin lesions; however, hearing loss is not a commonly associated finding.

9 A 3-week-old neonate born to a primiparous mother comes to the clinic for a health maintenance visit. The mother reports that the baby was delivered by cesarean section because "she was turned the wrong way." She has no complaints and states that the baby has been eating and growing well. On examination, the girl is a healthy-appearing infant and there is a sensation of a low-frequency clunk while abducting her left hip.

Of the following, what is the best treatment option for this patient?

(A) Triple diapers
(B) Prone sleeping position
(C) Surgical correction
(D) Vitamin D supplementation
(E) Reassurance

The answer is A: Triple diapers. The patient in the vignette has developmental dysplasia of the hip (DDH). DDH is an orthopedic condition resulting from poor association of the femoral head and acetabulum. This condition is often unilateral and is more common in female infants born in the breech position. The Ortolani and Barlow maneuvers evaluate for this disorder. The Ortolani maneuver is performed by abduction of the hips while placing a finger on the greater trochanter and feeling for a clunk that indicates relocation of the subluxed femoral head into the acetabulum. The Barlow maneuver is performed by placing a downward force on adducted hips and feeling for laxity at the hip joint that suggests subluxation or dislocation. Diagnosis is confirmed with a hip ultrasound in this age group and radiographs for children older than 3 months of age. **(A, E)** Initial management includes Pavlik harness or doubling or tripling the diapers as well as orthopedic consultation and follow-up.

(C) Surgery may be indicated if initial management fails. **(B)** Sleeping in the prone position does not improve DDH and is never recommended given the risk of sudden infant death syndrome. **(D)** There is no indication in the vignette that this child is vitamin D deficient and therefore supplementation will not improve her outcome.

10 A 4-hour-old newborn boy has had multiple episodes of nonbloody and nonbilious vomiting since birth. He was born at 38 weeks' gestation to a 38-year-old mother. On examination, he has poor overall tone, protruding tongue, and upward-slanting eyes. The skin between his head and shoulders is generous and he has a single transverse palmar crease on both hands. His abdominal radiograph is pictured in *Figure 2-6*.

Of the following, what is the most likely cause of this patient's vomiting?

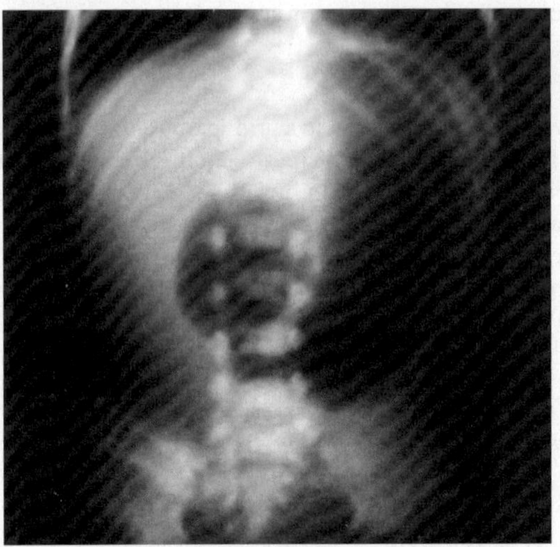

Figure 2-6

(A) Pyloric stenosis
(B) Duodenal atresia
(C) Esophageal stenosis
(D) Milk protein allergy
(E) Malrotation with midgut volvulus

The answer is B: Duodenal atresia. The infant described in the vignette has trisomy 21, or Down syndrome, with duodenal atresia. Trisomy 21 is a genetic disorder characterized by an extra copy of chromosome 21. It is the most common chromosomal disorder and the most common genetic cause of mental retardation. Patients with this disorder share similar features including a range of mental retardation; typical facies such as protruding tongue, upward-slanting eyes with epicanthal folds, flat nasal bridge, small ears, and neck skin folds; hypotonia and joint laxity; subendocardial cushion defects; hypothyroidism; increased risk of leukemia; and atlantoaxial instability. In addition, the gastrointestinal pathology associated with trisomy 21 includes duodenal atresia, Hirschsprung disease, and imperforate anus. **(B)** Duodenal atresia is the failure of the lumen of the first portion of the small intestine to recanalize following intestinal development. It presents as emesis that is frequently bilious within a few hours of birth, although the emesis may be nonbilious if the defect is proximal to the ampulla of Vater. The radiograph in the vignette shows the double-bubble sign, or air within the stomach and proximal duodenum that is separated by the pylorus.

(A) Pyloric stenosis presents with forceful or projectile nonbilious emesis typically after 3 weeks of age. Laboratory findings demonstrate a hypochloremic, hypokalemic metabolic alkalosis. **(C)** Esophageal stenosis is a narrowing of the esophagus often secondary to toxic ingestions and is rare in the neonatal period. **(D)** Milk protein allergy is rarely seen in the first few days of life; babies usually have an eczema-like rash and bloody stools. **(E)** Malrotation with midgut volvulus can present in the neonatal period with bilious emesis, but often presents within the first month of life rather than within the first few hours of life. Malrotation occurs when the intestines do not rotate normally in utero resulting in abnormal position and often with posterior fixation of the mesentery resulting in an increased risk of volvulus. Infants with trisomy 21 are not at an increased risk of malrotation.

A 4-day-old newborn is seen in the clinic for her first health maintenance visit. She was born by spontaneous vaginal delivery without vacuum assistance to a G2P2 mother. The delivery and initial hospital course were uneventful. Mother's and baby's blood types are both O–. The mother reports that the baby is exclusively breastfed approximately 10 minutes on each breast every 2 to 3 hours. The baby has had 5 to 6 voids and 1 to 2 soft stools per day since hospital discharge 2 days ago. She mentions that the baby's skin and eyes look yellow. Lingual, cutaneous, and scleral icterus is confirmed on examination. The baby otherwise looks very healthy. Laboratory tests confirm an unconjugated bilirubin level of 10.8 mg/dL.

Of the following, what is the most likely mechanism for this baby's unconjugated hyperbilirubinemia?

(A) Isoimmune hemolysis
(B) Neonatal hepatitis
(C) Inefficient bilirubin metabolism
(D) Biliary atresia
(E) Crigler-Najjar syndrome

The answer is C: Inefficient bilirubin metabolism. Unconjugated hyperbilirubinemia is the accumulation of indirect bilirubin and may be either physiologic or pathologic in nature. Infants with elevated unconjugated bilirubin are at risk for kernicterus because of the ability of indirect bilirubin to cross the blood–brain barrier. Physiologic jaundice is common in most neonates. It is caused by the increased bilirubin load and inefficient bilirubin metabolism. There is an increased bilirubin load secondary to increase in red blood cell number, corpuscular volume, and decreased life span resulting in increased hemoglobin degradation and increased bilirubin levels. In addition, neonates have poor hepatic uptake and conjugation as well as decreased bilirubin excretion. Therapy involves proper hydration and phototherapy.

(A) Isoimmune hemolysis is seen in neonates when the red cells of the newborn are destroyed by maternal-derived alloantibodies as seen with neonates who are Rh-positive born to Rh-negative mothers. This would also result in an unconjugated hyperbilirubinemia; however, the girl in the vignette is not at risk. **(B)** Infants with intrauterine cytomegalovirus infection may present with jaundice secondary to neonatal hepatitis but also frequently have microcephaly, intracerebral calcifications, intrauterine growth retardation, hepatosplenomegaly, and chorioretinitis. Neonatal hepatitis can cause an unconjugated or conjugated hyperbilirubinemia. **(D)** Neonates with biliary atresia have a conjugated, or direct, hyperbilirubinemia. Biliary atresia is a progressive disorder of the biliary tree and requires surgical intervention ideally within the first 6 weeks of life. **(E)** Crigler-Najjar syndrome is an autosomal recessive disorder characterized by unconjugated hyperbilirubinemia with levels over 20 mg/dL. This disorder should be suspected when jaundice persists and bilirubin levels are very elevated. Crigler-Najjar syndrome is rare, and much less likely than physiologic jaundice.

---

12 During a well-child visit, a new mother reports her 1-week-old son has developed a rash on his chest, back, and face that began prior to discharge from the hospital. The baby was born full term and he has had no other complaints besides this rash. On examination, the baby is a well-appearing 1-week-old newborn with multiple 2- to 3-cm blotchy erythematous macules with 1- to 4-mm central pustules as pictured in *Figure 2-7*. The rash spares his palms and soles. A Wright-stained preparation of the pustular material reveals numerous eosinophils.

Of the following, what is the most likely cause of this infant's rash?

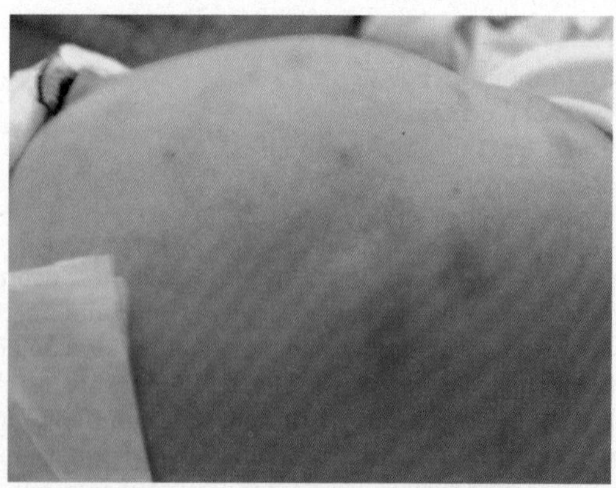

Figure 2-7

(A) Erythema toxicum
(B) Acne neonatorum
(C) Milia
(D) Miliaria rubra
(E) Transient neonatal pustular melanosis

The answer is A: Erythema toxicum. Erythema toxicum is a common neonatal rash usually present at 24 to 72 hours of life and can persist for several weeks. It presents with blotchy erythematous areas surrounding overlying white or yellowish pustules. Unroofing and staining reveals numerous eosinophils. This disorder is self-limiting and requires no specific therapy.

(B) Acne neonatorum is secondary to maternal hormones and typically peaks around 2 months of age. This rash has an appearance that is very similar to acne vulgaris seen during adolescence (see *Figure 2-8*). **(C)** Milia is caused by the retention of skin and oil within hair follicles and presents as white papules on the face, nose, and around the mouth. Milia typically resolves within the first month of life (see *Figure 2-9*). **(D)** Miliaria rubra is a heat rash caused by blockage of sweat glands. **(E)** Transient neonatal pustular melanosis presents as small pustules on a nonerythematous base and is more common in African-American infants (see *Figure 2-10*). Microscopic examination reveals numerous neutrophils rather than eosinophils.

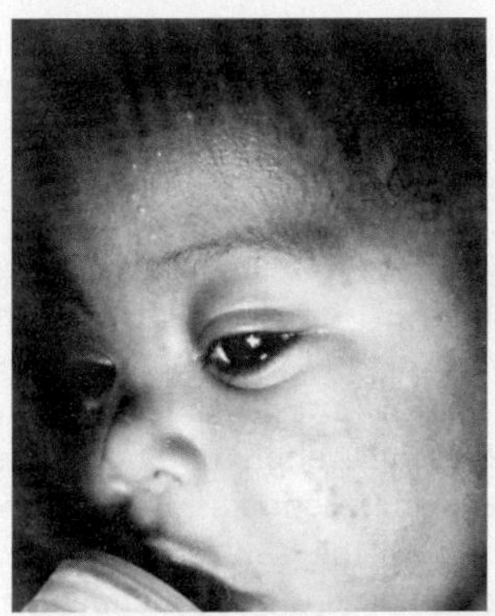
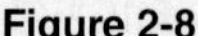

Figure 2-8

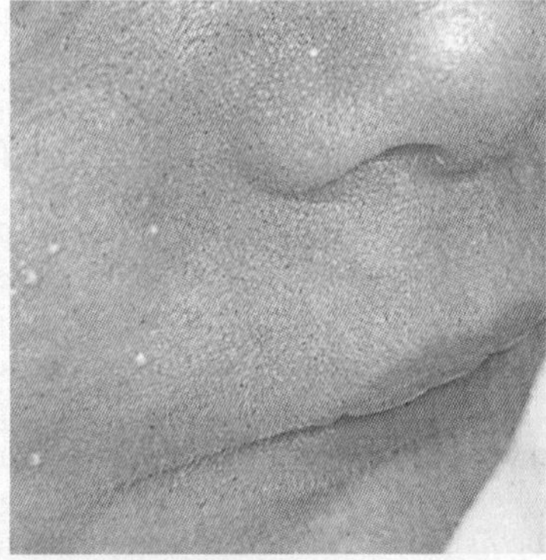

Figure 2-9

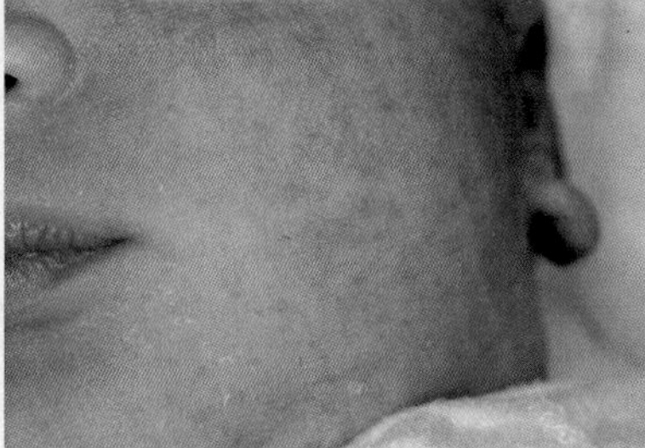

Figure 2-10

13 A mother brings her 2-week-old newborn to the emergency department for fever, fussiness, and poor feeding. She reports that the baby had a rectal temperature of 101.4°F this morning and that she has been more fussy than usual since yesterday. She states that the baby is very difficult to console and she is taking less than half of her normal formula intake. The baby was born vaginally at 37 weeks' gestation following prolonged rupture of membranes and she was monitored by a scalp probe during the prolonged labor process. There has been no follow-up since discharge from the nursery at day of life 3. On examination, the baby is irritable with a rectal temperature of 38.5°C, heart rate of 140 beats per minute, respiratory rate of 50 breaths per minute, and blood pressure of 82/46 mmHg. She has good pulses and adequate capillary refill. Her skin examination is normal except for a cluster of vesicles with an erythematous base at the site of the intrauterine scalp probe. In addition to admission to the inpatient ward and the appropriate diagnostic workup, the decision to begin empiric antibiotic treatment is made.

Of the following, what is the best option for the initial empiric intravenous antibiotic regimen?

(A) Vancomycin and acyclovir
(B) Ampicillin, cefotaxime, and acyclovir
(C) Ampicillin and gentamicin
(D) Gentamicin, acyclovir, and metronidazole
(E) Ampicillin, ceftriaxone, and fluconazole

The answer is B: Ampicillin, cefotaxime, and acyclovir. A febrile infant less than 2 months of age is at increased risk for life-threatening conditions, including urinary tract infections, sepsis, and meningitis. The baby described in the vignette is fussy, feeding poorly, febrile, and has a vesicular rash. A complete workup should be done including analysis and culture of blood, urine, and cerebrospinal fluid (CSF). A polymerase chain reaction assay for herpes simplex virus (HSV) should also be performed on the CSF. Group B *Streptococcus* (GBS) remains the major bacterial cause of sepsis and meningitis in neonates. Early-onset disease occurs in the first 6 days of life, while late-onset disease can present between 7 and 90 days of life. *Listeria monocytogenes* is an additional pathogen that can infect children during the first month of life. Infection with HSV is a concern for the baby in the vignette who is irritable and has vesicular lesions. HSV is typically passed to infants at the time of delivery and becomes symptomatic within the first 2 weeks of life. Neonatal HSV can present in three different forms: disseminated disease; localized central nervous system disease; or localized to skin, eyes, and mucosa. The optimal empiric antibiotic regimen should cover the most likely etiologies for the patient's presentation. Cefotaxime covers GBS and provides additional coverage for gram-negative pathogens. Ampicillin adds additional GBS coverage as well as specific activity against *Listeria*. Acyclovir is included for the specific concern of HSV infection and prevention of disseminated disease.

(A) Vancomycin offers broad-spectrum activity against gram-positive organisms, but does not cover gram-negative organisms, such as *Escherichia coli*. **(C)** Ampicillin and gentamicin together is an effective and traditional antibiotic regimen for neonatal sepsis, but does not provide any coverage for HSV. **(D)** Gentamicin and metronidazole together is a reasonable regimen for abdominal infections in older children. **(E)** There is no need to add fluconazole, as the baby in the vignette does not have any signs or symptoms suggesting a fungal etiology.

---

14 A 4-month-old infant comes to the clinic for a well-child visit. He was born full term and his nursery course was uneventful. His mother's only complaint is that the baby is constipated and passes stool every 2 to 3 days. She states that this has been his normal stooling pattern since birth and that "he didn't have a dirty diaper until he was 2 days old." His mother describes his stools as hard pellets without blood. He eats 4 to 5 ounces of cow's milk formula every 4 hours. His height is at the 5th percentile and his weight is below the 3rd percentile. On examination, the boy is small, but non–ill appearing. His abdomen is soft and he has no hepatosplenomegaly but a soft mass is felt along the left side of the abdomen. His rectal tone is increased and stool is absent from the rectal vault; however, he has a forceful expulsion of stool upon finishing the rectal examination. The image of a barium enema is included in *Figure 2-11*.

Of the following, what is the most likely mechanism for this baby's constipation?

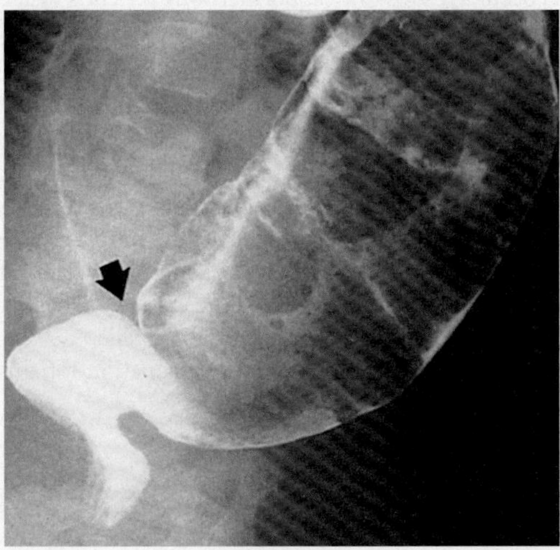

Figure 2-11

(A) Absence of ganglion cells from the rectal submucosal and myenteric plexuses
(B) Stool holding secondary to anal fissures
(C) Hypothyroidism
(D) Severe allergic reaction to milk proteins found in infant formula
(E) Spina bifida occulta

The answer is A: **Absence of ganglion cells from the rectal submucosal and myenteric plexuses.** The patient in the vignette has Hirschsprung disease, or congenital absence of ganglion cells in the myenteric plexus of the colon secondary to a failure of migration during development. This results in an abnormally innervated colon that does not contract naturally with the presence of stool and results in obstruction and constipation. The typical history reveals delayed passage of meconium beyond 24 hours, constipation, intermittent abdominal distention, and vomiting. The physical examination often reveals that stool is palpable throughout the colon but a rectal examination reveals an empty rectal vault. The blast sign may occur upon completion of the rectal examination with a forceful explosion of stool as described in the vignette. Diagnosis is confirmed by barium enema that reveals an increased sigmoid-to-rectum ratio, by rectal manometry, as well as by punch biopsy showing aganglionic megacolon. Treatment is surgical resection of the aganglionic colon.

(B) Anal fissures would be visible on the rectal examination and infants may show signs of constipation to avoid stooling secondary to pain. **(C)** Hypothyroidism does cause failure to thrive and constipation; however, the rectal examination would be expected to have normal tone and palpable stool within the vault. **(D)** Milk protein allergy may present with either constipation or diarrhea; infants often fail to thrive and have blood-streaked stools. Rectal tone is unaffected. **(E)** Spina bifida occulta results from abnormal bony vertebral fusion without herniation. This disorder is often asymptomatic during the infant period with neurologic compromise occurring later in life with growth of the vertebral column.

---

15 A 40 weeks' gestation infant is born by forceps-assisted vaginal delivery to a diabetic mother following a prolonged course of active labor. The infant is appropriately resuscitated and transferred to the nursery without issue. The nursery course over the next 2 days is uneventful; however, the baby develops diffuse bruising and petechiae on the scalp and lateral face. There is a large midline area on his scalp of soft edema that completely obscures the posterior fontanelle.

Of the following, what is the best explanation for this baby's scalp edema?

(A) Cephalohematoma
(B) Subgaleal hemorrhage
(C) Extradural hemorrhage
(D) Caput succedaneum
(E) Intraventricular hemorrhage

The answer is D: Caput succedaneum. Caput succedaneum is edema and ecchymotic swelling of the soft tissues of the head that results from birth trauma sustained during the birthing process. It presents as a diffuse swelling and fluid collection located superficial to the periosteum and characteristically crosses suture lines. Caput succedaneum usually resolves in the first 2 weeks of life. Infants are at increased risk for elevated bilirubin levels secondary to increased hemolysis.

(A) In contrast, a cephalohematoma is a subperiosteal hemorrhage that is limited to one cranial bone and therefore does not cross the suture lines. See *Figure 2-12* for a comparison of caput succedaneum and cephalohematoma. **(B)** Subgaleal hemorrhage is a life-threatening hemorrhage in infants that occurs beneath the aponeurosis and may be associated with significant blood loss and shock. **(C)** Extradural hemorrhage is usually the result of a skull fracture with a resultant bleed between the dura and skull and is often associated with trauma in children and adolescents. **(E)** Intraventricular hemorrhage is seen mostly in premature infants from bleeding of the germinal matrix secondary to immaturity of the vasculature.

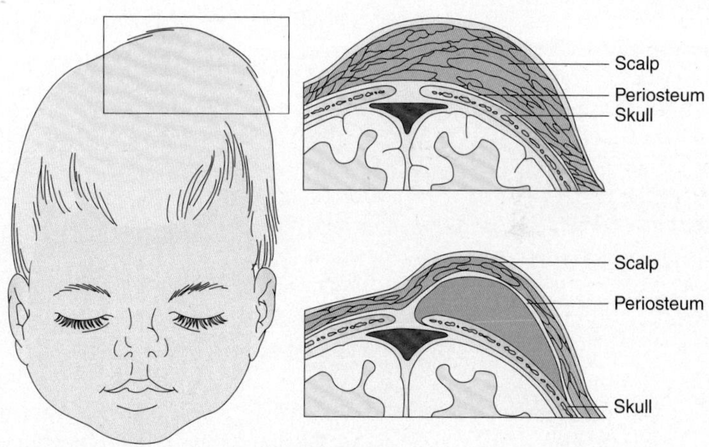

Figure 2-12

CHAPTER 3

Development

MARK M. BUTTERLY

1 A young boy displays the Moro reflex, holds his hands in fists most of the time, can lift his head while prone, startles to sound, and visually fixates on an object in his central gaze, tracking it to midline but not beyond.

Of the following, what is the youngest age this boy is most likely to be?

(A) 1 week
(B) 1 month
(C) 2 months
(D) 4 months
(E) 6 months

The answer is B: 1 month. At age 1 month, infants should be able to briefly lift their head while lying prone. The Moro reflex, as noted with bilateral and symmetric arm extension in reaction to extension of the neck, is still present, and hands are generally held in the fisted position. (**A**) Soon after birth, infants can visually fix on an object in their central field of gaze but will not track to midline until age 1 month. (**C**) Infants at age 2 months will track past midline and by age (**D**) 4 months to a full 180°.

2 A full-term 2-month-old presents for a well-child visit. While lying supine on the examination table with his head facing to the left, his left arm is held in extension and his right arm is in flexion. As his mother turns his head to face toward the right, his right arm extends and his left arm flexes.

Of the following, which is true of this child's reaction to head positioning?

(A) This infant demonstrates an appropriate rooting reflex
(B) This infant demonstrates an upper motor neuron abnormality
(C) This infant demonstrates an appropriate tonic neck reflex
(D) This infant demonstrates a lower motor neuron abnormality
(E) This infant demonstrates an inner ear or labyrinthine abnormality

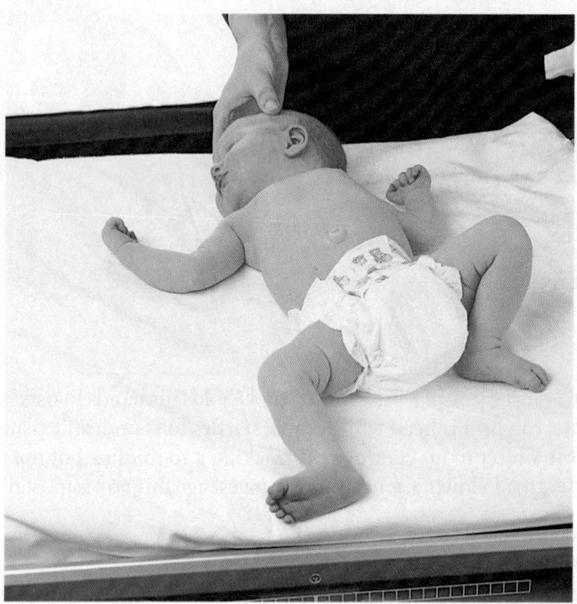

Figure 3-1

The answer is C: **This infant demonstrates an appropriate tonic neck reflex.** Newborn infants depend on neonatal reflexes to assist in passage through the birth canal in addition to survival in the first months of life. The infant in this scenario demonstrates an appropriate tonic neck reflex, also known as the fencing reflex (see *Figure 3-1*). When lying flat on his back the infant will extend the arm in the direction the head is facing, while flexing the contralateral arm. This reflex persists for up to 4 months while awake, though infants may sleep in this position for up to 12 months. **(A)** The rooting, or sucking, reflex is noted when the infant reflexively latches and sucks an object in or near the mouth. **(B, D, E)** As the tonic neck reflex is appropriate for a 2-month-old infant, there are no indications of upper or lower motor neuron or labyrinthine abnormalities in this child.

---

3 A term infant presents for her 2-month well-child visit. During the nutritional history the infant's mother notes that the baby feeds 2 to 3 oz of ready-made infant formula approximately every 2 to 3 hours. The mother states her previous children all ate more than this at age 2 months. Today, she appears well nourished, is vigorous on the examination table, and weighs 6,500 g. Her birth weight was 4,800 g.

Of the following, which is the most appropriate comment regarding infant nutrition and growth?

(A) Formula-fed infants need to eat more than breastfed infants to gain the same amount of weight
(B) Normal weight gain for an infant is dependent on birth weight
(C) Weight gain is not important if head circumference is advancing appropriately
(D) Healthy infants gain 50 to 60 g/d between ages 1 and 6 months
(E) Normal weight gain for an infant is 20 to 30 g/d

The answer is E: Normal weight gain for an infant is 20 to 30 g/d. Healthy term infants gain weight rapidly in the first year of life. **(D)** This weight gain is most marked in the first 6 months of life when the normal weight gain is between 20 and 30 g/d.

(A) Weight gain and growth velocity in both formula and breastfed infants are similar and **(B)** independent of initial birth weight. **(C)** Head circumference is an extremely important growth parameter in assessing brain growth; it is often preserved in states of malnourishment, making weight gain an important and earlier sign of potential nutritional problems.

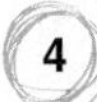

4 The father of a 2-year-old girl expresses distress over his daughter's behavior when she is upset. He notes when prompted to participate in activities she does not enjoy, like eating vegetables at dinner, sharing toys with her cousins, and getting dressed for church services, she often shouts, cries, and occasionally falls to the ground pounding her fists and feet on the floor.

Of the following, which is the most appropriate guidance regarding this patient's behavior?

(A) She should be disciplined by gently scolding the child immediately
(B) This behavior is a rare complication of extreme aggression in children
(C) This behavior is only concerning if the child holds her breath
(D) This behavior is most common in children 4 to 6 years old
(E) This behavior is best addressed by assuring the child's safety and ignoring the tantrum

The answer is E: This behavior is best addressed by assuring the child's safety and ignoring the tantrum. Anger is a normal and regular emotion. While older children and adults have the cognitive and language skills necessary to express anger in mature manners, infants and toddlers do not. Between the ages of 15 and 36 months, motor and cognitive skills, particularly the desire for autonomy, develop more astutely than language and speech skills. This relative discoordination leads toddlers to know what they want and how to get it, but leaves them unable to effectively express this want resulting in frustration and acting out in the form of a temper tantrum. **(B)** Thus, the typical and mild tantrums displayed by the girl in the vignette are normal developmental occurrences and not indicative of extreme aggression. **(C)** While breath-holding spells can be dramatic, even typical cyanotic breath-holding spells are within the spectrum of normal for temper tantrums. The most effective way to address these normally occurring events is to assure the child is in a safe environment so they will not hurt themselves or others, and ignore the event. **(A)** Scolding the child for a tantrum is ineffective and may exacerbate the tantrums' intensity and frequency. **(D)** As developmental progression occurs with age, tantrums become less frequent and generally subside by age 4 to 6 years.

5 Of the following, which is the most accurate statement regarding infant fontanelles?

(A) The anterior fontanelle closes between ages 9 and 18 months
(B) The posterior fontanelle closes between 32 and 40 weeks' gestation
(C) The posterior fontanelle closes between ages 6 and 12 months
(D) The anterior fontanelle is normally bulging
(E) The anterior fontanelle is located at the junction of the occipital and frontal bones

The answer is A: The anterior fontanelle closes between ages 9 and 18 months. The infant skull is composed of six separate bones connected along sutures. The intersection of three or more of these bones creates a fontanelle. **(E)** The anterior fontanelle is made up of the two frontal bones and two parietal bones, and the posterior fontanelle is made up of two parietal bones and the occipital bone (see *Figure 3-2*). These sutures allow for significant brain growth and intracranial expansion during infancy. **(D)** On palpation, the fontanelles should be soft and flat. Premature or delayed closures, as well as bulging or sunken positioning, of the fontanelles are important indicators of potential disease. **(B, C)** A healthy infant's posterior fontanelle closes between ages 1 and 2 months and the anterior fontanelle closes between ages 9 and 18 months.

6 A 6-month-old, full-term infant born at the 25th percentile for length, weight, and head circumference presents to the clinic for a health maintenance visit. The child's length, weight, and head circumference were all measured at the 20th percentile at the 4-month well-child visit. The teenage mother is working a full-time job and attending school. The father of the child is not involved in the child's care and she receives little support from her family. Though she is working very diligently, she does express concern for the cost of formula. On examination, the child is small appearing with little subcutaneous fat. His length is now at the 15th percentile, head circumference at the 20th percentile, and weight is just below the 3rd percentile. The remainder of the examination is unremarkable.

Of the following, which is the most appropriate next step in evaluating this child?

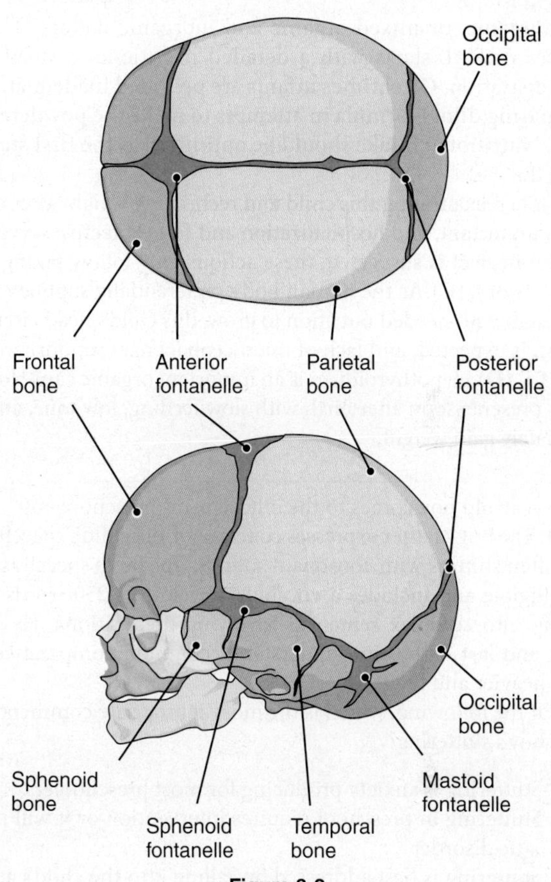

Figure 3-2

(A) Notify protective services regarding potential neglect
(B) Reexamine the child in 2 weeks and trend growth parameters
(C) Reassure the mother that her child's head circumference is appropriate
(D) Obtain thyroid function tests
(E) Obtain a detailed dietary history, including formula preparation

The answer is E: Obtain a detailed dietary history, including formula preparation. Failure to thrive (FTT) is defined as failure to grow at an expected rate, as noted by downward crossing of two percentile lines on a standardized growth curve, or weighing less than the 3rd percentile for age. The child in the vignette fits both parameters. FTT can be caused by organic, inorganic, or mixed organic and inorganic factors. The workup of all causes of FTT starts with a detailed nutritional history including formula preparation. Oftentimes infants are provided inadequate nutrition due to preparing dilute formula in attempts to make the powdered formula last longer. Nutritional intake should be optimized as the first step in treatment of FTT.

(B) While reexamining this child and rechecking weight after optimizing nutrition is important, and hospitalization and **(A)** protective services should be notified if neglect is suspected, these actions only follow taking a detailed nutritional history. **(C)** As the human body preferentially supplies the central nervous system with needed nutrition to grow, this child's head circumference preservation is expected, and lack of microcephaly may support an inorganic cause for FTT. **(D)** Hypothyroidism is an important organic cause for FTT, but it generally presents soon after birth with slow feeding, low tone, and inability to appropriately gain weight.

A 4-year-old boy comes to the office for his preschool entry well-child visit. The boy's father expresses concern for the child's speech and notes he often stutters with consonant sounds. The boy's speech is otherwise intelligible and includes a vocabulary well over 250 words combined easily into complex sentences involving prepositions. He knows his first and last name, and understands common comparative concepts like heavier and longer.

Of the following, which is the most appropriate comment regarding this boy's stuttering?

(A) Stuttering is anxiety producing for most preschoolers
(B) Stuttering in preschool requires intervention or it will progress to a tic disorder
(C) Stuttering is best addressed by calling it to the child's attention so he may concentrate on improving
(D) Stuttering is a normal experience affecting preschoolers
(E) Stuttering is a common sign of speech delay

The answer is D: **Stuttering is a normal experience affecting preschoolers.** Stuttering, as noted by repeating sounds, syllables, or even entire words with or without hesitation between words, is present in many healthy 5-year-olds. Stuttering is more common in boys. **(A)** Generally between the ages of 2 and 6 years, stuttering is not noticed by the child, **(C)** though calling attention to the stuttering, or scolding the child for stuttering, may cause anxiety and worsen symptoms. **(B)** In this age group, stuttering resolves with time. The best intervention is parental patience, allowing the child to finish his speech without interruption, while modeling effective speech strategies like speaking slowly to the child and providing encouragement. **(E)** Stuttering at this age is not a sign of speech delay or prognostic for future tic disorders.

8 A girl can reach for objects, rake them toward herself with her fingers and palm, and transfer them from hand to hand. She can shake toys and bang them together.

Of the following, what is the youngest age at which these fine motor skills are expected?

(A) 4 months
(B) 6 months
(C) 9 months
(D) 12 months
(E) 18 months

The answer is B: 6 months. At age 6 months, infants are rather object oriented and use multiple senses to investigate the objects in their surroundings. Like the young girl in the vignette, reaching for and raking at objects and then manipulating them by transferring from hand to hand and banging them together are actions consistent with the fine motor abilities of a 6-month-old infant. **(A)** A 4-month-old would be expected to reach for objects with both hands together, bat at objects, grab and retain objects, but does not transfer objects from hand to hand. **(C)** A 9-month-old uses a pincer grasp. **(D)** A 1-year-old child is expected to voluntarily release items. **(E)** An 18-month-old is expected to be able to build a three-block tower and spontaneously scribble.

9 The mother of an 8-month-old infant born at 32 weeks' gestation recalls introducing solid foods like rice cereal and oatmeal at about 6 months of age to her now 6-year-old, full-term son. She asks if it is time to begin solid foods for this 8-month-old infant.

Of the following, which developmental milestone is most critical to initiating solid foods in this child?

(A) Transfers object from hand to hand
(B) Brings hands to midline
(C) Bears weight on legs
(D) Pincer grasp
(E) Head steady while sitting

The answer is E: Head steady while sitting. Infant nutrition in the first 4 to 6 months of life should consist exclusively of breast milk or formula as these foods contain significant fat and protein needed for the extraordinary central nervous system growth during this timeframe. However, in order to help establish mastication, bolus formation, and swallowing mechanics, most infants begin taking soft or pureed solids at age 6 months. The most important developmental achievement prior to starting solid foods is excellent head control, as in spontaneously holding one's head steady while sitting. This indicates the child can effectively extend the neck, helping to protect the airway, and lessen the risk of aspiration. The infant in the vignette has a corrected age of 6 months. **(A, B, C, D)** While the additional developmental milestones listed may suggest the child is of an appropriate developmental age, head control is the critical milestone necessary for solid food initiation.

---

10 A family brings in their infant for a well-child visit. When the infant is placed on the table, the child's hands are fisted more than half the time and he lifts his head briefly when placed prone.

Of the following, which is the most likely additional milestone this infant has attained?

(A) Regards face
(B) Laughs out loud
(C) Rolls over
(D) Brings hands to midline
(E) Babbles

The answer is A: Regards face. The motor milestones described in the vignette are most consistent with an infant between ages 1 and 2 months. The social milestone consistent with this age is regarding a face in the infant's central line of vision when held at a close range. This allows the young infant to form appropriate bonding relationships with caregivers leading to associations of pleasure and comfort. These serve as a critical foundation for more advanced social milestones. **(B, C, D)** Infants roll over, laugh out loud, and bring their hands to midline starting at age 4 months, and **(E)** begin to babble at age 6 months.

---

11 A 30-month-old girl must be toilet trained in order to enter a preschool, according to her parents. The mother began toilet training 2 weeks ago and expresses that it is not going well. The girl is otherwise developmentally appropriate. The mother explains when she attempts to put the child on the toilet, the child refuses, attempts to escape the bathroom, and cries.

Of the following, which is the most appropriate approach to toilet training this child?

(A) Have parents gently scold her when she has an accident
(B) Remain consistent and have the parents insist she sit on the toilet every 2 hours during the day
(C) Recommend the family find a different preschool
(D) Tell the parents to transfer responsibility to the child for toilet training with no further prompting
(E) Develop a behavioral modification program to encourage her to use the toilet

The answer is E: Develop a behavioral modification program to encourage her to use the toilet. Physiologic and cognitive development, as well as parental preparedness, play key roles in toilet training success. Between ages 18 and 24 months, many children possess the cognitive combination of desiring autonomy, better appreciating cause and effect, and maintaining object permanence over long periods of time necessary to start toilet training. Though the majority of well children in the United States achieve daytime continence by age 36 months and full continence by age 48 months, toilet training readiness is highly variable. **(C)** Toilet training takes, on average, 3 to 6 months to achieve full continence. **(D)** Toilet training should be accomplished in conjunction with the child and responsibility should not be left solely to the child. Behavior modification programs, e.g., encouraged self-responsibility, including praise and reward for accomplishments, are the most successful methods for encouraging toilet training. **(B)** It is unrealistic that a toddler will comply with sitting on the toilet every 2 hours and may cause increased resistance. **(A)** Punishment leads to power struggle, stress, and resistance, prolonging time to success.

12 A child at a family picnic can balance on one foot for 1 to 2 seconds, draw a circle, and independently put on and take off costume clothing over her own clothes.

Of the following, which is most likely specifically representative of this child's language skills?

(A) Has a vocabulary of 25 to 50 words
(B) Essentially 100% of her speech is intelligible to strangers
(C) Knows her name, age, and gender
(D) Can count by 5s
(E) Can name all of the primary colors

The answer is C: Knows her name, age, and gender. The fine and gross motor milestones achieved by this child are consistent with the skills of a 3-year-old. The language skill most consistent with a 3-year-old is knowledge of concrete information such as her name, age, and gender. **(B)** Additionally, approximately three-quarters of her speech should be intelligible to strangers while 100% should be intelligible by 4 years of age. **(A)** Her vocabulary likely consists of over 250 words as opposed to 25 to 50 words, which is expected of a 2-year-old. **(D, E)** Counting in blocks of 5 to 10 and naming primary colors, however, are more abstract language skills not obtained until ages 4 and 5 years, respectively.

---

13 During a well-child visit with a 4-month-old infant, the mother inquires about her son's expected growth.

Of the following, which is the most accurate statement regarding normal infant growth?

(A) Infants double birth weight by age 6 months and double birth length by age 4 years
(B) Infants double birth weight by age 6 months and double birth length by age 2 years
(C) Infants double birth weight by age 2 weeks and double birth length by age 2 years
(D) Infants double birth weight by age 9 months and double birth length by age 4 years
(E) Infants double birth weight by age 2 months and double birth length by age 3 years

The answer is A: Infants double birth weight by age 6 months and double birth length by age 4 years. Healthy term infants may lose up to 10% of their birth weight in the first weeks of life, regaining birth weight by age 2 weeks. **(C, D, E)** Weight rapidly doubles in well-nourished infants by age 6 months and triples by age 12 months. Infants elongate more steadily. Healthy, well-nourished infants achieve 1 and 1½ times birth length at age 12 months and **(B, C, E)** do not double birth length until age 4 years.

14 A full-term 4-month-old infant presents for a well-child visit. He is at the 25th percentile for length, weight, and head circumference. The child can lift his head and shoulders while prone, but not while sitting supported. He tracks a rattle past midline, though he makes no attempt to grasp it. He spontaneously vocalizes with coos, but does not smile. When discussing these findings with the mother, she seems distant and unattached. She does not reach for the infant following the completion of his nonfocal examination.

Of the following, which statement best describes this infant?

(A) Developmentally appropriate infant
(B) Developmentally delayed due to physical abuse
(C) Developmentally delayed due to malnutrition
(D) Developmentally delayed due to cerebral palsy
(E) Developmentally delayed due to postpartum depression

The answer is E: Developmentally delayed due to postpartum depression. **(A)** The infant in this scenario displays the developmental age of a 2-month-old and is, thus, developmentally delayed. **(B)** Though all forms of abuse and neglect carry a high incidence of developmental delay in the affected child, there is no evidence of physical abuse described in this vignette. **(C, D)** Likewise, there are no risk factors or evidence for cerebral palsy or malnutrition in this infant. However, the mother's detachment may suggest postpartum depression. Postpartum depression leads to impaired maternal–infant bonding and decreased cognitive stimulation resulting in developmental delay. While formally screening this infant and referring for early intervention services is important, it is critical that this mother be screened for postpartum depression with a validated screening tool and referred for proper diagnosis and therapy as indicated.

---

15 A 4-month-old, full-term infant has a normal head circumference (50th percentile), but poor weight and length progression (weight and length both 50th percentile at birth, now both 10th percentile). His parents report he is a slow feeder. On examination, the child has low overall tone, with considerable head lag, and is not able to support his chest up on his arms while prone, and is unable to bear weight on his legs. Additionally, there is mild scleral icterus and a wide-spaced anterior fontanelle.

Of the following, which most likely accounts for this child's constellation of symptoms?

(A) Hypothyroidism
(B) Hyperthyroidism
(C) Congenital adrenal hyperplasia
(D) Inadequate caloric intake
(E) Congenital heart disease

The answer is A: Hypothyroidism. The infant in this vignette presents with failure to thrive (FTT), gross motor delays, mild icterus, and a wide-spaced anterior fontanelle, all consistent with untreated congenital hypothyroidism. Due to low neuromuscular tone, feeding is often slow and contributes to prolonged indirect hyperbilirubinemia and a persistently wide-spaced fontanelle. With rapid recognition, as is available through neonatal blood screening, therapy should be initiated in order to prevent the most concerning long-term consequence of hypothyroidism, namely, intellectual disability.

(D) Inadequate caloric intake is the most common, inorganic cause for FTT, but this does not account for many of the patient's abnormal physical examination findings including the wide-spaced fontanelle. **(B, C, E)** Additionally, while hyperthyroidism, congenital adrenal hyperplasia, and congenital heart disease all may contribute to organic causes for FTT, only hypothyroidism accounts for this child's entire constellation of symptoms.

---

16 A mother of a 6-year-old child is concerned about her child's school readiness. Though she reads to her child regularly and participates in imaginative play with her child, several of her friends' children were started in school programs much younger and this mother is worried that her child will be behind.

Of the following, which cognitive skills should be newly expected of this child and support that he is on track for school readiness?

(A) Copies a triangle
(B) Walks up and down stairs
(C) Knowing age and gender
(D) Tells a story
(E) Knows left from right

The answer is E: Knows left from right. Elements necessary for children to be ready for school are not only cognitive skills, but also motivation to learn and social–emotional readiness. Though early childhood programs help to improve socialization and set the stage for expectations in elementary school where reading and arithmetic will be taught, this mother's regular attention to reading and providing intellectual stimulation and emotional support for her child is critical. In addition to the ability to separate from parents, play well with others, take turns, follow directions in a group, and relate personal experiences, this 6-year-old child should have recently learned her left from right. **(A, C)** Knowing age, name, and gender, as well as copying a triangle is expected at age 5 years. **(B, D)** Walking downstairs and telling a story are milestones expected of 4-year-olds.

17 A boy presents to the clinic for a well-child visit. This boy can run, jump, walk upstairs and downstairs one step at a time, and kick a ball. He can also imitate horizontal lines with a crayon.

Of the following developmental milestones, which is most specifically consistent with his age?

(A) Dresses without assistance
(B) Brushes his teeth
(C) Drinks from a cup
(D) Plays pat-a-cake
(E) Washes and dries his hands

The answer is E: Washes and dries his hands. The boy in the vignette completes gross motor tasks consistent with that of a 2-year-old with more significant speed and strength such as running rather than walking. Additionally, fine motor skills emerge and begin to allow for more intentional use. The skills of a 2-year-old have gone beyond imitation of **(D)** pat-a-cake (age 9 months) or **(C)** drinking from a cup (age 15 months) and progressing to washing hands and using a spoon well. **(A)** Dressing without assistance occurs at age 4 years and **(B)** brushing one's own teeth at age 5 years.

18 A child in clinic is able to support his head while held, keep his chest up while prone using his arms as support, bring his hands to midline, turn laterally toward a sound, and laugh or squeal when excited.

Of the following, which additional milestone will this child most likely display?

(A) Stands alone for 10 seconds
(B) Rolls from front to back
(C) Raking grasp for objects
(D) Feeds self
(E) Uses "mama" and "dada" specifically

The answer is B: Rolls from front to back. The gross and fine motor functioning as well as language and personal social skills are consistent with those of a 4-month-old. Additional skills of 4-month-olds include rolling from front to back, briefly bearing weight on legs when the trunk is supported, beginning to reach and bat at objects, and smiling reciprocally with an examiner or in a mirror. The remaining milestones are more advanced than would be expected of a 4-month-old: **(C)** raking grasp (6-month-old), **(A, E)** stands alone for 10 seconds and using "mama" and "dada" specifically (12-month-old), and **(D)** feeding self (18-month-old).

19 A 4-month-old former 30 weeks' gestation infant is experiencing feeding difficulty. The infant's mother notes that the child was in the neonatal intensive care unit for the first 10 weeks of life. He was intubated twice, mechanically ventilated for 2 weeks, and fed through a nasogastric tube for 8 weeks. He has been gaining weight appropriately since discharge from the nursery. He feeds 2 ounces by bottle per feed though the mother notes that the child frequently gags and turns his head away from the bottle while sucking.

Of the following, which is the most appropriate next step in the management of this patient?

(A) Continue bottle feeding as directed by the neonatal intensive care unit
(B) Reinsert a nasogastric tube for feeding
(C) Start a H_2-receptor antagonist twice daily
(D) Reassure the mother that weight gain is appropriate and reexamine the child in 2 months
(E) Refer to speech therapy

The answer is E: Refer to speech therapy. The patient in the vignette is experiencing oral aversion, a complex disorder in which children experience difficulty sucking and swallowing, presumably due to a sensation of discomfort or pain during the feeding process. Though the etiology of oral aversion is not yet well understood, and oral aversion can happen to any child, it is more common in premature infants. This is possibly due to the increased likelihood of repetitive, relatively minor, oral and facial trauma associated with intubation, nasogastric tube insertion, and the facial taping and manipulation necessitated by such procedures. **(B)** The child in the vignette is gaining appropriate weight, so reinsertion of a nasogastric tube is not indicated. However, oral aversion often improves with appropriate speech therapy and **(A)** altering the feeding technique. **(D)** Further, improvement is greater and swifter the earlier the child starts therapy. **(C)** Though H_2 blockers are frequently used as first-line therapy for gastroesophageal reflux, they play no role in treating oral aversion.

20 The mother of a 9-month-old, full-term infant expresses distress that her son does not yet have any visible teeth.

Of the following, which statement regarding primary tooth eruption is most accurate?

(A) Upper teeth usually emerge before lower teeth
(B) Boys tend to show tooth eruption before girls, between 4 and 6 months of age
(C) Lower central incisors emerge first, between 6 and 12 months of age
(D) First molars emerge between 9 and 12 months of age
(E) Upper and lower incisors are necessary before starting solid foods

The answer is C: Lower central incisors emerge first, between 6 and 12 months of age. Primary teeth eruption is an important, but widely variable process in infancy. In general, primary teeth emerge in mirror image pairs on the left and the right sides of the jaw. **(A)** The bottom two central incisors erupt first **(B)** between ages 6 and 12 months. The upper central incisors generally follow. This paired eruption, with lower teeth preceding upper teeth, continues until all 20 primary teeth are present between ages 30 and 36 months. **(D)** First molars appear between ages 14 and 18 months. As with most growth processes, girls have a slight tendency to develop before boys. **(E)** Though teeth serve a distinct role in mastication later in life, soft solids may be started when a child displays appropriate head control whether or not teeth are present.

21 A 2-day-old, full-term neonate in the nursery has spontaneous movement of all four extremities, strong palmar and plantar grasps, a strong suck reflex when its cheek is lightly stroked, and a bilateral upgoing Babinski reflex. The infant is easily aroused from sleep.

Of the following, which statement is true regarding this infant's neurologic examination?

(A) Palmar grasp reflexes can persist for up to 12 months
(B) Plantar grasp reflexes can persist for up to 36 months
(C) Upgoing Babinski reflexes can persist for up to 12 months
(D) The suck reflex is also known as the Gallant reflex
(E) Neonatal reflexes resolve by age 2 months

The answer is C: Upgoing Babinski reflexes can persist for up to 12 months. Newborn infants depend on neonatal reflexes to assist in passage through the birth canal in addition to survival in the first months of life. Early absence or late extension of these neonatal reflexes may indicate significant problems with the infant's central nervous system. Upgoing Babinski reflexes can persist for up to 12 months. **(A)** Palmar grasp reflex generally persists for only 4 months, when a rudimentary pincer grasp begins to develop. **(B)** Plantar reflexes persist longer and may last up to 12 months. **(D)** The suck reflex is also known as the rooting reflex. The Gallant reflex is elicited by stroking along the flank of an infant causing ipsilateral contraction. This reflex persists until about 5 months of age.

---

22 A 7-day-old term neonate presents for a well-child visit. The neonate was born without complications weighing 3,200 g. The mother states that the neonate is exclusively breastfed. The neonate latches well, has been producing both urine and stool without difficulty, and spits up occasionally while burping after feeds. The neonate appears well today and weighs 3,000 g.

Of the following, which is the most appropriate statement regarding this neonate's weight?

(A) Healthy neonates regain their birth weight by age 2 weeks
(B) Healthy neonates may lose as much as 20% of their birth weight by age 2 weeks
(C) Exclusive breastfeeding is the primary cause of this neonate's weight loss
(D) Gastroesophageal reflux is the most likely cause of this neonate's weight loss
(E) This neonate should be reweighed on the nursery scale to confirm weight loss

The answer is A: Healthy neonates regain their birth weight by age 2 weeks. During physiologic adjustment from intrauterine to extrauterine existence, **(B)** healthy neonates may lose up to 10% of their birth weight during the first weeks of life. **(C)** Much of this weight is extracellular fluid lost through diuresis. However, with proper feeding of either breast milk or appropriately prepared commercial formula, healthy neonates should regain this weight, matching birth weight, by age 2 weeks. **(D)** This neonate's occasional spit-ups while burping after feeds are normal. **(E)** While weighing, neonates with abnormal weight gain or loss on the same scale may produce more accurate growth measurements for tracking, confirming normally expected weight loss in this neonate is unnecessary.

---

23 A 12-month-old neonate born at 28 weeks' gestational age can get to a sitting position, pull to stand, and has just begun cruising, though cannot walk with one hand for support. She can additionally bang two cubes, say "mama" and "dada" nonspecifically, and wave bye-bye.

In order to calculate this child's developmental quotient (DQ) (developmental age/chronologic age) × 100, which are the most appropriate ages to use?

(A) Developmental age—6 months; chronologic age—9 months
(B) Developmental age—6 months; chronologic age—12 months
(C) Developmental age—9 months; chronologic age—9 months
(D) Developmental age—9 months; chronologic age—12 months
(E) Developmental age—12 months; chronologic age—9 months

The answer is C: Developmental age—9 months; chronologic age—9 months. The DQ is a ratio of the child's developmental age in comparison to the chronologic age. This ratio helps quantify potential developmental delay. A DQ ≥ 85 is considered normal and not indicative of developmental delay. A DQ between 71 and 84 is indicative of mild-to-moderate delay. A DQ ≤ 70 denotes severe delay.

(A, B, D, E) The skills this child displays—sitting, standing, cruising, banging two cubes, using "mama" and "dada" specifically, and waving bye-bye, but not yet walking—are consistent with the developmental age of 9 months. The chronologic age of this child must be corrected for her 12 weeks of prematurity. Thus, this child's chronologic age is 12 months, minus 3 months for prematurity, resulting in 9 months. Overall, this child is developing appropriately with a DQ of (9 months/9 months) × 100 = 100.

24 A 6-year-old girl whose teachers are concerned about her ability to keep up with her classmates is found to have a Wechsler Intelligence Scale for Children (WISC)-IV intelligence quotient (IQ) of 70 with a verbal comprehension factor score of 65 and a perceptual reasoning factor score of 70.

Of the following, these results are most supportive of which diagnosis?

(A) Average intelligence
(B) General cognitive deficit
(C) Dyslexia
(D) Attention-deficit disorder
(E) Isolated nonverbal learning disability

The answer is B: General cognitive deficit. French psychologists Alfred Binet and Theodore Simon developed the first intelligence testing in the early 1900s. The Binet-Simon test for childhood intelligence was adapted by American researchers to the Stanford-Binet test which calculates a single number to reference intelligence; the IQ. A child's IQ is calculated by dividing the test taker's mental age by her chronologic age, and then multiplying this number by 100 with an average score being 100. Further research and attempts at improving the Stanford-Binet test led American researcher David Wechsler to develop the WISC, which has been updated several times since its creation. The WISC-IV provides scores in four major areas of intelligence: a Verbal Comprehension Index, a Perceptual Reasoning Index, a Working Memory Index, and a Processing Speed Index as well as a full-scale IQ score and General Ability Index. **(A)** The average value is again 100, with normal scores ranging from 75 to 115. **(E)** The young girl in the vignette scores below average on verbal comprehension and perceptual reasoning as well as overall IQ; thus, these results are most supportive of global or generalized cognitive deficit. **(C, D)** Dyslexia and attention-deficit disorder are independent of intelligence.

---

25 An 8-year-old boy is brought to the clinic for evaluation of worsening school performance and acting out. Both the mother and child note that although the child has always been active and outgoing, over the past several months the patient has had a more difficult time with speaking out of turn in class and sitting still. The child has attempted to control his outbursts, but claims he cannot. While in the examination room, he demonstrates intermittent ballistic movements of both arms as well as an occasional clearing of the throat.

Of the following, which is the most accurate statement regarding this condition?

(A) Affects women more often than men
(B) Peak age of onset is in the third decade of life
(C) Tics generally plateau with advancing age
(D) At onset, symptom-free periods can last for up to 6 months
(E) Involves both motor and vocal tics

The answer is E: Involves both motor and vocal tics. Tourette syndrome, as described in the child in the vignette, is a chronic tic disorder characterized by motor and vocal tics. **(B)** The peak age of onset is 7 to 10 years and **(A)** men are affected up to four times as frequently as women. A facial or neck tic is the most common presenting symptom. **(D)** Tics must be present for a period of 1 year with tic-free intervals no longer than 3 months. Tics can be either simple, involving a single muscle group, or complex, involving multiple muscle groups in coordination leading to the more distressing tics of Tourette syndrome: echolalia (repeating words) and coprolalia (uttering swear words). Motor tics precede vocal tics, and simple tics precede complex tics in the progression of Tourette syndrome. Though tics generally increase to peak in the teen years, **(C)** symptoms can improve, if not resolve, with advancing age and most patients do not require lifelong therapy.

26 The mother of a 30-month-old boy brought in for a well-child visit expresses concerns that her child does not respond to his name. On examination, the child inconsistently turns to the voice of his mother.

The external auditory canal, tympanic membrane, visible ossicles, and middle ear space appear normal.

Of the following, which is the most appropriate next step in assessing the mother's concern for her son?

(A) Refer the child for speech therapy
(B) Refer the child for brainstem audio-evoked response testing
(C) Refer the child for conditioned play audiometry testing
(D) Refer the child to a pediatric otolaryngologist
(E) Reassure mother her child's ears and hearing are normal

The answer is C: Refer the child for conditioned play audiometry testing. Infants and toddlers should be screened for hearing loss at each well-child visit. **(E)** Parental concern for abnormal hearing should be taken seriously and appropriately evaluated through audiometric testing by the primary care physician. Appropriate testing for hearing loss is dependent on the age and development of the child. **(B)** Brainstem auditory-evoked response testing tests electroencephalographic response to auditory stimuli and is most appropriate for testing infants from birth to age 6 months. Visually reinforced audiometry is when a child is conditioned to localize, or look at, an object near the emitted sound source and rewarded with a visual response. This form of testing is best used in children 7 months old to 2 years old. Conditioned play audiometry, when a child is conditioned to perform a specific play task in response to an emitted sound, is the most appropriate testing for children 2 to 3 years old. **(A, D)** This child may eventually need speech therapy or referral to a pediatric otolaryngologist. However, the most important priority at this time is to establish whether there is any hearing loss.

27 A previously healthy, full-term, 6-month-old infant presents for a well-child visit. On examination, she can reach for and take two objects and transfer them from hand to hand. She can roll over from both back to front and front to back. Though she smiles reciprocally and laughs, she does not babble, nor does she imitate speech when she is engaged during the examination. The remainder of the infant's examination, including otoscopic examination, is unremarkable.

Of the following, which is the most appropriate statement regarding this girl's developmental progress?

(A) Isolated language delay, refer for speech therapy
(B) Isolated gross motor delay, refer for physical therapy
(C) Isolated language delay, refer for audiology testing
(D) Isolated fine motor delay, refer for occupational therapy
(E) Mixed language and fine motor delay, refer to a behavior and developmental specialist

The answer is C: Isolated language delay, refer for audiology testing. The 6-month-old infant in this vignette displays appropriate **(B)** gross motor skills (rolls from front to back and back to front), **(D, E)** fine motor skills (reaches for objects, transfers from hand to hand), and personal/social skills (smiles reciprocally). She displays delayed language skills (laughs reciprocally, but does not imitate speech sounds or use single syllables). Isolated speech delay may indicate hearing loss and mandates evaluation. **(A)** While speech therapy may be an eventual referral for this child, this infant's hearing must first be objectively assessed. Thus, referral for audiology testing is the most appropriate next step.

---

28 A family notes no concerns of an 18-month-old girl at her well-child visit. On examination, the child climbs in and out of a chair, can throw a ball, has a vocabulary of 10 to 25 words, and is able to turn the pages of a board book. The child displays a rudimentary pincer grasp and can grasp two cubes when offered four. The child bangs them together, though cannot stack the cubes.

Of the following, which is the most accurate statement regarding this child's development?

(A) Normal gross motor, fine motor, and speech development; no referral necessary
(B) Normal fine motor and speech development with gross motor delay; refer for occupational therapy evaluation
(C) Normal fine motor and speech development with gross motor delay; refer for physical therapy evaluation
(D) Normal gross motor and fine motor development with speech delay; refer for speech therapy evaluation
(E) Normal gross motor and speech development with fine motor delay; refer for occupational therapy evaluation

The answer is E: Normal gross motor and speech development with fine motor delay; refer for occupational therapy evaluation. At age 18 months, infants have developed significant truncal strength and extremity dexterity. Cognitively, 18-month-old children have a greater appreciation of the individual parts of objects and enjoy investigating and manipulating them. The girl in the vignette is able to climb up and down simple structures like a chair. She has a vocabulary of 10 to 25 words and can point to pictures in a book while turning the pages of a board book. Additionally, self-care activities like feeding with utensils and changing clothes are common at this age. **(A, B, C, D)** However, at age 18 months, this child should have a well-developed pincer grasp and be able to stack three to four cubes in a tower. As the child in the vignette does not display these skills, she is at risk for fine motor delay and should be referred to occupational therapy for evaluation and treatment.

29 A 2-year-old boy is noted by his parents to have gained less weight than expected since the last well-child check. Upon reviewing this child's growth chart, his growth velocity from age 6 months to 12 months was greater than that from age 18 months to 2 years.

Of the following, which is the most accurate statement regarding this observation?

(A) Growth velocity normally decreases at age 2 years
(B) Growth velocity remains linear from birth to age 5 years
(C) A child doubles birth length before doubling birth weight
(D) Children lose weight between ages 15 and 24 months
(E) Failure to thrive (FTT) threshold is defined as weight below the 10th percentile

The answer is A: Growth velocity normally decreases at age 2 years. Beginning at age 9 months and rapidly progressing through age 2 years, autonomy is a crucial developmental skill in gaining independence. Between ages 9 and 24 months, children begin feeding themselves. At first, self-feeding is messy and exercising autonomy can be frustrating. Infants intermittently may refuse to eat a meal altogether and this can lead to slight decrease in caloric intake. **(B)** This developmental stage coincides with normally decreased growth velocity, **(D)** though no loss of weight. At age 2 years the rapid growth phase of infancy tapers off. **(E)** FTT is defined as weight less than the 3rd percentile for age or crossing two growth lines on the growth chart in children less than 3 years old. **(C)** Children double their birth weight by 6 months and they double their birth length by 4 years.

30 A boy can walk up the step at the base of the examination table while his hand is held, and climb into a chair after the examination's completion. When asked to stack cubes and then place them in the cup, he can stack three to four cubes and place them in the cup. His parents report he feeds himself with a spoon and fork, names three body parts, and can take off his shirt for bedtime.

Of the following, what is the youngest age at which these activities are expected?

(A) 9 months
(B) 12 months
(C) 18 months
(D) 24 months
(E) 36 months

The answer is C: 18 months. At age 18 months, children have developed significant truncal strength and extremity dexterity. **(A, B, D, E)** Cognitively, 18-month-old children have a greater appreciation of the individual parts of objects and enjoy investigating and manipulating them. The boy in the vignette is able to climb up and down simple structures as well as follow multiple-step commands. He knows and can distinguish multiple body parts and likely pictures of objects as in a book. Additionally, self-care activities like feeding with utensils and changing clothes are common.

31 A 3-year-old boy is in the examination room awaiting his well-child check and he is playing a game on his mother's smart phone.

Of the following, which is the most accurate recommendation for this mother regarding screen time for her child?

(A) Screen time should be limited to 3 hours per day
(B) Screen time should be limited to 5 hours per day
(C) Moving a television into the child's bedroom can help improve sleep
(D) Video games on computers, consoles, or smart phones all contribute to screen time
(E) Screen time includes only programming with advertisements

The answer is D: Video games on computers, consoles, or smart phones all contribute to screen time. The dramatically increased availability, variety, and portability of screened devices have been correlated with the significant epidemic of childhood obesity. For this reason, part of routine health advocacy should include education on a healthy lifestyle encouraging play and exercise, healthy nutrition, and limiting screen time. **(B)** Screen time includes all video games, movies, television, and smart phone activities. **(C)** Televisions should not be located in the child's bedroom and should not be turned on during mealtimes. **(A, B)** At age 2, all screen time should be limited to a total of 2 or fewer hours per day.

32 A 3-year-old child displays poor verbal communication and little or no eye contact. He also displays intermittent repetitive hand flapping.

Of the following which is the most accurate statement regarding additional resources for this patient?

(A) Vitamin therapy has been proven to cure some children of this disorder
(B) Zinc chelation in combination with antiepileptic therapy has proven effective
(C) Behavioral, speech, occupational, and physical therapies all assist in improving independent functioning
(D) There is no effective therapy for this disorder
(E) Withholding future routine immunizations will lessen symptoms

The answer is C: Behavioral, speech, occupational, and physical therapies all assist in improving independent functioning. The boy described in the vignette has autism spectrum disorder. Autism spectrum disorder is a group of disorders, more common in men, which includes classic autism; Asperger syndrome; and pervasive developmental disorder, not otherwise specified, also known as atypical autism. Classic autism is marked by verbal and nonverbal communication impairment. Nonverbal communication impairment may include not making eye contact, smiling, or pointing. Social development is also impaired as noted by difficulty sharing emotions and appreciating others' perspectives. Motor development is affected and may be marked by repetitive behaviors such as hand flapping. Autism spectrum disorder can be suspected as early as age 9 months through a validated screening questionnaire. All children should be screened for autism spectrum disorder at ages 9, 18, 24, and 36 months. **(D)** While there is no proven cure, some children do experience mild symptom improvement with time and behavioral, speech, occupational, and physical therapies all assisting to improve independent functioning and should be offered. **(A, B)** There is no proven efficacy to vitamin therapy, heavy metal chelation, or antiepileptic therapy in children with autism spectrum disorder. **(E)** There is no proven link that any routine childhood immunization, in any combination, leads to autism spectrum disorder or exacerbates its symptoms.

---

33 The parents of a 6-month-old infant born at 32 weeks' gestation note the infant is not yet sitting unassisted. On examination, the infant holds his head steady, rolls from front to back, follows an object 180°, and reaches for it while laughing.

Of the following, which is the most appropriate statement regarding this infant's developmental progress?

(A) The infant's development is at the level of a 4-month-old, consistent with his age corrected for prematurity
(B) The infant's development is at the level of a 4-month-old, delayed for his age corrected for prematurity
(C) The infant's development is at the level of a 6-month-old, consistent with his age corrected for prematurity
(D) The infant's development is at the level of a 6-month-old, advanced for his age corrected for prematurity
(E) The infant's development cannot be assessed due to his prematurity

The answer is A: The infant's development is at the level of a 4-month-old, consistent with his age corrected for prematurity. The human body is designed to grow and develop in utero for approximately 40 weeks of gestation. When an infant is born prematurely, though chronologic age advances with the days on the calendar, the infant's nervous system and body may still not yet have reached the maturity to match chronologic age. For this reason, the number of weeks infants were prematurely born is subtracted in order to set appropriate expectations for both growth and development. A chronologic age of 2 years marks the end of the period of adjusting for prematurity. **(B, C, D, E)** The infant in the vignette was born 8 weeks, or 2 months, prematurely, and therefore, should have attained all of the milestones expected of a 4-month-old, such as holding his head steady, rolling from front to back, following an object 180°, and laughing or squealing, but not yet those of a full-term 6-month-old. A 6-month-old would be expected to sit well unsupported, roll back to front, transfer objects between hands, babble, and recognize strangers.

34 A family brings their 2-month-old child in for his first well-child visit. He was born full-term and has been growing and developing appropriately. The child recently began regarding his hand and placing it in his mouth prompting sucking and leading to self-soothing. The parents have noted that the child is sleeping for longer stretches than he did just 2 weeks ago and is also wakeful for longer stretches.

Of the following, which is the most appropriate recommendation to promote proper sleep hygiene in this infant?

(A) Wake the child every 2 hours at night to feed
(B) Exhaust the child by keeping him awake as late as possible, leading to longer night-time sleep
(C) Put the child to sleep drowsy, but not yet asleep, on his back in a crib
(D) Place several soft toys in the child's crib allowing for distraction when the child wakes at night
(E) If the child wakes at night, stimulate the child until he is sleepy again

The answer is C: Put the child to sleep drowsy, but not yet asleep, on his back in a crib. Sleep is broadly classified into two types: REM (rapid-eye-movement) sleep and non-REM sleep (NREM). NREM sleep consists of several stages, ranging from drowsiness through deep sleep. In the early stages (stages I and II), one awakens easily and may not even realize sleep has occurred. In the deeper stages (III and IV), it is very difficult to wake up, and when aroused one is likely to be disoriented and confused.

REM sleep is more active. Breathing and heart rate become irregular, eyes move rapidly back and forth, and control of body temperature is impaired so sweating when hot or shivering when cold are absent. Infants pass more quickly into REM sleep than older children and adults. **(B)** Thus, to promote proper sleep associations of comfort and safety in bed, it is best to place a child in his crib drowsy, but not yet asleep, and on his back. Children should be allowed to pass in and out of sleep naturally at this age. **(E)** Stimulating a child to exhaustion is counterproductive and may promote difficulty sleeping. **(D)** A child should always be placed on its back to sleep, on a firm bedded surface, free of soft toys and blankets to reduce the risk of sudden infant death syndrome. **(A)** At 2 months, infants should be waking on their own to feed every 4 hours and do not need to be woken up every 2 hours if they are maintaining adequate weight gain.

35 The mother of a 2-month-old infant expresses concern that the child cries "all day long" and is intermittently difficult to console. Upon further history, while the infant sleeps and feeds well without issues passing bowels, the infant cries for up to 3 hours per day. On examination the child is sleeping and appears well nourished. When aroused for the examination, the infant cries. After approximately 2 minutes, the infant is consolable by mother's swaying and shushing. However, when the infant is placed back in her car seat, then she cries again.

Of the following, which statement is most accurate regarding this infant's crying?

(A) This infant displays excessive crying consistent with colic
(B) It is normal for infants this age to cry up to 3 hours per day
(C) Treating this infant with a proton pump inhibitor will reduce crying
(D) Crying is a sign of distress in this infant and must be investigated
(E) In addition to swaying and shushing the infant, the mother can employ additional aspects of the 5 S strategy, like shaking

The answer is B: It is normal for infants this age to cry up to 3 hours per day. Crying is a normal part of infant communication skills. Infants cry to express needs like hunger or discomfort. **(D)** However, not all crying is indicative of a want or need. **(A)** Infant crying normally peaks at age 6 to 12 weeks, lasting up to 3 hours per day. **(C)** Given the infant in the vignette has a normal pattern of crying, infantile colic and gastroesophageal reflux are less likely. The crying associated with colic is generally greater than 3 hours per day. Proven strategies of calming a crying infant include the 5 S: swaddling, shushing, swaying, nonnutritive sucking, and side-lying positioning. **(E)** Shaking is not one of the 5 S. An infant should never be shaken for the risk of severe and permanent neurologic damage or death.

Table 3-1 Commonly Quizzed Developmental Milestones

Age	Gross Motor	Fine Motor (Visual)	Language	Social/ Adaptive
Birth—1 mo	Raises head slightly in prone position	Follows with eyes to midline only; hands tightly fisted	Alerts/startles to sound	Fixes on face (at birth)
2 mo	Raises chest and head off bed in prone position	Regards object and follows through 180° arc; briefly retains rattle	Coos and vocalizes reciprocally	Social smile; recognizes parent

(continued)

Table 3-1 Commonly Quizzed Developmental Milestones *(continued)*

Age	Gross Motor	Fine Motor (Visual)	Language	Social/ Adaptive
4 mo	Lifts onto extended elbows in prone position; steady head control with no head lag; rolls over front to back	Reaches for objects with both hands together; bats at objects; grabs and retains objects	Orients to voice; laughs and squeals	Initiates social interaction
6 mo	Sits, but may need support; rolls in both directions	Reaches with one hand; transfers objects hand to hand	Babbles	Recognizes object or person as unfamiliar
9 mo	Sits without support; crawls; pulls to stand	Uses pincer grasp; finger feeds	Imitates speech sounds (nonspecific "mama," "dada"); understands "no"	Plays gesture games ("pat-a-cake"); understands own name; object permanence; stranger anxiety
12 mo	Cruises; stands alone; takes a few independent steps	Can voluntarily release items	Discriminative use of "mama," "dada," plus one to four other words; follows command with gesture	Imitates; comes when called; cooperates with dressing
15 mo	Walks well independently	Builds a two-block tower; throws ball underhand	four to six words in addition to above; uses jargon; responds to one-step verbal command	Begins to use cup; indicates wants or needs

(continued)

Table 3-1 Commonly Quizzed Developmental Milestones *(continued)*

Age	Gross Motor	Fine Motor (Visual)	Language	Social/ Adaptive
18 mo	Runs; walks up stairs with hand held; stoops and recovers	Builds a three-block tower; uses spoon; spontaneous scribbling	Uses 10–25 words; points to body parts when asked; uses words to communicate needs or wants	Uses words to communicate wants or needs; plays near (but not with) other children
24 mo	Walks unassisted upstairs and down stairs; kicks ball; throws ball overhand; jumps with 2 feet off the floor	Builds four- to six-block tower; uses fork and spoon; copies a straight line	Uses 50+ words, two- and three-word phrases; uses "I" and "me"; 50% of speech intelligible to stranger	Removes simple clothing; parallel play
36 mo	Pedals tricycle; broad jumps	Copies a circle	Uses five- to eight-word sentences; 75% of speech intelligible to stranger	Knows age and gender; engages in group play; shares
4 y	Balances on one foot	Copies a cross; catches ball	Tells a story; 100% of speech intelligible to stranger	Dresses self; puts on shoes; washes and dries hands; imaginative play
5 y	Skips with alternating feet	Draws a person with six body parts	Asks what words mean	Names four colors; plays cooperative games; understands "rules" and abides by them
6 y	Rides a bike	Writes name	Identifies written letters and numbers	Knows right from left; knows all color names

Reprinted from Marino BS, Fine KS. *Blueprints Pediatrics*. 5th ed. Baltimore, MD: Lippincott Williams & Wilkins; 2009.

CHAPTER

4

Adolescent Medicine

HEATHER DYER

1 A 14-year-old boy presents with acute onset of left-sided testicular pain. On examination, his testicle is tender to palpation with erythema, and there is a purple-bluish discoloration noted at the superior pole of the testicle. The cremasteric reflex is intact without any change in symptomatology after elevation of the testicle.

Of the following statements, which is the best next step in treatment for this patient?

(A) Surgical correction
(B) Abdominal ultrasound
(C) Administer diphenhydramine
(D) Administer ceftriaxone
(E) Administer ibuprofen

The answer is E: Administer ibuprofen. The patient in the vignette has physical examination findings consistent with torsion of the appendix testis. Torsion of the appendix testis is the most common cause of an acute scrotum in the pediatric population. The appendix testis is an embryologic remnant of the Müllerian duct that sits on the upper pole of the testis. This structure may twist and tort, resulting in infarction. The appendix testis does not serve any physiologic purpose, but may still cause a considerable amount of pain. Treatment for torsion of the appendix testes entails anti-inflammatory medication therapy and supportive care. The blue dot sign, when present, is diagnostic for this condition. It represents the infarcted tissue of the appendix testis, which may be visible through the scrotal skin. The cremasteric reflex is generally spared in cases of torsion of the appendix testis.

Other leading causes of testicular pain include testicular torsion and epididymitis. An acute scrotum may represent a urologic emergency due to concern for torsion of the testicle; however, torsion of the appendix testis is a benign and self-limited condition. **(B)** These can be differentiated with a testicular ultrasound with Doppler studies, rather than an abdominal ultrasound. **(A)** If testicular torsion is identified, emergent urology consultation and surgery are indicated. **(D)** Ceftriaxone is part of the therapy for epididymitis, which presents as fever, abdominal pain, and a painful swollen testicle. **(C)** Diphenhydramine would be indicated if there was a concern for allergic reaction or edema. There is no indication in the vignette that the patient is having reactive edema.

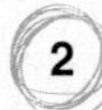

2 A previously healthy 13-year-old boy is brought to the office by his parents for a sports physical for the swim team. In a private discussion with the patient, he reveals he does not need a sports physical as he is not interested in participating this year. On further questioning, the patient reluctantly reveals he is concerned with breast tissue that he has developed over the summer. He reports that the left breast is larger than the right side with mild bilateral resolving tenderness. He denies fever, redness, or drainage from the area. His physical examination reveals a well-developed adolescent boy with height at the 60th percentile, weight at the 45th percentile, and sexual maturity rating stage 3. He has a small amount of firm glandular tissue palpable behind each nipple. His nipples are of normal size and color.

Of the following, which is the best initial plan in management for this patient?

(A) Recommend exercise and weight loss
(B) Referral to a surgeon
(C) Prescribe antibiotics
(D) Referral to endocrinology
(E) Provide reassurance

The answer is E: Provide reassurance. The boy in the vignette has physiologic gynecomastia, which is a common occurrence during male puberty. This condition is generally due to a minor imbalance of estrogen and testosterone during the hormonal fluctuations of puberty and is self-limited, lasting anywhere from a few months to 2 years. **(E)** For the majority of cases, reassurance to the patient and parents regarding the benign nature of the condition is sufficient. **(B)** If the breast tissue development is extreme or does not resolve over the expected time, surgical intervention is occasionally necessary.

(A) Pseudogynecomastia mimics physiologic gynecomastia in that it gives a similar appearance of developing breast tissue. However, this appearance is due to adipose tissue deposition, rather than true glandular development. Treatment includes lifestyle changes with diet and exercise as well as reassurance. The patient in the vignette is not overweight and glandular tissue is palpable on examination. **(C)** While cellulitis or abscesses may occur anywhere under the skin, simultaneous infections affecting both breasts would be extremely unlikely. The patient in the vignette also has no signs or symptoms of infection, such as fever, erythema, drainage, or fluctuance, and therefore antibiotic therapy is not indicated. **(D)** Testicular feminization is a condition in which androgen receptors fail to properly respond to testosterone during embryonic development and results in a child who is chromosomally male but phenotypically female. Such a patient would, indeed, develop breast tissue during puberty. Patients with testicular feminization generally present later due to lack of menarche. The patient in the vignette is a phenotypic male with normal development and therefore an endocrine referral is not indicated at this time.

---

3 A sexually active 17-year-old girl presents to the emergency department with complaints of fever of 101.2°F, dysuria, and lower abdominal pain. On examination, she has tenderness to palpation in the bilateral lower quadrants, left greater than right. Her last menstrual period began 5 days ago. Pelvic examination reveals a mucopurulent discharge and tenderness with cervical motion.

Of the following, which pathogen is the most likely cause of her symptoms?

(A) *Gardnerella vaginalis*
(B) *Chlamydia trachomatis*
(C) *Escherichia coli*
(D) *Yersinia pestis*
(E) *Staphylococcus saprophyticus*

The answer is B: *Chlamydia trachomatis*. The patient in the vignette has fever, abdominal pain, abnormal vaginal discharge, and cervical motion tenderness making pelvic inflammatory disease (PID) a likely diagnosis. PID is an infection of the upper genitourinary tract, including the uterus and fallopian tubes, and may spread to adjacent structures in the abdomen and pelvis. An ascending complication is perihepatitis, also known as Fitz-Hugh and Curtis syndrome. PID is a sexually transmitted disease and the most common organisms involved are *C. trachomatis* and *Neisseria gonorrhoeae.*

(C) Although *E. coli* has rarely been implicated in PID, it is more commonly associated with causing urinary tract infections (UTIs) and pyelonephritis. A UTI can present with abdominal pain and fever, but it would not explain the cervical motion tenderness described in the vignette. **(E)** *S. saprophyticus* causes UTIs in sexually active women.

(D) *Y. pestis* infection can mimic an acute appendicitis but is not implicated in PID. **(A)** Bacterial vaginosis is a bacterial overgrowth with pathogens including *G. vaginalis* and can cause foul-smelling abnormal vaginal discharge and pruritus. It is not a cause of PID.

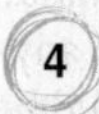

4 A 13-year-old girl presents to the office for evaluation of a rash. Her vital signs are within normal limits and both her height and weight are above the 97th percentile for age. She has no additional complaints, and on inspection of her skin, a 3 cm × 5 cm velvety, hyperpigmented lesion at the side of her neck is noted.

Of the following, which is the most likely explanation of the rash for this patient?

(A) Autoimmune destruction
(B) Allergic reaction
(C) Excess cortisol
(D) Insulin resistance
(E) Sun exposure

The answer is D: Insulin resistance. The description in the vignette is that of acanthosis nigricans. Acanthosis nigricans is a hyperpigmented (brown-to-black) velvety skin lesion, which is typically found in areas of skin folds, such as the axillae and neck. Acanthosis nigricans occurs secondary to increased circulating insulin levels causing hyperplasia of the skin. Thus, most patients with acanthosis nigricans are overweight or obese and identifying such a lesion in a patient should prompt a workup for insulin resistance and type II diabetes mellitus.

(A) Lesions of psoriasis are typically thick red plaques with silver-white scales and can be caused by an autoimmune predisposition. **(B)** Although allergic reactions are a very common explanation for skin lesions, the lesions described for the patient in the vignette are not typical of an allergic reaction. Atopic lesions are red in color and appear as urticarial lesions when generalized or localized over an area of contact with an offending item. **(C)** Cushing syndrome secondary to excessive cortisol is generally not associated with acanthosis nigricans, but would be associated with abdominal striae. **(E)** The plaque-like lesions described in the vignette are not typical of melanoma or sunburn, although lesions of melanoma are hyperpigmented. These lesions generally display variations of color and an irregular border.

5 A 15-year-old girl presents to the emergency department on Sunday evening for evaluation of abdominal pain. She reports nausea without vomiting, diarrhea, or fever. Her last menstrual cycle began 3 weeks ago and was unremarkable. Her symptoms began abruptly this evening, but the patient reports similar symptoms have occurred on three of the last five Sundays prior to presentation. She has been evaluated in three other emergency departments as well as at her primary pediatrician's office. Her mother is very concerned about the amount of school the patient has missed and presents her records from the previous visits, which reveal normal chemistry panels and complete blood cell counts. In addition, the records include a normal ultrasound of a well-visualized appendix, a normal endoscopy/colonoscopy, and an unremarkable computed tomography scan of the abdomen and pelvis. The nurse reports that the patient is feeling hungry and requests a dinner tray. On examination, her abdomen is soft and nondistended, with normal bowel sounds. The patient reports diffuse tenderness in all quadrants.

Of the following, which would be most likely to reveal the correct diagnosis in this patient?

(A) Repeat ultrasound of the appendix
(B) Amylase and lipase levels
(C) Confidential HEADDSSS history
(D) Stool sample for occult blood
(E) Urine pregnancy test

The answer is C: Confidential HEADDSSS history. HEADDSSS is the acronym for the social history taken in adolescents.

- H—Home and living situation: Questions should address who lives at home with the patient as well as their level of safety in home
- E—Education: Includes school performance and plans for career
- A—Activities: Includes discussions about what a patient does for fun
- D—Drugs: Questions should address any drug use, including illicit, over-the-counter, or inappropriate prescription drug use. Also, any of these activities by friends or acquaintances should be addressed
- D—Depression: Includes feelings of sadness or depression
- S—Sexuality: Questions should include a patient's own sexual activity as well as the sexuality they identify with
- S—Safety: Questions should include how safe a patient feels at home, as well as gun, helmet, and seatbelt safety
- S—Suicide: Adolescents should be questioned about ideas or attempts of suicide as well as if they have ever had feelings of harm toward others (homicide)

The presentation of the patient in the vignette with symptoms typically recurring just before the patient is about to return to school, combined with an extensive workup demonstrating normal clinical findings, suggests a non-organic etiology. Factitious, somatoform, and malingering disorders are valid considerations and a thorough history with regard to possible stressors and potential for secondary gain in assuming the sick role must be evaluated. Factitious disorders are those feigned or exaggerated in order to play the sick role, while malingering is continuation of symptoms even upon resolution to continue the external secondary gain. Somatoform disorders differ in that their symptoms are involuntary and unintentional.

(A) Although appendicitis is a leading concern in patients presenting with abdominal pain, the patient in the vignette's abdominal examination is not suggestive of appendicitis. **(B)** Amylase and lipase would be abnormal in patients with pancreatitis who present with nausea, vomiting, and abdominal pain that radiates toward the back. **(D)** There are many conditions that may cause both abdominal pain and blood in the stool; however, most of these would be accompanied by diarrhea and fever. **(E)** While pregnancy should remain a consideration in any girl of reproductive age who presents with abdominal pain, the patient in the vignette has undergone pelvic imaging which did not reveal an intrauterine or ectopic pregnancy, making factitious, somatoform, or malingering disorder more likely.

---

6 A 14-year-old boy with a history of seasonal allergies is brought to the office for evaluation of fatigue. His vital signs are within normal limits. He denies dizziness, chest pain, or palpitations. The patient's body mass index is 31 kg/m^2. On examination, the patient has significant tonsillar hypertrophy without erythema and a loud P2 on cardiac auscultation.

Of the following, which additional piece of history would most assist in establishing his diagnosis?

(A) Cardiac arrhythmias
(B) Recent weight loss
(C) Snoring or choking noises during sleep
(D) Sleepwalking
(E) Exposure to Epstein-Barr virus (EBV)

The answer is C: Snoring or choking noises during sleep. The patient in the vignette is obese, has tonsillar hypertrophy, and has a loud P2 on cardiac examination. The combination of these findings is concerning for obstructive sleep apnea (OSA). OSA is a common disorder among overweight children and adolescents and is characterized by brief, repeated episodes of airflow obstruction during sleep. Patients present with symptoms of fatigue, daytime sleepiness, and nocturnal enuresis, and may experience morning headaches related to carbon dioxide retention. The most frequently associated risk factor for OSA is adenotonsillar hypertrophy, as described for the patient in the vignette. A loud P2 sound suggests pulmonary hypertension, which may be present in severe cases.

(A) The presence of a cardiac arrhythmia might be associated with pulmonary hypertension and cause symptoms of fatigue, but it does not explain the presence of tonsillar hypertrophy. **(B)** While sudden rapid weight loss might be associated with feelings of fatigue, the additional symptoms of tonsillar hypertrophy and cardiac evidence of pulmonary hypertension would not be explained by weight loss. **(D)** Sleepwalking may contribute to disruptive sleep patterns and therefore fatigue, but it is not associated with tonsillar hypertrophy and pulmonary hypertension. **(E)** While EBV is an excellent consideration in the differential of an adolescent with symptoms of fatigue, the tonsils are likely to be inflamed, exudative, and erythematous, rather than simply hypertrophied.

7 A 13-year-old boy presents to clinic for a health maintenance visit. His mother voices concerns regarding his behavior. She states that he does not seem to have many friends, was recently caught stealing from the neighbor's garden, and ran away last summer and again last week. She

states that during the past few years he has been difficult to control and she fears being alone with him. She recently found him hanging the cat by a noose.

Of the following, which condition best explains his behavior?

(A) Oppositional-defiant disorder (ODD)
(B) Attention-deficit hyperactivity disorder (ADHD)
(C) Antisocial personality disorder
(D) Conduct disorder
(E) Schizotypal disorder

The answer is D: **Conduct disorder.** The patient in the vignette is displaying the disruptive and antisocial behavior typified by conduct disorder. Behaviors seen in patients with conduct disorder must be present for at least 6 months and include stealing, lying, fire setting, truancy, vandalism, cruelty to animals, armed robbery, and attempts to run away from home. **(A)** ODD is characterized by less severe disruptive behavior, including loss of temper, conflicts with authority figures, rule-breaking behavior, and frequent blaming of others. **(B)** Children with ADHD are more likely to meet criteria for ODD. ADHD includes difficulty focusing at school and at home with hyperactive, disruptive behaviors. **(C)** Antisocial personality disorder describes a person who disregards and violates the rights of others. Diagnosis of this personality disorder is often not made until late adolescence or early adulthood although symptoms commonly begin early in childhood or adolescence and many patients are diagnosed with conduct disorder prior to age 15. **(E)** Schizotypal personality disorder describes a person with a need for social isolation. Patients are not disruptive or aggressive but rather keep to themselves.

8 Which vaccines are routinely recommended for a healthy 11-year-old at the health maintenance visit?

(A) Tetanus, diphtheria, pertussis (Tdap) and hepatitis A vaccine
(B) Tdap, human papillomavirus vaccine, and meningococcal vaccine
(C) Diphtheria, tetanus, pertussis (DTaP), influenza vaccine, and meningococcal vaccine
(D) DTaP, human papillomavirus vaccine, and meningococcal vaccine
(E) Human papillomavirus vaccine and varicella vaccine

The answer is B: **Tdap, human papillomavirus vaccine, and meningococcal vaccine.** The Centers for Disease Control and Prevention recommended vaccine schedule for age 11 to 12 years includes a Tdap combination vaccine for patients who have completed the standard **(C, D)** DTaP series in early childhood. A three-dose series for human papillomavirus (HPV) is recommended (but not required) for both male and female patients at this age. The first meningococcal conjugate vaccine (MCV) is also recommended for

11- to 12-year-olds (with an MCV booster due at age 16 years). **(A, E)** Varicella and hepatitis A may be indicated if the patient needs to catch up on previously missed vaccines; however, **(B)** the recommended vaccines routinely scheduled for this age group are Tdap, MCV, and the HPV series. **(C)** Influenza vaccination should be recommended for all patients during flu season.

9 A 19-year-old young man is brought by ambulance to the emergency department after causing a disturbance on a nearby college campus. Police report that the patient was shouting incoherently about an upcoming apocalypse organized by the Red Cross and attempting to forcibly baptize passers-by in a large marble fountain on the college quad. The patient's emergency contact, his roommate, reports that the patient dropped out of classes the previous semester and has rarely left his room over the past 6 months, not even to shower. Prior to this time, the patient had been a successful pre-law student. On examination, he demonstrates agitation, disorganized speech, and admits to hearing three distinct disembodied voices, which he says, instructed him to warn his former classmates of the impending apocalypse. A toxicology screen and physical examination are unremarkable.

Of the following, which is the most likely diagnosis for this patient?

(A) Bipolar disorder
(B) Schizophrenia
(C) Schizoaffective disorder
(D) Major depression with psychotic features
(E) Antisocial personality disorder

The answer is B: Schizophrenia. The patient in the vignette is displaying symptoms consistent with schizophrenia. Criteria for the diagnosis of schizophrenia include the presence of two or more symptoms. Positive symptoms include delusions, hallucinations, disorganized speech, and grossly disorganized or catatonic behavior. Negative symptoms include flattened affect, lack of personal hygiene, and social withdrawal. The patient in the vignette displays multiple positive and negative symptoms that meet the criteria for a diagnosis of schizophrenia. The time duration of greater than 6 months, as well as the fact that the patient was previously high-functioning and does not currently seem to be under the influence of any substances, fulfills the remainder of the criteria for diagnosis.

(A) Bipolar disorder can be associated with psychotic symptoms; however, bizarre delusions and complex hallucinations are not typical for bipolar disorder. Patients typically present with symptoms of mood disorder (most commonly depressive symptoms). For diagnosis, the patient must have had at least one significant manic episode, which would be characterized by at least three of the following symptoms: grandiosity, decreased need for sleep, distractibility, excessive talking or pressured speech, flight of ideas or racing thoughts, increased goal-oriented behavior, or increased pleasurable activities. **(C)** Schizoaffective disorder is on the spectrum of schizophrenia; however, differing factors include mood disturbances, such as those seen with bipolar disorder. **(D)** While mood disorders such as depression can produce psychotic symptoms, it is not typical to experience the bizarre delusions and complex hallucinations present for the patient in the vignette. Delusions and hallucinations related to mood disorder are more accurately typified as feeling persecuted or watched, feeling punished for imagined misdeeds, or wrongly believing they suffer from a medical illness. **(E)** Antisocial personality disorder is characterized by a long-standing pattern of behavior of disregard for the rights and feelings of other people.

10 A 15-year-old boy presents to the pediatrician's office with concern regarding his complexion. On examination, the patient has many papules and pustules over his chest, face, and back, as well as numerous comedones, and two large, deep, nodular inflamed lesions.

Of the following pathogens, which is considered to be primarily implicated for this patient's condition?

(A) Virus
(B) Aerobic bacterium
(C) Anaerobic bacterium
(D) Fungus
(E) Yeast

The answer is C: Anaerobic bacterium. The patient in the vignette presents with acne vulgaris. The pathogen implicated in acne is *Propionibacterium acnes*, an anaerobic gram-positive bacterium. The organism is found in follicles and pores on the skin's surface. The bacteria use sebum and cellular debris as energy sources. Increased sebum production, as is seen commonly during puberty, can result in the proliferation of the *P. acnes* bacteria and formation of acne.

11 A 15-year-old girl presents because she has not reached menarche. Her mother's menarche was at age 13. She is a softball player and runs 2 miles twice a week. She reports no changes in her appetite or activity levels. On examination, her height is at the 75th percentile and her body mass index is at the 25th percentile. Her chart reveals that she had breast budding at age 11 and at age 13 had sexual maturity rating 3 of her breasts and pubic hair.

Of the following, what is the next best step in her evaluation?

(A) Measure gonadotropins
(B) Examine her external genitalia
(C) Provide reassurance
(D) Obtain a karyotype
(E) Assess thyroid function

The answer is B: Examine her external genitalia. The patient in the vignette is experiencing primary amenorrhea, or the lack of achieving menarche by age 16 or 4 years after the onset of thelarche. Thus, no pubertal development by age 13 or a halt in normal progression requires a further workup. Causes of primary amenorrhea include hypothalamic/pituitary etiologies, ovarian dysfunction, adrenal abnormalities, anatomic variants, and pregnancy. For the patient in the vignette, she achieved normal onset thelarche and normal progression up to age 13 years. However, 4 years after breast budding, she has still not obtained menarche, warranting further workup. **(A, E)** As she appears to be progressing through puberty appropriately without any other complaints, this is suggestive of an anatomic issue as opposed to thyroid or adrenal diseases. **(B)** Thus, the best next step would be to examine her for an imperforate hymen, presence of a vagina, and clitoral size. **(C)** Given she does have primary amenorrhea, reassurance cannot be given until a detailed workup into the etiology is complete. **(D)** There does not appear to be anything in her examination consistent with a genetic condition and her height is appropriate with no concern for Turner syndrome, another possible cause for amenorrhea in an adolescent girl.

12 A 12-year-old girl presents to the office for a routine school physical. On examination, a nontender asymmetric bulging deformity in the right scapular region of the back is noted when the patient bends forward at the waist. There is no history of trauma and the patient does not complain of any pain at the site. The remainder of the physical examination is unremarkable.

Of the following, which is the most likely diagnosis?

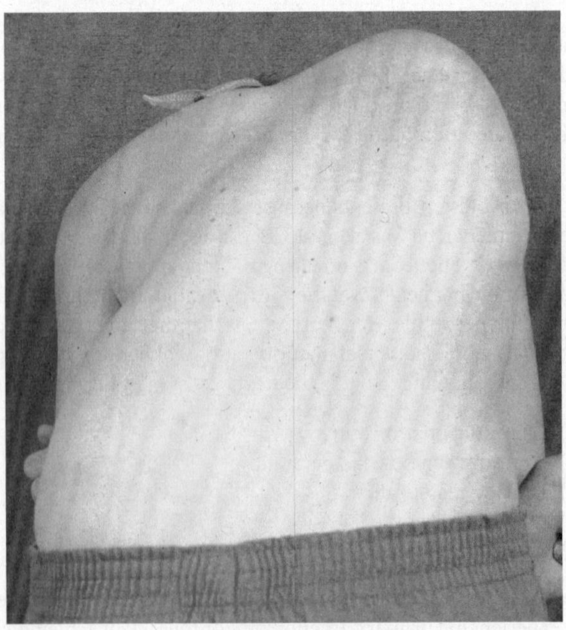

Figure 4-1

(A) Osteosarcoma
(B) Cushing hump
(C) Healing rib fracture
(D) Right shoulder dislocation
(E) Idiopathic scoliosis

The answer is E: Idiopathic scoliosis. Adolescent idiopathic scoliosis is characterized by a lateral deformity of the spine in the frontal plane, commonly affecting children during periods of rapid growth. The cause of idiopathic scoliosis is unknown. The earliest sign of this abnormality is asymmetry of the posterior chest wall on bending forward as presented in the vignette (see *Figure 4-1*). Treatment includes physical therapy, frequent monitoring, back brace, and surgery if the curvature is greater than 50°.

(A) Although osteosarcoma can occur in any bone, it most commonly presents with pain at the end of long bones. **(B)** Cushing syndrome, a result of prolonged exposure to elevated cortisol levels, can cause a hump-like deformity of the posterior back and neck; however, this deformity is composed of fat pads and generally is midline. **(C)** The callous of fracture repair might create some localized asymmetry, however, in the event of a fracture; it would be expected to elicit a history of trauma and pain at the fracture site. In addition, a rib fracture would more likely be anterolateral and would be significantly smaller than the deformity described in the vignette. **(D)** A patient with a dislocated shoulder would be expected to present with pain and limited mobility of the affected extremity.

A 15-year-old girl presents to the office with concern regarding irregular menstrual cycles, having had only three menstrual cycles in the past year and none at all in the last 6 months. She takes no medications. On physical examination, her vital signs are within normal limits with a body mass index of 36 kg/m^2. There are notable open and closed comedones on her face, back, and upper chest, as well as darker hair on her upper lip, face, and extremities. Her basic metabolic profile is unremarkable.

Of the following, which treatment option should be offered to this patient?

(A) Surgery
(B) Levothyroxine
(C) Insulin
(D) Oral contraceptives
(E) Reassurance

The answer is D: Oral contraceptives. The patient in the vignette has irregular menstrual cycles and physical examination findings consistent with polycystic ovary syndrome (PCOS). PCOS is a common disorder of hormone regulation, specifically with regard to the metabolism of androgens and estrogen. Presenting symptoms for PCOS include oligomenorrhea, hirsutism, and acne. PCOS is also associated with insulin resistance and obesity, **(C)** but rarely requires insulin therapy. **(D)** Treatment entails diet and lifestyle modification, as well as oral contraceptives. **(A)** While Cushing syndrome could explain the patient's symptoms of oligomenorrhea, hirsutism, and acne, the patient in the vignette does not exhibit other signs of cortisol overexposure, such as thinning of the skin, red or violet striae, hypertension, or electrolyte abnormalities. Treatment may involve reduction of corticosteroid use, medications, and possibly surgery. **(E)** Patients with androgen insensitivity are genotypically males, and therefore, do not experience menarche. Treatment for androgen insensitivity is generally supportive. **(B)** Hypothyroidism may present with irregular periods, dry skin, obesity, and hair changes, but is less likely to cause acne and therefore a less likely diagnosis than PCOS for the patient.

14 A 16-year-old girl presents to the emergency department with a sudden onset of nausea, vomiting, and abdominal pain. At her friend's prompting, the patient admits to taking 30 extra-strength Tylenol® tablets 8 hours ago after breaking up with her boyfriend. An acetaminophen level comes back elevated at 1,020 μmol/L, and her liver function tests are within normal limits.

Of the following options, which is the best management for this patient?

(A) Activated charcoal
(B) Syrup of ipecac
(C) Naloxone
(D) *N*-Acetylcysteine (NAC)
(E) Hemodialysis

The answer is D: *N*-Acetylcysteine (NAC). The patient in the vignette has ingested a large amount of acetaminophen and her 8-hour acetaminophen level places her well above the cutoff for high risk of hepatotoxicity. Acetaminophen is metabolized in the liver, and in an overdose situation the sulfonation and glucuronidation pathways are overwhelmed. Therefore, excess acetaminophen is metabolized by the p450 system and hepatotoxic metabolites are formed. In early acetaminophen toxic ingestion, liver enzymes will generally remain within normal limits. **(D)** Treatment with NAC should be started as soon as possible due to the high risk of liver failure. NAC is most effective when started 8 to 10 hours after the initial ingestion. Acetaminophen levels as well as liver function tests should be closely monitored.

(A) Activated charcoal is not the treatment of choice for this patient; however, when administered less than 2 hours following ingestion it can absorb some of the acetaminophen. **(B)** The induction of emesis with syrup of ipecac is never recommended. **(C)** Naloxone is the antidote for opioid overdose. **(E)** Hemodialysis may be indicated with salicylate toxicity.

---

15 A 14-year-old girl presents to the office with concerns that she has not yet experienced menarche. Her physical examination reveals an adolescent girl within the normal range for height and weight, and a sexual maturity rating 2. Follicle-stimulating hormone (FSH) and luteinizing hormone (LH) levels are checked and reported as low.

Of the following, which is her most likely diagnosis?

(A) Turner syndrome
(B) Androgen insensitivity
(C) Polycystic ovarian syndrome
(D) Constitutional delay
(E) Ovarian failure

The answer is D: **Constitutional delay.** Constitutional delay, or a relative delay of normal puberty, is a common cause of primary amenorrhea in young adolescent girls. FSH and LH levels are therefore expected to be low.

(A) Turner syndrome is characterized by a genotype of 45,X0 with a resulting phenotypic female appearance, but with short stature and a lack of ovarian function. Additional features may include a webbed neck, shield chest, heart defects, and lymphedema. Patients with Turner syndrome, as well as those with **(E)** ovarian failure, are expected to have high FSH and LH levels, as these hormones are futilely attempting to stimulate the nonfunctional ovaries. **(B)** Androgen insensitivity is a condition characterized by a genotype of 46,XY where receptors are resistant to the virilizing effects of testosterone, resulting in complete insensitivity to a phenotypic female appearance in a genotypic male. While patients with androgen insensitivity may present for evaluation of primary amenorrhea, the FSH and LH levels would be expected to be normal or high, rather than low, and breast development would be unlikely to be delayed, due to conversion of excess testosterone to estradiol. **(C)** Polycystic ovarian syndrome is a common cause of secondary amenorrhea. Expected additional features would include an elevated body mass index, excessive acne, and hirsutism. FSH and LH levels would not be expected to be low.

---

16 A 15-year-old girl presents to the adolescent clinic complaining of a foul-smelling vaginal discharge. She describes the discharge as thin and gray in color. She is sexually active. On further evaluation, a KOH whiff test is positive for a fishy odor and microscopic evaluation reveals the findings in *Figure 4-2*.

Of the following, which is the most appropriate treatment for this patient?

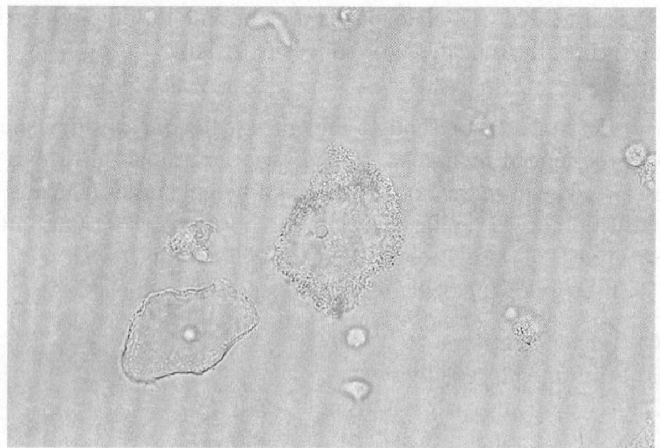

Figure 4-2

(A) Reassurance
(B) Fluconazole
(C) Azithromycin
(D) Ceftriaxone
(E) Metronidazole

The answer is E: Metronidazole. Bacterial vaginosis (BV) is a common condition typified by the symptoms described in the vignette: a thin and gray vaginal discharge with a fishy odor. BV may be asymptomatic in up to half of the cases and is not often associated with abdominal pain, significant pruritus, or dysuria. It occurs secondary to a change in the vaginal bacterial flora. The microscopic evaluation shown in the vignette demonstrates clue cells, a classic finding for BV. Clue cells are squamous vaginal epithelial cells covered with bacteria, which cause a stippled appearance and a ragged cellular border on microscopic examination. Bacterial involvement includes *Gardnerella vaginalis*, *Mycoplasma hominis*, *Ureaplasma* sp., and anaerobic species, along with a marked decreased in *Lactobacillus* sp. **(A, E)** Treatment for BV is metronidazole.

(B) Although vaginal candidal infections are quite common in adolescents, the patient in the vignette does not have the typical complaints including a white, clumpy discharge, vulvovaginal itching, and irritation. Treatment for vaginal candidiasis is with topical antifungal creams or oral fluconazole. **(C)** *Chlamydia trachomatis* is a sexually transmitted infection and may be characterized by vaginal discharge; however, patients are often asymptomatic. The description of the discharge and presence of clue cells is not consistent with *C. trachomatis* infection. Treatment for chlamydia is a single dose of 1 g of azithromycin or doxycycline BID for 1 week. **(D)** *Neisseria gonorrhoeae* infections are typified by vaginal discharge, dysuria, abnormal vaginal bleeding, and lower abdominal pain. It is treated with a single intramuscular injection with ceftriaxone.

17 A 16-year-old boy is dropped off at the emergency room by a group of friends. He is complaining of headache, diarrhea, and vomiting. He is unable to sit still, crying, and anxious to leave the hospital. He is unsure where his friends have gone. His physical examination is significant for a thin, agitated, perspiring man. He is yawning frequently and his pupils are dilated.

Of the following, which drug's withdrawal symptoms are most consistent with his findings?

(A) Alcohol
(B) Cocaine
(C) Mescaline
(D) Heroin
(E) Caffeine

The answer is D: Heroin. The patient in the vignette has signs and symptoms consistent with heroin withdrawal. Patients withdrawing from heroin addiction may begin experiencing withdrawal symptoms within as little as 3 hours, but symptoms generally reach their peak at 2 to 3 days after cessation of use. Withdrawal symptoms may include headaches, nausea, vomiting, diarrhea, muscle aches, anxiety, restlessness, diaphoresis, yawning, and dilated pupils. Medical treatment with clonidine or methadone can greatly reduce or even eliminate most of the symptoms of withdrawal.

(A) Findings associated with alcohol withdrawal include irritability, tremors, diaphoresis, hallucinations, and delirium tremens. Treatment for alcohol withdrawal includes benzodiazepines. **(B)** Cocaine withdrawal is not life-threatening and symptoms include constricted pupils, hunger, and anxiety. **(C)** Mescaline is a hallucinogenic and not associated with true withdrawal symptoms although patients may experience flashbacks later in life. **(E)** Caffeine withdrawal manifests with headaches, sleepiness, and nausea or vomiting. Pupillary size is unaffected.

18 A 16-year-old boy presents to clinic with a chief complaint of worsening rash despite therapy. He was diagnosed with pityriasis rosea the week prior and given supportive care. He is sexually active and reports using protection "most of the time."

Of the following, what laboratory test is most helpful to establish a diagnosis?

(A) Complete blood cell count
(B) Complete metabolic panel
(C) Enzyme-linked immunosorbent assay for human immunodeficiency virus (HIV)
(D) Rapid plasma reagin (RPR)
(E) Polymerase chain reaction for *Neisseria gonorrhoeae*/*Chlamydia trachomatis*

The answer is D: Rapid plasma reagin (RPR). The rash of secondary syphilis in teenagers can be confused with pityriasis rosea, as the distribution for each can be similar. Both rashes can be arranged along lines of skin stress on the back and looks like the boughs of a Christmas tree. Syphilis should be considered when the incorrectly diagnosed rash of pityriasis rosea does not resolve. The diagnostic test of choice for syphilis is RPR and fluorescent treponemal antibody absorption. **(C)** Skin findings associated with HIV are later manifestations of the disease and include the lesions associated with Kaposi sarcoma. **(A)** A complete blood cell count and complete metabolic panel are not diagnostic for the patient in the vignette. **(E)** Disseminated gonococcal infection can be associated with purpura, not the rash described in the vignette.

19 A 15-year-old girl is brought to the emergency department by her parents after she returned from a party "acting funny." On physical examination the patient is an anxious, restless adolescent who is extremely talkative. She laughs frequently and appears euphoric. Her vital signs are temperature 38.1°C, heart rate 120 beats/min, respiratory rate 18 breaths/min, and blood pressure 145/95 mmHg. Her pupils are dilated.

Of the following, what is the most likely causative agent of this girl's symptoms?

(A) Barbiturates
(B) Cannabis
(C) Amphetamines
(D) Ethanol
(E) Phencyclidine

The answer is C: Amphetamines. Amphetamine intoxication consists of euphoria, hyperactive reflexes, talkativeness, irritability, weakness, nausea, vomiting, and diarrhea. Prolonged use creates tolerance, requiring users to increase their dosages, thereby increasing their risk of toxicity. The patient in the vignette has low-grade fevers, hypertension, tachycardia, and dilated pupils all supportive of amphetamine ingestion. Severe overdose can result in seizures, coma, and stroke.

(A) Barbiturate ingestion results in a more sedative state, small or normal pupils, and hypotension. **(B)** Cannabis or marijuana would cause a more depressed mood, as opposed to being hyperactive. **(C)** While ethanol ingestion could explain the patient's symptom of agitation, it does not explain her hypertension, hyperthermia, or mydriasis. **(E)** Phencyclidine ingestion causes a more combative state and frequently presents with nystagmus, tachycardia, and can be potential hallucinogen.

20 A 16-year-old boy presents to clinic for his yearly physical examination. He has no current complaints and denies sexual activity or drug use. He is doing well in school and participates in sports year round. He has plans to go to college after graduation and is interested in studying computer science.

Of the following anticipatory guidance recommendations, which has the largest impact on this adolescent's overall morbidity and mortality risk?

(A) He should apply sunscreen daily
(B) He should receive the human papilloma virus vaccination
(C) He should increase his sports participation
(D) He should make sure his parents' handgun is loaded and stored in a locked case
(E) He should wear his seatbelt as a passenger in a motor vehicle

The answer is E: **He should wear his seatbelt as a passenger in a motor vehicle.** Teenagers are at a high risk of fatalities caused by motor vehicle accidents. Adolescents are less likely to wear a seatbelt while being a passenger in a vehicle than they are while driving. Teenagers and young adults have the lowest rates of wearing proper safety restraints compared with any other age group.

(A) Sunscreen use is beneficial, especially during the spring and summer season between the hours of 10 a.m. and 2 p.m. when the ultraviolet rays are the strongest. Although he should be encouraged to wear sunscreen at the appropriate times, appropriate seatbelt use is more likely to affect his overall mortality risk. **(B)** All children, starting as young as 9 years old, should be encouraged to receive the human papilloma virus vaccination. This vaccine can be life saving in women who are at risk for cervical cancer. **(C)** The patient in the vignette is already active in sports and there is no indication that he is obese or overweight. Diet and exercise can be life saving; however, for this otherwise healthy, active boy, appropriate seatbelt use is more important. **(D)** Handguns are involved in the vast majority of cases of criminal and accidental misuse. Having a gun in the house increases the risk of teenage suicide, homicide, or accidental injury. Firearms are the most common method of suicide attempt among men. Gun safety is essential and includes storing both the weapon and the ammunition locked in separate locations.

21 A 17-year-old girl with a past medical history significant for ovarian cysts presents to the emergency department with an acute onset of intermittent sharp right lower quadrant pain radiating to her right thigh. Her last menstrual period was 2 weeks ago. She has neither fever nor diarrhea, but does complain of nausea. Her last sexual encounter was 6 months prior with her boyfriend at that time. She states he has been her only sexual partner and she claims to always use condoms.

She denies any change in vaginal discharge or odor. On examination, her abdomen is tender in the right lower quadrant, and a bimanual examination reveals a tender adnexal mass. Her white blood cell count is $7.2 \times 10^3/\mu L$ with a hemoglobin of 11.5 g/dL. A urine pregnancy test is negative.

Of the following, which is the most likely diagnosis and treatment plan for this patient?

(A) Appendicitis; surgical removal
(B) Pelvic inflammatory disease (PID); intravenous antibiotics
(C) Ectopic pregnancy; administration of methotrexate
(D) Tubo-ovarian abscess; intravenous antibiotics
(E) Ovarian torsion; surgical repair

The answer is E: Ovarian torsion; surgical repair. The patient in the vignette is presenting with clinical symptoms of an ovarian torsion. Ovarian torsion typically presents as a sudden onset of unilateral lower abdominal pain, frequently with radiation to the back or thigh. Additional presenting complaints may include nausea and vomiting. A history of ovarian cysts and a tender adnexal mass palpable on examination is highly suggestive of ovarian torsion. Urgent surgical intervention is required to restore adequate blood flow and salvage the affected ovary.

(A) Appendicitis can present with localized right lower quadrant pain with fever and elevated white blood cell count. Treatment for nonperforated appendicitis includes surgical removal of the appendix. **(B)** PID is a frequent finding in sexually active teenagers. Symptoms include fever, suprapubic tenderness, as well as cervical motion and adnexal tenderness. Treatment is with antibiotics, including ceftriaxone, azithromycin, and doxycycline. **(C)** Ectopic pregnancy is a reasonable consideration in a reproductive-age woman presenting with unilateral lower quadrant pain. However, a pregnancy test would be expected to be positive. In the event an ectopic pregnancy is not ruptured, treatment by administration of methotrexate is an option. Symptoms of rupture include peritoneal signs as well as hypotension and dizziness. Prompt surgical intervention is appropriate in patients with a ruptured ectopic pregnancy. **(D)** Tubo-ovarian abscess is an inflammatory process that is located in the ovaries and/or fallopian tubes. It may arise as a complication of PID. Patients present similarly to those with PID, but have more extensive systemic signs including fever, leukocytosis, and chills.

A 17-year-old girl presents to the adolescent clinic for her routine annual examination and Papanicolaou smear. On vulvar examination, a 1-cm clean, ulcerated lesion with raised borders is identified on her labia (see *Figure 4-3*). The lesion is not tender to palpation. She also has painless inguinal adenopathy.

Of the following, which is her most likely diagnosis?

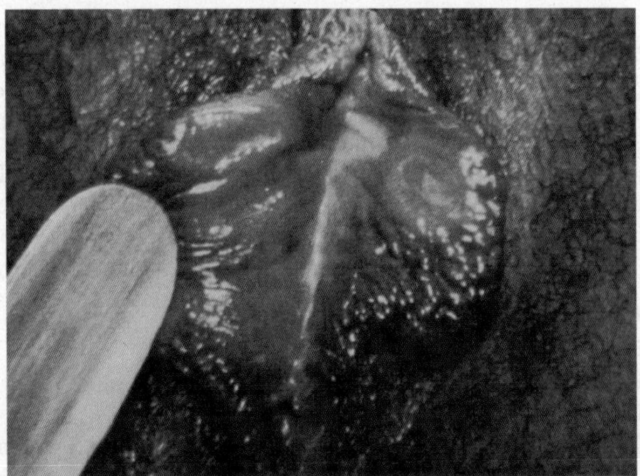

Figure 4-3

(A) Genital herpes
(B) Cervical cancer
(C) Chancroid
(D) Genital warts
(E) Primary syphilis

The answer is E: Primary syphilis. The lesion of primary syphilis as pictured in *Figure 4-3* is called a chancre and typically appears 2 to 4 weeks after exposure. It is characterized as a solitary, painless, and firm papule that is most commonly located on the genitalia. The lesions in female patients are often located in the vagina or on the cervix and therefore may go unnoticed. Patients are very contagious during the primary phase with an open and ulcerating lesion. The chancre will eventually heal regardless of treatment within 1 to 2 months. Regional lymph nodes are generally enlarged but nontender during this phase.

(A) The genital lesions of herpes are multiple, vesicular, and quite painful in nature. **(B)** Cervical cancer presents as a friable or ulcerated appearance of the cervix rather than a single clean-bordered lesion on the vaginal wall or vulva. **(C)** Chancroid is a sexually transmitted infection caused by *Haemophilus ducreyi* and presents with a painful erythematous ulcer with a friable base that may be covered with a gray, yellow, necrotic, or purulent exudate. **(D)** Genital warts, or condylomata acuminata, are skin-colored warts with a cauliflower-like surface and may be found on the vulvar or perianal areas. They are usually painless although may be associated with pruritus, burning, or bleeding.

23 A 16-year-old girl presents to the emergency department with an acute onset of nausea, vomiting, and shortness of breath. Her past medical history is unremarkable except for a recent diagnosis of bacterial vaginosis for which she is currently being treated. Her physical examination reveals a heart rate of 110 beats/min and facial flushing. Laboratory results reveal a blood ethanol level of 30 mg/dL (0.03%). The patient reports she was drinking alcohol just prior to the onset of symptoms.

Of the following, which is the most likely etiology of her symptoms?

(A) Alcohol poisoning
(B) Medication reaction
(C) Pregnancy
(D) Pelvic inflammatory disease (PID)
(E) Acetaminophen overdose

The answer is B: Medication reaction. The patient in the vignette is currently being treated with metronidazole, the first-line agent for bacterial vaginosis. Several medications, including metronidazole, include, as part of their side-effect profile, the potential to cause a disulfiram (Antabuse®) like reaction when combined with alcohol intake. Symptoms of the reaction include facial flushing, shortness of breath, tachycardia, nausea, and vomiting. For the patient in the vignette who exhibits all of these typical symptoms after exposure to alcohol in combination with her prescribed metronidazole, a presumptive diagnosis of disulfiram-like reaction can be made.

(A) While alcohol poisoning can cause symptoms including nausea and vomiting, her blood levels are relatively low. **(C)** Pregnancy is always a reasonable consideration in a reproductive-age girl presenting with nausea and vomiting; however, it does not explain the acute onset of shortness of breath and facial flushing. **(D)** Patients with PID can present with nausea and vomiting; however, additional findings include fever and tenderness with suprapubic palpation and cervical motion. **(E)** Adolescents often use more than one substance at a time and therefore suspicion should always be high for confounding substances. Although acetaminophen overdose can present with nausea, given the combined ingestion of ethanol and metronidazole, the diagnosis of a disulfiram-like reaction is more likely.

24 A 16-year-old girl presents to the emergency department with complaints of abdominal pain, nausea, and vomiting. She reports having normal menses of 5 to 6 days' duration occurring 30 days apart. She initially began menstruating at age 11 years. She has had two sexual partners with which she states she uses condoms most of the time. Her last menstrual period was 2 months prior, although she began to have vaginal bleeding today. She thinks this is different than her menses as it is accompanied by significant pain. She has never been tested for sexually transmitted

diseases before and complains of occasional vaginal pruritus and foul-smelling discharge. Her initial β-human chorionic gonadotropin (β-hCG) level is elevated and a repeat level 48 hours later is 25% higher.

Of the following, which historic point, if present, would have increased the risk of this patient's current presentation?

(A) Oral contraceptive use
(B) Pelvic inflammatory disease (PID)
(C) Turner syndrome
(D) Androgen insensitivity syndrome
(E) Emergency contraception use

The answer is B: Pelvic inflammatory disease (PID). The patient in the vignette has findings consistent with an ectopic pregnancy. Patients with an ectopic pregnancy can present with a history of amenorrhea or vaginal bleeding, abdominal pain, nausea, and vomiting. If the ectopic pregnancy ruptures, patients may present with signs of hypovolemic shock. **(B)** A history of PID, previous abdominal or pelvic surgery, and tobacco use increases a woman's risk of ectopic pregnancy. With intrauterine pregnancy, the β-hCG level doubles in 48 hours; however, in ectopic pregnancy it is associated with a slower rate of rise.

(A) Oral contraceptive use would decrease the patient's risk for pregnancy, ectopic or otherwise. **(C)** A patient with Turner syndrome has the absence of ovarian function and therefore is unable to become pregnant. **(D)** Patients with androgen insensitivity syndrome are genotypically male. **(E)** Use of emergency contraception has no effect on the ovulation process and would decrease the risk of any pregnancy, ectopic or otherwise. Although patients who have taken emergency contraception may experience abdominal pain, vaginal bleeding, and nausea, the β-hCG would be negative.

25 A 14-year-old girl presents to the adolescent clinic with complaints of heavy bleeding during her menstrual periods. The patient has regular 26-day cycles, with menses lasting 8 days per cycle. Her laboratory evaluation reveals a hemoglobin of 9 mg/dL, mean corpuscular volume of 72 fL, and platelets of $272 \times 10^3/\mu L$. Her prothrombin time is 12 seconds and activated partial thromboplastin time is 24 seconds. Her heart rate is 98 beats/min, respiratory rate is 18 breaths/minute, and blood pressure is 104/72 mmHg.

Of the following treatment options, which should be recommended to this patient?

(A) Transfusion of packed red blood cells
(B) Transfusion of platelets
(C) Infusion of factor VIII
(D) Assessment of lactate and uric acid levels
(E) Oral contraceptive pills

The answer is E: Oral contraceptive pills. The patient in the vignette has menorrhagia and microcytic anemia. Menorrhagia is characterized by a pattern of regular menstrual cycles but with prolonged duration of menses (greater than 7 days) and with excessive blood loss (greater than 80 mL). In addition to iron therapy, oral contraceptive pills are often a first-line treatment option in patients with menorrhagia. **(A)** Although the patient in the vignette has developed an iron-deficiency anemia, her vital signs are stable and she is asymptomatic. Therefore, there is no indication for transfusion at this time. **(B)** Without evidence of thrombocytopenia or impaired platelet function, a transfusion of platelets is unwarranted. **(C)** There is no evidence to support factor VIII deficiency given the normal coagulation studies; therefore, infusion of this factor is not indicated. **(D)** Lactate and uric acid levels would be indicated if there were a concern of an oncologic process, especially tumor lysis syndrome. At this point, the most likely diagnosis is menorrhagia and therefore iron therapy and oral contraceptive pills are indicated.

---

26 Of the following, what are the most common causes of death (in descending order) in the adolescent population?

(A) Suicide, accidental injury, homicide
(B) Homicide, suicide, accidental injury
(C) Accidental injury, suicide, homicide
(D) Homicide, accidental injury, suicide
(E) Accidental injury, homicide, suicide

The answer is E: Accidental injury, homicide, suicide. Accidental injury is the number one cause of death in the adolescent population, with motor vehicle collisions accounting for the greatest number of accidental fatalities. Homicides are the second most common cause of death in teenagers, followed by suicides. Up to a quarter of adolescents admit to having had suicidal ideation at some point. Suicidal patients have been shown to withhold their suicidal thoughts or depressive symptoms when seeking medical care unless they are specifically asked. Compassionate and confidential questioning during routine patient encounters is one of the more effective means of identifying at-risk teens and providing them with the necessary support to address the issue. Hospitalization would be recommended in the case of a patient who is experiencing current, active thoughts of suicide or who expressed intent to harm themselves or others. Female adolescents are three times more likely to attempt suicide than their male counterparts. However, male adolescents who attempt suicide are three times more likely to be successful.

27 A camp counselor brings three 13-year-old boys to the emergency department to be evaluated for alcohol intoxication. He found them behind the craft cottage laughing with slurred speech and unsteady gaits. Physical examinations 1 hour later show a return to baseline with no unusual findings. The boys deny alcohol or marijuana use. Urine toxicology screens and serum alcohol levels are negative.

Of the following, what is the most likely cause of the observed behavior in these patients?

(A) Organic solvents
(B) Morning glory seeds
(C) Oxycodone hydrochloride
(D) Phencyclidine (PCP)
(E) Ethanol

The answer is A: **Organic solvents.** Organic solvent abuse, often inhaled, presents with a short-lived toxidrome of immediate euphoria, drowsiness, slurred speech, ataxia, headache, nausea, vomiting, syncope, and seizure that can mimic ethanol intoxication. **(E)** However, ethanol intoxication does not resolve in a short period of time as described in the vignette. Death from organic solvent abuse can occur due to cardiac arrhythmia or asphyxia. Organic solvents are found in easily accessible items such as oil-based paints, varnishes, and dyes. Inhalant abuse is frequently a group activity and happens more frequently in younger teens.

(B) Morning glory seeds are flower seeds that have hallucinogenic properties when ingested and can present with nausea, dizziness, or diarrhea. The hallucinogenic effects would not wear off as quickly as described in the vignette. **(C)** Oxycodone is a prescription opioid with analgesic and euphoric properties that is a frequent drug of abuse. Opioid intoxication is characterized by central nervous system depression, respiratory depression, and pupillary miosis, or constriction. **(D)** PCP ingestion presents with aggression, and often nystagmus. This specific physical examination finding helps to differentiate PCP from other ingestions.

28 A sexually active 15-year-old girl presents to the office with a complaint of urinary frequency, urgency, and dysuria.

Of the following, which is the most likely pathogen responsible?

(A) *Enterococcus faecalis*
(B) *Klebsiella pneumoniae*
(C) *Staphylococcus saprophyticus*
(D) *Proteus mirabilis*
(E) *Pseudomonas aeruginosa*

The answer is C: ***Staphylococcus saprophyticus***. *S. saprophyticus* is a gram-positive cocci that is the second most common pathogen responsible for urinary tract infections (UTIs) in sexually active women. *Escherichia coli* is a gram-negative rod and is the single most common pathogen implicated in UTIs. **(A, B, D, E)** Although *E. faecalis*, *K. pneumoniae*, *Proteus mirabilis*, and *Pseudomonas aeruginosa* are pathogens implicated in UTIs, they are less likely than *S. saprophyticus* in sexually active women.

CHAPTER

5

Genetics and Metabolic Disorders

SONALI MEHTA PATEL

1 An 8-year-old boy presents to the clinic for evaluation of his school testing records, which demonstrate profound intellectual deficits. His physical appearance is significant for prominent ears and a high forehead and his testicular volume is increased.

Of the following, which is the most likely mechanism for this patient's condition?

(A) Translocation
(B) Imprinting
(C) Microdeletion
(D) Trinucleotide repeat
(E) Uniparental disomy

The answer is D: Trinucleotide repeat. The patient in the vignette has Fragile X syndrome. These patients present with macrosomia at birth, macroorchidism, a large jaw and ears, and mental retardation. They may also have autism, seizure disorder, strabismus, clubfeet, and scoliosis. This condition is secondary to a trinucleotide repeat of CGG, which occurs excessively in this population.

(A) Translocation can be associated with acquired oncologic conditions such as Burkitt lymphoma. **(B, E)** Imprinting is a genetic phenomenon that can arise secondary to uniparental disomy and is associated with Prader-Willi syndrome and Angelman syndrome. Most often, however, uniparental disomy causes no specific phenotypic abnormality. **(C)** DiGeorge syndrome is an example of a microdeletion on chromosome 22q11.

2 A 12-year-old boy comes to the pediatrician's office for a health maintenance visit. He has abnormally long legs, an increased arm span, gynecomastia, and small testes. He has been receiving special school services for learning disabilities for the past several years.

In addition to obtaining a karyotype, of the following, what is the next best course of treatment for this boy?

(A) Obtain karyotypes of parents
(B) Begin prednisone therapy
(C) Obtain a cardiac and ophthalmologic evaluation
(D) Refer to endocrinology for testosterone replacement therapy
(E) No further intervention is necessary

The answer is D: **Refer to endocrinology for testosterone replacement therapy.** The patient in the vignette has Klinefelter syndrome, characterized by hypogonadism, small testes, tall stature, female hair distribution, gynecomastia, learning disabilities, and decreased muscle mass. This chromosomal disorder is caused by the presence of an extra X chromosome in men, most frequently due to paternal nondisjunction. **(E)** Testosterone therapy replacement is recommended for these patients during puberty to improve secondary sexual characteristics. Complications of Klinefelter syndrome include osteoporosis, autoimmune disease, psychiatric conditions, and infertility secondary to primary testicular failure.

(A) Obtaining karyotypes of the parents may be beneficial regarding inheritance for future children, but will not assist in the treatment of this patient. **(B)** Prednisone therapy has not been used for the treatment of Klinefelter syndrome. **(C)** Obtaining a cardiac and ophthalmologic evaluation would be appropriate for Marfan syndrome, rather than Klinefelter syndrome. Marfan syndrome is inherited in an autosomal dominant fashion, with a defect in a fibrillin gene on chromosome 15. Marfan syndrome is characterized by cardiac anomalies, including aortic root dilation, and upward lens subluxation. Marfan syndrome patients possess normal intelligence and normal sized testicles.

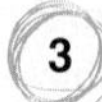

A patient with Down syndrome is brought into the clinic for his 6-month health maintenance visit. The patient had a normal complete blood cell count and echocardiogram at birth.

Of the following, which option correctly depicts the additional health supervision he needs at this visit?

(A) Thyroid function tests and referrals to ophthalmology and orthopedics
(B) Thyroid function tests and referrals to ophthalmology and audiology
(C) Complete blood cell count and audiology referral
(D) Complete blood cell count and ophthalmology referral
(E) Complete blood cell count and referrals to ophthalmology and audiology

The answer is B: **Thyroid function tests and referrals to ophthalmology and audiology.** According to the American Academy of Pediatrics Health Supervision Guidelines for Children with Down syndrome, children at the 6-month visit should be evaluated by an ophthalmologist and audiologist and have thyroid function testing. Ophthalmology referral is to evaluate for cataracts and strabismus. Patients with Down syndrome are at increased risk for hearing loss secondary to serous otitis media and stenotic external ear canals and should be screened by audiology every 6 months. Thyroid testing should be performed every 6 months until 1 year of age, then annually.

(C, D, E) If a complete blood cell count was noted to be normal at birth, this lab does not need to be repeated until the 1-year visit, and then annually afterward. Patients with Down syndrome are at increased risk for hematologic and oncologic processes, such as anemia and leukemia. **(A)** Though there is an increased risk of joint laxity, short stature, and atlantoaxial dislocation for patients with Down syndrome, there is not an indication for orthopedic referral at the 6-month visit in the absence of complaints.

4 A neonate in the nursery area is diagnosed shortly after birth with tetralogy of Fallot. Chest radiography demonstrates an absent thymus, and physical examination reveals a bifid uvula, cleft palate, low set ears, and a small jaw.

Of the following microdeletions, which is most likely to be found in this patient?

(A) 5p-
(B) 11p13
(C) 15q11
(D) 17p11.2
(E) 22q11

The answer is E: 22q11. The patient in the vignette has DiGeorge syndrome, characterized by congenital heart disease, an absent thymus, dysmorphia, and palatal abnormalities. These patients can also present with signs and symptoms of hypocalcemia, secondary to hypoparathyroidism. The microdeletion most commonly associated with this condition is 22q11.

(A) The microdeletion 5p- is the deletion that would be found in cri-du-chat syndrome, which presents in the early infancy period with failure to thrive, developmental delay, and a cat-like cry. **(B)** The 11p13 microdeletion is associated with the WAGR sequence, which stands for Wilms tumor, aniridia, genitourinary abnormalities, and mental retardation. **(C)** The microdeletion 15q11 can be found in either Prader-Willi syndrome or Angelman syndrome, depending on whether the deletion was maternal or paternally derived. **(D)** The microdeletion 17p11.2 is the deletion that would be found in Smith-Magenis syndrome, characterized by mental retardation, self-mutilating behavior, aggressive behavior, and dysmorphic facies.

5 A 15-year-old tall, lanky boy presents with downward lens dislocation and a low intelligence quotient.

Of the following, which additional condition is this patient at risk for?

(A) Pectus excavatum
(B) Vascular thrombosis
(C) Multicystic dysplastic kidney
(D) Dural ectasia
(E) Mitral valve prolapse

The answer is B: Vascular thrombosis. The patient in the vignette has signs and symptoms characteristic of homocystinuria. Homocystinuria is an aminoacidopathy caused by a defect in cystathionine B-synthetase enzyme, which results in a patient with a Marfanoid body habitus, developmental delay, downward lens dislocation, and increased risk of thromboembolism in arteries and veins.

(A, C, D, E) Pectus excavatum, multicystic dysplastic kidney, dural ectasia, and mitral valve prolapse would all be expected findings for a patient with Marfan syndrome. Patients with Marfan syndrome have normal intelligence and an upward lens dislocation.

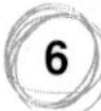
6 A 38-week-gestation neonate is born to a 23-year-old mother and found to have upward slanting eyes, small, low-set ears, a single palmar crease in both hands, and epicanthal folds (see *Figure 5-1*).

Of the following, which mechanism of inheritance is increased for this patient's condition given the mother's age?

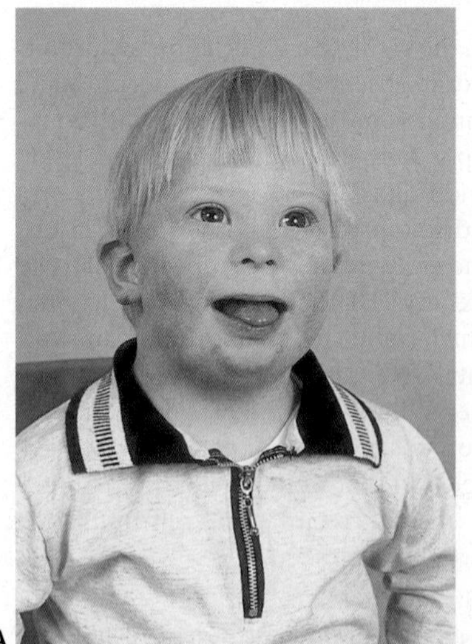
A

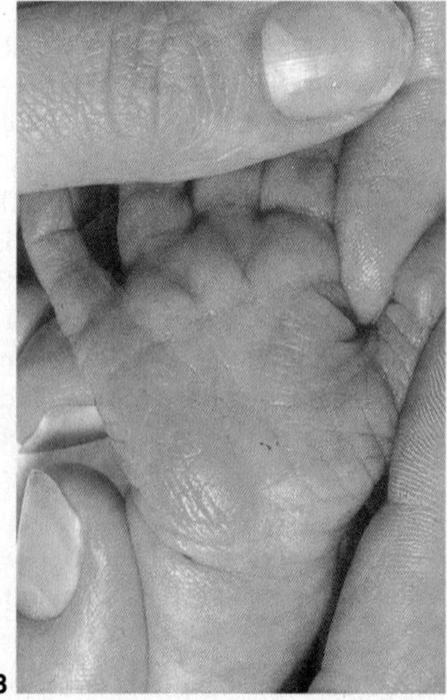
B

Figure 5-1

(A) Meiotic nondisjunction of homologous chromosomes
(B) Imprinting
(C) Mosaicism
(D) Robertsonian translocation
(E) Trinucleotide repeat

The answer is D: Robertsonian translocation. The patient in the vignette has trisomy 21 or Down syndrome which is characterized by several clinical manifestations including epicanthal folds, upward slanting eyes, small upturned nose, low nasal bridge, hypotonia, simian crease, clinodactyly (curved shape) of the fifth finger, prominent tongue, extra neck skin folds, short stature, joint laxity, Brushfield spots on irises, endocardial cushion defects, duodenal atresia, Hirschsprung disease, atlantoaxial instability, and mental retardation.

(A) The most common inheritance pattern is that of parental nondisjunction, generally maternally derived secondary to advanced maternal age. **(D)** Given that the mother in the vignette is only 23 years old, her daughter has an increased chance to have inherited trisomy 21 because of a Robertsonian translocation. This translocation is the second most common cause of Down syndrome and can be inherited as a result of spontaneous mutations. **(C)** A small percentage of Down syndrome can also be due to mosaicism, in which there are two or more populations of cells present in one individual. **(B)** Imprinting entails a genetic process by which certain deletions are either maternally or paternally derived, with different clinical manifestations that develop accordingly. Imprinting is not associated with Down syndrome. **(E)** Trinucleotide repeat is not the genetic mutation associated with Down syndrome, but is associated with Huntington disease.

7

A 6-week-old infant presents to the emergency department with vomiting and failure to thrive. His past medical history is significant for neonatal hyperbilirubinemia with a total bilirubin of 20 mg/dL. He was hospitalized at 2 weeks of age for a fever and found to have *Escherichia coli* urosepsis. On presentation, he is thin, ill-appearing, and noted to have hepatosplenomegaly.

Of the following, which additional finding is associated with his underlying condition?

(A) Macular cherry red spot
(B) Cataracts
(C) Blue sclera
(D) Lisch nodules
(E) Retinal hemorrhages

The answer is B: Cataracts. The patient in the vignette has galactosemia. Galactosemia is associated with neonatal *E. coli* urosepsis, liver disease, cataracts, jaundice, vomiting, and diarrhea. These patients can present with cataracts in the newborn and infancy period. It is caused by a deficiency of galactose-1-phosphate uridyl transferase (GALT), causing the enzymatic precursors to accumulate in the kidneys, liver, and brain because of deficient galactose metabolism. This disorder is inherited in an autosomal recessive fashion and can be diagnosed by newborn screening. Diagnosis can be confirmed by measuring GALT activity and with an elevated galactose-1-phosphate level.

Treatment is to remove all galactose from the diet. Lactose is a disaccharide that is broken down to glucose and galactose. In the newborn/infancy period, formula should be changed to a soy-based formula, which contains sucrose as the primary carbohydrate. Sucrose does not contain galactose and is broken down to glucose and fructose. **(E)** Retinal hemorrhages can be found in abuse as well as a metabolic disorder called glutaric acidemia. **(A)** A cherry red spot on the macula is found in some lysosomal disorders such as Tay-Sachs disease and Niemann-Pick syndrome. **(C)** Blue sclera can be found in osteogenesis imperfecta. **(D)** Lisch nodules are hamartomas or connective tissue growths found in neurofibromatosis.

8 A 32-week-gestation neonate is born to a 26-year-old mother and found to have a cleft lip and palate, polydactyly, a holosystolic murmur, holoprosencephaly, and feet as shown in *Figure 5-2*.

Of the following, which is this patient's most likely diagnosis?

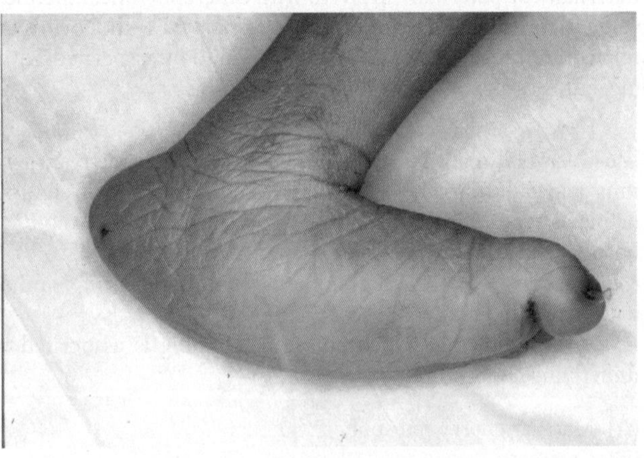

Figure 5-2

(A) Trisomy 13
(B) Trisomy 18
(C) Trisomy 21
(D) Cri-du-chat
(E) DiGeorge syndrome

The answer is A: Trisomy 13. The patient in the vignette has trisomy 13, otherwise known as Patau syndrome, which is characterized by midline facial defects, polydactyly, congenital heart disease, and rocker-bottom feet. **(B)** A key distinguishing factor from trisomy 18, or Edwards syndrome, is the presence of holoprosencephaly, a condition in which the forebrain of the embryo fails to divide into two hemispheres. Trisomy 18 may also have the presence of a trigger finger (fixed in flexion), or a clenched hand with overlapping fingers (see *Figure 5-3*). **(D)** Cri-du-chat syndrome is due to a partial deletion of the short arm of chromosome 5. Typical clinical manifestations include a cat-like cry, feeding problems, low birth weight, mental retardation, cardiac defects, hypertelorism, and low set ears. **(E)** DiGeorge syndrome is caused by a 22q11 deletion, with common manifestations being congenital heart disease, hypocalcemia, immunodeficiency, and facial dysmorphia. **(C)** Trisomy 21 is characterized by epicanthal folds, upward slanting of eyes, small upturned nose, low nasal bridge, hypotonia, and a prominent tongue.

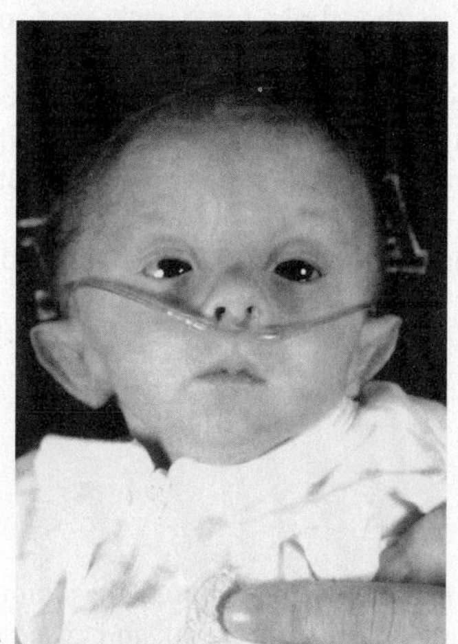
A

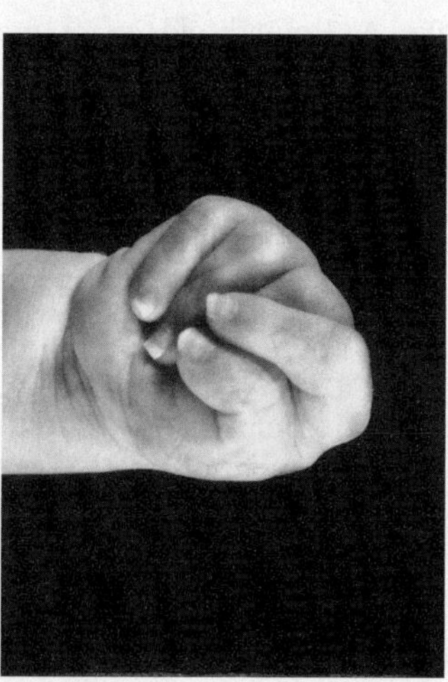
B

Figure 5-3

9 A 5-week-old infant in the pediatric intensive care unit is intubated, lethargic, and on hemodialysis for treatment of a urea cycle defect, ornithine transcarbamylase (OTC) deficiency.

Of the following, what is the risk of OTC deficiency in a male child whose mother is a carrier and whose father is unaffected?

(A) 0%
(B) 25%
(C) 50%
(D) 75%
(E) 100%

The answer is C: 50%. The urea cycle is responsible for removal of nitrogenous waste from the body. Amino acid catabolism produces free ammonia, which is detoxified to urea through the urea cycle. The majority of these disorders are inherited in an autosomal recessive fashion, with the exception of OTC deficiency, which has an X-linked inheritance pattern. Clinical manifestations occur shortly after the ingestion of dietary protein, in which the newborn develops lethargy, coma, and/or seizures. These patients have high ammonia levels, and definitive diagnosis is made by finding elevated levels of orotic acid in the urine. **(A, B, D, E)** The risk of a male child to be afflicted with this disease as described in the vignette is 50%. A son receives an X chromosome from the mother and Y chromosome from the father. A daughter receives an X chromosome from both the mother and the father. Thus, half of the sons born to these parents would have OTC deficiency, while half of the daughters born to them would be carriers.

---

10 A 2-month-old infant presents to the clinic for a sick visit and poor weight gain. Upon reviewing the growth chart and performing the physical examination, he is noted to have failure to thrive, hepatomegaly, macroglossia, and significant central hypotonia with head lag. On further evaluation, chest radiography demonstrates cardiomegaly.

Of the following inborn errors of metabolism, which does this patient most likely have?

(A) Hurler disease
(B) Pompe disease
(C) Krabbe disease
(D) Farber disease
(E) Niemann-Pick disease

The answer is B: Pompe disease. The patient in the vignette has Pompe disease, which is an inherited disorder of glycogen metabolism caused by a deficiency of lysosomal acid 1,4-glucosidase. This disorder presents in the infantile period with glycogen deposition in the cardiac and skeletal muscle tissue. Clinical manifestations include cardiomegaly, hypotonia, and hepatomegaly. Electrocardiogram reveals a shortened PR interval and high-voltage QRS waves. Treatment is supportive with enzyme replacement. Death generally occurs in the first year of life secondary to cardiac complications.

(E) Niemann-Pick disease is a lysosomal storage disorder caused by deficiency of sphingomyelinase. It presents with hepatosplenomegaly, jaundice, and signs of neurologic deterioration. These patients may have a cherry red spot on their macula. **(A)** Hurler disease is also a type of lysosomal storage disease, but a mucopolysaccharidosis. These patients present with corneal clouding, mental retardation, obstructive airway disease, organomegaly, coarse facial features, and cardiac disease. **(C)** Krabbe disease is a type of lysosomal storage disease in which the hallmark of its presentation is progressive central nervous system degeneration. **(D)** Farber disease, also a lysosomal storage disease, presents with nodules on joints, vocal cords, and severe mental and motor retardation.

---

11 A couple recently adopted an 8-month-old infant from another country. On examination, she has fair skin, light hair, and a musty odor. She is not rolling over or sitting with support.

Of the following tests, which would be most helpful to diagnose her underlying condition?

(A) Magnetic resonance imaging of the brain
(B) Echocardiogram
(C) Renal ultrasound
(D) Newborn screen
(E) Karyotype

The answer is D: Newborn screen. The patient in the vignette has phenylketonuria (PKU), an autosomal recessive amino acid disorder in which phenylalanine cannot be converted to tyrosine secondary to a defect in the enzyme phenylalanine hydroxylase. These patients can present with vomiting, an eczematoid rash, developmental delay, and a peculiar musty odor, due to phenylacetic acid in the urine. They are fair-haired, fair-skinned, and blue-eyed. PKU is universally included in newborn screening panels in the United States. All positive newborn screens should then be confirmed with a metabolic specialist for a more thorough, quantitative analysis of phenylalanine and tyrosine levels. Therapy is lifelong, which includes a phenylalanine-restricted diet, although not complete elimination, as some phenylalanine is essential for normal growth and development. It is important for women of childbearing years to continue to abide by this diet as well, as untreated PKU can act as a potential teratogen resulting in microcephaly, intellectual disability, and cardiac defects. If caught early, PKU has an excellent prognosis on appropriate therapy. Elevated levels of phenylalanine are neurotoxic and result in irreversible behavioral intellectual disabilities. **(A, B, C, E)** For the patient in the vignette, magnetic resonance imaging, echocardiogram, renal ultrasound, and karyotype are nondiagnostic for PKU.

---

12 A 6-month-old infant is brought to the emergency department for fever and poor oral intake for 2 days. Prior to this illness, the patient was doing well with no concerns, per his parents. His mother states he is not acting like himself, not playing, and is sleeping more. Family history is significant for a sister who died in her crib after a similar incident at 4 months age.

Of the following metabolic disorders, which is most consistent with this patient's presentation?

(A) Galactosemia
(B) Tay-Sachs
(C) Alkaptonuria
(D) Maple syrup urine disease
(E) Medium-chain acyl-CoA dehydrogenase deficiency (MCAD)

The answer is E: **Medium-chain acyl-CoA dehydrogenase deficiency (MCAD).** The patient in the vignette most likely has a fatty acid oxidation defect, such as MCAD. This condition typically begins to manifest when infants begin to sleep longer periods of time or with illnesses that lead to decreased oral intake. Patients with MCAD are unable to metabolize glucose from fat during periods of stress or fasting. These patients may have vomiting, lethargy, seizures, and coma secondary to a defect in appropriate utilization of fatty acids by the mitochondria. MCAD is treated with frequent feeding, carnitine, and cornstarch.

(A) Galactosemia presents earlier with hyperbilirubinemia, *Escherichia coli* sepsis, and poor feeding. **(B)** Tay-Sachs disease presents with a loss of skills at roughly 4 to 8 months, hyperacusis, and a cherry red spot on the macula. Tay-Sachs is due to a lack of hexosaminidase A and is an autosomal recessive genetic disorder more common in those of Ashkenazi Jewish descent. **(C)** Alkaptonuria is a rare genetic disorder, inherited in an autosomal recessive fashion, and is associated with disorders of phenylalanine and tyrosine metabolism. These patients may present with black urine, joint, and cardiac problems. **(D)** Maple syrup urine disease is a disorder of branched amino acids in which the urine, hair, and skin smell similar to maple syrup. There is central nervous system disease early in the first week of life with rapid progression to death if untreated. Treatment consists of acute dialysis and long-term dietary restriction of isoleucine, leucine, and valine.

A 12-month-old infant presents to the inpatient wards with hypoglycemia, lactic acidosis, hyperuricemia, and seizures. On physical examination, he has thin extremities and his liver is palpable 3 cm below the costal margin. The mother reports that he has had seizures before, although usually overnight.

Of the following, which treatment option is best for this patient's likely underlying condition?

(A) Anticonvulsant therapy
(B) Chemotherapy
(C) Frequent feedings
(D) Enzyme replacement therapy
(E) Bone marrow transplant

The answer is C: Frequent feedings. The patient in the vignette presents with signs and symptoms concerning for a glycogen storage disorder. Patients with type 1 glycogen storage disease, otherwise known as Von Gierke disease, present with hypoglycemia, seizures, hepatomegaly, dolls facies, and thin extremities secondary to a defect of glucose-6-phosphatase activity. Treatment for these patients entails avoiding fasting with frequent feedings during the day, and continuous feedings overnight. Treatment may also involve lipid-lowering agents and allopurinol for hyperuricemia. **(A)** Anticonvulsant therapy would not treat the underlying cause of seizures in this patient, namely hypoglycemia. **(B)** Chemotherapy would not be indicated for patients with glycogen storage disease, unless independently diagnosed with an oncologic process. **(D, E)** Enzyme replacement therapy and bone marrow transplant may be therapy options for patients with lysosomal storage disorders, but are not helpful in the treatment of glycogen storage disorders.

---

14 A 6-year-old girl presents to the clinic with short stature, aortic coarctation, and horseshoe kidneys.

Of the following choices, which combination corresponds to her most likely diagnosis and karyotype?

(A) Noonan syndrome, XY
(B) Noonan syndrome, XO
(C) Turner syndrome, XY
(D) Turner syndrome, XO
(E) Turner syndrome, XX

The answer is D: Turner syndrome, XO. The patient in the vignette has Turner syndrome, which is caused by an absence of an X chromosome, **(C, E)** giving a karyotype of XO. This leads to oocyte degeneration in utero and results in gonadal dysgenesis. Therefore, Turner syndrome is only seen in girls. Common clinical manifestations include short stature (which may be the only presenting sign), lymphedema of hands and feet in newborns, cystic hygromas in newborns, primary amenorrhea, coarctation of the aorta, bicuspid aortic valves, broad chest with widely spaced nipples, low posterior hairline, webbed neck, normal intelligence, and renal anomalies including horseshoe kidneys (see *Figure 5-4*).

(A, B) Noonan syndrome patients resemble Turner syndrome patients in appearance; however, this syndrome is secondary to a defect of genes on chromosome 12 and can be found in either men (XY) or women (XX). Clinical manifestations of Noonan syndrome include short stature, webbed neck, lymphedema of hands/feet, mild mental retardation, learning disabilities, renal anomalies, and cardiac abnormalities. Pulmonary stenosis, rather than aortic coarctation, is more commonly associated with Noonan syndrome.

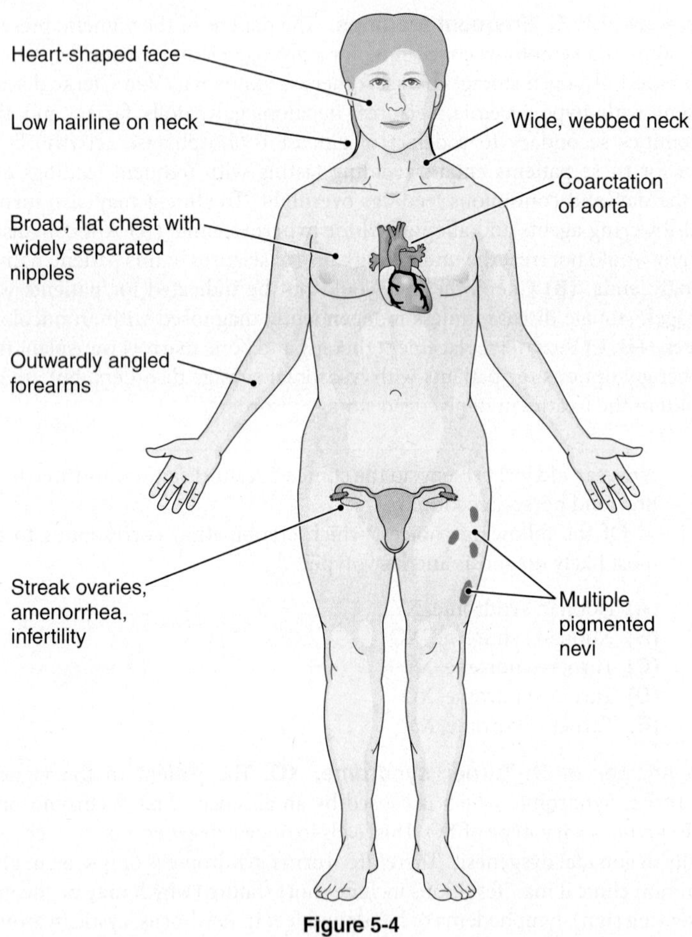

Figure 5-4

15 A 2-month-old infant with a prenatal diagnosis of achondroplasia presents to the office for a checkup. She has been feeding and growing well, and the parents report no complaints.

As part of the anticipatory guidance for this patient, which of the following topics should be included in discussion with this family?

(A) The patient is unlikely to achieve normal intelligence
(B) The patient will have a short trunk, but normal long bones
(C) Recognition of signs and symptoms of hydrocephalus
(D) The patient's children are unlikely to have achondroplasia
(E) The patient will achieve normal motor milestones

The answer is C: **Recognition of signs and symptoms of hydrocephalus.** Patients with achondroplasia possess a defect in the gene for fibroblast growth factor receptor, located on the short arm of chromosome 4. This condition is inherited in an autosomal dominant manner; however, there are cases of spontaneous mutations as well. **(D)** Children with only one affected parent have a 50% chance of having this disorder as well. Clinical manifestations include disproportionate short stature with a **(B)** normal-sized trunk but shortening of the long bones, a large head with a small foramen magnum, frontal bossing, and trident hand (wide and plump digits of equal length) (see *Figure 5-5*). **(A, E)** Patients with achondroplasia have normal intelligence, delayed motor milestones, and recurrent otitis media secondary to short Eustachian tubes and nasopharyngeal cavities. These patients' complications include sleep apnea, hydrocephalus secondary to a small foramen magnum, thoracolumbar kyphosis secondary to unsupported sitting without adequate muscular strength, and hearing loss secondary to chronic otitis. Thus, it is important for the pediatrician to counsel regarding the signs and symptoms of hydrocephalus and to follow head circumference growth closely, especially in the first year of life.

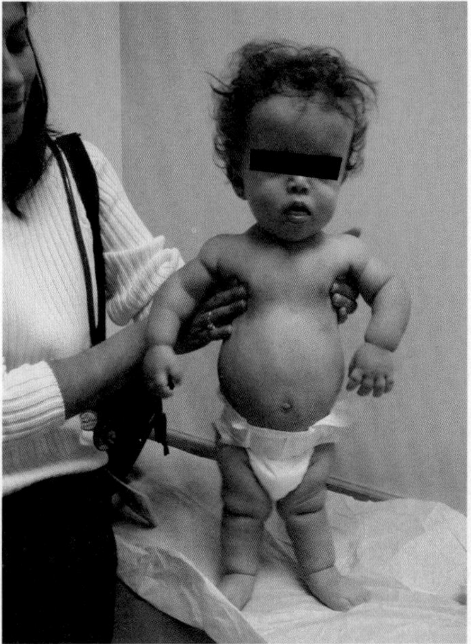

Figure 5-5

CHAPTER

6

Cardiology

JASON MITCHELL

1 A 14-year-old boy complains of intermittent episodes of chest discomfort for the past 2 months. These episodes usually occur while he is sitting in class at school or watching television at home. He says that they happen once or twice a day, usually out of the blue and last for 3 to 5 minutes before stopping. One of the episodes lasted over 10 minutes. His electrocardiogram (ECG) while asymptomatic is included in *Figure 6-1*). While in the office, he experiences another episode, and the rhythm strip is obtained (see *Figure 6-2*).

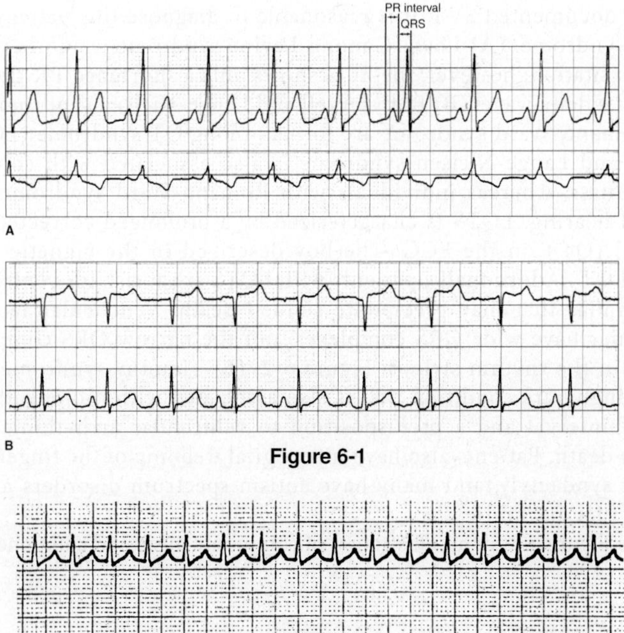

Figure 6-1

Figure 6-2

Of the following, what is this patient's diagnosis?

(A) Lown-Ganong-Levine syndrome
(B) Jervell and Lange-Nielsen syndrome
(C) Wolff-Parkinson-White (WPW) syndrome
(D) Romano-Ward syndrome
(E) Timothy syndrome

The answer is C: Wolff-Parkinson-White (WPW) syndrome. The adolescent in the vignette has WPW syndrome. WPW is diagnosed when patients have evidence of ventricular preexcitation on an ECG as well as documented episodes of supraventricular tachycardia (SVT). Ventricular preexcitation occurs due to the presence of an accessory conduction pathway between the atria and ventricles. This accessory pathway does not include the atrioventricular (AV) node and is able to conduct much more rapidly than the AV node would normally permit. The ECG of the patient in the vignette shows evidence of the presence of such a pathway by the shortened PR-interval and slurring of the initial part of the QRS complex, termed a delta wave (see *Figure 6-1*). Second, the rhythm strip taken during an episode of palpitations shows a regular, narrow tachycardia, a typical description of SVT (see *Figure 6-2*). With evidence of an accessory pathway and ventricular preexcitation as well as documented SVT, it is reasonable to diagnose this patient with WPW syndrome. **(A)** Lown-Ganong-Levine syndrome is another form of preexcitation; however, the ECG shows only a shortened PR-interval without a delta wave. **(B)** Both Jervell and Lange-Nielsen syndrome and **(D)** Romano-Ward syndrome are forms of long QT syndrome (LQTS). Jervell and Lange-Nielsen syndrome is also associated with congenital deafness, whereas individuals with Romano-Ward syndrome have normal hearing. LQTS is characterized by a prolonged corrected QT-interval (QT_c) on the ECG. The boy described in the vignette has a normal QT_c. Additionally, patients with LQTS are at risk for ventricular arrhythmias that may precipitate sudden death. Ventricular tachyarrhythmias have wide QRS complexes, not the narrow QRS complexes shown in the rhythm strip in Figure 6-2. **(E)** Timothy syndrome is an exceedingly rare condition that is also associated with prolongation of the QT-interval and a predisposition to ventricular arrhythmias and sudden death. Patients also have interdigital webbing of the fingers and toes or syndactyly, and many have autism spectrum disorders and/or intellectual disabilities.

See Figure 6-3 for an illustration of commonly measured components of ECGs.

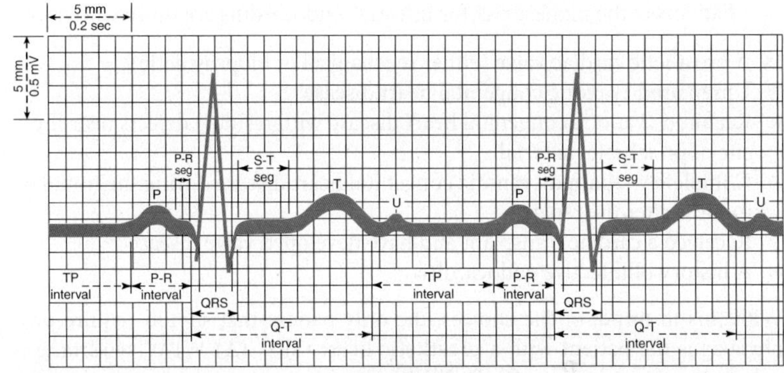

Figure 6-3

2 Of the following, which children should receive prophylaxis against bacterial endocarditis?

(A) A 13-year-old with Wolff-Parkinson-White (WPW) syndrome receiving fluoride treatments

(B) A 14-year-old with pulmonary stenosis undergoing placement of orthodontic braces

(C) A 15-year-old with a prosthetic pulmonary valve undergoing routine dental cleaning

(D) A 16-year-old with a patent foramen ovale undergoing root canal oral surgery

(E) A 17-year-old with repaired coarctation of the aorta undergoing wisdom tooth extraction

The answer is C: **A 15-year-old with a prosthetic pulmonary valve undergoing routine dental cleaning.** The American Heart Association recommends prophylactic antibiotics for patients who are considered at risk prior to any procedure that causes bacteremia with an organism likely to cause infective endocarditis. Previous guidelines recommended prophylaxis for a greater number of procedures, but the most recent guidelines published in 2007 take into account that the bacteremia from most dental procedures is less likely to result in endocarditis than the bacteremia from normal daily activities. Prophylaxis is not required for routine dental cleaning, placement or adjustment of orthodontic braces, fluoride treatment, dental radiography, and the normal shedding of deciduous teeth that occurs in young childhood. Other dental procedures that involve manipulation of the gingivae or perforation of the oral mucosa, such as dental extraction or oral surgery, may require prophylaxis for at-risk patients.

Patients at the highest risk for infective endocarditis are those who have:

- A prosthetic cardiac valve (either mechanical or bioprosthetic)
- Unrepaired cyanotic congenital heart disease
- Repaired cyanotic congenital heart disease with residual defects near the site of prosthetic material
- Completely repaired cyanotic congenital heart disease during the initial 6 months after the repair
- Received a cardiac transplant and have developed valve disease
- A history of infective endocarditis

With this in mind, of the choices, the only patient that should require prophylaxis is the patient with a prosthetic heart valve. **(A)** WPW syndrome is a disorder of conduction. **(B, D, E)** Pulmonary valve stenosis, patency of the foramen ovale, and coarctation of the aorta are not cyanotic heart defects. As such, they do not meet the criteria for endocarditis prophylaxis.

A neonate is cyanotic, tachycardic, and tachypneic. Upon inspection, there is no chest wall deformity. Auscultation of the chest reveals a loud, harsh systolic murmur at the left upper sternal border. The murmur is louder than S1 and S2, but palpation is unremarkable as the point of maximum impulse is not displaced and there is no palpable thrill. An echocardiogram demonstrates right-to-left shunting across a patent foramen ovale due to critical pulmonary valve stenosis. Balloon valvuloplasty in the cardiac catheterization lab restores adequate pulmonary blood flow, and the infant is discharged home a few days later.

Of the following, which category best describes the infant's murmur prior to the procedure?

(A) Grade I
(B) Grade II
(C) Grade III
(D) Grade IV
(E) Grade V

The answer is C: Grade III. Murmurs should be described based on characteristics such as timing, pitch, and where they are heard best (or clearest) on the chest. Systolic murmurs should also be graded from I to VI based on the intensity. **(A)** Grade I murmurs are quiet and barely audible. **(B)** Grade II murmurs have a medium intensity. **(C)** As described for the patient in the vignette, grade III murmurs are loud but there is no palpable thrill on the chest wall. **(D)** Grade IV murmurs are loud with a thrill. **(E)** Grade V murmurs are quite loud, but still require placement of the stethoscope on the patient's chest. Murmurs that are so loud that they can be heard without a stethoscope are grade VI.

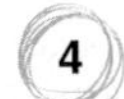

4 A neonate is emergently transported to a pediatric cardiac center hours after his birth at an outlying hospital. Prior to transport he was intubated, and umbilical arterial and venous lines were placed. In spite of appropriate ventilator settings and fluid management, he is acidotic, cyanotic, and poorly perfused. There is no murmur and pulmonary crackles are heard. His pulses are weak in all extremities and his capillary refill time is prolonged. A chest radiograph shows a small heart with pulmonary edema. A brief, limited echocardiogram is done at the bedside and reveals an atrial septal defect (ASD) with flow from an enlarged right atrium into the left atrium. The left ventricle (LV) also appears small. The right ventricle (RV) and main pulmonary valve are also enlarged.

Of the following which is his most likely diagnosis?

(A) Tetralogy of Fallot (TOF)
(B) Truncus arteriosus
(C) Total anomalous pulmonary venous return (TAPVR)
(D) D-transposition of the great arteries (D-TGA)
(E) Tricuspid atresia

The answer is C: Total anomalous pulmonary venous return (TAPVR). The infant described in the vignette is critically ill and has signs of circulatory shock (acidosis, weak pulses, and prolonged capillary refill) and cyanosis. Obstruction of anomalous pulmonary veins is responsible for the cyanosis and for the low cardiac output. The anomalous pulmonary veins connect to the right side of the heart by way of alternate venous pathways either above, at the level of, or below the heart. Obstructed TAPVR results in the backup of blood within the pulmonary vasculature, the increased pulmonary markings on chest radiography, and the increase in right-sided pressures that result in right-to-left shunting across the ASD. Because there is no return of oxygenated blood to the left atrium, it is typically smaller than normal. The only flow into the left atrium is blood from the right atrium, which contains deoxygenated systemic venous return as well as oxygenated pulmonary venous return. Flow across the atrial septum is the only source of blood available for systemic perfusion.

(A) TOF would present with the murmur of pulmonary stenosis (PS), and there would not be increased pulmonary venous markings on chest radiograph. **(B, D)** Truncus arteriosus and D-TGA do not present with circulatory shock, but rather with congestive heart failure. **(E)** In tricuspid atresia, the RV would not be enlarged, but be small and underdeveloped.

5 A term male neonate is tachycardic, tachypneic, and cyanotic with peripheral oxygen saturations in the 70s in all four extremities. He has a quiet precordium with a harsh 3/6 holosystolic murmur across the left chest and a gallop rhythm. A plain radiograph of the chest demonstrates cardiomegaly with slightly decreased pulmonary vascular markings.

Pregnancy was complicated by inadequate prenatal care and maternal diagnoses of bipolar disorder and schizophrenia. The mother was treated with lithium carbonate along with an antipsychotic medication until she was lost to follow up. Measures are taken to stabilize the infant, and echocardiography is ordered to guide further management.

Of the following, which is the most likely finding on echocardiography?

(A) Pulmonary stenosis, hypertrophy of the right ventricle (RV), and a ventricular septal defect (VSD) with an overriding aortic valve

(B) A common arterial trunk from which the aorta and pulmonary artery both arise

(C) Atresia of the mitral and aortic valves with hypoplasia of the aorta and left ventricle (LV)

(D) Drainage of the pulmonary veins into the systemic circulation below the diaphragm

(E) Downward displacement of the tricuspid valve with atrialization of the RV

The answer is E: Downward displacement of the tricuspid valve with atrialization of the RV. In the 1970s, maternal use of lithium was strongly associated with development of Ebstein anomaly in the fetus, but more recent data indicate that the risk of congenital heart disease is lower than reported previously. Ebstein anomaly involves abnormal development of the tricuspid valve. It is displaced toward the cardiac apex and into the ventricle, dividing the RV into two portions. The thin-walled atrialized part above the valve is continuous with the atrium. Normal myocardium lies below the valve; however, the chamber is often smaller and poorly contractile. The severity of the tricuspid valve regurgitation varies, and an intra-atrial communication is necessary to decompress the excess volume of blood in the enlarged right atrium into the left atrium. This shunting of deoxygenated blood into the systemic circulation explains the cyanosis.

(A) Pulmonary valve stenosis, right ventricular hypertrophy, and a misaligned VSD with overriding of the aortic valve are the hallmarks of tetralogy of Fallot. **(B)** A common arterial trunk from which the aorta and pulmonary artery both arise is the description of truncus arteriosus, which has been associated with maternal use of isotretinoin. **(C)** Atresia of the mitral and aortic valves with hypoplasia of the aorta and LV is the description of hypoplastic left heart syndrome. **(D)** Drainage of the pulmonary veins into the systemic circulation below the diaphragm describes total anomalous pulmonary venous return.

6 An 8-year-old girl presents as a new patient for evaluation. She was recently adopted from South Central Asia. Her parents visited her there 2 months ago and state that she was a happy, healthy little girl, but they are now concerned that she is regressing developmentally and may have a psychiatric illness. The girl sits quietly and appears to be alert, but she has continuous writhing movements of her fingers on both hands. She also displays lip smacking, facial twitches, and her tongue occasionally darts in and out of her mouth. Her parents say that she was able to brush her teeth and write, but that now she seems to have lost those skills. They say she sometimes laughs inappropriately as well. On examination her lungs are clear and she has a pansystolic murmur at the left sternal border. Her muscle tone, strength, and deep tendon reflexes are normal, but her gait is unsteady. Serum electrolytes, blood urea nitrogen, creatinine, and liver function tests are normal. Her throat culture is negative. An electroencephalogram shows no epileptiform activity.

Of the following, what additional test result is required to confirm the diagnosis?

(A) First-degree atrioventricular (AV) block
(B) Elevated erythrocyte sedimentation rate (ESR)
(C) Two blood cultures positive for *Streptococcus viridans*
(D) Elevated antistreptolysin O titer (ASO)
(E) Presence of vegetations on an echocardiogram

The answer is D: Elevated antistreptolysin O titer. The physical examination findings described in the vignette are consistent with chorea and carditis making a diagnosis of acute rheumatic fever (ARF) most likely. The diagnosis of ARF is guided by the Jones criteria. Diagnosis is made by establishing the presence of a recent infection with group A β-hemolytic *Streptococcus* (GAβHS) along with the presence of either: (1) two major Jones criteria or (2) one major criterion + two minor criteria. These criteria are listed below:

Major Jones criteria

- Migratory polyarthritis—often affecting large joints and responds to nonsteroidal anti-inflammatory drugs
- Carditis—may present as endocarditis, myocarditis, or pericarditis; rarely patients with carditis have congestive heart failure (CHF) at presentation; when chronic valvular disease is present, this is often termed rheumatic heart disease
- Subcutaneous nodules—nontender nodules over tendons and bony prominences of the extremities and back
- Erythema marginatum—transient, pink, macular, nonpruritic rash typically on the arms, trunk, and thighs (see *Figure 6-4*)
- Chorea—a late manifestation of ARF that may appear more than 3 months after the initial illness; involuntary movements of the face and limbs; may accompany emotional lability

Minor Jones criteria

- Arthralgia—may not be used to diagnose ARF when arthritis is used as a major criterion
- First-degree AV block—prolonged PR-interval; may not be used to diagnose ARF when carditis is used as a major criterion

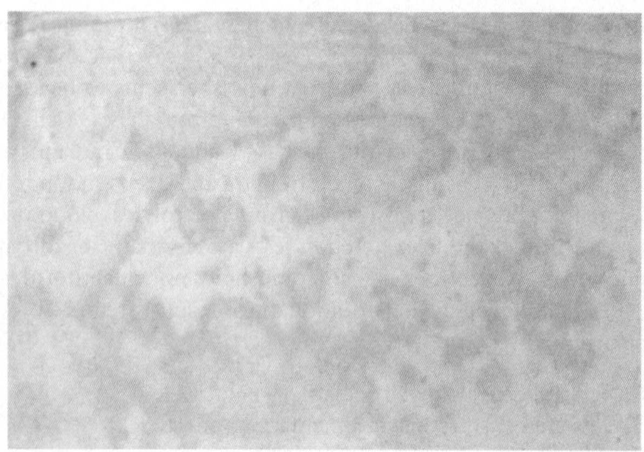

Figure 6-4

- Fever
- Elevated ESR or C-reactive protein (CRP)

The pansystolic murmur at the left sternal border is indicative of significant mitral regurgitation. Additional signs of carditis include a murmur of aortic regurgitation, pericarditis, cardiomegaly, and/or CHF. Because two of the major Jones criteria are already present, the only condition not met for diagnosis is evidence of GAβHS infection. GAβHS infection is usually established either by throat culture or a rapid antigen test. Because chorea is a late manifestation of ARF and occurs weeks after GAβHS infection, a throat culture may be negative. Therefore, GAβHS infection may also be documented by the presence of elevated (or rising) streptococcal antibody titers, either ASO or anti-DNase B antibodies. **(A, C, E)** First-degree AV block, evidence of two blood cultures positive for *S. viridans*, as well as the presence of vegetations on an echocardiogram are all part of the Duke criteria for diagnosis of infective endocarditis. **(B)** ESR is one of the minor Jones criteria and certainly may be present; however, evidence of a preceding GAβHS infection is necessary.

7 A 13-year-old girl is taken to the emergency department by ambulance after a syncopal event that occurred while she was jogging. Her only memory of the event is waking up on the sidewalk with others around her. She denies any chest pain, palpitations, lightheadedness, or dizziness prior to passing out. She was born at term after an uncomplicated pregnancy. Profound hearing loss was diagnosed after she failed a neonatal hearing screen. She has no prior history of syncope and denies any other medical problems. Her family history includes a maternal grandfather who was also deaf and died suddenly in his early 30s.

Of the following, what is her cardiac evaluation likely to reveal?

(A) Fall in systolic blood pressure greater than 20 mmHg after standing
(B) Harsh ejection murmur that decreases when she squats
(C) QT-interval greater than 500 milliseconds
(D) Short PR-interval with initial slurring of the QRS complex
(E) Wide, deep Q-waves and T-wave inversion in leads I and aVL

The answer is C: QT-interval greater than 500 milliseconds. The patient in the vignette most likely has prolonged QT or a QT-interval greater than 500 milliseconds. The patient's personal history of hearing loss as well as the history of sudden death in a family member who was deaf must raise suspicion for a form of long QT syndrome called the Jervell and Lange-Nielsen syndrome. This syndrome is characterized by bilateral sensorineural hearing loss and a corrected QT-interval (QT_c) longer than 500 milliseconds. The formula for calculation of the QT_c is as follows: $QT_C = QT \div \sqrt{RR}$. The upper limit of normal for QT_c is often cited as 440 milliseconds. A prolonged QT_c predisposes the patient to ventricular arrhythmias that can lead to sudden death.

(A) A fall in blood pressure of more than 20/10 mmHg (systolic/diastolic) within 3 minutes of standing is indicative of orthostatic hypotension, particularly when the heart rate does not increase. **(B)** The murmur of subaortic stenosis that changes with certain maneuvers is a classic examination finding in patients with hypertrophic obstructive cardiomyopathy (HCM). Actions that increase systemic vascular resistance, for example, squatting, handgrip, and/or phenylephrine administration, decrease the murmur intensity. Maneuvers that lower the systemic vascular resistance, for example, Valsalva or nitroglycerin, increase the intensity of the murmur. Although HCM can be a cause of exercise-related syncope, patients often complain of chest pain or dyspnea with strenuous activity or exercise. **(D)** Wolff-Parkinson-White (WPW) syndrome may be suspected from the presence of a short PR-interval and a delta wave, or initial slurring of the QRS complex on an electrocardiogram. WPW syndrome may predispose patients to tachyarrhythmias as well as precipitate episodes of presyncope or syncope. **(E)** The electrocardiographic findings of anomalous origin of the left coronary artery from the pulmonary artery (ALCAPA) are indicative of myocardial ischemia or infarction in the area of the left coronary artery (anterolaterally). This manifests as prominent Q-waves with ST-segment and/or T-wave changes in leads I and aVL. ALCAPA is typically diagnosed in the first few months of life as the infant begins to experience episodes of chest pain.

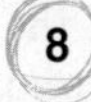

A 13-year-old is referred to cardiology for a murmur and an abnormal electrocardiogram (ECG). He originally presented complaining of fever with pain and inflammation in his left knee and both elbows. He denies any recent upper respiratory symptoms, sore throat, or skin rashes. On examination he is tachypneic, is tachycardic, and has a 3/6 holosystolic murmur at the apex with a gallop rhythm. His liver is palpable 3 to 4 cm below the costal margin. The ECG shows a tachycardic sinus rhythm with no evidence of ischemia or hypertrophy, but there is an increased PR-interval of 280 milliseconds. Serum chemistries, blood urea nitrogen, and creatinine are unremarkable. A complete blood count shows leukocytosis, his erythrocyte sedimentation rate (ESR) and C-reactive protein (CRP) are elevated, and antistreptolysin O titer (ASO) titers are positive.

Of the following, which must be included in this patient's management?

(A) Echocardiographic confirmation of the diagnosis
(B) Surveillance for post–streptococcal glomerulonephritis
(C) 4 to 6 weeks of intravenous antibiotics to eradicate the infection
(D) Corticosteroids and diuretics
(E) Antibiotic prophylaxis until the age of 21

The answer is D: Corticosteroids and diuretics. The patient in the vignette certainly fulfills the necessary criteria for a diagnosis of acute rheumatic fever (ARF), which were reviewed earlier (see Question 6). He has evidence of group A β-hemolytic streptococcal (GAβHS) infection with a markedly elevated ASO titer as well as two major Jones criteria: migratory polyarthritis (knee and bilateral elbow inflammation) and carditis (evidenced by the presence of the murmur of mitral regurgitation) with signs of congestive heart failure (CHF) (the gallop rhythm). Even if the carditis was not recognized, the patient still fulfills the Jones criteria by the presence of a major criterion (migratory polyarthritis) and two minor criteria (first-degree atrioventricular block and elevated CRP or ESR).

Bedrest is important for all patients with ARF. The management of ARF also involves three additional points: treating the GAβHS infection, relief of symptoms, and prophylaxis against recurrence. First, eradication of GAβHS may be accomplished by a 10-day course of either oral penicillin V potassium (VK) or amoxicillin or a single intramuscular injection of penicillin G. Second, the symptoms of ARF must be treated. Arthralgia and fever may be treated with nonsteroidal anti-inflammatory drugs. For patients with evidence of carditis, steroids are indicated, and those with signs of CHF (as is the case for the patient in the vignette) must be managed with diuretics with or without inotropic support if needed. Patients with chorea are typically managed with medications such as haloperidol, valproic acid, or phenobarbital. **(E)** Prophylaxis against recurrence is essential. Either a daily dose of oral penicillin or a monthly intramuscular injection of penicillin is chosen; however, daily oral doses of erythromycin or sulfadiazine are acceptable as well. The duration of prophylaxis depends upon the presence of carditis. Patients who never develop carditis require prophylaxis for either 5 years after ARF has resolved or until the age of 21, whichever is longer. Patients who have carditis, but do not develop residual heart disease require prophylaxis for either 10 years after ARF has resolved or until the age of 21, whichever is longer.

Patients with carditis who do develop residual heart disease require prophylaxis against recurrence for either 10 years after ARF has resolved or until the age of 40, whichever is longer unless they live in an endemic area, had severe carditis, or have recurrence of carditis after the acute phase of the illness has been treated. Those patients should receive prophylaxis for the rest of their lives. The patient described in the vignette should receive either daily penicillin VK, erythromycin, or sulfadiazine prophylaxis or a monthly injection of penicillin G until he is 40 years of age.

(D) The presence of carditis with CHF mandates that he receives corticosteroids and diuretics. **(A)** Neither the Jones criteria nor guidelines for treatment require an echocardiogram. **(B)** Treatment of streptococcal infection does not prevent the risk of post–streptococcal glomerulonephritis. **(C)** Intravenous antibiotics for 4 to 6 weeks is the appropriate treatment for infective endocarditis. GAβHS, however, is a highly sensitive organism and may be eradicated with a 10-day oral course or single intramuscular dose of penicillin.

9 A 13-year-old presents for a well-child evaluation. His medical history is significant for two hospitalizations, one at 5 years of age for dehydration following a prolonged gastrointestinal virus, and another 2 years ago for a spontaneous pneumothorax. He takes no medications, has no allergies, and his immunizations are up to date. His weight is at the 50th percentile, and his height is greater than the 99th percentile. Examination of the chest and abdomen is unremarkable. His hands are shown in Figure 6-5. He also demonstrates that when he places his arms behind his back he can nearly touch his elbows together. A slit lamp examination reveals the findings shown in Figure 6-6.

Of the following, which echocardiographic finding is most likely to be found in this patient?

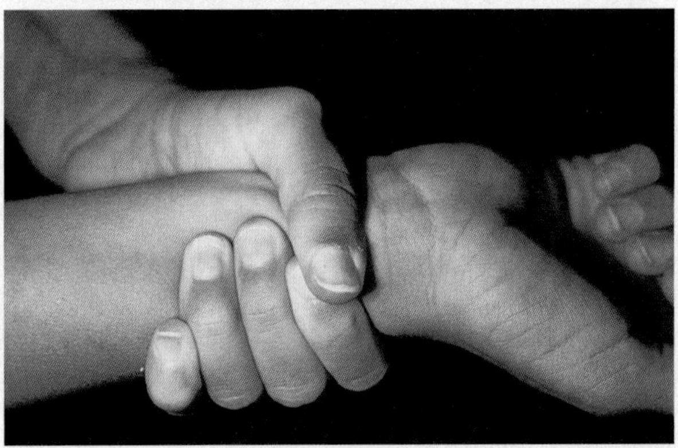

Figure 6-5

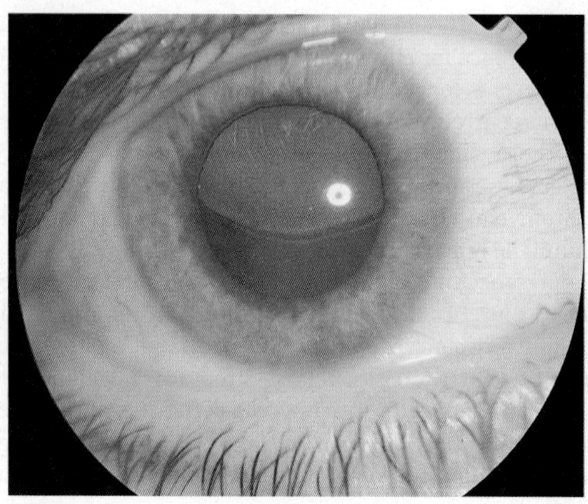

Figure 6-6

(A) Interrupted aortic arch
(B) Cardiac rhabdomyoma
(C) Peripheral pulmonary artery stenosis
(D) Coarctation of the aorta
(E) Dilation of the ascending aorta

The answer is E: Dilation of the ascending aorta. The boy in the vignette has characteristic findings of Marfan syndrome. The revised Ghent criteria list major and minor findings of Marfan syndrome divided according to organ system (i.e., cardiovascular, ocular, integumentary, respiratory, etc.). The only major cardiovascular manifestation is dilation of the aortic root and/or the ascending aorta. Minor manifestations include mitral valve prolapse, calcification of the mitral annulus, dilation of the pulmonary artery in the absence of pulmonary valve stenosis, and dissection of the thoracic aorta in patients younger than 50. **(A)** Patients with DiGeorge syndrome more frequently have truncus arteriosus or interrupted aortic arch. **(B)** Rhabdomyomata may be associated with tuberous sclerosis. **(C)** Peripheral pulmonary artery stenosis is associated with Alagille syndrome. **(D)** Coarctation of the aorta is more common in Turner syndrome.

---

10 A 2-day-old term newborn has cyanosis that does not respond to supplemental oxygen. Pregnancy and vaginal delivery were uncomplicated. On examination, his respiratory rate is 72 breaths/min with nasal flaring and a 3/6 harsh systolic ejection murmur at the mid- and upper left sternal border. A chest radiograph is included in Figure 6-7. An electrocardiogram (ECG) shows right axis deviation and right ventricular hypertrophy (RVH). The infant's symptoms improve after an infusion of prostaglandin E_1 (PGE_1) is initiated.

Of the following, which is the most likely diagnosis?

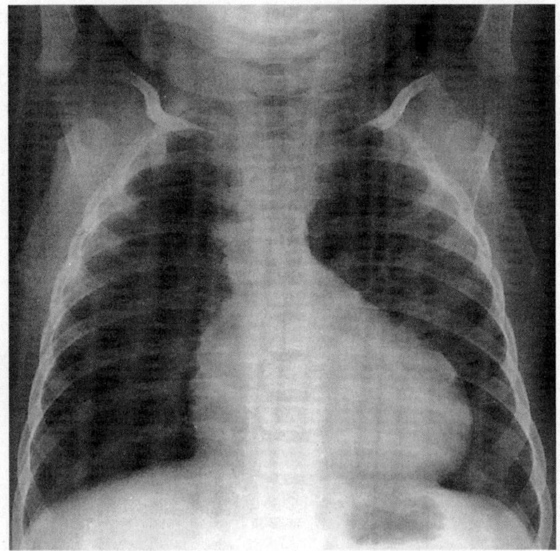

Figure 6-7

(A) Truncus arteriosus
(B) Tricuspid atresia
(C) Tetralogy of Fallot (TOF)
(D) Total anomalous pulmonary venous return (TAPVR)
(E) D-transposition of the great arteries (D-TGA)

The answer is C: Tetralogy of Fallot (TOF). The patient in the vignette has TOF. TOF consists of four abnormalities: (1) right ventricular outflow tract (RVOT) obstruction from pulmonary stenosis, (2) RVH, (3) a ventricular septal defect (VSD) with (4) an overriding aorta. The severity of presentation depends on the degree of RVOT obstruction. For infants with mild degrees of RVOT obstruction, cyanosis may not be apparent immediately after delivery. They may present later with signs and symptoms of heart failure secondary to the left-to-right shunt through the VSD. Infants with more severe RVOT obstruction are symptomatic at birth or within the first few hours or days of life, as the ductus arteriosus begins to close. The murmur of the infant in the vignette is due to turbulent flow through the RVOT and not due to the VSD. The large VSD of TOF is not associated with turbulent flow, so a murmur is not heard. Radiography of the chest shows the classic boot-shaped heart due to upturning of the cardiac apex from RVH and decreased pulmonary vascular markings from reduced blood flow through the RVOT. The infant in the vignette developed cyanosis and respiratory distress due to reduced pulmonary blood flow. With more severe degrees of RVOT obstruction, pulmonary blood flow becomes dependent on the ductus arteriosus. Thus, the immediate treatment is PGE_1, to open the ductus and reestablish adequate pulmonary blood flow.

(A) Newborns with truncus arteriosus usually have cardiomegaly and increased pulmonary vascular markings due to unrestricted flow into the pulmonary artery (see *Figure 6-8*). **(B)** In tricuspid atresia, there is underdevelopment of the right ventricle. The ECG shows left ventricular hypertrophy and right atrial enlargement. **(D)** The chest radiograph in TAPVR with pulmonary vein obstruction typically shows increased markings from pulmonary venous congestion (see *Figure 6-9*). **(E)** D-TGA also has increased pulmonary vascular markings, and an egg-shaped heart with a narrowed mediastinum.

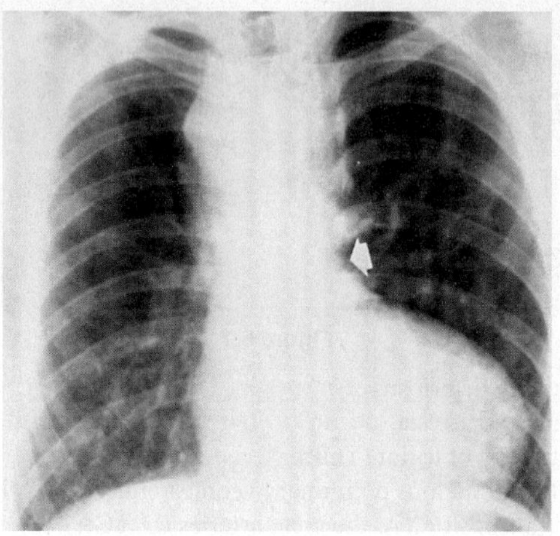

Figure 6-8

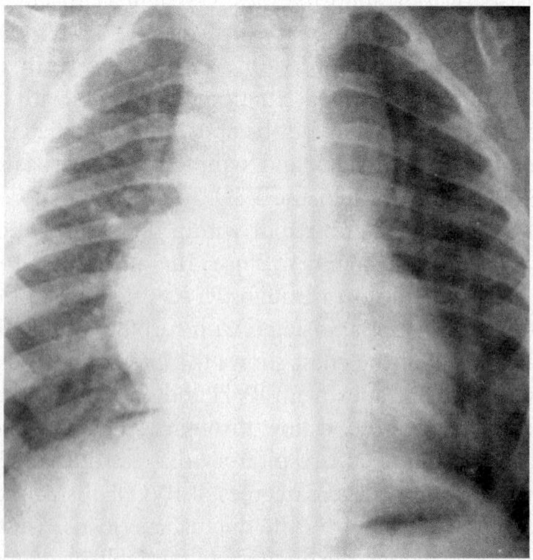

Figure 6-9

---

11 A 5-year-old girl is found to be hypertensive on a routine health assessment. She was born at term and has had normal growth and development. Her blood pressure is 130/68 mmHg in the right arm, 100/62 mmHg in the left arm, and 104/66 mmHg in the left leg. There is a systolic ejection click and a I/VI early systolic murmur at the upper sternal border. The right radial pulse is 3+. Her right femoral pulse is 1+ and is felt after the radial pulse when they are palpated simultaneously. Additional testing to confirm the diagnosis is ordered.

Of the following, which findings are most likely?

(A) Electrocardiogram (ECG) demonstrating a sinus rhythm, left axis deviation, and increased voltage in the left lateral leads
(B) Echocardiogram showing a discrete coarctation of the aorta between the left common carotid and left subclavian arteries
(C) Plain radiography of the chest showing an enlarged cardiac silhouette and notching of the inferior border of the ribs
(D) Abdominal ultrasound showing stenosis of the right renal artery
(E) Increased concentration of vanillylmandelic acid in a 24-hour urine collection

The answer is B: **Echocardiogram showing a discrete coarctation of the aorta between the left common carotid and left subclavian arteries.** The patient described in the vignette has physical examination findings characteristic of coarctation of the aorta. Normally, blood pressure in the lower extremities is 10 to 20 mmHg higher than in the upper extremities. In coarctation of the aorta this is reversed. For a discrete juxtaductal coarctation, blood pressure is higher in the right arm than in the left arm and in the right and left legs because the coarctation is distal to the origin of the right subclavian artery, but proximal to the origin of the left subclavian and the femoral arteries. **(A)** While older patients with unrecognized coarctation may have evidence of left ventricular hypertrophy on ECG as well as cardiomegaly and rib notching on chest radiography, this is not typically seen in young children within the first decade of life. **(C)** Rib notching occurs over years due to pressure erosion by enlarged collateral vessels that develop in order to offset diminished blood flow from the descending aorta. The cause of the systolic click in the patient described in the vignette is likely due to a bicuspid aortic valve. Bicuspid aortic valve is associated with coarctation of the aorta in the majority of cases. **(D)** Renal artery stenosis **(E)** and pheochromocytoma may be causes of hypertension in children; however, neither would cause a blood pressure gradient between upper and lower extremities. Blood pressure in all four extremities would be uniformly elevated.

12 A term newborn in the nursery is noted to be tachypneic. Pregnancy, labor, and vaginal delivery were unremarkable. Vital signs are pulse 180 beats/min, respirations 60 breaths/min, right arm blood pressure

72/30 mmHg, and O_2 saturation 84% on room air. There is a somewhat dusky appearance of the lips and tongue, along with a bluish coloration of the hands and feet. Auscultation reveals tachycardia with a regular rhythm. S1 is normal, and S2 is prominent and single. Brachial and femoral pulses are normal. The abdomen is soft. The liver is palpable 4 cm below the right costal margin; the spleen is not palpable. The infant is given 100% FiO_2 by nasal cannula for 15 minutes. Vital signs, including O_2 saturation, remain unchanged. A chest radiograph shows an enlarged cardiothymic silhouette with a slender anterior mediastinum and hyperemic lung fields.

Of the following, what is the most likely diagnosis?

(A) Tetralogy of Fallot (TOF)
(B) Hypoplastic left heart syndrome (HLHS)
(C) Obstructed total anomalous pulmonary venous return (TAPVR)
(D) Critical pulmonary stenosis
(E) D-transposition of the great arteries (D-TGA)

The answer is E: D-transposition of the great arteries (D-TGA). The patient in the vignette has D-TGA. This newborn has central cyanosis with signs of congestive heart failure (CHF). The bluish color of the hands and feet, or acrocyanosis, is not abnormal and can be found in most newborns. However, a blue or dusky coloration of the lips, gingiva, or tongue may be due to central cyanosis and is indicative of hypoxia. Signs of CHF in the infant include tachycardia, tachypnea, cardiomegaly, and hepatomegaly. It is not unusual to feel the liver edge in newborns, but 4 cm below the costal margin is excessive. This infant also failed to respond to supplemental oxygen given by nasal cannula. The findings with auscultation are due to the abnormal positioning of the semilunar valves in D-TGA. S2 is often described as single and loud. Finally, the description of the cardiac silhouette on the chest film is the characteristic "egg on a string." The mediastinum is narrowed due to the abnormal position (often nearly anterior–posterior) of the great vessels. The lung fields are hyperemic, with increased pulmonary vascular markings due to excess pulmonary blood flow into the main pulmonary artery from the left ventricle.

(A) Patients with TOF would have a characteristic pulmonary stenosis (PS) murmur and oligemic lung fields. **(B)** Newborns with HLHS may also have a single, loud S2, but this is due to atresia of the aortic valve. They may also have increased pulmonary vascular markings due to excess pulmonary blood flow; however, this increased pulmonary flow is at the expense of systemic flow. Neonates with HLHS may then have decreased systemic output leading to decreased perfusion and poor peripheral pulses. **(C)** TAPVR occurs when all four pulmonary veins connect and drain into the right heart rather than to the left atrium. Obstructed TAPVR presents as cyanosis and tachypnea due to backup of blood into the pulmonary vasculature. Auscultation demonstrates a widely split and fixed S2 because there is increased return to the right heart and, therefore, a constant increase in flow across the pulmonary valve. There is typically a diastolic rumble at the left lower sternal border as well. This represents increased flow across the tricuspid valve. Radiography of the chest shows congested, hyperemic lung fields. **(D)** Auscultation with PS should reveal an ejection murmur at the left upper sternal border. Patients with mild PS are usually asymptomatic. With critical PS, patients are cyanotic and tachypneic, but often without a murmur due to inadequate blood flow across the valve. The chest radiograph would show a normal cardiac silhouette with post-stenotic dilation of the main pulmonary artery as well as oligemic lung fields.

13 A 3-month-old infant is seen in clinic for fever and listlessness that began a week ago and has progressed over the past several days. His parents initially believed he had "a cold" that would improve with time. Today, though, they noticed a rash and decided to seek medical attention. He was born with hypoplastic left heart syndrome and has had one surgery thus far, done at 4 days of life. Following surgery, he was in the pediatric cardiac intensive care unit for several days, but was transitioned to the general pediatric floor after he was extubated and indwelling central venous catheters were removed. Vital signs are temperature 38.2°C, pulse 136 beats/min, respiratory rate 28 breaths/min, and blood pressure 82/65 mmHg. Oxygen saturation on room air is 80%, which is normal for his heart defect at this stage of the surgical repair. He has a 1/6 continuous murmur at the upper sternal border and a single S2. His breath sounds are clear. His spleen is palpable about 1 cm below the left costal margin, and he has several small, nontender, erythematous macules on the soles of his feet bilaterally.

Of the following, which if present, would establish a definite diagnosis?

(A) Blood culture positive for coagulase-negative staphylococcus
(B) History of previous bacterial endocarditis
(C) Improvement in symptoms within 4 days of antibiotic therapy
(D) Presence of atrioventricular (AV) block
(E) Echocardiographic presence of vegetations

The answer is E: Echocardiographic presence of vegetations. The patient in the vignette has infective endocarditis. Duke criteria assist in the diagnosis of infective endocarditis. Diagnosis may be made if a patient meets two major criteria, one major and three minor criteria, or five minor criteria. The criteria are as follows:

Major Duke criteria

- Two separate blood cultures positive for a usual organism (*Streptococcus viridans, Streptococcus bovis, Haemophilus* spp., *Actinobacillus, Cardiobacterium hominis, Eikenella corrodens, Kingella kingae*)

- Evidence of endocardial involvement (echocardiogram showing an oscillating intracardiac mass, an abscess, or new dehiscence of a prosthetic valve)

Minor Duke criteria

- Fever
- Predisposing cardiac condition or intravenous drug use
- Microbiologic evidence (positive blood culture that does not meet the major criterion)
- Echocardiographic evidence (findings consistent with infective endocarditis that do not meet the major criterion)
- Vascular phenomena (Janeway lesions, conjunctival or intracranial hemorrhages, pulmonary infarct, arterial emboli)
- Immunologic phenomena (Osler nodes, Roth spots, glomerulonephritis)

The infant in the vignette has three of the minor Duke criteria. He has fever, a predisposing cardiac condition (cyanotic heart disease status post–surgical intervention), and Osler nodes (the painless erythematous macules noted on his soles). See Figures 6-10 and 6-11 for examples of Janeway lesions and Osler nodes. The diagnosis of infective endocarditis may be made for the patient in the vignette with the presence of either (1) one major criterion or (2) two more minor criteria. **(E)** The only answer choice that fits this requirement is echocardiography showing vegetations. That would provide evidence of endocardial involvement. **(A)** Positive blood cultures would satisfy another minor requirement, but only four minor criteria are not sufficient for diagnosis. **(B)** History of previous bacterial endocarditis is important to know for deciding upon the need for prophylaxis against future episodes of endocarditis; however, it is not

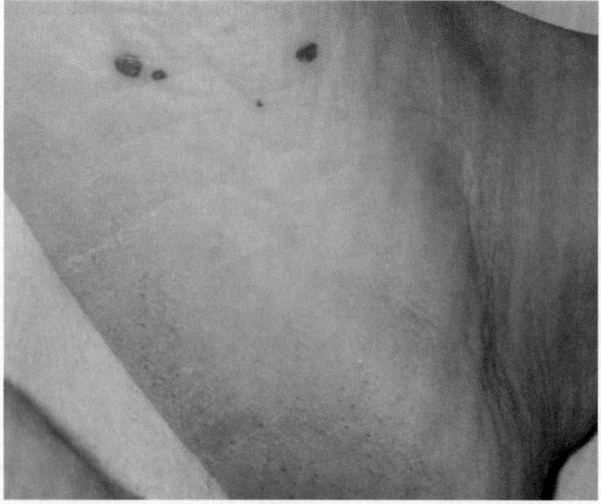

Figure 6-10

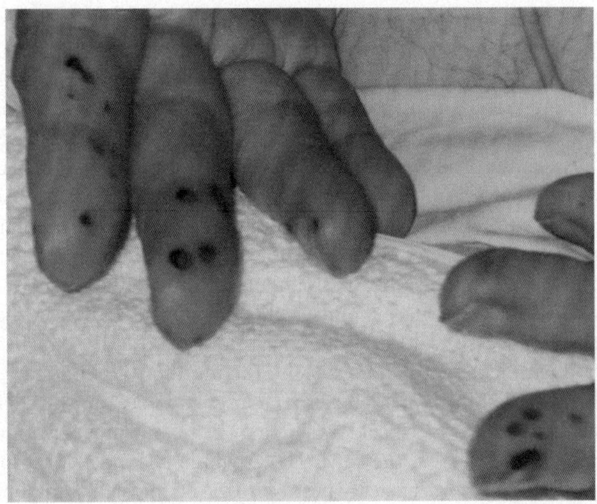

Figure 6-11

a major or minor Duke criteria. **(C)** Improvement in symptoms after initiating antibiotics cannot be evidence of a bacterial infection and is not part of the Duke criteria. If antibiotics are given toward the end of a viral illness, the symptoms will improve; however, the antibiotic agent is not responsible for the resolution of symptoms. Even if a bacterial etiology were still strongly suspected, the administration of antibiotics does not necessarily indicate that the bacterial infection was endocarditis. **(D)** Presence of AV block is incorrect because heart block of any degree is not part of the Duke criteria. First-degree AV block is a minor criterion for the diagnosis of ARF, not infective endocarditis.

14 A 3-week-old presents for a health maintenance visit. She was born at 39 weeks' gestation after an uncomplicated pregnancy. Her parents have no concerns and say she has done well since her visit 2 weeks earlier. Her respiratory rate is 38 breaths/min, and her heart rate is 130 beats/min. Breath sounds are clear, but there is a 2/6 systolic crescendo-decrescendo murmur at the second intercostal space on the left that is also heard in both axillae and when auscultating the patient's back. Her abdomen is soft. Femoral and brachial pulses are normal bilaterally.

Of the following, what is the most likely cause of her murmur?

(A) Patent ductus arteriosus (PDA)
(B) Total anomalous pulmonary venous return (TAPVR)
(C) Critical pulmonary valve stenosis
(D) Vibratory innocent murmur
(E) Peripheral pulmonary artery stenosis

The answer is E: Peripheral pulmonary artery stenosis. The presentation of the patient in the vignette is consistent with findings of peripheral pulmonary artery stenosis. The murmur of peripheral pulmonary artery stenosis is usually heard in the pulmonary area and transmits to the axillae and back. It is caused by turbulent flow within the branch pulmonary arteries. **(A)** In otherwise normal infants, the murmur of a PDA is continuous because the left-to-right shunting of blood occurs in both systole and diastole as pressure in the aorta is greater than pressure in the pulmonary artery throughout the cardiac cycle. An infant with a large, hemodynamically significant PDA may also have bounding pulses due to the wide pulse pressure caused by diastolic run off through the patent ductus. **(B)** Infants with TAPVR may have a midsystolic murmur heard best in the second left intercostal space. **(C)** Critical pulmonary valve stenosis presents in the neonatal period with tachypnea and cyanosis. The murmur of pulmonary stenosis (PS) is often heard at the upper left sternal border and may transmit to the back and axillae; however, with critical PS there may be no murmur due to markedly decreased blood flow across the valve. **(D)** A vibratory innocent murmur, also known as a Still murmur, is usually best heard at the mid-left sternal border or the lower left sternal border. It is often characterized as musical, vibratory, or groaning and is more common in the preschool or early school age population.

15 Amniocentesis diagnoses trisomy 21 in a second-trimester fetus. The parents are concerned about the possibility of a heart defect and have asked for advice regarding testing after the baby is born.

Of the following, what is the most appropriate response?

(A) Echocardiography is indicated only if there are signs of congestive heart failure
(B) A screening echocardiogram should be performed within the first year of life
(C) Unless symptomatic, screening echocardiography is not indicated until 5 years of age
(D) Echocardiography is only indicated if corrective cardiac surgery is required
(E) Routine echocardiography is indicated after delivery, even if the infant is asymptomatic

The answer is E: Routine echocardiography is indicated after delivery, even if the infant is asymptomatic. Approximately one-half of infants with Down syndrome have some form of congenital heart defect. Of those, a complete atrioventricular (AV) septal defect occurs in a significant portion. This lesion is also called an "AV canal" or an "endocardial cushion defect." Isolated atrial septal defects, ventricular septal defects, patent ductus arteriosus, and tetralogy of Fallot are also more common in infants with Down syndrome. Infants with a complete AV septal defect may initially be asymptomatic, but as the pulmonary vascular resistance naturally falls in the weeks and months after delivery, signs and symptoms of excess pulmonary blood flow such as tachypnea, fatigue, and poor weight gain begin to develop. This typically occurs during the first year of life. **(A, B, C, D)** Despite the absence of symptoms in the neonatal period, routine screening echocardiography should be performed for all infants with Down syndrome at the time of diagnosis because of the increased incidence of heart defects. This allows time for the infant to be evaluated by a pediatric cardiologist well before symptoms develop and cardiac surgery is required.

16 A 9-month-old is born abroad and presents for a health assessment evaluation after immigrating to the United States with her adoptive parents. Reportedly, she was born at term and lived at an orphanage until approximately 8 weeks of age. The only known medical history is that she has been treated for several pulmonary infections and is up to date with all recommended immunizations. On examination, she is mildly tachycardic and tachypneic with a normal blood pressure and normal oxygen saturations. She is between the third and fifth percentiles for weight, and she is at the 25th percentile for length. She is given 2 ounces of formula by bottle and takes it slowly, stopping multiple times and falling asleep prior to finishing. There is a holosystolic blowing murmur along the lower sternum and a mid-diastolic rumble at the apex that is best heard with the stethoscope bell. A chest radiograph is shown in Figure 6-12.

Of the following, which is her most likely diagnosis?

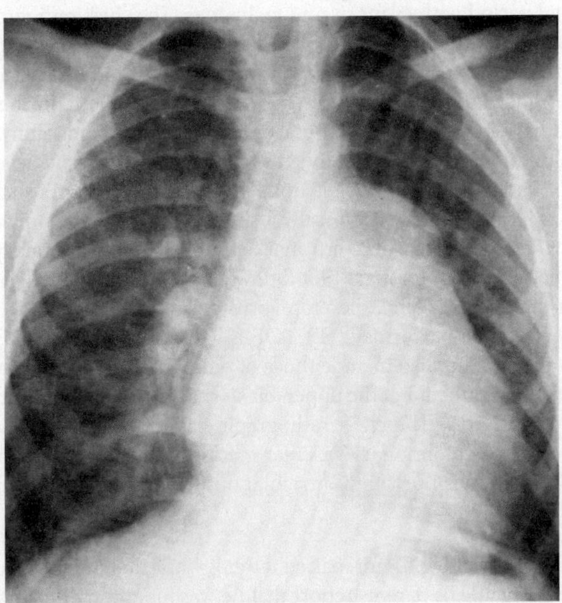

Figure 6-12

(A) Tricuspid atresia
(B) D-transposition of the great arteries (D-TGA)
(C) Pulmonary atresia with intact ventricular septum
(D) Ventricular septal defect
(E) Tetralogy of Fallot (TOF)

The answer is D: Ventricular septal defect. The infant in the vignette most likely has a moderate-to-large ventricular septal defect (VSD). The clinical manifestations of a large VSD are related to pulmonary overcirculation, which leads to congestive heart failure. There may also be a history of repeated pulmonary infections. Poor weight gain with failure to thrive is classically accompanied by poor or difficult feeding with respiratory distress and/or diaphoresis. The left-to-right shunting that occurs with a moderate-to-large VSD places a burden on the left heart, not the right. This is because the right ventricle (RV) contracts at the same time as the left ventricle (LV), so the volume shunted into the RV is ejected into the pulmonary circulation as it is shunted into the right heart. Therefore, it is the pulmonary vasculature, left atrium, and LV that receive the volume burden. This is the reason for the apical diastolic rumble. This murmur represents increased flow across the mitral valve. Plain radiography of the chest reveals increased pulmonary vascular markings and cardiomegaly due to enlargement of the left atrium and LV (and later, the RV).

The other choices are less likely because the patient described has normal oxygen saturations. Additionally, **(A)** tricuspid atresia often presents early in the neonatal period with cyanosis and tachypnea. The chest radiograph would show oligemic lung fields instead of increased pulmonary vasculature. Most infants with tricuspid atresia do not survive beyond 6 months without surgical intervention. Infants with **(B)** D-TGA would be cyanotic in the newborn period and have increased vascular markings on a chest radiography. **(C)** Neonates with pulmonary atresia and intact ventricular septum have severe cyanosis at birth. The pulmonary valve is not stenotic; it is atretic. As such, there is no murmur, although there is typically a single S2 because the only semilunar valve is the aortic valve. There are markedly decreased pulmonary vascular markings because all pulmonary blood flow comes from the ductus arteriosus. Closure of the ductus is fatal; therefore, prostaglandin E_1 infusion is necessary until surgery can be performed. **(E)** TOF is associated with a VSD; however, clinical manifestations also include those of pulmonary stenosis. There is often a systolic ejection murmur at the upper left sternal border, corresponding to the pulmonary valve area. The chest radiograph classically shows a boot-shaped heart and decreased pulmonary vascular markings due to the decrease in pulmonary blood flow via the right ventricular outflow tract and pulmonary valve.

17 A 3-month-old with unrepaired tetralogy of Fallot (TOF) is admitted to the hospital. His parents report that he was fussy and difficult to console earlier in the day. In the emergency department, he is irritable and crying after his blood is drawn. While crying, he becomes blue and efforts to calm him are unsuccessful. As he continues crying, he becomes progressively more cyanotic.

Of the following, which of these interventions is the best choice for treating acute hypoxic spells associated with TOF?

(A) Inhaled nitric oxide
(B) Intravenous enalaprilat
(C) Intravenous furosemide
(D) Emergency surgical repair
(E) Bringing the knees to the chest

The answer is E: Bringing the knees to the chest. Hypoxic spells (also known as "tet spells") are the result of a cycle that involves crying and hyperpnea that increases systemic venous return. Due to the fixed obstruction or spasms of the right ventricular outflow tract (RVOT), increased systemic venous return increases the amount of desaturated blood that shunts right-to-left through the ventricular septal defect and makes the infant more cyanotic and hypoxic. Hypoxia and acidosis cause hyperpnea, creating the cycle.

Treatments are directed at breaking the cycle. **(E)** The best choice is to place the infant in the knee–chest position. This will increase the systemic vascular resistance and promote blood flow into the pulmonary circulation. Supplemental oxygen is often given; however, it has a limited role because the main problem is decreased pulmonary blood flow, not oxygenation. **(A)** Similarly, inhaled nitric oxide will not reverse the fixed obstruction at the RVOT and is less useful. **(B)** Enalaprilat is an intravenous angiotensin-converting enzyme inhibitor that causes vasodilation by inhibiting the conversion of angiotensin I to angiotensin II. Systemic vasodilation is counterproductive during a hypoxic spell, as it would lower systemic vascular resistance and further increase the right-to-left shunt, worsening the hypoxia. **(C)** Furosemide is a loop diuretic commonly used in the treatment of congestive heart failure. In contrast to diuretic use, volume expansion is sometimes helpful during a hypoxic spell by increasing preload. **(D)** Urgent surgery is required when all medical efforts have failed. Additional medical treatments for patients' having a tet spell include subcutaneous or intramuscular morphine sulfate (for respiratory suppression and sedation), sodium bicarbonate (as acidosis stimulates the respiratory center), ketamine (for respiratory suppression and sedation), intravenous propranolol (for negative chronotopy), and phenylephrine (to increase systemic vascular resistance and promote pulmonary blood flow).

---

18 A 17-year-old previously healthy boy presents with severe pain located in the center of his chest that radiates to the left shoulder and upper arm. He is nauseated and feels short of breath. His vital signs are heart rate 110 beats/min and blood pressure 130/88 mmHg. Other than pallor and diaphoresis, his examination is normal. He has clear breath sounds and no murmurs. A chest radiograph is normal and his electrocardiogram (ECG) is included in Figure 6-13.

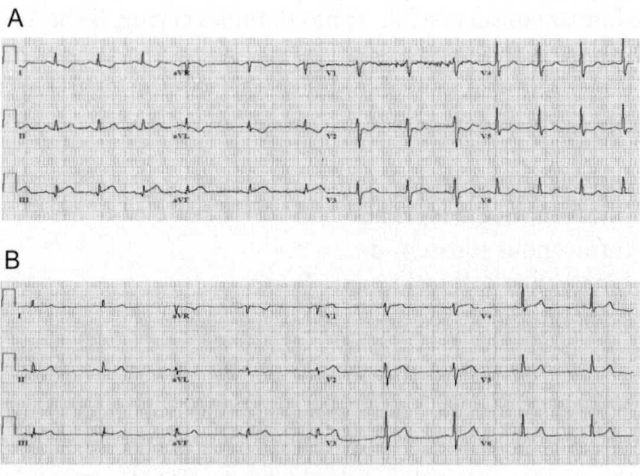

Figure 6-13

Of the following, what is the most likely ingestion responsible for this adolescent's symptoms and ECG findings?

(A) Phencyclidine
(B) Cocaine
(C) Methamphetamine
(D) Amyl nitrite
(E) Anabolic steroids

The answer is B: Cocaine. Cocaine is a vasoconstrictor that has several damaging cardiovascular effects. The ST-segment elevation in this patient is indicative of myocardial ischemia due to coronary vasospasm, a well-reported effect of the drug. **(A)** Phencyclidine is a hallucinogen with toxic effects of myocardial irritation that may be similar to cocaine, for example, tachycardia, hypertension, and diaphoresis; however, it is not known for its vasoconstricting effects and is less likely to cause myocardial ischemia. **(C)** Methamphetamine is a stimulant that has been shown to prolong the corrected QT-interval, and can worsen existing myocardial ischemia by increasing the heart rate. It does not typically cause acute myocardial ischemia. **(D)** Amyl nitrite is a potent vasodilator with effects that include lower blood pressure, tachycardia, headache, and dizziness. With overdose, side effects of severe hypotension, dyspnea and hypoventilation, and syncope may occur. Inhalation of amyl nitrite may cause flattening of the T-wave and/or prominence of U-waves, but elevation of ST-segments has not been described. **(E)** Exogenously administered anabolic steroids increase skeletal muscle growth and are also likely to have effects on cardiac muscle. Although not extensively studied, hypertrophy and reduced diastolic function, or impaired relaxation, of the left ventricle have been reported in long-term abusers of anabolic steroids. Acute myocardial ischemia is an unlikely presentation of anabolic steroid use.

19 A healthy 15-year-old boy is hit in the chest with a baseball during a game, collapses, and remains unresponsive. Several spectators begin resuscitative efforts that continue as he is taken to a nearby hospital where he is ultimately pronounced dead.

Of the following, what best describes the part of the cardiac cycle at the time the ball hits his chest?

(A) Atrial depolarization
(B) Atrial repolarization
(C) Ventricular depolarization
(D) Ventricular repolarization
(E) Interval between ventricular repolarization and atrial depolarization

The answer is D: **Ventricular repolarization.** The description in the vignette is that of commotio cordis, sudden death that results from nonpenetrating chest trauma. It primarily affects adolescents and children and classically occurs during sporting events. Fortunately, it is a rare event. **(A, B, C, E)** The blow to the chest must occur during a short period of ventricular repolarization that corresponds to the first few milliseconds during the upstroke of the T-wave. The result is that the ventricle begins to fibrillate. Unfortunately, the majority of cases are fatal even in spite of prompt initiation of cardiopulmonary resuscitation.

20 An adolescent with polycystic kidney disease and chronic renal failure is evaluated in the emergency department. She missed her last two dialysis appointments and is brought for evaluation by her boyfriend after passing out. Blood analysis shows several electrolyte derangements including severe hyperkalemia.

Of the following, which electrocardiographic changes are consistent with severe hyperkalemia?

(A) Shortened PR-interval, widened QRS duration, increased T-wave amplitude
(B) Shortened PR-interval, widened QRS duration, decreased T-wave amplitude
(C) Prolonged PR-interval, widened QRS duration, increased T-wave amplitude
(D) Prolonged PR-interval, widened QRS duration, decreased T-wave amplitude
(E) Prolonged PR-interval, shortened QRS duration, decreased T-wave amplitude

The answer is C: **Prolonged PR-interval, widened QRS duration, increased T-wave amplitude.** As the potassium level rises, there are a series of electrocardiographic changes that become apparent (see *Figure 6-14*). **(A, B, D, E)** T-waves increase in amplitude, becoming peaked, or taller. At higher potassium

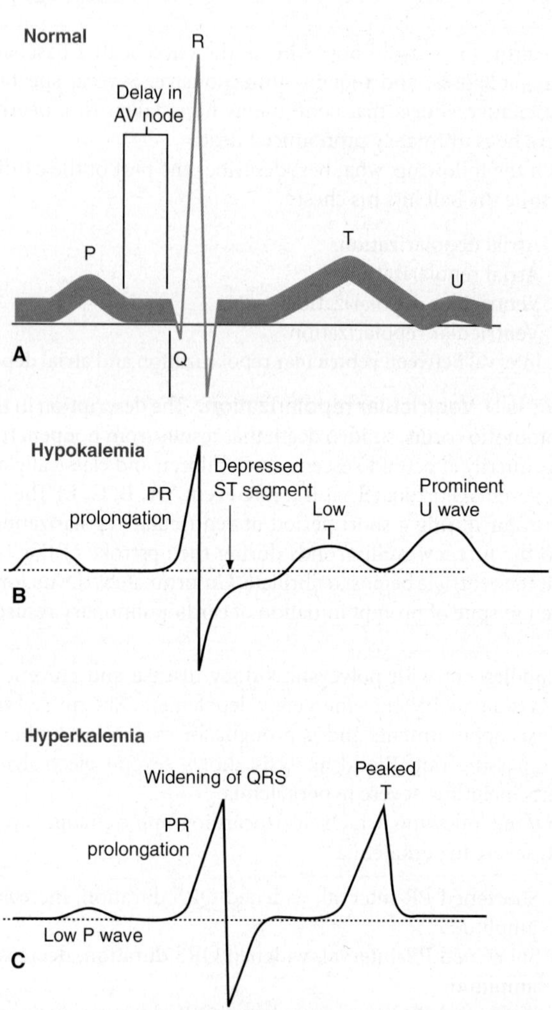

Figure 6-14

concentration, the QRS duration prolongs and becomes wider. Prolongation of the PR-interval follows. At extremely high potassium levels, the P-wave may disappear and the QRS can become so prolonged that they appear diphasic, also called a sine wave or sinusoidal. If not treated quickly and aggressively, asystole occurs.

---

21 A term neonate presents at 3 days of life with tachycardia, tachypnea, and cyanosis. He has a single, loud second heart sound with no murmur, a gallop rhythm, and diminished femoral and brachial pulses.

His capillary refill time is longer than 5 seconds. The infant is urgently intubated, and a chest radiograph demonstrates pulmonary edema. An arterial blood gas shows a pH of 7.1, pCO_2 40, and HCO_3^- of 16.

Of the following, which is his most likely diagnosis?

(A) Pulmonary atresia
(B) L-transposition of the great arteries (L-TGA)
(C) Aortic stenosis
(D) Hypoplastic left heart syndrome (HLHS)
(E) Tricuspid atresia

The answer is D: Hypoplastic left heart syndrome (HLHS). The infant in the vignette has HLHS. This infant has developed symptoms due to closure of the ductus arteriosus and a decrease in the pulmonary vascular resistance. The large dilated right ventricle (RV) can no longer provide output to the systemic circulation through the descending aorta via the ductus, causing severe metabolic acidosis and signs of shock. The single S2 is due to closure of the lone semilunar valve, the pulmonary valve, as the aortic valve is atretic. The chest radiograph shows pulmonary edema because as the ductus closes there is obstruction to systemic flow, leaving flow to the lungs unbalanced. **(A)** Infants with pulmonary atresia may also present as the ductus closes with no murmur and a single S2 (from the aortic valve instead of the atretic pulmonary valve). Pulmonary atresia is also a ductal-dependent lesion as affected infants rely on left-to-right shunting for pulmonary blood flow. The chest radiograph in pulmonary atresia would show decreased pulmonary vascular markings and oligemic lung fields due to reduced pulmonary blood flow as opposed to the pulmonary edema seen for the infant in the vignette. **(B)** Newborns with L-TGA may also have a single, loud S2 due to the anterior–posterior relationship of the great arteries; however, they are asymptomatic unless there are other associated defects. Neonates with mild or moderate aortic stenosis are often asymptomatic. **(C)** Critical aortic stenosis presents immediately after delivery with weak or thready pulses. The obstruction to systemic flow does not depend on the ductus, so symptoms are noted immediately. **(E)** Tricuspid atresia is a cyanotic heart disease in which the systemic venous return is redirected into the left heart and into the systemic circulation again. If there are no other associated lesions, blood reaches the pulmonary circulation either via the ductus arteriosus (from the aorta into the pulmonary artery) or after entering the left heart, blood crosses through a ventricular septal defect into the RV and through the pulmonary valve into the pulmonary artery. As pulmonary blood flow is reduced, pulmonary vascular markings on chest radiograph are often decreased.

22 A 6-hour-old newborn is transferred from the nursery to the neonatal intensive care unit (NICU) after a seizure is witnessed by several members of the medical staff. Pregnancy and term delivery were uncomplicated.

On examination, he appears dysmorphic, with a short philtrum and increased distance between the eyes. He is slightly cyanotic. Cardiovascular examination reveals a 2/6 systolic murmur and bounding brachial and femoral pulses. Chest radiograph shows cardiomegaly, an absent thymic shadow, and congested pulmonary vasculature. NICU staff sends blood for culture and analysis and initiate intravenous antibiotics for presumed sepsis secondary to the seizure. His chemistry panel shows the following: sodium 140 mEq/L, potassium 3.6 mEq/L, and calcium 4.8 mg/dL.

Of the following, which is this infant's most likely congenital heart lesion?

(A) Downward displacement of the tricuspid valve with atrialization of the right ventricle (RV)
(B) Drainage of the pulmonary veins into the systemic circulation below the diaphragm
(C) Common arterial trunk from which the aorta and pulmonary artery both arise
(D) Common atrioventricular (AV) valve with atrial ventricular septal defect (VSDs)
(E) Atresia of the mitral and aortic valves with hypoplasia of the aorta and left ventricle (LV)

The answer is C: Common arterial trunk from which the aorta and pulmonary artery both arise. The infant in the vignette has clinical features that are suspicious for DiGeorge syndrome. Dysmorphic facies that include a short philtrum and hypertelorism, an absent thymus, hypocalcemia (due to hypoparathyroidism), and cyanotic congenital heart disease are all indicative of the 22q11 deletion. DiGeorge syndrome is associated with anomalies of the conotruncus, particularly interrupted aortic arch, tetralogy of Fallot, and truncus arteriosus. The only choice consistent with a conotruncal defect is a truncus arteriosus. **(C)** In the most common form of truncus arteriosus, the aorta and pulmonary artery arise from a common arterial trunk with a single truncal valve that overrides a defect in the ventricular septum. In this form, there is increased pulmonary blood flow, resulting in increased pulmonary vascular markings on chest radiography. Examination may reveal the systolic murmur of the VSD. If there is insufficiency of the truncal valve, a diastolic murmur may be heard as well.

(A) Downward displacement of the tricuspid valve with atrialization of the RV describes an Ebstein anomaly, which has been associated with maternal lithium use. **(B)** Drainage of the pulmonary veins into the systemic circulation below the diaphragm is synonymous with infracardiac total anomalous pulmonary venous return. **(D)** A common AV valve with an atrial septal defect and VSD describes a complete AV septal defect, also known as an endocardial cushion defect. This is commonly associated with Down syndrome. **(E)** Atresia of the mitral and aortic valves with hypoplasia of the aorta and LV describes hypoplastic left heart syndrome.

---

23 A healthy 15-year-old girl complains of episodes of a rapid heartbeat that occur at least once per day. These episodes begin suddenly, last less than 1 minute, and end abruptly. None have been associated with exercise or activity.

Of the following, what is the most likely mechanism of this patient's episodes of tachycardia?

(A) Reentry circuit involving the atrioventricular (AV) node
(B) Reentry circuit within atrial muscle
(C) Localized automatic focus within the atrium
(D) Enhanced automaticity of the AV node
(E) Reentry circuit within ventricular muscle

The answer is A: **Reentry circuit involving the atrioventricular (AV) node.** Reentrant forms of supraventricular tachycardia characteristically start and terminate abruptly and typically occur when the patient is at rest. The most common mechanism is reentry involving an accessory pathway and the AV node. Tachycardia is initiated when a premature atrial impulse is unable to travel down the AV node because it is still refractory from the previous sinus beat. The presence of an accessory pathway allows the premature impulse to reach the ventricle. By this time, the AV node is no longer refractory, and the impulse travels up the normal conduction pathway in a retrograde fashion and back to the atrium where the accessory pathway is available to conduct again, continuing the circuit. **(B)** A reentry circuit located within atrial muscle describes the etiology of atrial flutter. Atrial flutter manifests as a saw-tooth pattern (F-waves) on electrocardiogram and most commonly occurs in older pediatric patients with underlying heart disease. **(C)** Ectopic atrial tachycardias originate from a locus within the atrium that has abnormal automaticity. These tachycardias are often described as "warming-up" rather than starting abruptly, but many patients do not notice palpitations at all. **(D)** Junctional ectopic tachycardia is caused by enhanced automaticity of the AV node. It is rare in the pediatric population and most commonly seen in younger patients following surgery for congenital heart disease. **(E)** Reentry circuits within ventricular muscle cause various forms of ventricular tachycardia. Ventricular tachycardia may be present in children without an obvious form of structural heart disease; however, ventricular tachycardia is also associated with dilated cardiomyopathy, myocardial ischemia, myocarditis, and various metabolic/pharmacologic derangements.

24 A 3-year-old boy presents for a well-child evaluation. His mother describes him as a picky eater and states he will only eat candy, sweets, and fatty foods and refuses fruits and vegetables. She is concerned that he has only gained 4.5 lb (2 kg) since his checkup 1 year ago. His 60-year-old paternal grandfather takes medication for both atrial fibrillation and hypercholesterolemia. During the examination, he is playful and cooperative. His pulse is 80 beats/min and respiratory rate is 25 breaths/min. His cardiac examination reveals a normal S1, splitting of S2 that is wider with inspiration and disappears with expiration, and no murmur. The remainder of his examination is normal.

Of the following, what additional screening is required for this child?

(A) Blood pressure measurement
(B) Fasting lipid panel
(C) 12-Lead electrocardiogram (ECG)
(D) Echocardiogram
(E) Chest radiography

The answer is A: Blood pressure measurement. Although systemic hypertension is uncommon in children, blood pressure should be routinely measured beginning at 3 years of age. It should be considered part of the standard screening that all children receive during their annual physical examinations. Like other vital signs, the normal ranges of systolic and diastolic pressure vary by age, but normal blood pressure is also indexed to gender and height. Systemic hypertension in young children is often due to a secondary cause that must be investigated. Adolescents, like adults, are more likely to have primary (essential) hypertension although other causes must be ruled out.

(B) A fasting lipid profile is unnecessary for this patient. A high-fat diet is not unusual for this age group, and while a family history of dyslipidemia is important, current guidelines only mandate lipid screening for a child whose parent or grandparent has evidence of coronary disease at an age younger than 55 years. **(C)** Routine ECG screening is not recommended during well-child visits in the United States. **(D)** Screening echocardiography is recommended for children and adolescents with certain conditions, for example, Down syndrome, Marfan syndrome, and Kawasaki disease. The child described in the vignette is healthy and developing normally without signs of failure to thrive or any medical condition that requires echocardiographic screening. **(E)** Similarly, chest radiography is recommended for children with certain conditions, but is not necessary for this patient.

---

25 A 5-year-old presents for a well-child evaluation. He has no significant past medical or surgical history, and neither he nor his parents have any complaints. He is afebrile with a heart rate of 100 beats/min and respiratory rate of 22 breaths/min. He remains at the 50th percentile for height and weight. Upon auscultation, he has a 2/6 nonradiating, crescendo-decrescendo, midsystolic murmur best heard at the left sternal border. The murmur does not change with a Valsalva maneuver, but increases in intensity when the patient is supine. Records indicate that he had no murmur at any previous evaluation. The remainder of his examination is unremarkable.

Of the following, which best explains this child's cardiac findings?

(A) Venous hum
(B) Still murmur
(C) Peripheral pulmonary artery stenosis
(D) Aortic stenosis
(E) Mitral regurgitation

The answer is B: Still murmur. The murmur described in the vignette is consistent with a Still murmur. Still vibratory murmur is an innocent murmur most commonly heard in toddlers and young school-aged children, typically between 3 and 7 years of age. Its intensity often changes with respiration and position, and there is often no radiation of the murmur. **(A)** A venous hum is also a common innocent murmur of childhood caused by turbulent flow in the jugular veins. However, venous hum is a low-pitched, continuous murmur and best heard at the lower portion of the neck or in the infraclavicular region. **(C)** The murmur of peripheral pulmonary artery stenosis is also known as a pulmonary flow murmur of infancy. It is an innocent systolic ejection murmur often heard at the left upper sternal border that radiates to the axillae and back. It is typically noted during the newborn period, more common in preterm infants, and should disappear by 6 months of age. **(D)** Children with mild forms of aortic stenosis may be asymptomatic and have normal development. Examination findings of mild aortic stenosis include an early systolic ejection click that is often absent in severe obstruction. Severe obstruction generates a more intense and longer murmur, heard at the right upper sternal border and radiating into the neck. **(E)** Children with significant mitral regurgitation often exhibit symptoms of congestive heart failure such as tachypnea, tachycardia, failure to thrive, and exercise intolerance far earlier than adults with the same degree of regurgitation. The murmur of mitral regurgitation varies with severity and is often described as a harsh holosystolic murmur at the apex that radiates to the axillae and back.

26 An 8-year-old boy undergoes surgical repair of an atrial septal defect that was deemed too large to close in the cardiac catheterization lab. There are no intraoperative complications and he is transferred to the pediatric cardiac intensive care unit (PCICU) on minimal ventilatory and inotropic support. He is appropriately extubated the following day. Over the next 12 hours, the trend in his vital signs shows progressively worsening tachycardia and decreasing systolic blood pressure. The pressure reading from an indwelling central venous line is significantly higher than what it was upon his admission to the PCICU. His heart sounds are muffled, there are no murmurs present, and his neck veins appear to be distended. His peripheral pulses are 1+. A chest radiograph shows an enlarged cardiac silhouette and small bilateral pleural effusions. His vital signs are pulse 118 beats/min, respirations 30 breaths/min, blood pressure 86/68 mmHg, and central venous pressure 12 mmHg.

Of the following, which is the best next step to improve this patient's hemodynamics?

(A) Bolus 20 mL/kg 0.9% (normal) saline intravenously (IV)
(B) Reintubation with mechanical ventilation
(C) Dopamine infusion at 10 μg/kg/min
(D) Furosemide infusion at 0.5 mg/kg/h
(E) Pericardiocentesis or surgical drainage

The answer is E: Pericardiocentesis or surgical drainage. The boy in the vignette has likely had rapid accumulation of pericardial fluid leading to the worrisome hemodynamic changes described. A small amount of pericardial fluid is usually tolerated in most patients. A large volume of fluid within the pericardial space, especially that which collects over a short time period, can result in restriction of cardiac filling and narrowing of the pulse pressure. Physical examination findings include distant or muffled heart sounds. The neck veins may become distended as the pressure within the pericardium begins to limit drainage of the superior vena cava into the right atrium. Similarly, the central venous pressure, or right atrial pressure, rises as the external pressure increases due to the accumulation of fluid. **(E)** The appropriate treatment for tamponade is either pericardiocentesis or surgical drainage of the pericardial fluid. **(A)** In this case, a bolus of isotonic saline will only further raise the central venous pressure. There is not likely to be any effect on systolic pressure or perfusion. **(B)** While reintubation may be indicated, the institution of positive pressure ventilation will increase the intrathoracic pressure and place additional external pressure on the heart. **(C)** Dopamine is a chronotrope and inotrope. While it is often an appropriate choice for hypotension due to decreased stroke volume or vasodilatory shock, this is not the case for the patient described. With an increased heart rate there will be less diastolic filling time, and therefore reduced blood volume ejected. This may actually worsen the patient's hemodynamics. **(D)** Furosemide is an appropriate treatment for fluid overload, including pleural effusions; however, it will not reduce the extravascular fluid collection that exists within the pericardium. It would also not be advisable to administer a continuous infusion of a diuretic to a patient with a dangerously low blood pressure.

27 Which of the following correctly describes the cardiovascular effects of milrinone?

	Systolic Function	Diastolic Function	Systemic Vascular Resistance	Pulmonary Vascular Resistance	Myocardial O_2 Demand
(A)	↑	↔	↑	↓	↑
(B)	↑	↑	↓	↓	↑
(C)	↑	↑	↓	↓	↓
(D)	↑	↔	↑	↑	↓
(E)	↑	↔	↓	↑	↓

The answer is B: Systolic function: improves; diastolic function: improves; systemic vascular resistance: decreases; pulmonary vascular resistance: decreases; myocardial O_2 demand: increases.

Milrinone inhibits phosphodiesterase 3 and exerts its effect by preventing the degradation of cyclic adenosine monophosphate. It is generally used as adjunctive therapy along with another inotrope such as dopamine or dobutamine. Milrinone is both a positive inotrope, improving systolic function, and a vasodilator, reducing systemic vascular resistance and left ventricular afterload. To a lesser effect, it also dilates the pulmonary vasculature, reducing pulmonary vascular resistance as well. Like all inotropes, it does increase myocardial oxygen demand; however, other inotropes (epinephrine, norepinephrine, and high-dose dopamine) have a far greater effect and may significantly increase myocardial oxygen demand as compared to milrinone. Finally, a unique property of milrinone is its ability to improve cardiac relaxation, diastolic function. This is known as a positive lusitropic effect.

28 A 15-year-old girl presents to the emergency department with chest pain and shortness of breath. History is obtained from her track coach who accompanied her in the ambulance. She had been feeling well until attending track practice after school. After several warm-up sprints, she began running with other members of the team. Approximately 10 minutes into the exercise, she began to complain of chest discomfort and difficulty breathing. Several minutes later, she stopped running and sat on the side of the track. The coach states that she was breathing rapidly and holding her chest. She was unable to speak more than one to two words at a time, but indicated that her chest felt heavy, and that she could not breathe. In the ambulance, she is placed on 100% FiO_2 by face mask at 8 L/min and attached to cardiorespiratory monitors. Her pulse is 88 beats/min, and the monitor shows a sinus tachycardia with no ST-segment or T-wave changes. Her respiratory rate is 40 breaths/min, and her breaths are shallow. There is no murmur appreciated. Her air exchange is poor and there is no wheezing. When asked if she still feels the chest discomfort, she nods yes.

Of the following, what is the next best course of action?

(A) Oral aspirin and sublingual nitroglycerin
(B) Obtain a plain radiograph of the chest and echocardiography
(C) Cardiac catheterization for coronary angiography
(D) Nebulized bronchodilators and intravenous steroids
(E) Observation

The answer is D: **Nebulized bronchodilators with intravenous steroids.** The patient in the vignette most likely has exercise-induced asthma or bronchospasm. As opposed to adults, the causes of chest pain in children and adolescents are far less likely to be cardiac in origin. Musculoskeletal, respiratory, and gastrointestinal etiologies account for the vast majority of chest pain or discomfort in otherwise healthy children. Of course, children with congenital heart disease, a history of cardiac surgery, or Kawasaki disease have a higher likelihood of cardiac etiologies of chest pain. For the girl described in the vignette, nebulized bronchodilators and intravenous steroids may begin to alleviate her symptoms. Because this patient is in moderate distress, treatment should be initiated as soon as possible. **(A)** Oral aspirin and sublingual nitroglycerin are appropriate initial treatments for patients with chest pain and a higher likelihood of a cardiac cause. **(B)** While chest radiography may help confirm a diagnosis, imaging studies should not take precedence before initiating treatment. Echocardiography is not likely to be useful in this patient. Even in patients with acute myocardial ischemia, echocardiography would be inappropriate. **(C)** Electrocardiography is a more appropriate initial test versus echocardiography or cardiac catheterization to diagnose an acute ischemic event. **(E)** Observation alone is inappropriate for this patient who is clearly in distress.

29 A 6-hour-old newborn is in the newborn nursery. She was born by spontaneous vaginal delivery at 39 weeks' gestation to a 25-year-old primigravida woman with unremarkable prenatal serologies. Pregnancy was complicated by a maternal urinary tract infection at 22 weeks' gestation. Labor and delivery were uncomplicated. The infant cries throughout the evaluation, but the examination is otherwise normal. Her temperature is 37.2°C, and her pulse is 185 to 195 beats/min while crying. When swaddled and held, she calms immediately, and her heart rate slows to 130 to 140 beats/min. Her parents are quite concerned that her heart rate is very high, even while she is calm.

Of the following, what is the most appropriate course of action?

(A) Obtain a detailed maternal history for autoimmune disorders
(B) Perform a 12-lead electrocardiogram and echocardiogram
(C) Immediately administer 0.1 mg/kg adenosine IV
(D) Order maternal and neonatal thyroid function tests
(E) Reassure her parents that her heart rate is normal

The answer is E: Reassure her parents that her heart rate is normal. Unlike adults, vital signs in pediatric patients are not fixed. There is a range of normal that changes as infants grow and develop into older children, adolescents, and finally into adults. The normal heart rate for a term infant at rest may range between 100 and 160 beats/min. Because they cannot easily increase stroke volume, infants and young children increase their heart rate in order to increase cardiac output in times of stress. Heart rates approaching 200 beats/min are not uncommon for an infant that is crying, febrile, anxious, or excited. The neonate described in the vignette has normal vital signs that vary appropriately with her mood and environment. The parents should be reassured that her heart rate and behavior are normal.

Autoimmune disorders such as systemic lupus erythematosus and Sjögren syndrome are known to affect the developing conduction system in the fetus, and affected newborns may present with bradycardia due to atrioventricular block. **(A)** The infant in the vignette has a normal heart rate, and obtaining a more detailed maternal history is unnecessary. **(B)** Cardiac evaluation by electrocardiography and echocardiography is also unnecessary in the setting of normal vital signs and a normal physical examination. **(C)** Adenosine is useful in the diagnosis and treatment of various forms of supraventricular tachycardia but would be inappropriate for the infant described in the vignette. **(D)** Tachycardia can certainly be a sign of abnormal thyroid function; however, hyperthyroidism in the newborn period is quite rare. There is no need to assess thyroid function for the infant in the vignette, in the setting of a normal heart rate.

---

30 A 20-month-old girl is discovered minutes after falling into a swimming pool. She is unresponsive and apneic. Emergency medical services are called while resuscitative efforts are started.

For a single rescuer, of the following, what is the correct ratio of chest compressions to rescue breaths (until an advanced airway is established)?

(A) 30 compressions:1 breath
(B) 30 compressions:2 breaths
(C) 20 compressions:1 breath
(D) 15 compressions:2 breaths
(E) 15 compressions:1 breath

The answer is B: 30 compressions:2 breaths. For infants and children, it is recommended that single rescuers provide chest compressions and rescue ventilation at a ratio of 30:2. In situations with two rescuers the ratio is changed to 15:2. Adults requiring cardiopulmonary resuscitation should receive 30 chest compressions for every two rescue breaths, regardless of the number of rescuers.

31 An adolescent girl is brought to the emergency department by ambulance after ingesting an unknown medication in an attempt to commit suicide. An electrocardiogram (ECG) shows a sinus rhythm with a wide QRS complex and prolonged QT-interval.

Of the following, which medication is she most likely to have ingested?

(A) Digoxin
(B) Atenolol
(C) Verapamil
(D) Paroxetine
(E) Amitriptyline

The answer is E: Amitriptyline. The electrocardiographic changes described in the vignette are most consistent with the effects of a tricyclic antidepressant (TCA) overdose. Amitriptyline is a TCA. Toxic effects on the cardiovascular system include slowing of conduction that manifests on the ECG with widened QRS complexes and prolongation of the QT-interval. **(A)** Digoxin is a cardiac glycoside and toxicity affects the ECG by prolonging the PR-interval, shortening the QT-interval, and causing ST-depression with a downsloping appearance. **(B)** β-Blockers like atenolol may cause bradycardia and widening of the QRS complex. **(C)** Verapamil is a calcium channel blocker and ECG findings associated with calcium channel blocker toxicity include PR prolongation and bradyarrhythmias. **(D)** Selective serotonin reuptake inhibitors, such as paroxetine, may be therapeutic over a wide dosage range, so their toxic effects are typically mild. The most common cardiac effect is tachycardia, but conduction defects are rare.

32 A 16-year-old girl has had frequent episodes of lightheadedness and dizziness for the past year. She lost consciousness on several occasions, but recovered spontaneously after 20 to 30 seconds in the supine position. Neurocardiogenic syncope was diagnosed, she increased her salt and water intake, and treatment with fludrocortisone was initiated. In spite of strict compliance, her symptoms have not resolved, and treatment with a β-blocker is now indicated.

Of the following, which medical history is a contraindication to β-blocker therapy?

(A) Anxiety disorder
(B) Migraine headaches
(C) Asthma
(D) Supraventricular tachycardia
(E) Congestive heart failure

The answer is C: Asthma. Treatment with a β-blocker is contraindicated in patients with a history of asthma or bronchospasm. Sympathetic activation of β_2-receptors is responsible for bronchodilation. When nonselective β-blockers are present, bronchodilation is prevented and bronchoconstriction may result.

(A, B, D, E) The remaining choices are conditions for which β-blockers have been found to be useful.

33 A 12-year-old girl complains of chest pain when she runs during her gym class at school. She describes the pain as if someone is pushing on her. She has no associated shortness of breath or wheezing, but has become dizzy and lightheaded if she ignores the pain and attempts to continue running. Her pulse and oxygen saturations are within normal limits, and she has a slightly narrow pulse pressure. She has a 4/6 harsh systolic ejection murmur and a click heard at the right upper sternal border. The murmur radiates to the neck. A thrill is palpable in the suprasternal notch. Her electrocardiogram shows a left axis deviation and is suggestive of left ventricular hypertrophy.

Of the following, which is her most likely diagnosis?

(A) Coarctation of the aorta
(B) Aortic valve insufficiency
(C) Interrupted aortic arch
(D) Aortic valve stenosis
(E) Aortic valve atresia

The answer is D: Aortic valve stenosis. The signs and symptoms of the girl in the vignette are most consistent with moderate-to-severe valvular aortic stenosis. Patients with mild aortic stenosis may have no symptoms, but the description of anginal chest pain with exertion is consistent with more severe aortic stenosis. Her dizziness and lightheadedness are presyncopal symptoms that may also occur during exertion in patients with severe aortic stenosis. A narrowed pulse pressure, reflected by a lower systolic blood pressure, is due to the increased pressure gradient across the aortic valve in systole. Upon auscultation, patients may have an ejection click with a harsh ejection murmur in the aortic area. The murmur often radiates to the suprasternal area and carotid arteries, and there may be a palpable thrill in these areas as well.

(A) The hallmark of coarctation of the aorta is differential pulses and blood pressures in the extremities. This suggests a pressure differential in vessels proximal to the coarctation versus those distal to the coarctation. In the absence of associated defects, there may be no murmur at all. **(B)** Aortic valve insufficiency would cause an early diastolic decrescendo murmur. **(C)** Interruption of the aortic arch is a rare congenital heart defect where the ascending aorta arises normally from the heart but is not continuous with the descending aorta, which arises from the ductus arteriosus. The head and neck vessels that normally arise from the top of the aortic arch arise from either the ascending portion or the descending portion, depending upon the location of the interruption. Like coarctation, infants present with poor peripheral pulses and signs of low cardiac output early in the neonatal period. Again, like coarctation of the aorta, unless there are associated defects, there may be no murmur. **(E)** Atresia of the aortic valve is associated with hypoplasia of the left ventricle and other forms of hypoplastic left heart syndrome. Neonates with aortic atresia depend on the ductus arteriosus to provide systemic blood flow and present in shock early in the neonatal period as the ductus begins to close.

34 A 7-month-old infant presents with a large abdominal mass that is identified as a hepatoblastoma. She acutely decompensates in the operating room during surgical resection of the mass. The monitoring electrocardiogram shows increased amplitude of the T-waves with widening of QRS complexes. Her serum potassium level is measured at 7.0 mEq/L.

Of the following, what is the best immediate treatment for this infant?

(A) 1 mL/kg 10% calcium gluconate IV over 3 minutes
(B) 0.1 units/kg regular insulin and 1 mL/kg 50% glucose, IV over 1 hour
(C) Sodium polystyrene sulfonate
(D) 1 mEq/kg sodium bicarbonate IV over 5 minutes
(E) 1 mg/kg furosemide intravenous push

The answer is A: 1 mL/kg 10% calcium gluconate IV over 3 minutes. The initial treatment for life-threatening hyperkalemia is intravenous calcium. Both calcium gluconate and calcium chloride solutions are effective at decreasing the myocardial irritability caused by hyperkalemia. Calcium does not act to decrease the potassium level; it functions only in a cardioprotective capacity. In addition to identifying and discontinuing sources of potassium intake, the next step in management is lowering potassium to a safe level. **(B, D)** Sodium bicarbonate and insulin counteract hyperkalemia by moving potassium from the extracellular into the intracellular space. It is necessary to give glucose along with insulin to facilitate the entry of potassium ions into the cell as well as to maintain normal glucose levels after giving insulin. The serum level is lower after treatment with sodium bicarbonate or with insulin and glucose, but the total body potassium level remains constant. **(C, E)** Furosemide and sodium polystyrene sulfonate function to remove potassium from the body through the urinary tract and gastrointestinal tract, respectively. While lowering serum potassium levels and removal of potassium are certainly important, it is vital to provide the cardioprotective effects of calcium as a first step in the management of life-threatening hyperkalemia.

35 A developmentally delayed 3-year-old boy is referred to interventional pediatric cardiology for transcatheter closure of a moderately sized atrial septal defect (ASD). He has required furosemide and digoxin therapy to manage symptoms of congestive heart failure for several months. His picture is included in Figure 6-15.

Of the following, which intrauterine exposure is the most likely cause of his constellation of signs and symptoms?

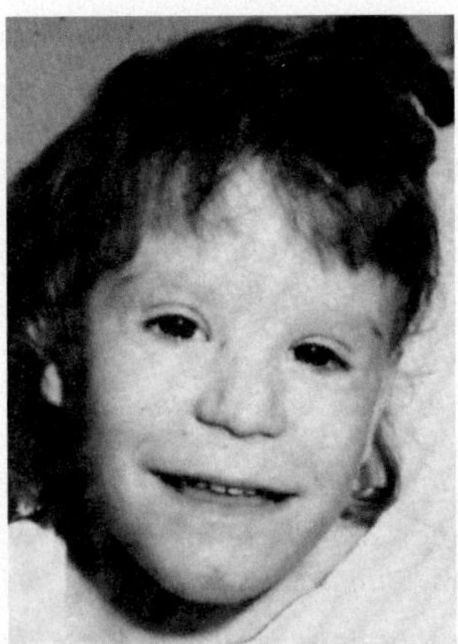

Figure 6-15

(A) Alcohol
(B) Retinoic acid
(C) Valproic acid
(D) Lithium
(E) Warfarin

The answer is A: Alcohol. The patient in the vignette has the characteristic facies of fetal alcohol syndrome. Fetal alcohol syndrome constitutes a specific constellation of malformations that includes growth deficiency, characteristic facies (short palpebral fissures, flat nasal bridge, thin lips, and smooth philtrum), cardiac defects (typically ASDs or ventricular septal defects), limb anomalies, and varying degrees of developmental delay and intellectual disability.

The remaining options are associated with characteristic teratogenic syndromes, but none explain the constellation of signs as described in the vignette. **(B)** Retinoic acid derivatives can disrupt formation and septation of the right and left ventricular outflow tracts. **(C)** Valproic acid use in pregnancy has been associated with an increase in neural tube defects, cleft lip and palate, cardiac abnormalities, and developmental delays. **(D)** Lithium use has been associated with Ebstein anomaly in the fetus. **(E)** Warfarin use during pregnancy may result in the fetal warfarin syndrome, which is characterized by facial dysmorphism (hypoplasia of the nasal bridge), congenital heart defects (ASDs and patent ductus arteriosus), stippled epiphyses, and growth retardation.

---

36 A 19-year-old young man was born with critical aortic stenosis and has undergone several procedures to correct the aortic valve, which left him with some degree of aortic insufficiency. He recently began to complain of dyspnea and chest pain with exertion and the decision was made to perform a pulmonary root autograft. He presents for a postoperative checkup. He has had several days of a low-grade fever, abdominal pain, and a rash.

On examination, his temperature is 38.8°C. He has a 2/6 systolic murmur, clear lung sounds, and a palpable spleen. He also has scattered petechiae on his trunk. His echocardiogram in clinic shows normal cardiac function with no obstruction across the left ventricular outflow tract or aortic valve. There is, however, a 2- to 3-mm mobile, echogenic mass attached to the anterior mitral valve leaflet. Blood cultures are drawn.

Of the following, which of these organisms is the most common etiology of his current findings?

(A) *Staphylococcus* and *Cardiobacterium*
(B) *Streptococcus* and *Haemophilus*
(C) *Streptococcus* and *Cardiobacterium*
(D) *Haemophilus* and *Cardiobacterium*
(E) *Streptococcus* and *Staphylococcus*

The answer is E: *Streptococcus* and *Staphylococcus*. The patient in the vignette has bacterial endocarditis. The diagnosis of infective endocarditis is guided by the Duke criteria. Please see the explanation for Question 13 for more information about the Duke criteria. The most common causative organism for infective endocarditis is α-hemolytic streptococci (*Streptococcus pneumoniae* and *Streptococcus viridians*). The second most common infective organism is *Staphylococcus aureus*. In the past, *Streptococcus*, *Staphylococcus*, and *Enterococcus* were responsible for the vast majority of cases of endocarditis. **(A, B, C, D)** While these organisms still predominate, cases attributed to organisms of the HACEK group (*Haemophilus*, *Actinobacillus*, *Cardiobacterium*, *Eikenella*, and *Kingella*) have increased in frequency in the past several years.

37 A 2-year-old girl is referred to pediatric cardiology for a murmur and cardiomegaly. Referral had been made for the same murmur after her 6-month and 12-month well-child evaluations, but the family did not follow up until now. At her 2-year evaluation, the murmur was noted again and she was tachypneic, but in no apparent distress. A chest radiograph demonstrated cardiomegaly. At the cardiologist's office, she is shy, but playful. She is slightly tachypneic and tachycardic. Her systolic blood pressure is normal, while her diastolic pressure is lower than expected. She has a 2/6 harsh, continuous murmur at the upper left sternal border and the left infraclavicular area. The cardiologist also notes an apical diastolic rumble and bounding peripheral pulses. Her ECG is indicative of biventricular hypertrophy.

Of the following, which is her echocardiogram most likely to reveal as the etiology of these findings?

(A) Patent ductus arteriosus (PDA)
(B) Peripheral pulmonary artery stenosis
(C) Pericarditis
(D) Pulmonary valve insufficiency
(E) Patent foramen ovale (PFO)

The answer is A: Patent ductus arteriosus (PDA). The tachycardia, tachypnea, and cardiomegaly described in the vignette are indicative of congestive heart failure (CHF). That, along with the wide pulse pressure, bounding pulses, and the description of the murmurs point toward a PDA as the etiology. With a large PDA, there is a large and continuous left-to-right shunt that reduces diastolic blood pressure due to run off from the aorta to the pulmonary artery during diastole. Because systolic blood pressure is not affected, the pulse pressure widens and bounding pulses may be present. The continuous shunt is also the cause of the continuous murmur, which may be described as harsh or machinery sounding. The apical diastolic murmur is due to relative mitral stenosis from increased flow from increased pulmonary venous return.

(B) The murmur of peripheral pulmonary artery stenosis may be best heard transmitting to the back and/or axillae, and signs of CHF are not typical. **(C)** The auscultatory findings of pericarditis are of a friction rub and cardiac murmurs are often absent. **(D)** The murmur of pulmonary valve insufficiency may indeed be best heard at the upper left sternal border, but it is a diastolic murmur. The pulmonary artery diastolic pressure will be lower with pulmonary valve insufficiency; the systemic diastolic pressure would not be affected. **(E)** An isolated PFO would not be responsible for the signs and symptoms of CHF as described.

---

38 A 4-month-old infant presents for a well-child evaluation. Her growth and development have been normal, and her parents have no concerns. Examination reveals a normal first heart sound (S1), and a widely split second heart sound (S2) that does not vary during respiration. An echocardiogram demonstrates a 4-mm defect in the atrial septum.

Of the following, which is the best explanation for the abnormality of the second heart sound (S2) in this patient?

(A) Left ventricular diastolic volume is increased throughout the respiratory cycle, prolonging the ventricular ejection time and delaying closure of the aortic valve

(B) Increased flow across the tricuspid valve throughout the respiratory cycle results in earlier closure of the mitral valve and delayed closure of the tricuspid valve

(C) Right ventricular diastolic volume is increased throughout the respiratory cycle, prolonging the ventricular ejection time and delaying closure of the pulmonary valve

(D) Increased flow across the aortic valve throughout the respiratory cycle reduces the intra-aortic pressure causing delayed closure of the aortic valve

(E) Increased flow constricts the pulmonary vasculature throughout the respiratory cycle, increasing pressure in the main pulmonary artery and delaying pulmonary valve closure

The answer is C: **Right ventricular diastolic volume is increased throughout the respiratory cycle, prolonging the ventricular ejection time and delaying closure of the pulmonary valve.** The second heart sound (S2) is caused by closure of the semilunar valves. The aortic valve component (A2) occurs before closure of the pulmonary valve (P2). There is a normal physiologic splitting of S2 that normally varies with the respiratory cycle. Inspiration decreases intrathoracic pressure and augments venous return to the right heart. This increases the blood volume entering the right ventricle (RV) during diastole and, in turn, extends the right ventricular ejection time and delaying closure of the pulmonary valve. For patients with an atrial septal defect (ASD), right ventricular diastolic volume is continuously increased due to the left-to-right shunt at the atrial level, thus continuously delaying pulmonary valve closure.

(A) Left ventricular diastolic volumes would not be increased in the setting of an uncomplicated ASD as the shunt is left-to-right, not right-to-left. **(D)** Similarly, there would not be increased flow across the aortic valve because volumes and blood flow is increased on the right, not through the left heart. **(B)** While increased flow across the tricuspid valve is certainly associated with ASDs and may, in some cases, result in a diastolic murmur heard at the lower left sternal border, closure of the atrioventricular valves constitutes the first heart sound (S1) and does not explain a change in S2. There is indeed increased blood flow into the main pulmonary artery and into the pulmonary vascular bed. **(E)** However, the pulmonary vasculature initially dilates in response. This also contributes to delayed closure of the pulmonary valve as it takes longer for the pressure within the main pulmonary artery to overcome the pressure within the RV during systole.

---

39 A 6-week-old infant presents with a 2-day history of fussiness and irritability. In the past 8 hours, he has been feeding poorly and has been more listless. Examination shows a quiet, lethargic infant who is minimally responsive. His breaths are rapid and shallow, and his heart rate is reported as too rapid to count. Peripheral pulses are weak, and the capillary refill time is approximately 5 seconds. The electrocardiogram (ECG) is shown in Figure 6-16.

Of the following, what is the most likely diagnosis?

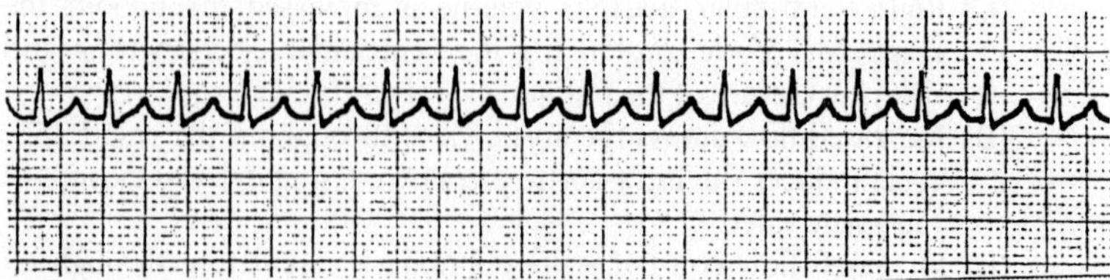

Figure 6.16

(A) Supraventricular tachycardia (SVT)
(B) Atrial flutter
(C) Ventricular tachycardia
(D) Ventricular fibrillation
(E) Sinus tachycardia

The answer is A: **Supraventricular tachycardia (SVT).** The infant in the vignette has signs of respiratory distress and poor perfusion from inadequate cardiac output due to his tachyarrhythmia. The ECG shows a rapid, regular, and narrow waveform, consistent with SVT. P-waves are usually absent. The most common form of SVT involves conduction along a circuit that includes both an accessory pathway connecting the atria and ventricles and the normal conduction pathway through the atrioventricular node. Conduction proceeds down one limb of this circuit and reenters the atria retrograde through the other limb. SVT may be tolerated in infants for longer periods of time compared to older children and adults.

(B) Atrial flutter appears as a rapid atrial rate with a slower ventricular rate (see *Figure 6-17*). The multiple atrial signals are classically called a saw tooth pattern, and the QRS complexes occur at a slower rate. QRS complexes are usually at a multiple of the atrial signals, representing a block in the conduction of atrial impulses to the ventricle (for example, 3:1 block, 4:1 block). **(C)** Ventricular tachycardia occurs when impulses originate in the ventricle. This causes wide QRS complexes, and the rate is usually somewhat slower than SVT, typically not greater than 200 beats/min in children (see *Figure 6-18*). **(D)** Similarly, ventricular fibrillation appears as wide, bizarre QRS complexes (see *Figure 6-19*). While the rate is rapid, the rhythm is irregular and disorganized. **(E)** Sinus tachycardia should certainly appear as a narrow QRS complex tachycardia. Neonates and infants can increase their heart rates substantially, even greater than 200 beats/min. The newborn described in the question stem is presenting with signs and symptoms of poor cardiac output. SVT is more likely compared with sinus tachycardia.

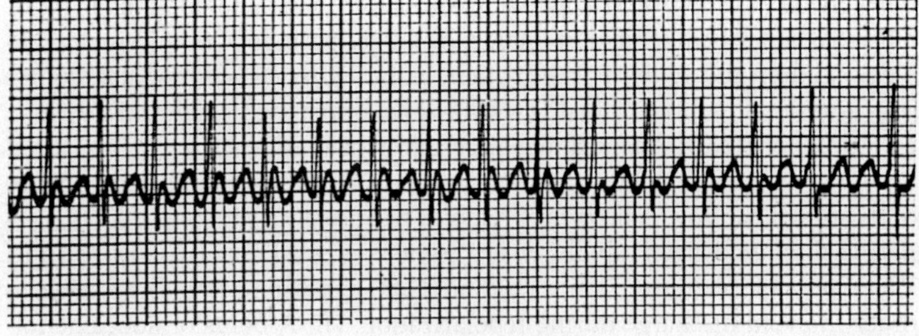

Figure 6.17

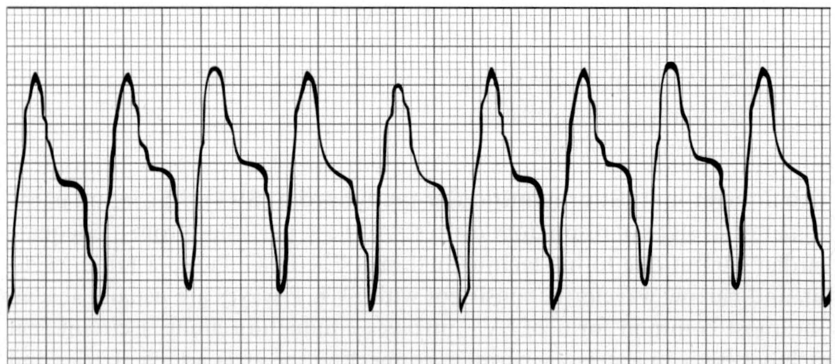

Figure 6.18

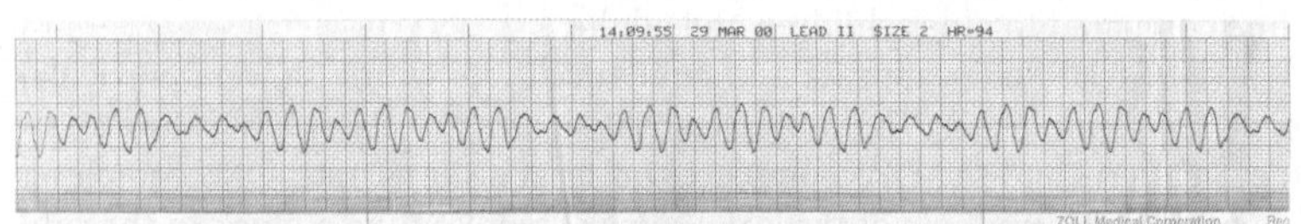

Figure 6.19

40 Of the following, what is the most appropriate treatment for the arrhythmia of the infant in the previous vignette (39)?

(A) Adenosine 0.1 mg/kg intravenous push
(B) Adenosine 0.1 mg/kg intravenous bolus over 20 minutes
(C) Unsynchronized cardioversion at 12 J/kg
(D) Synchronized cardioversion at 0.5 J/kg
(E) Lidocaine 1 mg/kg intravenous over 1 to 2 minutes

The answer is D: Synchronized cardioversion at 0.5 J/kg. The patient in the vignette has supraventricular tachycardia (SVT) with hemodynamic instability. SVT may be tolerated in infants for longer periods of time compared to older children and adults. For the patient in the vignette, the immediate course of action should be to terminate the tachyarrhythmia with synchronized direct cardioversion. **(A,B)** Adenosine may certainly be used when a patient in SVT is hemodynamically stable; however, the infant in the vignette shows evidence of shock and cardioversion is the preferred treatment. For stable patients, adenosine should be given rapidly, by intravenous push, due to its short half-life. When possible, cardioversion should be **(C,D)** synchronized to the R-wave in order to avoid discharge during repolarization. **(E)** A bolus of lidocaine followed by a continuous infusion of lidocaine may be attempted for hemodynamically stable patients with ventricular arrhythmias.

41 A 16-year-old soccer player presents with a 1-month history of intermittent chest pain. He describes the pain as a dull ache in the center of his chest that sometimes radiates to his shoulder. The pain only occurs when he is inactive. It is worse when he takes a deep breath or lies down, and sitting or leaning forward tends to relieve it. He is afebrile with a heart rate of 88 beats/min, respiratory rate 16 breaths/min and blood pressure 105/72 mmHg. His chest is nontender with palpation and his breath sounds are clear. There is no murmur, but he has a faint, low-pitched rubbing sound and his neck veins are not distended. A plain radiograph of the chest is unremarkable, and an electrocardiogram is included in Figure 6-20. His mother is very concerned because she has heard of several athletes who have died suddenly due to unexpected, sudden cardiac events. She asks that cardiac imaging be done.

Of the following, what is the most appropriate response?

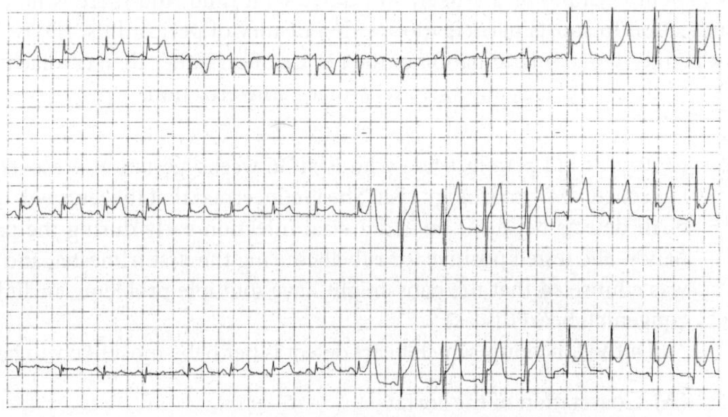

Figure 6.20

(A) His condition is noncardiac, and imaging is not likely to demonstrate any heart defect or structural abnormality

(B) His condition is not life-threatening and can be treated successfully with over-the-counter anti-inflammatory medications

(C) Cardiac imaging is not indicated, but an exercise stress test is necessary to determine whether sports participation is safe

(D) He should be admitted for a full evaluation, including imaging, due to the possibility of acute cardiac ischemia

(E) He should undergo cardiac catheterization for coronary angiography as well as possible revascularization with stent placement.

The answer is B: His condition is not life-threatening and can be treated successfully with over-the-counter anti-inflammatory medications. (A) The young man described in the vignette has physical examination and electrocardiographic findings consistent with pericarditis. Bacterial or purulent pericarditis is far less common and presents with high fevers, chest pain, dyspnea, and signs of pericardial tamponade. The most common causes of pericarditis in the United States are viral illnesses. Acute rheumatic fever and tuberculosis are more common in other parts of the world. Pericarditis may also be part of the presentation of collagen vascular diseases or it may result after cardiac surgery. Viral pericarditis is usually self-limited and can be treated supportively with rest and over-the-counter anti-inflammatory medications. Echocardiography may reveal a pericardial effusion, which would resolve as his condition improves. Large pericardial effusions may present with signs of tamponade and may be seen in patients with more severe disease. Those patients would, however, typically have signs and symptoms of tamponade.

(C) An exercise stress test will not aid in diagnosis or management of pericarditis. Stress testing is indicated for some patients with exercise-induced symptoms or to determine electrocardiographic changes at high heart rates. This patient's symptoms are likely to resolve with time, and there is no contraindication to sports participation with a history of pericarditis. **(D, E)** The chest pain is due to inflammation of the pericardium rather than cardiac ischemia and therefore does not warrant cardiac catheterization.

42 A 20-year-old primigravida who is at 36 weeks' gestation presents for her scheduled gynecology visit. She is concerned that the fetus will have birth defects because she had a viral infection early during the pregnancy. She tested positive for rubella during the first trimester, and she was counseled that the baby might have multiple problems, including congenital heart disease.

Of the following, which heart defect is her baby most likely to have?

(A) Coarctation of the aorta
(B) Supravalvar aortic stenosis
(C) Dextrocardia
(D) Patent ductus arteriosus (PDA)
(E) There is no increased risk unless the infection occurred in the third trimester

The answer is D: Patent ductus arteriosus (PDA). The triad of congenital cataracts, deafness, and congenital heart defects characterizes congenital rubella syndrome. **(E)** Infection during the first trimester is the most damaging for the fetus. Additional manifestations include microcephaly, microphthalmia, thrombocytopenic purpura (skin manifestations of extramedullary hematopoiesis), and hepatitis. Several forms of congenital heart disease have been reported. The most common are PDA and stenosis of the pulmonary arteries. **(A)** An increased incidence of coarctation of the aorta along with bicuspid aortic valve is associated with Turner syndrome. **(B)** Williams syndrome is associated with supravalvar aortic stenosis. **(C)** Kartagener syndrome is associated with dextrocardia and situs inversus.

43 A 34-year-old woman is admitted to obstetrics with the onset of active labor. Her first child was delivered via scheduled cesarean section due to placenta previa. She wants a vaginal delivery, and she consents to regular examinations by the obstetrician and transabdominal fetal monitoring during labor. During the second stage of labor, she experiences a sudden, sharp abdominal pain. Minutes later, frank blood is expelled from the birth canal and the fetal heart rate begins to fall rapidly. Emergent cesarean delivery is performed. A male infant is delivered and he is pale, limp, and nonresponsive. He is immediately intubated, and positive pressure ventilation is initiated. The heart rate is between 40 and 50 beats/min. Chest compressions are started, as intravenous access is being attempted. The neonatologist orders a dose of epinephrine, and that the additional doses are drawn up and ready.

Of the following, which is true regarding administration of epinephrine during resuscitation?

(A) Epinephrine may only be given intravenously (IV) or via endotracheal tube in infants

(B) By any route, the 1:1,000 concentration of epinephrine should be used for neonates

(C) Endotracheal epinephrine is associated with higher blood levels of the medication

(D) If epinephrine is given endotracheally, ventilation should be held for 10 to 15 seconds so that the drug can be absorbed

(E) Epinephrine may be given via an endotracheal tube if other access is unavailable

The answer is E: **Epinephrine may be given via an endotracheal tube if other access is unavailable.** (**A**) Epinephrine may be given IV, via endotracheal tube, or intraosseously (IO) during the resuscitation of any patient. Intraosseous access is used in emergencies in pediatric resuscitation when IV access is difficult or impossible to establish. Medications, fluids, and blood products may be given IO, and samples may be drawn for laboratory analysis. Additionally, there is no age restriction; however, like all medications, doses of epinephrine are weight based in children and neonates. (**B**) Either the 1:1,000 or 1:10,000 concentration of epinephrine may be used, although the Neonatal Resuscitation Program recommends that only the 1:10,000 concentration be used for neonates. This helps to eliminate the possibility of dilution errors. (**C**) Epinephrine administered via the endotracheal route has been associated with lower blood concentrations of the drug, not higher. (**D**) Endotracheal administration of epinephrine should be followed by several positive-pressure breaths to ensure adequate distribution within the lungs and improved absorption.

44 A 4-month-old full-term girl is brought to the pediatrician by her parents with a 2-day history of poor feeding and fevers to 38.6°C. She has

had an uncomplicated pregnancy and routine pediatric care. Newborn metabolic screening was normal. She is not febrile in the office and minimally reactive during the examination. Her heart rate is 180 beats/min and respiratory rate is 68 breaths/min. She has distant heart sounds, but no murmur. Her breath sounds are clear with shallow respirations and subcostal and intercostal retractions. Peripheral pulses are diminished, and the capillary refill time is 5 seconds. The infant is stabilized after intubation and mechanical ventilation. Echocardiography demonstrates a structurally normal heart with normal coronary arteries and severely depressed function of both ventricles.

Of the following, what is the most common causative agent for this infant's condition?

(A) *Listeria monocytogenes*
(B) *Streptococcus viridans*
(C) Rubella
(D) Epstein-Barr virus
(E) Coxsackievirus B

The answer is E: Coxsackievirus B. The infant described in the vignette is quite ill with signs of impending respiratory failure and shock. While fever and dehydration from poor feeding may cause tachycardia, the infant is afebrile in the office. Her tachycardia is out of proportion to her temperature. This along with prolonged capillary refill time, diminished pulses, and lethargy are signs of poor or insufficient cardiac output. Poor ventricular function in the absence of congenital heart disease or anomalous coronary arteries may be evidence of myocarditis. Viral myocarditis is more common than other infectious causes. **(C, D)** Adenovirus and coxsackievirus B are more common than rubella or Epstein-Barr virus. **(A)** The early form of neonatal listeriosis presents in the first few days of life with septicemia. The late-onset form occurs after the first week of life, typically as a form of meningitis. Beyond the neonatal period, listeriosis is rare in the absence of immunosuppression or malignancy. Again, central nervous system involvement is the typical presentation. **(B)** Bacterial myocarditis is less common than viral myocarditis, and α-hemolytic *Streptococcus* such as *S. viridans* is the most common cause of endocarditis, not myocarditis.

45 A term neonate with a congenital ductal-dependent heart defect diagnosed in utero by fetal echocardiography is being delivered. A prostaglandin E1 (PGE_1) infusion has already been prepared and is at the bedside. The infant is delivered and passed to the neonatology team. He is cyanotic and tachypneic. There is a single S2 appreciated upon auscultation. Umbilical lines are quickly placed and the PGE_1 infusion is started. Chest and abdominal radiographs are obtained. The heart size is normal to slightly increased, and the pulmonary vascular markings are decreased.

Of the following what will the echocardiography most likely show?

(A) Intact atrial septum, atresia of the tricuspid valve, and an enlarged left ventricle (LV)
(B) Intact atrial septum, atresia of the tricuspid valve, and an enlarged right ventricle (RV)
(C) Intact atrial septum, atresia of the tricuspid valve, and biventricular enlargement
(D) Atrial septal defect (ASD), atresia of the tricuspid valve, and an enlarged RV
(E) ASD, atresia of the tricuspid valve, and an enlarged LV

The answer is E: ASD, atresia of the tricuspid valve, and an enlarged LV. The description of the infant in the vignette is that of tricuspid atresia. In tricuspid atresia, an ASD is necessary for survival. **(A)** Because the normal outlet from the right atrium is absent, an ASD must be present in order to decompress the right atrium. Deoxygenated blood flows into the left atrium where it mixes with the pulmonary venous return before traversing the mitral valve into the LV. The LV enlarges due to this increase in flow. A ventricular septal defect is also often present, and a small amount of blood may cross the ventricular septum back into the right heart. **(B, C, D)** In the most common form of tricuspid atresia, the RV, pulmonary valve, and pulmonary artery are hypoplastic due to reduced flow. Therefore, there would not be an enlarged RV. The majority of the left ventricular output is ejected through the aortic valve. Most blood continues forward into the systemic circulation, but some blood must cross the ductus arteriosus, as it is the primary source of pulmonary blood flow.

46 A 4-day-old girl presents to the emergency department with a 1-day history of poor feeding and fussiness. She is afebrile, tachycardic, tachypneic, and cyanotic. Examination reveals a normal S1 and a single loud S2 with no murmur. A plain radiograph of the chest shows well-expanded lungs, increased pulmonary vascular markings, and a mildly enlarged cardiac silhouette with a narrow mediastinum. The infant is intubated and supplemental oxygen is given, but fails to improve oxygen saturations.

Of the following, which is the next best step in the management of this patient?

(A) Echocardiography
(B) Direct cardioversion
(C) Intravenous adenosine
(D) Cardiac catheterization
(E) Prostaglandin E_1 (PGE_1)

The answer is E: Prostaglandin E_1 (PGE_1). The age at presentation, cyanosis, and inability of supplemental oxygen to improve oxygenation are indicative of a ductal-dependent congenital heart defect. The presence of a single S2 and the description of the chest radiograph are suggestive of D-transposition of the great arteries. The most important step is to reopen the ductus arteriosus with intravenous PGE_1. **(A)** While echocardiography is integral in the ongoing management and surgical planning, treatment with PGE_1 will be lifesaving, and should not be delayed. **(D)** Infants with a restrictive foramen ovale have severely limited mixing of saturated and desaturated blood; thus, emergent cardiac catheterization at birth is necessary to perform a balloon atrial septostomy. The infant in the vignette is tachycardic due to hypoxia and impaired systemic cardiac output. **(B, C)** Neither adenosine nor cardioversion will reestablish mixing between the desaturated blood recirculating through the systemic circulation and the saturated blood recirculating through the pulmonary vasculature.

47 A patient is diagnosed with endocarditis. Echocardiography shows a small echogenic mass attached to the mitral valve. Blood cultures are positive for *Staphylococcus aureus*.

Of the following, what is the most appropriate treatment regimen?

(A) Penicillin G 200,000 units/kg/d orally for 4 weeks
(B) Amoxicillin 50 mg/kg/d orally for 6 weeks
(C) Nafcillin 200 mg/kg/d IV for 6 weeks
(D) Gentamicin 7.5 mg/kg/d IV for 14 days
(E) Ceftriaxone 50 mg/kg/d IV once

The answer is C: Nafcillin 200 mg/kg/d IV for 6 weeks. The most common causative organism for infective endocarditis is α-hemolytic *Streptococcus*, followed by *S. aureus*. The correct treatment for staphylococcal endocarditis includes a penicillinase-resistant penicillin like oxacillin or nafcillin. **(A)** Many strains of *S. aureus* produce β-lactamases, rendering them penicillin resistant. **(B)** Intravenous therapy is required to achieve high serum levels. **(D, E)** Prolonged therapy is necessary because organisms have a relatively low rate of cell division and vegetations are often encased within a fibrin matrix. **(D, E)** Ceftriaxone or gentamicin may be added to some antibiotic regimens to treat streptococcal endocarditis, but again, the duration of treatment is far too brief.

48 A 17-year-old girl needs cardiology clearance prior to surgical repair of pectus excavatum. Her medical history is benign. Her vital signs are within normal limits. She is nondysmorphic with a slender build and an obvious pectus deformity of the chest wall. She has a regular rate and rhythm with a midsystolic click that is followed by a soft, 1/6 late systolic murmur best heard at the apex. The click and the murmur are more prominent when she leans forward. When she strains and expires against a closed epiglottis, the click is heard earlier in systole, and the murmur is longer. Her chest radiograph is unremarkable except for a slight degree of scoliosis. Her electrocardiogram is within normal limits. Due to her physical examination findings, an echocardiogram is ordered before she is cleared for surgery.

Of the following, which is the most likely echocardiogram finding in this patient?

(A) Bicuspid aortic valve
(B) Hypertrophic cardiomyopathy (HCM)
(C) Mitral valve stenosis
(D) Supravalvar aortic stenosis
(E) Prolapse of the mitral valve

The answer is E: Prolapse of the mitral valve. Mitral valve prolapse (MVP) occurs when the leaflets of the mitral valve protrude into the annulus of the valve, backward into the left atrium, when the valve closes during ventricular systole. MVP is associated with Marfan syndrome, Ehlers-Danlos syndrome, and other connective tissue disorders. In most cases, though, it is a primary disease of the mitral valve with autosomal dominant inheritance pattern. Patients may complain of chest pain at rest or palpitations, but MVP is often asymptomatic. It is more common in older adolescents and adults, and it appears more frequently in women than in men. Pectus excavatum and skeletal anomalies have also been associated with MVP. The classic auscultatory finding is a click in midsystole that may be followed by the murmur of mitral regurgitation. The timing of the click is affected by the blood volume within the left ventricle (LV). Actions that increase LV volume such as bradycardia, squatting, and handgrip tend to push the click later in systole, or toward S2, and shorten the murmur of mitral regurgitation, if present. Actions that decrease LV volume such as tachycardia, straining, and/or Valsalva maneuvers bring the click closer to S1, or earlier in systole, and prolong the murmur. Asymptomatic patients with MVP require no treatment. However, as MVP may be associated with mitral regurgitation, which can worsen with time, patients with severe regurgitation may require mitral valvuloplasty or valve replacement.

(A) Bicuspid aortic valve is associated with a systolic click and often an early systolic murmur at the upper sternal border. **(B)** HCM is associated with a murmur that increases with Valsalva maneuvers; however, it is not increased in patients with pectus excavatum. **(C)** Mitral valve stenosis is most often associated with a history of rheumatic heart disease and physical examination does not reveal a mid-systolic click. In addition, the murmur would be more significant. **(D)** Supravalvar aortic stenosis is associated with Williams syndrome and the murmur would be more significant without a click.

49 A 25-year-old woman presents to the emergency department with a 2-month history of worsening fatigue and shortness of breath with exertion. She has no primary care physician, stating that she has been healthy all her life. She reports no chronic medical problems, takes no medications, and has never been hospitalized nor had surgery. She originally attributed her symptoms to "being out of shape," but she now finds it difficult to climb stairs and even walk long distances. Her vital signs are unremarkable. Breath sounds are clear bilaterally. Her cardiac examination is significant for a normal S1 with a prominent S2 and a short 1/6 diastolic murmur at the left upper sternal border. A plain radiograph of her chest shows a prominent main pulmonary artery and increased pulmonary vascularity at the hilum. An echocardiogram demonstrates hypertrophy of the right ventricle (RV), tricuspid and pulmonary insufficiency, and blood shunting from the RV to the left ventricle across a ventricular septal defect (VSD).

Of the following, what is the best explanation of these findings for this patient?

(A) This is the natural history of the acyanotic form of tetralogy of Fallot (TOF)
(B) Critical pulmonary valve stenosis is responsible for the VSD shunt
(C) She has primary pulmonary hypertension from a congenital heart defect
(D) Her symptoms are the result of hypertrophic cardiomyopathy (HCM)
(E) She has developed pulmonary vascular obstructive disease

The answer is E: She has developed pulmonary vascular obstructive disease. Eisenmenger syndrome is the reversal of a left-to-right shunt into a right-to-left shunt due to the development of pulmonary vascular obstructive disease that develops over time due to excess pulmonary blood flow. It is seen in patients with a communication between the left and right heart, for example, in patients with a VSD, atrial septal defect, patent ductus arteriosus, atrioventricular septal defect, and/or aortopulmonary window, that goes unrepaired. In normal infants, pulmonary vascular resistance falls and the RV becomes more compliant in the initial weeks after birth. This accounts for the left-to-right flow of blood across a VSD. Excess blood enters the pulmonary circulation, and the pulmonary vasculature dilates in order to accommodate the excess volume. Over years, hypertrophy occurs within the medial and intimal layers of the muscular pulmonary arteries and arterioles, raising the pulmonary vascular resistance. Ultimately, right-sided pressures become greater than those in the left heart, and flow across the VSD reverses.

(A) The patient in the vignette does not have TOF. The murmur is not one of pulmonary stenosis (PS), but of pulmonary insufficiency that has developed due to increased pressure within the pulmonary arteries. Similarly, the RV has hypertrophied in response to increasing pulmonary pressures. The acyanotic form of TOF occurs when the RV outflow tract obstruction is mild and does not severely limit pulmonary blood flow. Affected infants may be asymptomatic and maintain adequate oxygen saturations. Over time, they may present with signs of heart failure due to the left-to-right VSD shunt. Infants with the acyanotic form of TOF eventually become cyanotic as hypertrophy of the RV infundibulum increases as they grow. This typically occurs in the first year of life. **(B)** A VSD in the setting of critical pulmonary valve stenosis may shunt right-to-left; however, critical PS requires attention in the newborn period. **(C)** The patient in the vignette does not have primary pulmonary hypertension. Her pulmonary disease progressed over years as a result of excess pulmonary blood flow due to the VSD. If her VSD had been treated early in life, this patient would not have developed Eisenmenger syndrome. **(D)** As described earlier, the RV hypertrophy developed in response to increasing pulmonary pressures and does not represent HCM.

50 On her initial physical examination, a term female neonate is noted to have a 3/6, harsh, low-pitched, crescendo-decrescendo, systolic murmur at the right upper sternal border. Echocardiography demonstrates narrowing of the aorta above the aortic valve but only minimal obstruction to blood flow. The infant is discharged home and followed regularly over the next several years. At 6 years of age, she has a friendly, outgoing personality and is quite talkative. She also has signs of developmental delay and mild mental retardation. On examination, she has a round face with full cheeks and lips, and a short, upturned nose. Other than a mildly elevated blood pressure, her vital signs are normal. Her cardiac examination and echocardiogram are unchanged.

Of the following, which condition is this patient most likely to have?

(A) Turner syndrome
(B) Marfan syndrome
(C) DiGeorge syndrome
(D) Williams syndrome
(E) Noonan syndrome

The answer is D: Williams syndrome. The girl described in the vignette has several characteristic features of Williams syndrome. Williams syndrome is caused by a microdeletion of 7q11.23. Affected individuals are often described as having an overtly friendly and outgoing personality but may also have difficulties with hyperactivity and inattentiveness. There is typically some degree of mental retardation and developmental delay as well. Facial features common to Williams syndrome include a short round face, flat nasal bridge, long philtrum, and an upturned nose with a wide mouth and full lips (see *Figure 6-21*). Patients may also have widely spaced teeth and micrognathia. Patients with Williams syndrome have associated supravalvar aortic stenosis as described by the echocardiogram in the vignette.

(A) Turner syndrome is associated with coarctation of the aorta and bicuspid aortic valve. **(B)** Marfan syndrome is associated with aortic and mitral valve regurgitation, and patients with Marfan syndrome are predisposed to aneurysms of the aorta due to dilation of the aortic root and/or ascending aorta. **(C)** DiGeorge syndrome is associated with truncus arteriosus and interrupted aortic arch. **(E)** Noonan syndrome is associated with valvar pulmonary stenosis.

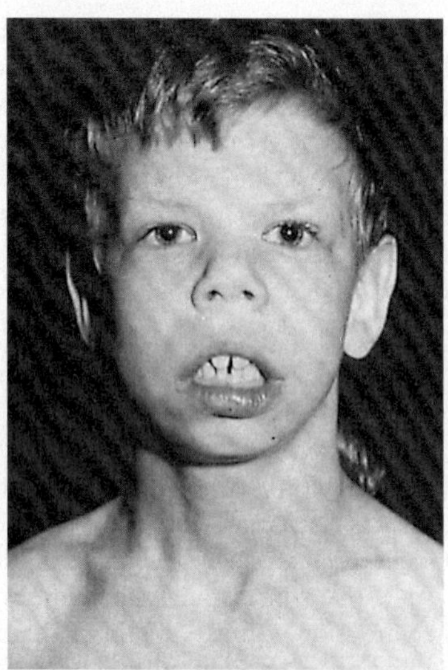
A

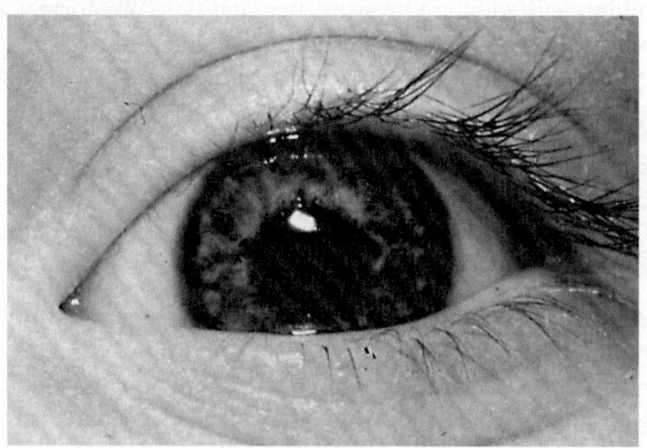
B

Figure 6-21

51 Of the following, which should prompt screening for dyslipidemia in children?

(A) A 50-year-old grandparent with documented coronary artery disease
(B) A 40-year-old parent with a total cholesterol level of 200 mg/dL
(C) A 30-year-old parent with obesity and inactivity
(D) A 20-year-old sibling with a triglyceride level of 70 mg/dL
(E) A 10-year-old sibling with complex congenital heart disease

The answer is A: A 50-year-old grandparent with documented coronary artery disease. Guidelines from the National Cholesterol Education

Program for Children and Adolescents recommend obtaining a fasting lipid profile for children with a family history of coronary artery disease prior to the age of 55 in a grandparent or parent. **(B)** Children with a parent who has a cholesterol level greater than 240 mg/dL should have their total cholesterol level measured as well. No intervention is recommended if the level is less than 170 mg/dL; however, the child should be reevaluated within 5 years. Children with borderline elevations in their cholesterol level (171 to 199 mg/dL) should have the level repeated and the values averaged. Those with persistent borderline levels should have a fasting lipid profile, and the level of low-density lipoprotein (LDL) helps guide further management. Along with hypertension, diabetes, and smoking, obesity and inactivity are significant risk factors for coronary heart disease. **(C)** Children with any of these risk factors should receive counseling, but screening for dyslipidemia is not mandatory and is performed according to the judgment of the provider. **(D)** A total triglyceride level of 70 mg/dL in a first-degree adult relative would not require screening. This is a normal triglyceride level in adults, but would be considered elevated in a school-aged child. **(E)** A family history of congenital heart disease does not increase the risk of familial dyslipidemia and does not mandate screening.

52 A 17-year-old competitive soccer player complains of anterior chest pain and difficulty breathing with exercise. He had no complaints last season, but he is now becoming fatigued after only 30 to 45 minutes of practice. He has also experienced lightheadedness and dizziness associated with this pain. On examination, he has a medium-pitched systolic ejection murmur along the left sternal border. The murmur becomes more prominent when he bears down. An electrocardiogram shows increased voltage and nonspecific T-wave changes in the left precordial leads.

Of the following, which is the most likely echocardiographic finding in this patient?

(A) Patent foramen ovale (PFO) with left-to-right shunting
(B) Interventricular septal thickness above normal
(C) Origin of the left coronary artery from the pulmonary artery
(D) Thickened, poorly mobile aortic valve leaflets
(E) Origin of the left common carotid from the brachiocephalic trunk

The answer is B: Interventricular septal thickness above normal. A murmur that increases with a Valsalva maneuver, or bearing down, is characteristic of hypertrophic cardiomyopathy (HCM). HCM is the leading cause of sudden cardiac death in young athletes and is most often related to a mutation in a gene that codes for proteins of the sarcomere. It results in abnormal thickening of cardiac muscle that may obstruct flow out of the left ventricle and produce symptoms that include shortness of breath, anginal chest pain during exertion, and presyncope or syncope.

(A) A PFO may be seen in a small percentage of patients beyond childhood. When a shunt is present, left-to-right flow is normal and patients typically have no symptoms. A right-to-left shunt indicates increased right-sided pressures and would warrant further investigation. **(C)** Anomalous left coronary artery from the pulmonary artery is a congenital heart disease typically diagnosed in the first few months of life as blood from the pulmonary artery provides an insufficient oxygen supply to the myocardium for infants in times of stress. **(D)** A thickened and poorly mobile (or immobile) aortic valve leaflet is a description of valvar aortic stenosis. The murmur of aortic stenosis is typically heard at the right second intercostal space and may radiate into the neck. As opposed to the murmur of HCM, which becomes more prominent, it becomes less prominent with Valsalva. **(E)** The aortic arch is normally left-sided with the following branching sequence: brachiocephalic arterial trunk, which divides into the right subclavian artery and right common carotid; then the left common carotid; and last the left subclavian. A small minority of individuals have a normal variation in branching of the head and neck vessels from the aortic arch that is sometimes called a bovine arch, in which the left common carotid arises from the brachiocephalic arterial trunk as well as the right subclavian and right common carotid. It is a variant of normal anatomy that causes no symptoms.

53 A 12-year-old girl presents for a well-child examination. Her mother is concerned about behavioral changes that have occurred in the past 3 to 4 months. She states that her daughter has become irritable and emotional and that she has difficulty concentrating. Her school performance has suffered, and she barely sleeps. On examination her pulse is 98 beats/min and her blood pressure is 140/70 mmHg. Her eyes are prominent, and her upper eyelids appear retracted. There is a mild fullness in the anterior neck. Her cardiac examination reveals a 1/6 systolic murmur at the apex and she has a faint tremor when her arms are outstretched. An electrocardiogram demonstrates a sinus rhythm at 100 beats/min with no evidence of ischemia or hypertrophy.

Of the following, which is the most appropriate treatment for the patient's sinus tachycardia?

(A) Digoxin
(B) Propranolol
(C) Levothyroxine
(D) Adenosine
(E) Methimazole

The answer is E: Methimazole. The patient in the vignette has a history and physical examination concerning for hyperthyroidism. Sinus tachycardia is managed by searching for and treating its underlying cause. Both methimazole and propylthiouracil are antithyroid agents used in pediatric patients.

(A) When used as an antiarrhythmic, digoxin is given for atrial flutter, atrial fibrillation, and supraventricular tachycardia (SVT) in the absence of Wolff-Parkinson-White syndrome. Digoxin may certainly slow the heart rate; however, the best treatment for this patient is to control her thyroid dysfunction. **(B)** Propranolol is important in the treatment of congenital hyperthyroidism and is sometimes used as a supplemental therapy for older patients with severe thyroid toxicity. It may help decrease the catecholaminergic symptoms of tachycardia, lid lag, and tremor in this patient, but that would not adequately treat her hyperthyroidism, the underlying cause of her sinus tachycardia. **(C)** Levothyroxine is an appropriate treatment for hypothyroidism rather than hyperthyroidism. **(D)** Adenosine transiently blocks conduction through the atrioventricular (AV) node and is useful in the diagnosis and treatment of SVT. A patient with sinus tachycardia will also experience a transient AV block when given adenosine, but the rhythm will continue after the effect wears off.

54 An 8-year-old girl presents with a 2-day history of fever, abdominal pain, and sore throat. Her oropharynx is erythematous, and a rapid antigen test confirms the diagnosis of group A β-hemolytic *Streptococcus* (GAβHS) pharyngitis. A 10-day course of penicillin V is prescribed.

Of the following, what is the primary benefit of antibiotic treatment for streptococcal pharyngitis?

(A) Prevention of mitral and aortic valve disease
(B) Prevention of tricuspid and pulmonary valve disease
(C) Prevention of isolated pericarditis
(D) Prevention of coronary artery aneurysms
(E) Prevention of third-degree (complete) heart block

The answer is A: Prevention of mitral and aortic valve disease. The best indication for antibiotic treatment of pharyngitis caused by GAβHS is the prevention of rheumatic heart disease and acute rheumatic fever (ARF). Cardiac involvement is responsible for the majority of morbidity and mortality of ARF. There is a wide spectrum of cardiac involvement that can range from asymptomatic inflammatory changes to a fatal pancarditis. Valvulitis is found in almost all cases of rheumatic carditis. The left-sided valves are most commonly involved with either isolated mitral disease or disease of both the mitral and aortic valves. **(B)** Involvement of the right-sided valves is less common. **(C)** Pericarditis as an isolated finding is also rare, typically occurring in the setting of left-sided valve disease. **(D)** While a generalized vasculitis involving the coronaries has been reported, it rarely results in long-term vessel damage. Aneurysms of the coronary arteries and occasionally other small- and medium-sized arteries are more commonly associated with Kawasaki disease, not ARF. First-degree heart block (a prolonged PR-interval) is a minor Jones criterion for diagnosis and not a sequela of ARF. **(E)** Second- and third-degree heart blocks are less commonly noted in patients with rheumatic heart disease.

CHAPTER

7

Pulmonology

JOANA BENAYOUN

1 A 2-week-old neonate presents to the clinic for his first visit after birth. The baby was born full term without any complications. His mother notes that he has been breastfeeding very well, but she is concerned because he is a very noisy breather and the noise is worsened with crying. He has regained his birth weight and his physical examination is significant for a hemangioma on his chin, extending to his left cheek. Otherwise, he is well appearing.

Of the following, what is the next best step in the management of this neonate?

(A) Referral to a dermatologist
(B) Referral to an otolaryngologist
(C) Chest radiography
(D) Magnetic resonance imaging (MRI) of his brain
(E) Reassurance

The answer is B: Referral to an otolaryngologist. Hemangiomas are common cutaneous findings in children and most resolve without intervention by age 10 years. However, hemangiomas in certain locations can be associated with serious problems. The patient in the vignette has a hemangioma with a beard-like distribution, defined as involvement of lower lip, chin, anterior portion of the neck, and preauricular areas. Patients with hemangiomas in this distribution have a much higher occurrence of airway hemangiomas and should be referred to an otolaryngologist for diagnosis and monitoring. The patient in the vignette has evidence of airway involvement and therefore requires immediate referral to an otolaryngologist.

(E) If the presentation did not suggest an airway hemangioma, tracheomalacia would be his most likely diagnosis and reassurance would be the next best step in management. **(C)** A chest radiograph would not clearly aid in the diagnosis of an airway hemangioma. **(A)** Referral to a dermatologist is not indicated until airway pathology is ruled out. **(D)** MRI of the brain is not indicated, as the distribution of his hemangioma is more concerning for airway, not intracranial pathology. Patients who have a port-wine birthmark in the upper eyelid and forehead do require an MRI to rule out intracranial anomalies, as is the case in patients with Sturge-Weber syndrome.

2 A 1-month-old neonate presents to the emergency department following an episode during which she stopped breathing and her parents performed rescue breaths. She was born full term without any complications and has been growing well since birth. Her parents deny any cold symptoms or fever. They cannot recall how long she stopped breathing but deny any blue coloring to her mouth or face. They note she started crying once they called out to her and gently slapped her back. On examination, her temperature is 37°C, heart rate is 120 beats/min, respiratory rate is 30 breaths/min, blood pressure is 82/54 mmHg, and oxygen saturation is 99% on room air. She is well appearing and the remainder of her physical examination is within normal limits.

Of the following, what is the most likely cause of this patient's presentation?

(A) Congenital heart disease
(B) Sudden infant death syndrome (SIDS)
(C) Apparent life-threatening event (ALTE)
(D) Apnea of prematurity
(E) Pertussis

The answer is C: Apparent life-threatening event (ALTE). The presentation described in the vignette is consistent with an ALTE. An ALTE is defined as an episode that involves apnea, change in tone, color change, choking, or gagging that is frightening to the observer. Although the etiology of half of ALTEs is idiopathic, it is important to attempt to determine the cause of the event. The differential diagnosis for an ALTE is broad and includes gastroesophageal reflux as well as apnea, congenital heart disease, infections, seizures or other neurologic diseases, cardiac dysrhythmias, airway anomalies, and nonaccidental trauma.

(A) Though congenital heart disease can be the cause of an ALTE, it is unlikely in a currently stable, previously healthy infant with normal physical examination and vital signs as described in the vignette. **(B)** SIDS is a diagnosis given to an infant who had died suddenly without any identifiable cause. Only a small minority of victims of SIDS had a history of an ALTE. **(D)** Given that the patient in the vignette was not born prematurely, a diagnosis of apnea of prematurity does not apply. **(E)** Without a history of upper respiratory infection symptoms, a diagnosis of pertussis is unlikely.

3 A 3-year-old unimmunized boy presents to the emergency department with a sudden onset of labored breathing, drooling, and fever. On examination, he is toxic appearing and drooling, and stridor is present on lung auscultation.

Of the following, what organism is most likely responsible for his presentation?

(A) *Staphylococcus aureus*
(B) *Streptococcus viridans*
(C) *Haemophilus influenzae* type b
(D) *Streptococcus pneumoniae*
(E) *Streptococcus pyogenes*

The answer is C: *Haemophilus influenzae* type b. The symptoms of the patient in the vignette are consistent with acute epiglottitis. Epiglottitis is a medical emergency. Children with epiglottitis are at risk for airway obstruction due to swelling of the epiglottis and supraglottic structures. Epiglottis is caused most commonly by *H. influenzae* type b (Hib), though routine vaccination against Hib has markedly reduced the incidence. **(D)** *Streptococcus pneumoniae* can cause epiglottitis and would be the most likely bacterial etiology in an immunized immunocompetent patient. Patients with epiglottitis have a sudden onset and rapid progression of symptoms including high fever, muffled voice, drooling, and anorexia. In order to receive better air entry, patients often sit leaning forward with their jaw thrust forward and mouth open, better known as the sniffing position. Lateral neck radiographs reveal the thumb print sign, due to a large and bulging epiglottis and swelling of the epiglottic folds (see *Figure 7-1*). Diagnosis is confirmed with direct visualization of the epiglottis, which should only be

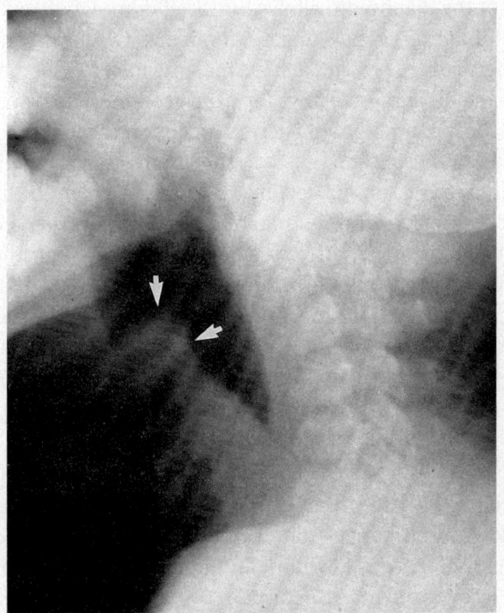

Figure 7-1

done in the operating room with an anesthesiologist and surgeon prepared for intubation or tracheostomy if required. Children with epiglottitis require endotracheal intubation to maintain airway patency as well as antibiotic therapy.

(A, B, E) *Staphylococcus aureus* and several subtypes of *Streptococcus* have been implicated in epiglottitis, but Hib remains the most likely cause in an unvaccinated child.

---

4 A 1-hour-old newborn boy is being evaluated for tachypnea. His prenatal history is unremarkable and the delivery was uncomplicated. On examination, he has a respiratory rate of 65 breaths/min and auscultation reveals the absence of breath sounds on the left side of the chest and his abdomen is scaphoid in shape.

Of the following, which is the most likely cause for this patient's respiratory distress?

(A) Neonatal respiratory distress syndrome (RDS)
(B) Meconium aspiration syndrome
(C) Dextrocardia
(D) Pulmonary hypoplasia
(E) Pneumothorax

The answer is D: Pulmonary hypoplasia. The likely cause of the respiratory distress for the patient in the vignette is pulmonary hypoplasia due to a diaphragmatic hernia. A diaphragmatic hernia is a congenital abnormality in which a malformation of the diaphragm allows for the abdominal organs to move into the chest cavity inhibiting proper lung development. The most common kind of diaphragmatic hernia is the Bochdalek hernia, in which a defect in the posterolateral corner of the diaphragm allows for passage of the abdominal organs into the chest cavity. Most diaphragmatic hernias occur on the left side. Infants present with tachypnea and respiratory distress shortly after birth. On physical examination, the abdomen is scaphoid secondary to displacement of the abdominal organs into the chest cavity. Lung auscultation demonstrates markedly decreased or absent breath sounds on the affected side. Diagnosis is confirmed with chest radiography, which demonstrates bowel in the chest. Treatment is surgical.

(A, B, E) Neonatal RDS, meconium aspiration syndrome, and pneumothorax all present with varying degrees of respiratory distress but are not accompanied by the physical examination findings described in the patient in the vignette. **(C)** In dextrocardia, lung sounds should be normal, but heart sounds are auscultated on the right side of the chest.

5 A 10-week-old infant presents to the emergency department with persistent cough and congestion. The parents are concerned because he has been sick for 8 days without an improvement of symptoms. He has not had a fever during this time. His appetite has decreased without associated vomiting or diarrhea. On examination, his temperature is

37.9°C, his respiratory rate is 45 breaths/min, and he appears mildly dehydrated but nontoxic. Lung auscultation reveals fine rales throughout without stridor or wheezing. A chest radiograph is significant for hyperinflation with mild diffuse interstitial infiltrates.

Of the following, what is the most likely organism responsible for this patient's symptoms?

(A) Respiratory syncytial virus (RSV)
(B) *Streptococcus agalactiae*
(C) *Escherichia coli*
(D) *Chlamydia trachomatis*
(E) *Listeria monocytogenes*

The answer is D: *Chlamydia trachomatis*. The patient in the vignette is presenting with signs of a pneumonia caused by *C. trachomatis*. One of the most salient features of this infection is that there is no associated fever. This condition occurs in infants aged 1 to 3 months and presents with prolonged cough and congestion. Radiographic findings include hyperinflation and interstitial infiltrates without focal consolidations. Cytomegalovirus, *Mycoplasma hominis*, and *Ureaplasma urealyticum* can produce a similar respiratory syndrome. The likely source of chlamydia in affected infants is their mother. Treatment is with oral erythromycin or azithromycin.

(A, B, C, E) RSV, *S. agalactiae, E. coli,* and *L. monocytogenes* are all associated with pneumonias; however, more systemic symptoms, such as fever, should be present.

6 The parents of a newborn present to the clinic with questions regarding immunizations.

Of the following, which is recommended for prevention of *Bordetella pertussis* infection?

(A) The newborn should be immunized against pertussis at his post-hospital discharge office visit
(B) Both parents and household members should receive the DTaP (diphtheria-tetanus-acellular pertussis) vaccine as soon as possible
(C) Both parents and other adult household members should receive the Tdap (tetanus-diphtheria-acellular pertussis) vaccine as soon as possible
(D) Only household members without a history of a recent tetanus booster should be immunized with Tdap
(E) Siblings who are up-to-date on their immunizations should receive a booster against pertussis, regardless

The answer is C: Both parents and other adult household members should receive the Tdap (tetanus-diphtheria-acellular pertussis)

vaccine as soon as possible. Cases of whooping cough, caused by *B. pertussis*, are on the rise in the United States. Several factors contribute to this, including decreasing vaccination rates and waning immunity in adolescents and adults. Recent studies have indicated that the peak age of incidence of pertussis is less than 4 months. These infants are too young to be fully immunized and also have the most severe complications and highest mortality rates.

(A) Routine vaccination of all children with the DTaP vaccine should occur at 2 months, 4 months, 6 months, 15 to 18 months, and 4 to 6 years. A booster of Tdap is also recommended at 11 to 12 years of age. **(C)** All adult household members who have not received the Tdap vaccine should be immunized in the immediate postpartum period or before the baby is born. Pregnant women can be vaccinated with Tdap in the second and third trimesters. **(B)** The difference between DTaP and Tdap is that the Tdap vaccine has a decreased dose of the diphtheria and pertussis elements.

Parents of newborns should be highly encouraged to receive the Tdap booster before leaving the hospital, if they have not received it before. **(D)** All other household members should verify their immunization status with their primary care physicians to ensure that they have received the Tdap vaccine as most adults typically get only tetanus boosters every 10 years. **(E)** If a sibling's immunizations are up-to-date, a booster is not indicated.

A 4-month-old infant presents to the emergency department (ED) with cough, rapid breathing, and inability to take her bottle. The parents note that she has had congestion and cough for 2 days that has worsened since this morning. They brought her to the ED when they noticed she was breathing fast and was using her abdominal muscles to breathe. On arrival, her respiratory rate is 50 breaths/min, her oxygen saturation is 92% on room air, and her heart rate is 140 beats/min. On physical examination, she has subcostal retractions, and slight wheezing throughout her lung fields. She received a respiratory treatment with an inhaled β_2-agonist without any improvement in oxygen saturation, respiratory rate, or examination findings.

Of the following, what is the next best step in the management of this patient?

(A) An hour-long treatment with a nebulized β_2-agonist
(B) Oral corticosteroids
(C) Supplemental oxygen via nasal cannula
(D) Racemic epinephrine nebulization
(E) Intravenous ampicillin

The answer is C: Supplemental oxygen via nasal cannula. The infant in the vignette has symptoms consistent with an infection with respiratory syncytial virus (RSV). Patients with RSV bronchiolitis can present in mild-to-severe respiratory distress. Infants and neonates are at risk for respiratory failure and death. Treatment is mostly supportive and the mainstays are oxygen supplementation and frequent nasopharyngeal suctioning. Several pharmacologic agents have been tried, most with little to no proven benefit. **(A)** An hour-long treatment with a nebulized β_2-agonist (albuterol) would only be indicated in a patient who had shown improvement with a prior treatment or who has a history of asthma. **(B, D)** Racemic epinephrine and corticosteroids have not been shown to improve symptoms of RSV bronchiolitis. **(E)** Antibiotics should be used only if there is concurrent bacterial infection.

---

8 A 13-year-old boy presents to the clinic with complaints of fever, neck pain, and throat pain for 5 days. He notes that he has had mild difficulty swallowing due to the pain which is more pronounced on the left side of his neck and radiates toward his ear. On examination, he is not drooling, his oropharynx is erythematous, and his tonsils are enlarged with the soft palate on the left side displaced anteriorly (see *Figure 7-2*).

Of the following, what is his most likely diagnosis?

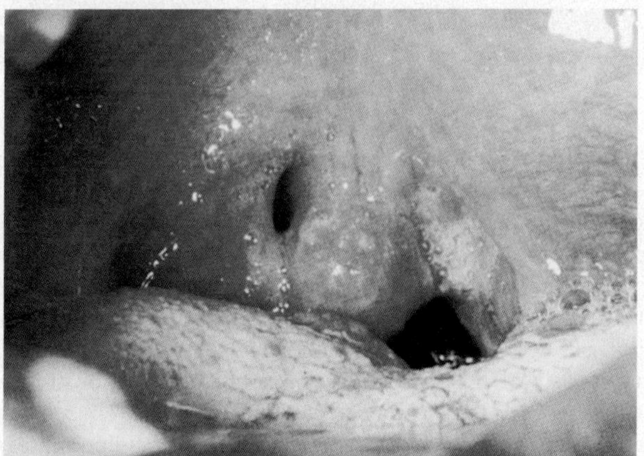

Figure 7-2

(A) Retropharyngeal abscess
(B) Meningitis
(C) Mumps virus infection
(D) Peritonsillar abscess
(E) Adenovirus infection

The answer is D: Peritonsillar abscess. The presentation and physical examination findings described for the boy in the vignette are consistent with a left peritonsillar abscess. A peritonsillar abscess develops from direct infiltration from a bacterial tonsillitis. Clinical diagnosis is generally sufficient but computed tomography demonstrates a low-attenuation mass with an

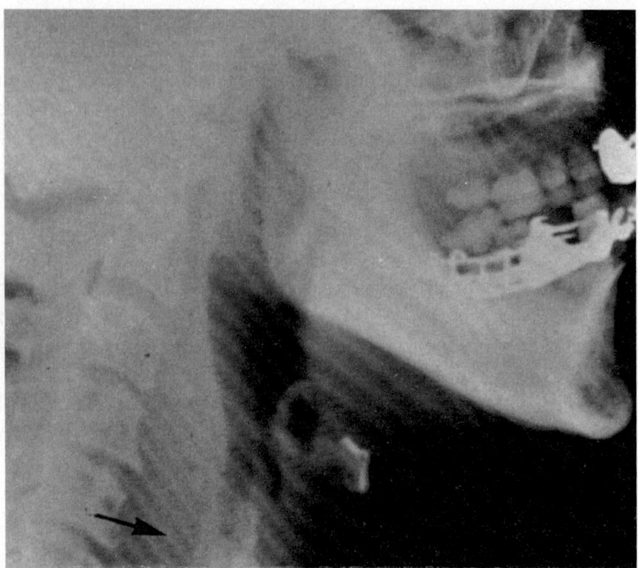

Figure 7-3

enhancing wall in the peritonsillar region with ipsilateral lymphadenopathy. The best treatment for a peritonsillar abscess involves antibiotics and drainage. Several organisms have been implicated in peritonsillar abscesses including *Streptococcus pyogenes, Staphylococcus aureus*, and anaerobic organisms.

(A) Retropharyngeal abscesses present with constitutional symptoms as well as dysphagia, muffled voice, neck stiffness, and difficulty opening the mouth, or trismus. Physical examination may demonstrate a bulge in the posterior pharyngeal wall. Lateral radiographs of the neck demonstrate widening of the tissues between the airway and the spine (see *Figure 7-3*). A computed tomography scan of the neck is the diagnostic test of choice and demarcates the extent of the abscess. Retropharyngeal abscesses are more common in the toddler age group and less likely in teenagers as the connection between the retropharyngeal space decreases with age and is less likely to become infected.

(B) Meningitis presents with neck stiffness, headache, and vomiting. Although patients with peritonsillar abscesses may have neck stiffness secondary to pain, their meninges are not affected. **(C, E)** Neither the mumps virus nor adenovirus has been implicated in a peritonsillar abscess.

9 A 15-year-old girl with no significant past medical history presents to the emergency department with chest pain for 1 day. She reports she woke up with the pain and it is localized to her sternum. It is constant in nature and does not radiate but is aggravated by deep inspiration. She denies shortness of breath, palpitations, or recent trauma.

Of the following, which physical examination finding best fits with her presentation?

(A) Heart rate of 200 beats/min
(B) Tenderness to palpation of the chest wall
(C) Blood pressure of 145/90 mmHg
(D) Decreased air entry and wheezing at the lung bases
(E) Oxygen saturation of 92% on room air

The answer is B: **Tenderness to palpation of the chest wall.** Chest pain is a common complaint in pediatrics, especially among adolescents. There are many causes for chest pain in children, though the most common are costochondritis, pneumonia, and asthma. Cardiac causes should be ruled out, but, in general, are not as common in children when compared with adults. **(B)** Costochondritis is a benign inflammation of the rib cartilage and is characterized by reproducible chest pain on examination. Treatment of choice is anti-inflammatory medications.

(D, E) Asthma is a common cause for chest pain in the pediatric population. However, asthmatic pain is not reproducible on examination. Wheezing, decreased breath sounds, tachycardia, and low oxygen saturation are common findings in an acute asthma exacerbation.

(A) Arrhythmias, myocardial infarction, myocarditis, and pericarditis are cardiac etiologies associated with chest pain. Myocardial infarction is not common in children or adolescents, unless associated with congenital coronary anomalies or cocaine use. **(C)** Given that the patient in the vignette is otherwise well appearing, it is less likely that she is tachycardic and hypertensive.

10 A 12-year-old boy presents to the clinic for the first time. His history reveals that he has had multiple episodes of pneumonia, and he notes that he has a hard time recovering from upper respiratory infections. He has also had multiple ear and sinus infections since childhood. On examination, his heart sounds are present, without murmurs and are best heard along the right sternal border.

Of the following, what is the most likely underlying cause of this patient's condition?

(A) Elevated immunoglobulin E (IgE) levels
(B) Mutation in the cystic fibrosis transmembrane regulator (CFTR) gene locus
(C) Abnormal IgG levels
(D) Ciliary dyskinesia
(E) Absence of all circulating immunoglobulins

The answer is D: **Ciliary dyskinesia.** The patient in the vignette likely has a form of primary ciliary dyskinesia, an autosomal recessive disorder that causes dysmotile cilia. When primary ciliary dyskinesia is accompanied by situs inversus, bronchiectasis, and chronic sinusitis, it is classified as Kartagener syndrome. Since the patient in the vignette has findings of situs inversus as suggested by his cardiac examination as well as chronic sinusitis, he likely has Kartagener syndrome. The dysmotile cilia cause impaired clearance of mucus in the respiratory epithelium leading to repeat pulmonary, sinus, and ear infections. There is also associated infertility, due to immotile sperm flagella.

(A) Elevated IgE level is associated with Job syndrome. Patients with Job syndrome are susceptible to recurrent staphylococcal and candidal infections, pneumonias, and an eczema-like rash. **(B)** Cystic fibrosis (CF) is caused by a mutation in the CFTR gene and is not associated with situs inversus. **(C, E)** Patients with common variable immunodeficiency have low levels of IgG as well as variably low levels of IgA and IgM. These patients have recurrent infections of the lungs, sinuses, ears, and skin, but they do not have situs inversus. X-linked agammaglobulinemia is also associated with recurrent respiratory infections but not situs inversus.

11 A 40-week-gestation infant is delivered in the presence of meconium-stained amniotic fluid. The baby has poor tone and color, and immediate tracheal suctioning yields 1 mL of meconium-stained fluid. She is dried and stimulated and yet she continues to have poor tone, color, and a weak cry. Her heart rate of 80 beats/min remains unchanged. Appropriate resuscitation is initiated with improvement in color, tone, and heart rate. Despite this improvement, the baby has a respiratory rate of 75 breaths/min with nasal flaring and intercostal retractions.

Of the following, which radiographic findings are most consistent with this baby's presentation?

(A) Consolidation in the right upper lobe
(B) Radiopaque line along the horizontal fissure in the right lung
(C) Bibasilar consolidations
(D) Ground glass appearance throughout the lung fields
(E) Hyperinflation with areas of patchy opacities

The answer is E: Hyperinflation with areas of patchy opacities. The baby in the vignette has meconium aspiration syndrome. Meconium is a baby's first bowel movement. It is composed of intestinal secretions, mucous, and swallowed amniotic fluid components. Normally, babies do not pass meconium until after birth; however, when a baby is under stress in utero, passage can occur. Some causes for in utero meconium passage include placental insufficiency, oligohydramnios, maternal hypertension, preeclampsia, and other sources of fetal hypoxic stress. Meconium fluid aspiration can occur before, after, or during birth and can lead to severe symptoms due to obstruction, chemical pneumonitis, surfactant dysfunction, and pulmonary hypertension. Obstruction can lead to air trapping and hyperinflation. The components of meconium also deactivate surfactant leading to inadequate gas exchange due to atelectasis and irritate the lung parenchyma causing a chemical pneumonitis. Persistent pulmonary hypertension of the newborn results from constriction of the pulmonary vasculature, resulting in significant right-to-left shunting with resultant severe hypoxemia. Prior to resuscitation, tracheal suctioning should be performed with an endotracheal tube. Symptoms of meconium aspiration can be mild, requiring only supportive care, or severe, requiring extracorporeal membrane oxygenation. Chest radiography demonstrates hyperinflation with patchy opacities due to atelectasis and chemical pneumonitis.

(A, C) Meconium aspiration syndrome does not show focal consolidations (either bibasilar or in the right upper lobe), such as a bacterial pneumonia would on chest radiography. **(B)** A radiopaque line along the horizontal fissure in the right lung is consistent with transient tachypnea of the newborn. **(D)** Ground glass appearance of the lungs is most consistent with neonatal respiratory distress syndrome.

---

12 A 10-year-old victim of a hit and run is evaluated in the emergency department. He is tachypneic and agitated. On examination, there is an obvious right humeral deformity and he has multiple lacerations and bruising. He has equal breath sounds bilaterally and a segment of his chest moves inward with inspiration.

Of the following, what best describes this patient's condition?

(A) Flail chest
(B) Hemothorax
(C) Pneumothorax
(D) Pulmonary contusion
(E) Pleural effusion

The answer is A: Flail chest. The patient in the vignette exhibits flail chest. Flail chest is characterized by paradoxical movement of a segment of the chest, in which the detached segment moves in the opposite direction of the chest wall during inspiration and expiration. Flail chest occurs following trauma to the chest and is often associated with at least two fractured ribs occurring in two different places. The paradoxical movement typically disappears with positive pressure ventilation. Flail chest is usually accompanied by pulmonary contusion and can lead to respiratory failure.

The other answer choices do not lead to paradoxical movement of the chest wall. **(B, C, D, E)** When a hemothorax, pleural effusion, pulmonary contusion, or pneumothorax is present, breath sounds are expected to be diminished on the affected side.

---

13 A 6-year-old Caucasian girl is admitted to the hospital with pneumonia. A thorough history reveals multiple hospitalizations for recurrent respiratory infections, as well as a chronic cough. On examination, her weight is less than the third percentile and her nasopharyngeal examination reveals the finding in Figure 7-4.

Of the following tests, what is best indicated in this patient to help establish a diagnosis?

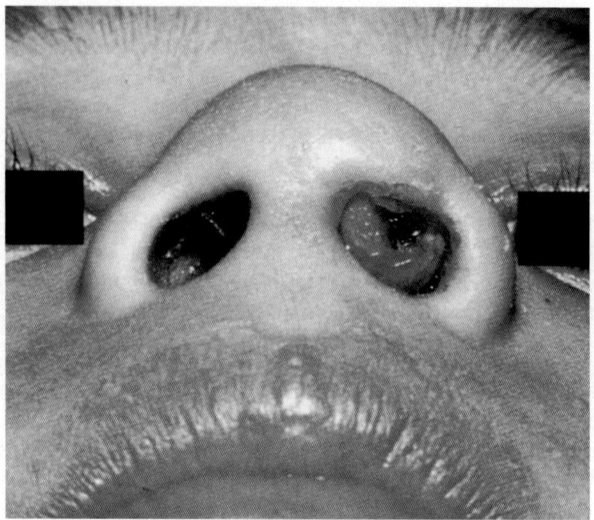

Figure 7-4

(A) Neutrophil burst assay
(B) Serum *Mycoplasma pneumoniae* immunoglobulin (Ig)G and IgM
(C) Epstein-Barr virus IgG and IgM
(D) Sweat chloride test
(E) Serum α-1-antitrypsin levels

The answer is D: Sweat chloride test. The patient in the vignette has symptoms concerning for cystic fibrosis (CF). CF should be suspected in any patient with a chronic cough, recurrent lung infections, growth restriction, and nasal polyps. **(D)** Diagnosis is confirmed by performing a sweat chloride test. Patients with CF have impaired chloride transport. Sweat chloride concentration is measured in collected sweat after stimulation of the skin with pilocarpine and patients with CF have elevated concentrations of chloride in their sweat.

(A) The neutrophil burst assay is used to diagnose chronic granulomatous disease (CGD). CGD is an inherited immunodeficiency disorder that leads to chronic infections, such as pneumonias, skin infections, bacteremia, and osteomyelitis. The patient in the vignette would be expected to have a history of prior abscesses if CGD were her diagnosis. **(B, C)** *M. pneumoniae* and Epstein-Barr virus do not cause chronic symptoms although both can present acutely with upper respiratory symptoms. **(E)** α-1-Antitrypsin deficiency is typically suspected in children with liver disease of unknown etiology. These patients do not develop lung problems until adulthood, and thus would be highly unlikely for the patient in the vignette.

14 A 9-year-old boy was intubated in the pediatric intensive care unit for the 30 days following a severe motor vehicle accident. He was successfully extubated 2 weeks ago but has residual hoarseness and episodes of shortness of breath on exertion despite treatment with corticosteroids.

Of the following, what is the most likely cause for his symptoms?

(A) Vocal cord nodule
(B) Vocal cord dysfunction (VCD)
(C) Subglottic stenosis
(D) Residual effects of a pulmonary contusion
(E) Exercise-induced asthma

The answer is C: Subglottic stenosis. The boy in the vignette has subglottic stenosis. Subglottic stenosis can be congenital or caused by prolonged intubation. The subglottic area is the narrowest area of the airway because unlike the trachea and the larynx, it has a complete cartilaginous ring that does not expand and is not pliable. Acquired subglottic stenosis is typically caused by trauma from an endotracheal tube (ET) due to prolonged intubation, repeated intubations, or improperly sized ET. Acquired subglottic stenosis is more common in premature infants, who require long periods of intubation. Mild acquired subglottic stenosis leads to hoarseness and shortness of breath with exercise. Severe cases may require tracheostomy and tracheal reconstruction.

(A) Vocal cord nodules are usually not caused by prolonged intubation, and though they present with hoarseness and dysphonia, they are not associated with shortness of breath. Vocal cord nodules are usually caused by phonotrauma, from overuse of the vocal cords during talking or singing. **(B)** VCD occurs with abnormal adduction of the vocal cords during the respiratory cycle. **(D, E)** It is unlikely that the patient in the vignette is still suffering from the effects of a pulmonary contusion or exercise-induced asthma.

15 A 6-year-old patient presents to the emergency department with fever and cough. Her mother notes that she has been sick for 3 weeks and has finished a course of cefdinir and azithromycin for pneumonia that was diagnosed 2 weeks ago. She notes that she is still having daily fevers and night sweats and her cough has not improved despite antibiotic treatment. Her summer was spent at their lake house on Lake Erie where her father was building an addition to the house. A chest radiograph reveals a right lower lobe infiltrate, unchanged from 2 weeks ago. She is admitted to the inpatient pediatric unit due to her persistent pneumonia and fevers.

Of the following, empiric therapy should be started for which disease?

(A) Human immunodeficiency virus
(B) Pulmonary tuberculosis
(C) Influenza
(D) Atypical pneumonia
(E) Pulmonary blastomycosis

The answer is E: Pulmonary blastomycosis. The presentation of the patient in the vignette is consistent with a fungal pneumonia. The persistent fevers, right lower lobe infiltrate, and night sweats are indicative of a chronic pneumonia. **(D)** The patient in the vignette received adequate treatment for bacterial pneumonia without improvement; thus, other causes of chronic pneumonia need to be investigated. In the United States, the most common fungal pathogens that cause pneumonia in immunocompetent hosts are *Histoplasma capsulatum*, *Coccidioides immitis*, *Blastomyces dermatitidis*, and *Paracoccidioides brasiliensis*. Opportunistic infections for immunocompromised patients include *Candida* sp., *Aspergillus* sp., *Mucor* sp., and *Cryptococcus neoformans*.

H. capsulatum is a dimorphic fungus endemic to the Ohio, Missouri, and Mississippi river valleys. It is found in the soil and infection is associated with construction and renovations that alter the soil. Treatment is done with itraconazole, though amphotericin B is indicated in severe infections. *B. dermatitidis* is a dimorphic fungus endemic to the Mississippi and Ohio rivers as well as the Great Lakes region. It is also found in soil and the diagnosis is made through urine antigen detection. *C. immitis* is endemic to California's San Joaquin valley and is contracted through aerosolized soil. Treatment for both fungi is itraconazole.

(E) If there is a high suspicion of fungal pneumonia, empiric treatment should be initiated pending results. The patient in the vignette has a history of living in the Great Lakes region as well as exposure to soil through construction, making **(A)** fungal pneumonia the most likely diagnosis. **(B)** She has no risk factors for tuberculosis and therefore empiric therapy is not indicated. **(C)** Empiric treatment with oseltamivir for suspected influenza is only effective if given within 24 to 72 hours of symptom development.

---

16 A 14-year-old girl presents with fever and cough for 7 days' duration. She denies exposure to travel, pets, or sick contacts and is otherwise healthy. On physical examination, auscultation reveals diffuse crackles throughout all lung fields. Chest radiography reveals diffuse interstitial infiltrates without focal consolidations.

Of the following, which organism is the most likely cause of this patient's illness?

(A) *Streptococcus pneumoniae*
(B) *Staphylococcus aureus*
(C) *Mycobacterium tuberculosis*
(D) *Mycoplasma pneumoniae*
(E) *Pneumocystis jiroveci*

The answer is D: *Mycoplasma pneumoniae.* The symptoms and radiographic findings described for the patient in the vignette are consistent with an atypical pneumonia. (**D**) In this age group, the most common etiology is *Mycoplasma pneumoniae*. Symptoms usually appear gradually and are similar to those of a viral upper respiratory tract infection. *Mycoplasma pneumoniae* should be suspected in a patient with malaise, protracted cough, fever, headache, and chills. Diagnosis is made on clinical symptoms and a chest radiograph can be useful to exclude lobar pneumonias.

(**A, B**) *Streptococcus pneumoniae* and *Staphylococcus aureus* cause focal consolidations in the lungs as opposed to the diffuse interstitial findings described in the vignette. (**C**) *Mycobacterium tuberculosis* should be suspected in any patient with a pneumonia that fails conventional antibiotic treatment or in any patient with cavitary lesions in the lungs. (**E**) *Pneumocystis jiroveci* pneumonia, previously known as *Pneumocystis carinii* pneumonia, is an opportunistic infection that occurs in immunocompromised patients and is commonly associated with human immunodeficiency virus infection. It presents with nonspecific symptoms such as malaise, cough, and fever, and chest radiography reveals diffuse bilateral infiltrates.

17 A 3-year-old patient presents to the emergency department with a sudden onset of cough. Her mother denies any history of fever or cold symptoms. On examination, her lungs are clear to auscultation. Chest radiography reveals hyperinflation of the right lung.

Of the following, which is the most likely cause of this patient's symptoms and radiographic findings?

(A) Foreign body aspiration
(B) Hydrocarbon aspiration
(C) Acute asthma exacerbation
(D) Pneumonia
(E) Acute pneumothorax

The answer is A: Foreign body aspiration. The presentation and clinical findings of the girl in the vignette are most consistent with a foreign body aspiration. Often children present without a history of choking, as the episode of choking is not witnessed or not recalled. Some foreign body aspirations are not detected for days to weeks and may present with chronic cough or recurrent pneumonias. Most foreign bodies are aspirated into the right mainstem bronchus because of the shallower branching angle from the trachea versus the left bronchus. Chest radiography reveals hyperinflation on the ipsilateral side of the aspiration. Treatment is removal of the foreign body.

(B) Hydrocarbon aspiration produces a chemical pneumonitis and radiography of the chest would reveal bibasilar infiltrates with patchy atelectasis. **(C)** An acute asthma exacerbation would be associated with wheezing on examination and diffuse nonfocal hyperinflation on chest radiography. **(D)** Pneumonias are associated with fever and focal consolidations. **(E)** A pneumothorax may present similarly as described in the vignette, but physical examination would reveal decreased breath sounds on the affected side and chest radiography would demonstrate a demarcation indicating the visceral pleura with lack of lung markings peripheral to it.

18 A 4-month-old infant presents with cough and increased work of breathing for 1 day. According to his parents, he has had a runny nose and cough for 2 to 3 days, associated with a fever to 39.2°C. On examination, the patient has a respiratory rate of 50 breaths/min, is using his abdominal muscles to breathe, has mild wheezing and coarse breath sounds throughout all lung fields on auscultation.

Of the following, which is his most likely diagnosis?

(A) Bronchitis
(B) Pharyngitis
(C) Tracheitis
(D) Bronchiolitis
(E) Pneumonia

The answer is D: Bronchiolitis. The symptoms of the patient in the vignette are consistent with bronchiolitis. Acute bronchiolitis is the most common cause of lower respiratory infections in children under 1 year of age. Respiratory syncytial virus infection is often the causative agent. Viral invasion of the lower airways causes increased mucus production leading to bronchial obstruction, atelectasis, air trapping, and decreased ventilation. Symptoms range from mild to severe and may be fatal. Patients with bronchiolitis present with a history of a few days of cold-like symptoms followed by a worsening cough and increased work of breathing. Physical examination can demonstrate wheezing, rales, retractions, and crackles. Chest radiographs are highly variable in patients with bronchiolitis but may reveal hyperinflation with areas of atelectasis that are commonly in the right upper lobe. Treatment is supportive.

(A) Bronchitis is an inflammation of the bronchi, as opposed to the bronchioles. Most cases of bronchitis are viral in etiology as well. Patients usually present with a history of cold-like symptoms which progress to a worsening cough. Bronchitis is a self-limited illness in healthy children, typically lasting 7 to 10 days. The patient in the vignette presents with a more severe respiratory course than would be expected for a child with bronchitis. **(B)** Acute pharyngitis presents with a sore throat and cold-like symptoms. Acute pharyngitis does not lead to the respiratory symptoms described in the vignette. **(E)** Pneumonia can present in a similar manner as described in the vignette; however, physical examination would typically reveal focal finding in the lungs and chest radiography would reveal a consolidation. **(C)** Bacterial tracheitis is an inflammatory process of the airway, including the larynx, trachea, and bronchi. Patients with bacterial tracheitis can present as a croup-like illness with stridor, barking cough, and fever; however, symptoms do not respond to any of the treatments for croup and require antibiotic therapy. Laryngotracheobronchoscopy is indicated for diagnosis which typically reveals an adherent mucopurulent membrane. The most common cause of bacterial tracheitis is *Staphylococcus aureus.*

---

19 A 12-year-old girl presents to her pediatrician's office with complaints of mild cough productive of blood-tinged sputum. The cough started 2 days ago and she noticed the blood this morning. She denies any fever, night sweats, chills, fatigue, or weight loss. Her past medical history is significant for allergic rhinitis and allergies to penicillin and eggs. She is generally well appearing and her vital signs are temperature 37.2°C, heart rate 75 beats/min, respiratory rate of 18 breaths/min, and oxygen saturation of 99% on room air. Her physical examination reveals pink, moist oral mucosa with some streaks of blood visible in the posterior pharynx. She has good air entry with no wheezing or crackles.

Of the following, what is the most likely source of her blood-tinged sputum?

(A) Hematemesis
(B) Bronchiectasis
(C) Epistaxis
(D) Pneumonia
(E) Damage to the bronchi from forceful coughing

The answer is C: Epistaxis. Hemoptysis is a term generally applied to the expectoration of blood originating in the airway and lungs, while **(A)** hematemesis refers to blood that originates in the gastrointestinal tract. Patients often report coughing up blood, but it is essential to differentiate the blood's true origin. The patient in the vignette is most likely coughing up blood from her epistaxis, or nose bleed, as evidenced by streaks of blood in the posterior oropharynx and her history of allergic rhinitis.

(B) The patient in the vignette does not have a history of chronic lung disease and thus likely does not have bronchiectasis. **(D)** Pneumonia is unlikely with a normal physical examination along with a lack of fever. **(E)** Damage to the airway from forceful coughing can cause blood-streaked sputum, but the cough described in the vignette is mild and therefore she is unlikely generating enough force to damage the airway.

---

20 A mother brings her 12-year-old daughter for evaluation of her snoring. She is concerned because her daughter's snoring has worsened over the past year and now is associated with several episodes of cessation of respiration during the night. Her daughter is also more irritable than usual and has had a few episodes of nocturnal enuresis. Pertinent findings on examination include obesity and a normal-appearing oropharynx. The remainder of her examination is unremarkable.

Of the following, what is the most severe complication of this patient's disorder?

(A) Reactive airway disease
(B) Eisenmenger syndrome
(C) Recurrent pneumonia
(D) Left ventricular hypertrophy
(E) Cor pulmonale

The answer is E: Cor pulmonale. The patient in the vignette is suffering from obstructive sleep apnea (OSA). OSA presents with snoring and distress during sleep and is associated with episodes of gasping, respiratory pauses, and hypoxia. This condition is due to partial or complete upper airway obstruction. Intermittent hypoxia leads to elevation of pulmonary arterial pressures due to pulmonary vasoconstriction. **(E)** The chronic hypoxemia leads to pulmonary hypertension and cor pulmonale, which is defined as **(D)** right ventricular hypertrophy secondary to increased pulmonary pressures.

(B) Eisenmenger syndrome occurs when a previously untreated congenital heart defect leads to pulmonary hypertension and subsequent reversal of shunt flow. The previously left-to-right shunt becomes a right-to-left shunt. This patient does not have any signs or symptoms to indicate she has a congenital cardiac defect. **(A, C)** OSA is not associated with reactive airway disease or recurrent pneumonia.

21 A 2-day-old neonate in the nursery has had five episodes of yellow emesis and has not passed meconium. On examination, his abdomen is markedly distended and rectum is prolapsed. An abdominal radiograph and contrast enema are obtained and have findings consistent with a distal obstruction (see *Figure 7-5*).

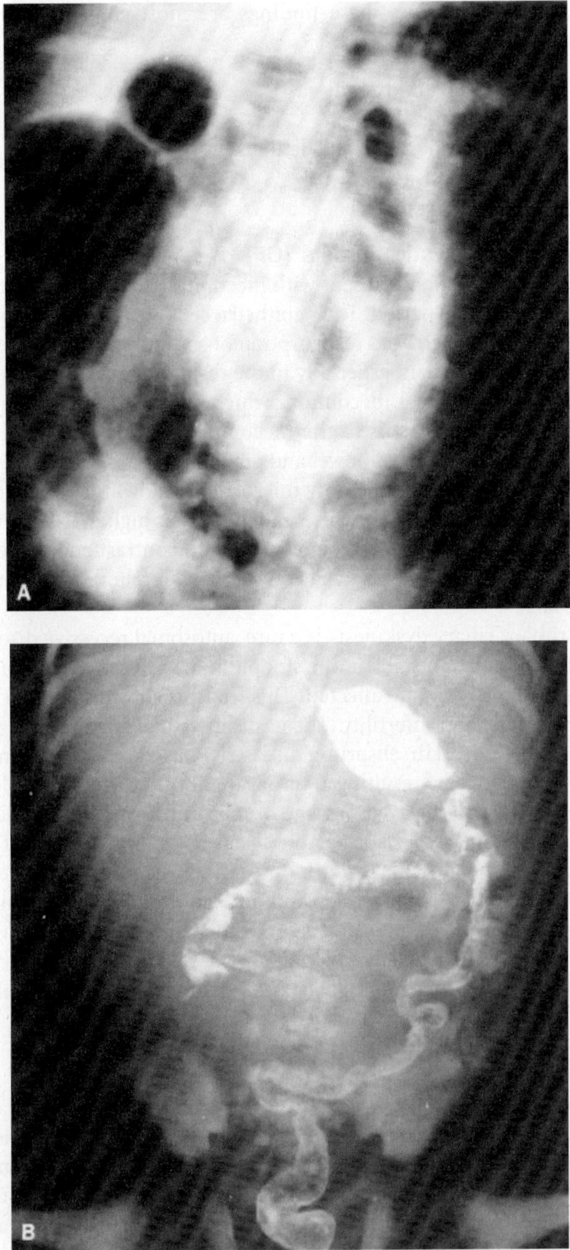

Figure 7-5

Of the following, these findings are most consistent with which condition?

(A) Primary ciliary dyskinesia
(B) Situs inversus
(C) Chromosome 22q11.2 deletion syndrome
(D) Cystic fibrosis (CF)
(E) Hirschsprung disease

The answer is D: **Cystic fibrosis (CF).** Patients with CF have impaired chloride transport and may present with meconium ileus or rectal prolapse in the immediate neonatal period. Their epithelial cells are relatively impermeable to chloride and have increased reabsorption of sodium, leading to dehydrated secretions and thick mucus, especially in the respiratory system. Patients with CF also produce abnormal meconium, which can lead to a blockage of the intestines due to inspissations of the meconium in the distal ileus. Imaging may reveal distended loops of bowel and air-fluid levels above the level of the obstruction and a narrow and empty microcolon below it. Meconium ileus is a life-threatening emergency because patients are at higher risk for intestinal perforation. Meconium ileus can be relieved with contrast enemas, which are also diagnostic; however, surgery may be required to relieve the obstruction if the enema fails.

(A) Primary ciliary dyskinesia is a rare, autosomal recessive disorder that causes immotile cilia. The cilia in the sinopulmonary tree, the fallopian tubes, and the flagella of sperm are affected. This leads to chronic respiratory infections, hearing loss, and infertility. The gastrointestinal tract is typically unaffected in this disorder. Hirschsprung disease is caused by failure of migration of the neural crest cells, resulting in an aganglionic segment of colon. Neonates can present with delayed passage of meconium and abdominal distension. Contrast enema reveals a narrow distal colon with proximal dilation. Diagnosis is confirmed with rectal biopsy, which demonstrates the absence of ganglion cells. **(E)** Rectal prolapse is uncommon in the presentation of Hirschsprung disease. **(B)** Situs inversus is a congenital condition in which the visceral organs form contralaterally to their expected positions. This condition is not associated with meconium ileus. **(C)** Chromosome 22q11.2 deletion, or DiGeorge syndrome, is also not associated with meconium ileus.

22 A 10-year-old patient with a history of sickle cell disease was admitted to the inpatient ward 2 days ago with an acute pain crisis in his chest. A chest radiograph at the time of admission was unremarkable. On day 2 of admission, he developed a fever and blood cultures were ordered. On examination, he has a respiratory rate of 40 breaths/min, and decreased air entry over the right lower lung field. His oxygen saturation is 90% on room air. A repeat chest radiograph is remarkable for a right lower lobe consolidation.

If given at the time of admission, which of the following would have decreased the risk of development of his current condition?

(A) Prophylactic antibiotics
(B) Incentive spirometry
(C) Inhaled β_2-agonist therapy upon admission
(D) Adequate pain control
(E) Inhaled corticosteroids

The answer is B: Incentive spirometry. The patient in the vignette has developed acute chest syndrome, a vaso-occlusive crisis within the lungs of patients with sickle cell anemia. Patients with acute chest syndrome often initially complain of chest pain, and shortly thereafter develop a cough, respiratory distress, tachycardia, and hypoxia. Physical examination is significant for decreased breath sounds over affected areas of the lungs and chest radiography findings with consolidation in the same area. This is a serious complication of sickle cell disease and typically involves infection and infarction. The patient in the vignette was admitted with an acute pain crisis without signs of respiratory distress. One of the risk factors for developing acute chest syndrome is poor air exchange. When a patient with sickle cell disease is admitted with a pain crisis, their respiratory effort is diminished secondary to splinting from pain and use of narcotic medications. Incentive spirometry has been shown to decrease the risk of developing acute chest syndrome. Treatment of acute chest syndrome involves intravenous fluids, oxygen, analgesics, antibiotics, bronchodilators, and red blood cell transfusions. Exchange transfusions may be required in severe cases.

(A, C, E) Prophylactic antibiotics, β_2-agonist, or corticosteroid therapies do not prevent episodes of acute chest syndrome. However, β_2-agonist therapy is indicated if a patient is wheezing, but should not be used prophylactically. **(D)** Adequate pain control should always occur with sickle cell patients. Studies show decreased hospitalizations and length of stay when pain control is adequate; however, for this patient incentive spirometry use would better prevent acute chest syndrome.

23 A 30-day-old, ex-26-week premature neonate is in the neonatal intensive care unit. He was extubated to nasal cannula yesterday. The nurse reports repeated episodes of apnea associated with bradycardia. During these episodes, he responds to tactile stimulation. Aside from these episodes, he maintains his saturation well and is not tachypneic nor showing any other signs of respiratory distress.

Of the following, what is the most likely cause for these episodes?

(A) Premature extubation
(B) Respiratory distress syndrome (RDS)
(C) Sepsis
(D) Periodic breathing
(E) Immaturity of the central respiratory drive

The answer is E: Immaturity of the central respiratory drive. The neonate in the vignette is exhibiting signs of apnea of prematurity. Apnea is defined as cessation of breathing for longer than 20 seconds or for less time if accompanied by desaturation or bradycardia. Premature neonates having an immature respiratory drive may exhibit apnea. Apnea of prematurity should resolve by the time the neonate reaches a postconceptual age of 37 to 40 weeks. Apnea of prematurity is treated with caffeine, either orally or intravenously. In some infants, the apnea is severe enough that intubation or continuous positive airway pressure may be required until the caffeine is at a therapeutic level.

(A, B) The fact that the patient in the vignette is otherwise doing well without signs of respiratory distress indicates that he was ready for extubation and does not have RDS. **(C)** Though sepsis should always be a concern for premature infants, the patient in the vignette is not exhibiting any other signs of sepsis, for example, ill appearance or fever. **(D)** Periodic breathing is a normal occurrence in neonates and is not associated with apnea and bradycardia.

24 A 10-year-old boy is brought to the office by his mother secondary to wheezing. He is new to the practice and his past medical history reveals frequent emergency department (ED) visits for the same complaint. His mother states that he always improves after the breathing treatment in the ED and frequently is discharged on an oral medication. She reports that he has woken up coughing four times in the past month. Upon examination, his respiratory rate is 35 breaths/min, he does not have retractions, but does have diffuse bilateral expiratory wheezing on auscultation.

After initiating treatment with inhaled albuterol and oral corticosteroids in the office, of the following, what is the next best step in management?

(A) Referral to a pulmonologist for uncontrolled asthma
(B) Advise the mother to give him a daily dose of albuterol
(C) Follow up with the child in 1 week to assess for improvement
(D) Begin daily treatment with an inhaled corticosteroid
(E) Begin a long-acting β_2-agonist along with albuterol as needed

The answer is D: Begin daily treatment with an inhaled corticosteroid. The history and presentation of the patient in the vignette are consistent with poorly controlled asthma. One of the most important interventions for children with uncontrolled asthma is appropriate teaching regarding the diagnosis, which should include an explanation of symptoms associated with asthma, proper use of medications, as well as completion of an asthma action plan. Discussion should include possible triggers such as smoking, pets, perfumes, and carpet, as well as recognizing respiratory distress.

An acute asthma exacerbation is managed with the use of inhaled albuterol and a brief course of oral corticosteroids. **(D)** Patients with poorly controlled asthma should additionally be prescribed daily inhaled corticosteroid therapy to prevent future exacerbations. **(C)** The patient in the vignette needs proper therapy and following up in 1 week would not correct his poorly controlled asthma symptoms. **(B)** β_2-Agonists such as albuterol should not be used prophylactically. **(A)** Pulmonology referral should be delayed until the patient fails appropriate management. If compliance to the appropriate therapy is established but the patient continues to be symptomatic, a referral may be warranted at that time. **(E)** Addition of a long-acting β_2-agonist could be considered if the patient in the vignette fails primary inhaled corticosteroid therapy.

---

25 A 14-year-old boy presents to the clinic with chest tightness, shortness of breath, and coughing for 2 weeks. The cough is usually worse at night. The patient recently moved to a new home, started a new school, and welcomed a new sibling along with a Chihuahua puppy. On physical examination, wheezing is audible on auscultation and his skin has a scaly rash on the flexor surfaces of the arms bilaterally.

Of the following, what pulmonary function test (PFT) results are most consistent with his most likely diagnosis?

(A) Increased forced expiratory volume in 1 second (FEV_1)/forced vital capacity of the lungs (FVC) with decreased diffusional lung capacity of carbon monoxide (DLCO)
(B) Decreased FEV_1/FVC with decreased DLCO
(C) Increased FEV_1/FVC with increased or normal DLCO
(D) Normal FEV_1/FVC with normal DLCO
(E) Decreased FEV_1/FVC with increased or normal DLCO

The answer is E: **Decreased FEV_1/FVC with increased or normal DLCO.** The symptoms and physical examination of the boy in the vignette are most consistent with a diagnosis of asthma. Asthma is a disease characterized by IgE-mediated hypersensitivity and chronic inflammation of the airways leading to bronchospasm. The etiology of asthma is currently unknown but is attributable to both genetic and environmental factors. There is a strong correlation between asthma and atopic disease such as allergic rhinitis or eczema. The rash of the patient in the vignette suggests a diagnosis of eczema. Patients suspected to have asthma are often treated empirically, but PFTs can be used to assess asthma severity and may play a role in assessing risk of recurrence of asthma exacerbation.

Patients with asthma are unable to exhale forcefully secondary to increased airway resistance from bronchospasm. Therefore, their FEV_1 is reduced. Usually the total volume on forced exhalation called the FVC is unchanged in asthma resulting in a reduced FEV_1/FVC ratio. DLCO is reduced in patients with decreased alveolar surface area as seen in restrictive lung diseases. Patients with asthma, however, have normal alveolar spaces, so the DLCO is typically normal. **(C, E)** Increased DLCO can be seen in patients who have increased air trapping and hyperinflation of the lungs. When testing for asthma using PFTs it is customary to repeat the measurements after administering a bronchodilator. Improvement of FEV_1/FVC following bronchodilator use is a strong indication of asthma as the diagnosis. In general, the FEV_1/FVC ratio is often used to divide lung diseases into **(B, E)** obstructive lung diseases (decreased FEV_1/FVC) versus **(A, C)** restrictive lung diseases (increased FEV_1/FVC). Examples of obstructive lung diseases include asthma and bronchiectasis, while restrictive lung diseases include interstitial lung disease, muscular dystrophies, sarcoidosis, and idiopathic pulmonary fibrosis.

26 A 3-hour-old newborn is being evaluated for an increased respiratory rate. His respiratory rate was 70 breaths/min at birth and has remained 60 to 80 breaths/min. Oxygen saturation is 92% on pulse oximetry. On physical examination, the patient is tachypneic with nasal flaring. His lungs are clear to auscultation, though there is decreased air entry on the left side. Cardiac examination does not reveal a murmur. A chest radiograph reveals a large, radiolucent cavity in the upper to middle regions of the left lung and a mediastinal shift toward the right side.

Of the following, what is the most likely diagnosis?

(A) Congenital pulmonary adenomatoid malformation (CPAM)
(B) Bronchogenic cyst
(C) Pneumothorax
(D) Congenital lobar overinflation
(E) Diaphragmatic hernia

The answer is D: Congenital lobar overinflation. The presentation and findings of the baby in the vignette are consistent with congenital lobar overinflation, previously known as congenital lobar emphysema. In this disorder, there is overinflation of a segment of the lung, usually the left upper lobe. The etiology is not identified in most cases, though some are due to bronchial obstruction. Patients often present with respiratory distress of varying degrees. Chest radiography reveals a large, space-occupying, radiolucent area with a mediastinal shift (see *Figure 7-6*). A lateral film demonstrates a clear mediastinum. Treatment is surgical with a lobectomy.

(A) CPAM, previously known as congenital cystic adenomatoid malformation (CCAM), is caused by adenomatous overgrowth of terminal bronchioles. Children with CPAM can present in many ways, ranging from severe respiratory distress in the neonatal period to recurrent pneumonias as older children. Chest radiography reveals a mass containing air-filled cysts (see *Figure 7-7*). Treatment is surgical resection.

(B) Bronchogenic cysts present as recurrent infections. Patients can present with respiratory distress in the neonatal period, but that is usually due to the cyst being located near the carina, and impinging on the airway. Chest radiography demonstrates a sharply demarcated spherical mass in the mediastinum (see *Figure 7-8*). It is important to note that patients with

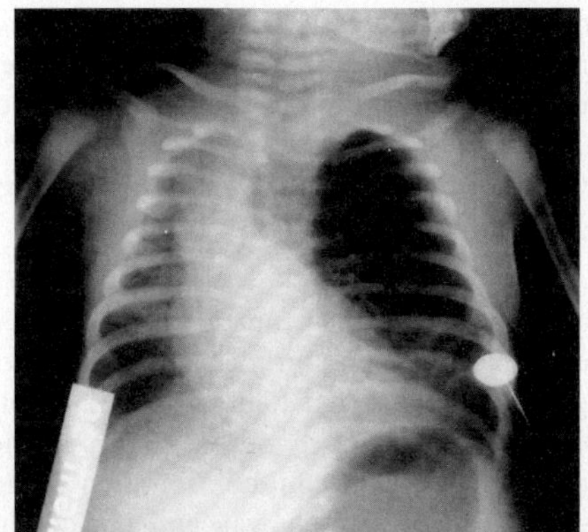

Figure 7-6

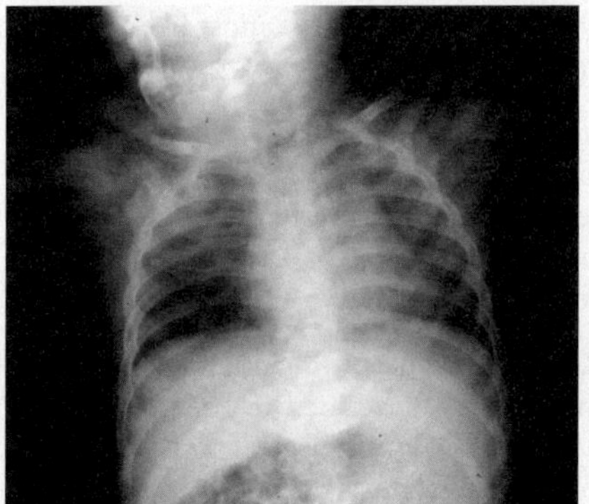

Figure 7-7

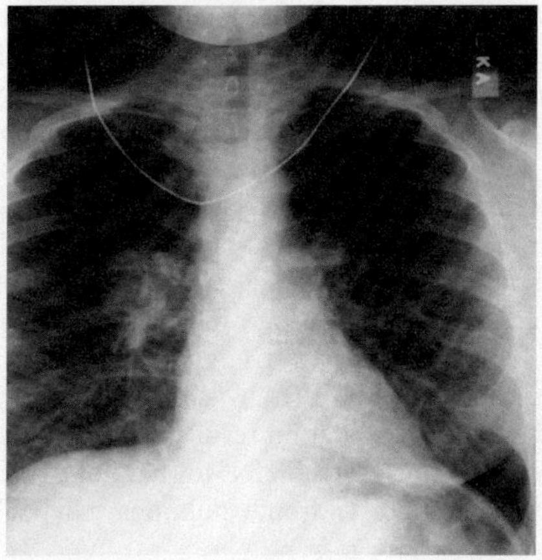

Figure 7-8

bronchogenic cysts are at an increased risk for cancerous changes within the cystic tissue and therefore surgical removal is recommended. **(E)** Diaphragmatic hernias present with respiratory distress and chest radiography findings of bowel in the chest cavity. **(C)** A pneumothorax would reveal a line indicating the visceral pleura with lack of lung markings peripheral to it on chest radiograph.

27 A 12-hour-old neonate is in the neonatal intensive care unit due to persistent cyanosis. Despite being on mechanical ventilation, 100% oxygen, and aggressive efforts, the patient's oxygen saturation ranges from 80% to 85%, he is still cyanotic, and has poor perfusion. Chest radiography is consistent with meconium aspiration syndrome. Echocardiogram reveals a patent foramen ovale and a patent ductus arteriosus (PDA) with right-to-left shunting without evidence of congenital heart defects.

Of the following, which is the most likely reason for this patient's poor oxygenation?

(A) Neonatal pneumonia
(B) Respiratory distress syndrome
(C) Persistent pulmonary hypertension of the newborn (PPHN)
(D) Sepsis
(E) Pulmonary hypoplasia

The answer is C: **Persistent pulmonary hypertension of the newborn (PPHN).** The findings described in the vignette are consistent with PPHN. PPHN, as the name implies, refers to the persistence of hypertension of the pulmonary vasculature leading to a persistent fetal circulatory state. In utero oxygenated blood received from the placenta bypasses the fetal lungs through the ductus arteriosus and then returns through the pulmonary veins to the left atrium to be circulated systemically. High pulmonary pressures ensure that oxygenated blood does not flow distally down the pulmonary arteries but is rather preferentially shunted through the ductus arteriosus. Under normal physiologic conditions, after the baby is born and the lungs fill with air, pulmonic resistance drops favoring blood flow from the pulmonary arteries past the ductus arteriosus to the lungs. Over a short time, the ductus arteriosus closes as less blood is shunted down this pathway. In PPHN, the pulmonary resistance remains high despite the presence of air in the lungs and blood continues to shunt through the ductus arteriosus, bypassing the lungs, and remains unoxygenated. The continued blood flow down the ductus results in a PDA with deoxygenated blood entering the left atrium and systemic circulation resulting in hypoxia.

There are many reasons for PPHN to develop, including neonatal asphyxia, meconium aspiration syndrome, pulmonary hypoplasia, congenital pneumonia, congenital cyanotic heart disease, hypothermia, and hypoglycemia. Meconium aspiration syndrome is one of the most common causes of PPHN. **(A, B, D, E)** Though the other choices can all cause PPHN, they are typically separate entities and not associated with meconium aspiration syndrome.

---

28 A 9-year-old girl is brought to the emergency department after being hit by a car while crossing the street. She has altered mental status and a laceration to her left temple. She was placed in a cervical spine collar in the ambulance. Cervical radiographic studies are pending. Currently the patient opens her eyes to verbal command, does not respond verbally, and withdraws her limbs to painful stimuli.

Of the following, what is the next best step in her management?

(A) Do not intubate the patient until the cervical radiographs have been reviewed
(B) Immediately intubate the patient using the head tilt technique
(C) Immediately intubate the patient using the jaw thrust technique
(D) Emergent tracheostomy
(E) Place the patient on a nonrebreather mask and consult a neurosurgeon

The answer is C: **Immediately intubate the patient using the jaw thrust technique.** The altered mental status for the patient in the vignette makes her a prime candidate for immediate intubation. **(A)** Intubation should not be delayed while awaiting radiography results, as an airway must be secured before potential complications occur. **(B)** In most situations, the head tilt maneuver is the most common method for intubation; however, this technique places increased strain on the spinal cord. The patient in the vignette's neck should be maintained in a neutral position until a cervical spine injury is ruled out. **(C)** For this reason, a jaw thrust maneuver is preferred for intubation in the case in the vignette. **(D)** Tracheostomy is warranted in cases of severe damage to the face and suspected fractures to the face that would complicate safe intubation. **(E)** A nonrebreather mask is inappropriate in an altered patient such as the patient in the vignette who cannot protect her airway.

---

29 A 15-year-old patient presents with a productive cough and fever for 5 days. A chest radiograph reveals a right lower lobe consolidation with pleural effusion as seen in Figure 7-9. Gram-stain of the sputum shows gram-positive cocci in pairs.

Of the following, which organism is most likely responsible for this patient's pneumonia?

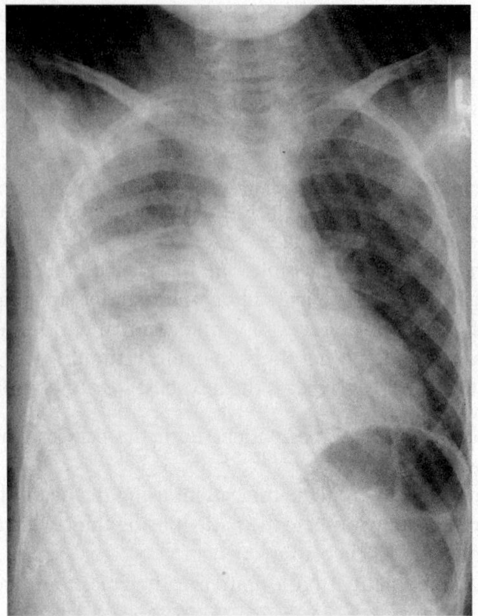

Figure 7-9

(A) *Moraxella catarrhalis*
(B) *Streptococcus pneumoniae*
(C) *Staphylococcus aureus*
(D) *Haemophilus influenzae*
(E) *Escherichia coli*

The answer is B: *Streptococcus pneumoniae.* The patient in the vignette has a bacterial lobar pneumonia. Common pathogens include *Streptococcus pneumoniae, M. catarrhalis, Staphylococcus aureus*, and *H. influenzae. E. coli* can cause a lobar pneumonia usually through aspiration of gastrointestinal contents. **(B)** *Streptococcus pneumoniae* is characterized by gram-positive cocci in pairs or chains. **(A)** *M. catarrhalis* is characterized by gram-negative diplococci. **(C)** Gram-positive cocci in clusters are characteristic of *Staphylococcus aureus.* **(D)** *H. influenzae* is characterized by gram-negative coccobacilli and **(E)** *E. coli* is characterized by gram-negative bacilli.

30 A 9-month-old infant presents to the clinic for the first time. His parents report that he has a history of noisy breathing since birth and gastroesophageal reflux for as long as they can remember. His previous pediatrician was treating him with ranitidine for his reflux. The parents have not noticed any improvement in his noisy breathing or reflux, but are concerned that his reflux is worsening. According to his parents, he has never had any studies performed to evaluate either condition. A barium swallow study reveals an indentation in the esophagus, with no evidence of gastroesophageal reflux.

Of the following, what is the most likely cause of this patient's symptoms?

(A) Tracheoesophageal fistula
(B) Asthma
(C) Tracheomalacia
(D) Laryngomalacia
(E) Vascular ring

The answer is E: Vascular ring. The presentation and history described for the patient in the vignette are most consistent with a vascular ring. Vascular rings present with stridor secondary to tracheal compression, and emesis, choking, or dysphagia due to esophageal compression. The most common type of vascular ring is a right-sided aortic arch with a persistent left-sided ductus arteriosus and aberrant left subclavian artery, which complete a ring around the trachea. A double aortic arch causes another type of vascular ring. Diagnosis may be delayed for some time due to relatively mild symptoms. Imaging studies confirm the presence of a vascular ring. A right-sided aortic arch may be visible on plain chest radiography due to the location of the aortic knob. Chest computed tomography and magnetic resonance imaging can accurately delineate the type of vascular ring present. A video swallow or a barium swallow, as described in the vignette, suggests the presence of a vascular ring due to the indentation seen in the esophagus. Treatment is surgical.

(A) Most tracheoesophageal fistulas (TEF) present shortly after birth. The most rare type, a type H TEF, may present with recurrent pneumonias and a chronic cough later in life. **(B)** Asthma does not present at birth and would be unlikely in the patient in the vignette given his history and radiographic findings. **(C, D)** Tracheomalacia and laryngomalacia produce stridor that typically improves with age.

---

31 Of the following, which is expected to shift the oxygen dissociation curve to the right?

(A) Decreased body temperature
(B) Increased blood levels of 2,3-diphosphoglyceric acid
(C) Alkalotic states
(D) Methemoglobinemia
(E) Carbon monoxide poisoning

The answer is B: Increased blood levels of 2,3-diphosphoglyceric acid. The oxygen dissociation curve shows the percentage of oxygenated hemoglobin (Hb) as a function of the partial pressure of oxygen in the blood. The normal curve is shown in Figure 7-10. Note then when the curve is shifted

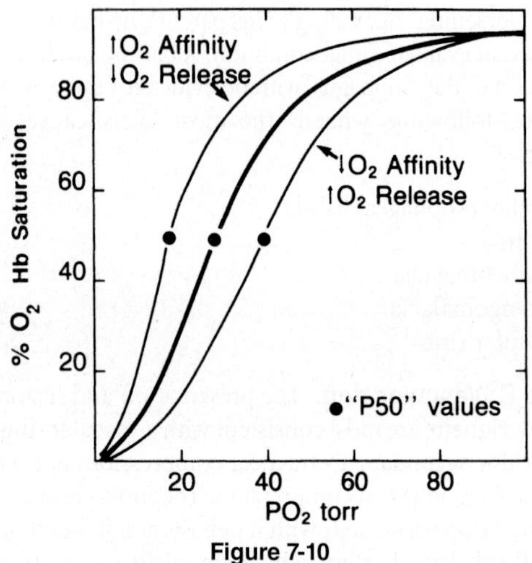

Figure 7-10

to the right, the percentage of Hb decreases for a given partial pressure of oxygen indicating decreased affinity of Hb for oxygen. This decreased affinity for oxygen allows more oxygen to be delivered to tissues that need it rather than remaining tightly bound to Hb. Oxygen bound to Hb cannot interact with metabolically active tissues and provide oxygen for cellular respiration. Several factors can shift the normal oxygen dissociation curve left or right, but perhaps the easiest way to remember at least some of them is to consider the exercise state.

During exercise, the tissues need increased oxygen and are aided by a shift of the curve to the right. The body's temperature increases and lactic acid builds up. Not surprisingly, decreased pH, increased body temperature, increased CO_2 (which leads to an acidotic state) all shift the oxygen dissociation curve to the right. **(A, C)** Contrarily, increased pH, decreased CO_2, or decreased body temperature shift the O_2-dissociation curve to the left.

Other important factors that influence the curve are carbon monoxide poisoning and methemoglobinemia. **(E)** Carbon monoxide binds Hb changing its shape and increasing the affinity for O_2 (hence a left shift in the curve). This results in less peripheral oxygen unloading and physiologic hypoxic states.

(D) Methemoglobinemia occurs when the iron atom in the heme molecule is oxidized to the ferric state. This results in increased affinity of Hb for oxygen and decreased unloading of O_2 into the periphery (hence a left shift in the O_2-dissociation curve). Interestingly, the ferric state of Hb binds cyanide with high affinity, so one method for treating cyanide poisoning is to induce a state of methemoglobinemia.

The red blood corpuscles of the body produce a chemical called 2,3-diphosphoglyceric acid (2,3-DPG), which binds to the β-subunit of Hb and decreases the Hb affinity for oxygen (shifts the curve to the right).

This increases oxygen unloading to the tissues. Fetal Hb is composed of two α-subunits and two γ-subunits and is not affected by 2,3-DPG; however, adult Hb (composed of two α- and two β-subunits) is affected. During pregnancy, the placenta produces 2,3-DPG which increases oxygen unloading from adult Hb at the placenta, aiding in the oxygenation of fetal Hb (which is naturally shifted to the left as compared to adult Hb) allowing for oxygen delivery to the developing fetus.

32 A 10-year-old girl is in the emergency department with an acute asthma exacerbation. She is wheezing audibly and is unable to speak in full sentences. She has already received 3-hour-long nebulizer treatments, each with 10 mg albuterol, 60 mg of corticosteroid, and has not improved. The patient's respiratory rate is 40 breaths/min and shallow and she is using accessory muscles to breath. Her oxygen saturation is 81% and she is somnolent and does not respond to questions.

Of the following, what is the next step in her management?

(A) Begin theophylline therapy
(B) Place an endotracheal tube (ET)
(C) Intravenous corticosteroid therapy
(D) Magnesium sulfate 50 mg/kg IV
(E) Increase albuterol dose to 20 mg instead of 10 mg

The answer is B: Place an endotracheal tube (ET). The patient in the vignette is rapidly going into respiratory failure as evidenced by her decreasing oxygen saturation and altered mental status. In addition to her accessory muscle use and her inability to speak in full sentences, she has altered mental status and is becoming somnolent. When a patient's mental status begins to deteriorate secondary to poor gas exchange with hypoxia and hypercarbia, their ability to maintain an open airway becomes compromised. No matter how much therapy is given for an acute asthma exacerbation, if a patient cannot maintain an open airway, they will not recover proper gas exchange.

(A, C, D, E) The patient in the vignette is likely to continue receiving albuterol treatments through the ET and possibly will receive adjunctive therapies such as magnesium sulfate, corticosteroids, and theophylline; however, intubating the patient in the vignette in order to maintain a secure airway must be a priority in this scenario.

33 A 15-year-old boy presents with fever, malaise, and worsening cough for 8 days. On examination, his vital signs are respiratory rate 24 breaths/min, heart rate 95 beats/min, and he has a temperature of 40.1°C orally. On auscultation, there are diffuse crackles. His chest radiograph is pictured in Figure 7-11.

Of the following, his presentation is most consistent with which infectious agent?

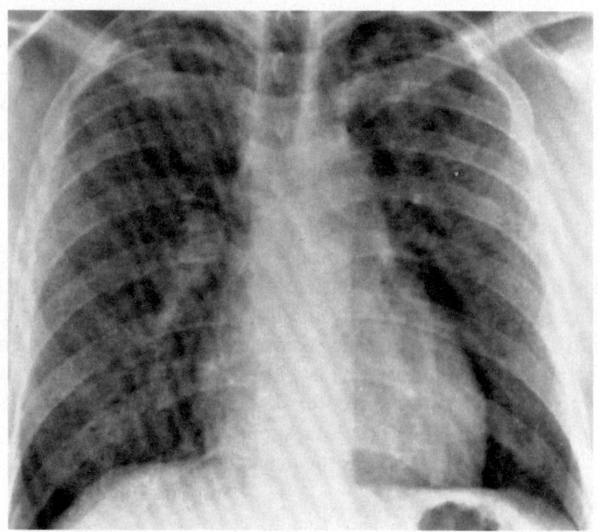

Figure 7-11

(A) *Streptococcus pneumoniae*
(B) *Staphylococcus aureus*
(C) *Mycoplasma pneumoniae*
(D) Adenovirus
(E) Influenza

The answer is C: *Mycoplasma pneumoniae.* *M. pneumoniae* is a common cause of community-acquired pneumonia. It is often referred to as atypical pneumonia or walking pneumonia. Patients typically present with fever and dry cough of days to weeks in duration, as well as fatigue and malaise. Development of symptoms is insidious, and patients can have symptoms for weeks before seeking medical help. **(A, B)** Pneumonias caused by *Streptococcus pneumoniae* and *Staphylococcus aureus* are also associated with fever, cough, and malaise; however, the symptoms are more abrupt and severe in presentation. Chest radiographic findings reveal lobar consolidations.

(D, E) Viral infections such as influenza and adenovirus are typically self-limited. While presentation can be similar to an infection with *M. pneumoniae*, symptoms improve after several days without therapy.

---

34 An 18-month-old boy presents to the clinic with complaints of cough, runny nose, fever, and red eyes for the past 2 days. His mother notes that the boy's symptoms have not improved and he developed a diffuse, red rash. On examination, he is nontoxic appearing with a temperature of 38.8°C, heart rate of 125 beats/min, and respiratory rate of 20 breaths/min. He has a diffuse, erythematous, blanching rash.

Of the following, which virus is the most likely cause of his constellation of symptoms?

(A) Rhinovirus
(B) Coxsackie virus
(C) Influenza virus
(D) Respiratory syncytial virus (RSV)
(E) Adenovirus

The answer is E: Adenovirus. The boy in the vignette has findings consistent with infection with adenovirus. Adenovirus is characterized by cough, rhinorrhea, erythematous rash, conjunctivitis, erythema of the oropharynx, and can cause cystitis and gastroenteritis. **(A)** Rhinovirus is the virus responsible for the illness often referred to as the common cold and is characterized by fever, rhinorrhea, and cough. **(B)** Coxsackie virus is responsible for hand-foot-and-mouth disease, which presents with sores in the mouth and a rash on the hands and feet as seen in Figure 7-12. **(C)** Influenza presents with high fevers, fatigue, and malaise, as well as cough and rhinorrhea. **(D)** RSV produces symptoms of the common cold, although can cause severe respiratory distress in infants.

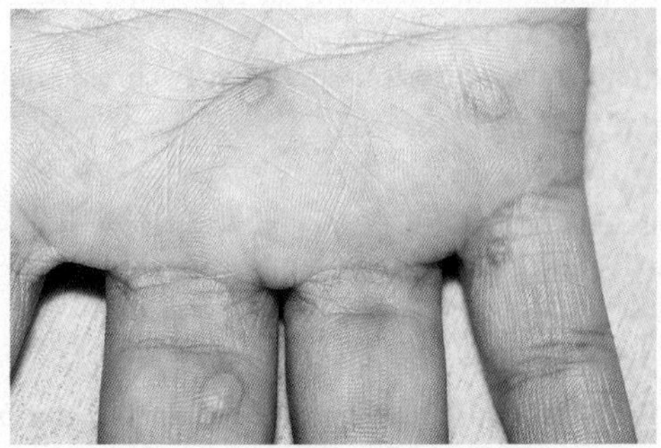

Figure 7-12

---

35 The parents of a 7-year-old boy bring him to the office for concern of white spots in his mouth. The spots began 2 days ago and are not associated with fever or pain. Aside from a history of asthma for which he uses a daily inhaled corticosteroid and a β_2-agonist as needed, he has no other significant medical history.

Of the following, what is the best advice to give his parents?

(A) Recommend the patient undergo immunodeficiency testing
(B) Supervise the patient's teeth-brushing sessions
(C) Discontinue use of the inhaled corticosteroids and albuterol
(D) Begin preventative antifungal oral rinses
(E) Recommend the patient rinse his mouth after every administration of inhaled corticosteroid

The answer is E: **Recommend the patient rinse his mouth after every administration of inhaled corticosteroid.** Prolonged use of inhaled corticosteroid can cause oral candidiasis, or thrush. Chronic use of steroids causes impaired immunity against microbes in the mouth, including viruses, bacteria, and fungi. Rinsing the mouth after inhaled corticosteroid dosing and the use of a spacer have been shown to decrease rates of oral candidiasis.

(A) Though thrush is uncommon at this age, the patient in the vignette is otherwise healthy and takes a medication that is associated with oral candidiasis; thus, he does not warrant immunodeficiency testing. **(B)** While proper tooth brushing should always be encouraged, improper tooth brushing is not associated with thrush. **(C)** The patient in the vignette should continue his asthma medications, as they are extremely important to his health. **(D)** Preventative antifungals are not used to prevent thrush in patients with asthma.

---

36 A 10-year-old boy with a history recurrent sinusitis and chronic productive cough presents with an acute worsening of his cough. On examination, his height and weight are less than the third percentile. Pulmonary examination reveals fair air exchange and coarse breath sounds throughout with crackles in the right lower lobe. His distal phalanges are rounded and bulbous.

Of the following, which is the most likely chronic finding on chest radiography?

(A) Solitary cavitary lesion
(B) Diffuse dilation and thickening of the bronchi
(C) Focal dilation and thickening of the bronchi
(D) Perihilar infiltrates
(E) Multiple cysts

The answer is B: **Diffuse dilation and thickening of the bronchi.** The patient in the vignette presents with signs and symptoms consistent with Cystic fibrosis (CF). Patients with CF commonly have radiographic signs of chronic bronchiectasis, an abnormal dilation of the airways. This is caused by scarring of the airway and lung parenchyma. The differential diagnosis for bronchiectasis is divided based on the type of bronchiectasis, either diffuse or focal. **(C)** Focal bronchiectasis can be found after an infection such as pneumonia or tuberculosis (TB) infection. **(B)** Diffuse bronchiectasis is seen in diseases like CF, primary ciliary dyskinesia, human immunodeficiency virus, and recurrent aspiration syndromes.

(A) Fungal pneumonia and TB may cause local bronchiectasis from scarring, but do not typically cause diffuse bronchiectasis. **(E)** Congenital pulmonary adenomatoid malformation (CPAM) is a congenital anomaly of the lung, in which a part of the lung is replaced by cystic, nonfunctional lung tissue. CPAM appears as a large cystic lesion on computed tomography scan. **(D)** Perihilar infiltrates are changes on chest radiography often associated with viral pneumonia. The description of the patient in the vignette is chronic and not consistent with an acute viral pulmonary infection.

37 A healthy 13-month-old infant presents to the clinic for his well-child visit. He is up-to-date on his immunizations but has never received the influenza vaccine due to a history of hives associated with egg ingestion.

Of the following which is the best recommendation for this patient regarding influenza vaccination?

(A) Single intramuscular dose of the inactivated influenza vaccine or a single intranasal dose of the live attenuated influenza vaccine (LAIV)
(B) Single intranasal dose of the LAIV followed by a second dose 28 days later
(C) Single intramuscular dose of the inactivated influenza vaccine followed by a second dose 28 days later
(D) The influenza vaccine is contraindicated in this patient
(E) Defer vaccination in this patient until he is 4 years old

The answer is C: Single intramuscular dose of the inactivated influenza vaccine followed by a second dose 28 days later. **(E)** Starting at 6 months of age, children should receive yearly influenza vaccination. There are two formulations of the influenza vaccine approved for use in children in the United States, the inactivated influenza vaccine and the LAIV. These vaccines are targeted against strains of influenza that research indicates will be prevalent in a specific season, and usually include strains from influenza B and influenza A (e.g., H1N1 and H3N2).

The inactivated influenza vaccine is approved for use in children aged 6 months to 18 years. **(B)** The LAIV is approved for use in children aged 2 to 18 years. **(A)** In children under 8 years of age who have not previously received the influenza vaccine, 2 doses of the vaccine must be given at least 28 days apart. The LAIV cannot be given to children with a history of asthma, chronic ear or lung disease, patients who are severely immunocompromised, or patients with chronic medical conditions.

The contraindications to the influenza vaccine are severe egg allergy or prior allergic reaction to the influenza vaccine. Patients reporting any of the following after egg consumption should not receive the vaccine: respiratory distress, angioedema, recurrent emesis, and lightheadedness; or patients who have required epinephrine for stabilization after egg ingestion (anaphylaxis). **(D)** Hives after egg ingestion are not considered a contraindication to the influenza vaccine. These patients should receive the vaccine administered by a healthcare professional and be monitored for at least 30 minutes after the vaccination.

38 A mother brings her 13-year-old son to the pediatrician for a school physical. The family recently emigrated from Mexico where they

resided with his grandfather. He states that he has been having a productive cough for several weeks for which a purified protein derivative (PPD) skin test is placed. On the return visit his skin test is indurated to 17 mm and a chest radiograph shows a right upper lobe infiltrate.

Of the following, what is the most appropriate treatment protocol for him?

(A) Isoniazid for 9 months
(B) Isoniazid, rifampin, ethambutol, and pyrazinamide for 2 months followed by 6 months of isoniazid and rifampin
(C) Isoniazid, rifampin, streptomycin, and pyrazinamide for 2 months followed by 6 months of isoniazid and rifampin
(D) Rifampin for 4 months
(E) Isoniazid plus rifampin for 3 months

The answer is B: **Isoniazid, rifampin, ethambutol, and pyrazinamide for 2 months followed by 6 months of isoniazid and rifampin.** The patient in the vignette has active tuberculosis (TB) as evidenced by the presence of symptoms, abnormal chest radiograph, and positive tuberculin PPD skin test. The treatment protocol for active TB, unlike latent TB infection, is a three- or four-drug regimen. Latent TB infection presents with a positive PPD without clinical symptoms or chest radiograph findings. Treatment for active TB is isoniazid, rifampin, ethambutol, and pyrazinamide for 2 months followed by 6 months of isoniazid and rifampin.

(C) Streptomycin is reserved for refractory TB or TB meningitis and is never used as an initial treatment option. **(A, D, E)** Treatment with isoniazid for 9 months, rifampin for 4 months, or isoniazid plus rifampin for 3 months are options for treatment of latent TB.

A 6-month-old born at 26 weeks' gestation presents to the emergency department with increased work of breathing. He was discharged home from the neonatal intensive care unit requiring supplemental oxygen. His parents report he has had a cough and rhinorrhea for 2 days that has been worsening since the morning of presentation, requiring more oxygen to maintain adequate saturation. On physical examination, he has nasal flaring, retractions, and tachypnea. Chest radiograph reveals many small cystic areas throughout, with areas of hyperinflation and atelectasis.

Of the following, which is the most likely cause for these findings?

(A) Respiratory syncytial virus (RSV) infection
(B) Chronic pneumonia
(C) Severe chronic asthma
(D) Bronchopulmonary dysplasia (BPD)
(E) Fungal pneumonia

The answer is D: Bronchopulmonary dysplasia (BPD). The description of the chest radiograph of the patient in the vignette is consistent with BPD. BPD is a clinical diagnosis given to neonates that are oxygen dependent past 36 weeks postconceptual age and have characteristic clinical and radiographic findings. The clinical findings of BPD are a continual oxygen requirement, hypercapnia with compensatory metabolic alkalosis, poor growth, pulmonary hypertension, and development of right-sided heart failure. The radiographic findings typically include cystic areas with hyperinflation and atelectasis, which give the lung parenchyma a sponge-like appearance. BPD develops as a result of lung injury following treatment for respiratory distress syndrome (RDS). Treatment for RDS includes oxygen and mechanical ventilation. High concentrations of oxygen are damaging to the lungs and generate free radicals, superoxides, and hydrogen peroxide, all of which disrupt membrane lipids. Mechanical ventilation with increased pressures causes barotrauma, worsening the effect of the oxygen toxicity.

Infants with BPD are particularly susceptible to respiratory infections that can often trigger respiratory distress, especially infections caused by RSV. RSV infection in patients with BPD has a high morbidity and mortality rate. **(A, B, E)** While RSV or any other respiratory illness, like pneumonia, can trigger acute respiratory distress in patients with BPD, the radiographic findings of the patient in the vignette are most consistent with changes from BPD. **(C)** Severe chronic asthma is an unlikely diagnosis for a patient who is younger than 1 year of age.

40 A 3-year-old boy presents with cough and difficulty breathing. As per his parents, he has had a cough and cold symptoms for 2 days, which have gradually worsened. On the morning of presentation, they noticed that he was wheezing and his cough was severe, prompting an emergency department visit for evaluation. On examination, his respiratory rate is 45 breaths/min with no retractions or nasal flaring. On auscultation, there is a harsh noise on inspiration, heard best over the neck.

Of the following, what is his most likely diagnosis?

(A) Acute bronchospasm due to a viral illness
(B) Foreign body aspiration
(C) Epiglottitis
(D) Laryngotracheobronchitis
(E) Pneumonia

The answer is D: Laryngotracheobronchitis. The patient in the vignette has laryngotracheobronchitis, or croup. The harsh noise heard on physical examination is consistent with stridor. Stridor is heard best near the upper airways and is usually caused by obstruction of the extrathoracic airway. Wheezing is a high-pitched noise produced by partial obstruction of the lower airways and is heard best during exhalation.

(B) Croup, foreign body aspiration, and epiglottitis can all cause stridor; however, the patient in the vignette has associated cough and cold symptoms that point to croup as the most likely diagnosis. **(C)** Epiglottitis is an acute inflammation of the glottis resulting from a bacterial infection with *Haemophilus influenzae* or *Staphylococcus aureus*. Patients present with severe symptoms of airway obstruction, such as drooling, sitting forward, or gasping for air. Epiglottitis is a pediatric emergency. **(A, E)** While pneumonia and acute bronchospasm are associated with wheezing, neither is expected to produce stridor.

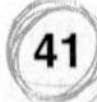

41 A 16-year-old boy with cystic fibrosis (CF) presents with a prolonged nose bleed. He reports a diet consisting of fast food, soda, and frequent high-fat snacks. He has been hospitalized four times in the past 6 months for CF exacerbations.

Of the following, which vitamin is most likely responsible for his chief complaint?

(A) Vitamin A
(B) Vitamin D
(C) Vitamin E
(D) Vitamin K
(E) Thiamine

The answer is D: Vitamin K. Patients with CF have a mutation in the gene encoding a transmembrane chloride ion channel. Inability to excrete chloride results in thicker secretions than usual. In the lungs, this leads to the classic symptoms of cough with thick, sticky secretions and repeated lung infections. In the pancreas, it leads to CF-related diabetes and decreased production of exocrine pancreatic enzymes such as pancreatic lipase necessary for breaking down ingested fat. This inability to breakdown and absorb fat in the diet leads to poor weight gain and fat-soluble vitamin deficiency. Fat-soluble vitamins therefore need to be supplemented in patients with CF. Vitamins A, D, E, and K are fat soluble.

The patient in the vignette appears poorly controlled and likely has a deficiency in all fat-soluble vitamins. **(A, B, C)** Only vitamin K plays a role in coagulation and is therefore the most likely cause of his prolonged epistaxis. **(E)** Thiamine does not participate in the clotting cascade.

42 A neonate is having breathing difficulties. The baby was born via normal spontaneous vaginal delivery 2 hours prior with Apgar scores that were 9 and 9, at 1 and 5 minutes, respectively. The nurse notes that the baby seems to gasp for air when lying down but appears well when picked up or lying in the prone position. On examination, he has a small cleft in his palate and his mandible is small. The remainder of his physical examination is unremarkable.

Of the following, what disorder best describes this patient?

(A) Goldenhar syndrome
(B) Pierre-Robin sequence
(C) Mandibulofacial dysostosis
(D) Beckwith-Wiedemann syndrome
(E) Fetal alcohol syndrome

The answer is B: Pierre-Robin sequence. The presentation of the patient in the vignette is consistent with Pierre-Robin sequence. The defects in Pierre-Robin are due to failure of the mandible to grow during the first weeks of gestation resulting in micrognathia. This in turn causes the tongue to be in an abnormal position during development leading to a U-shaped cleft. Infants with Pierre-Robin typically have feeding problems, obstructive apnea, and airway obstruction. The airway obstruction is relieved when lying in the prone position; however, infants often require nasal tube to maintain a patent airway. Feeding difficulties are common and require special feeding instruments. Once the airway and feeding issues are resolved in infancy, patients with Pierre-Robin can lead normal lives.

(A) Goldenhar syndrome is characterized by improper unilateral development of the ear, mandible, nose, lip, and palate. Affected patients have similar problems to those with Pierre-Robin but have other visible anomalies, such as lip anomalies, microtia, and preauricular skin tags. **(C)** Mandibulofacial dysostosis, also known as Treacher-Collins syndrome, is a rare, autosomal dominant disorder. It is characterized by craniofacial abnormalities that include absence of cheek bones, downward slanting eyes, micrognathia, conductive hearing loss, and malformed or absent ears. **(D)** Beckwith-Wiedemann syndrome is characterized by macroglossia, macrosomia, midline abdominal wall defects such as umbilical hernia or omphalocele, ear anomalies, and neonatal hypoglycemia. **(E)** Fetal alcohol syndrome has typical facial features that include a smooth philtrum, thin upper lip, and small palpebral fissures.

A 17-year-old boy was found unresponsive in his room by his parents. When emergency medical system (EMS) arrived, they noted he had a pulse of 60 beats/min, was unresponsive to light touch, and had decreased respiratory effort. EMS initiated bag mask resuscitation. Upon presentation to the emergency department, he is still unresponsive. His examination reveals pinpoint pupils.

Of the following, which medications will most likely restore his respiratory drive?

(A) Flumazenil
(B) Naloxone
(C) *N*-Acetylcysteine
(D) Physostigmine
(E) Syrup of ipecac

The answer is B: **Naloxone.** The presentation of the patient in the vignette is consistent with an opioid overdose. Patients with an opioid overdose present with pinpoint pupils, respiratory depression, hypotension, hyporeflexia, and coma. Naloxone antagonizes opioid receptors and, as such, helps restore respiratory drive.

(A) Flumazenil is the antidote for benzodiazepine toxicity by antagonizing benzodiazepine receptors. Benzodiazepine toxicity can present with depressive symptoms such as apnea, sedation, hypotension, and depressed myocardial function. **(C)** *N*-Acetylcysteine is an agent that protects the liver by acting as a glutathione substitute and enhancing the nontoxic conjugation of acetaminophen. Acetaminophen overdose presents with nausea, vomiting, and delayed hepatic failure. **(D)** Physostigmine inhibits the destruction of acetylcholine by acetylcholinesterase and is the antidote for anticholinergic toxicity. Anticholinergic toxicity can present with delirium, fever, dry skin/mucosa, mydriasis, tachycardia, and urinary retention. **(E)** Syrup of ipecac induces emesis and is no longer recommended given the risk of aspiration and esophageal burns when vomiting harmful substances.

44 The parents of a 4-year-old girl are concerned about her chest. On examination, her chest is as pictured in Figure 7-13. She reports no respiratory complaints and is doing well otherwise.

Of the following, which is the best advice for her parents?

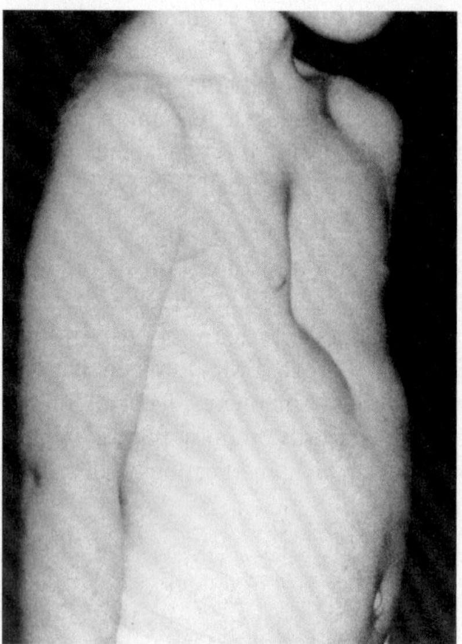

Figure 7-13

(A) Surgical correction is indicated if there is cardiopulmonary compromise
(B) She will outgrow this and there is no need for any intervention
(C) An external brace should be applied when the patient is over 6 years old
(D) Surgical correction is indicated immediately
(E) Sleeping in a prone position has been shown to be beneficial in reducing the deformity

The answer is A: **Surgery is indicated if there is cardiopulmonary compromise.** The patient in the vignette has pectus excavatum, the most common deformity of the chest wall. It is usually diagnosed at birth, and almost all cases are diagnosed within the first year of life. Cardiopulmonary compromise is the most important indication for surgical repair. Patients with cardiopulmonary compromise can present with shortness of breath and inability to perform physical activities. These symptoms usually appear during the teenage years. **(D)** Immediate surgical correction is not indicated for the patient in the vignette as she shows no signs of cardiopulmonary compromise. Another indication for surgical repair is cosmetic concern especially as it can lead to low self-esteem. This complication is often worse in women, whose breasts may develop asymmetrically because of the deformity. These patients may undergo elective repair prior to, during, or after puberty. **(C)** Bracing has not been shown to reduce the deformity and **(B)** pectus excavatum is not outgrown, in fact, it tends to worsen with age. **(E)** Infants should not be placed in the prone position to sleep, as prone sleeping has been associated with sudden infant death syndrome and will not change the pectus excavatum deformity.

45 A mother brings her 14-year-old son to the clinic. He has a past medical history significant for asthma and he reports he has been taking albuterol as needed. He describes having asthma exacerbations approximately twice per week with one of these episodes often occurring during the day and the other at night. He does not use his inhaler outside of these episodes and does not feel that he is having difficulty with normal physical activity.

Of the following, what is the best classification of his asthma?

(A) Mild persistent
(B) Mild intermittent
(C) Moderate persistent
(D) Severe persistent
(E) Severe intermittent

The answer is A: Mild persistent. For children older than 12 years of age, the National Asthma Education and Prevention Program (NAEPP) has categorized asthma severity as either intermittent (sometimes called mild intermittent) or persistent disease. Those with persistent disease can then be subdivided based on the level of severity into mild, moderate, or severe. The categorization depends upon several major factors including (1) the frequency of daytime symptoms, (2) the frequency of nighttime awakenings, (3) the frequency of rescue inhaler use for symptoms, (4) the level of interference with normal daily activities, and (5) the forced expiratory volume in 1 second/forced vital capacity of the lungs percent of predicted.

Based on the presence of nightly awakenings more than twice per month, the patient in the vignette meets criteria for mild persistent disease. See Table 7-1 for the specific classification of asthma severity.

Table 7-1 Classification of Asthma Severity

Components of Severity	Intermittent	Persistent: Mild	Persistent: Moderate	Persistent: Severe
Symptoms	≤2 d/wk	≥2 d/w but not daily	Daily	Throughout the day
Nighttime awakenings	≤2×/mo	3–4×/mo	>1×/wk but not nightly	Often 7×/wk
Short-acting β_2-agonist use for symptom control	≤2 d/wk	≥2 d/wk but not daily, and not more than once on any day	Daily	Several times per day
Interference with normal activity	None	Minor limitation	Some limitation	Extremely limited
Lung function	• Normal FEV_1 between exacerbations • FEV_1 > 80% predicted • FEV_1/FVC normal	• FEV_1 > 80% predicted • FEV_1/FVC normal	• FEV_1 > 60% but < 80% predicted • FEV_1/FVC reduced 5%	• FEV_1 < 60% but • FEV_1/FVC reduced > 5%

FEV_1, forced expiratory volume in 1 second; FVC, forced vital capacity of the lungs.

45 Of the following, what is the best treatment plan for the patient in the previous question?

(A) Long-acting β_2-agonist in addition to his rescue inhaler
(B) No change in medical management but follow-up in 3 months
(C) Leukotriene inhibitor and a medium-dose inhaled corticosteroid
(D) Low-dose inhaled corticosteroid in addition to his rescue inhaler
(E) Systemic corticosteroid

The answer is D: **Low-dose inhaled corticosteroid in addition to his rescue inhaler.** The patient in the vignette has poorly controlled mild persistent asthma. **(B)** He requires advancement of his treatment regimen with the addition of a low-dose inhaled corticosteroid as a controller medication.

(A) If he continues to have symptoms on the above regimen, addition of a long-acting β_2-agonist would be indicated. **(C)** Leukotriene inhibitor and a medium-dose inhaled corticosteroid is an appropriate regimen for moderate persistent asthma. **(E)** Systemic corticosteroids are given during an acute asthma exacerbation.

47 A 12-year-old patient presents for a new patient visit. His mother reports that he has a history of wheezing that has been managed with albuterol since the age of 5. On further history, his mother notes that he uses the albuterol two to three times per week and has been hospitalized once per year for wheezing, though he has never been admitted to the intensive care unit. He also wakes up at night two to three times a month with wheezing symptoms. On examination, he is well appearing and he has mild wheezing bilaterally, but says he does not feel short of breath.

Of the following, which best describes this patient's clinical course?

(A) The patient has asthma with some airway structural damage due to chronic, improperly treated symptoms
(B) The patient has exercise-induced asthma and has been adequately treated
(C) The patient has moderate persistent asthma with adequate treatment
(D) The patient does not have asthma; he likely has vocal cord dysfunction since he has never been placed on an inhaled corticosteroid
(E) The patient does not have asthma since he is not short of breath despite the wheezing auscultated on examination

The answer is A: **The patient has asthma with some airway structural damage due to chronic, improperly treated symptoms.** The patient in the vignette has a long history of improperly treated asthma. Asthma is an inflammatory process of the airways resulting from activation of inflammatory cells such as eosinophils, mast cells, neutrophils, and T lymphocytes, and inflammatory factors such as leukotrienes, histamine, bradykinin, and cytokines. This inflammation makes patients susceptible to attacks by allergens, viral infections, exercise, and irritants. These attacks cause constriction of the airways as well as edema, increased mucus production, and entry of inflammatory cells into the airways. If untreated, this process can lead to chronic inflammation and airway remodeling as well as irreversible structural changes in the lung and worsening pulmonary function.

(C, D, E) The patient in the vignette is classified as having mild persistent asthma. Treatment for patients with mild persistent asthma includes controller therapy with inhaled corticosteroids. **(B)** The patient in the vignette does not report that his symptoms worsen with response to exercise or stress.

48 A 17-year-old girl presents to the emergency department (ED) with acute shortness of breath. On examination, she appears to be in severe distress and is tachycardic and tachypneic, and her oxygen saturation is 100% on room air. She has some wheezing and stridor on auscultation. There are no retractions or accessory muscle use. She receives several inhaled β_2-agonist treatments. Her symptoms eventually resolve after prolonged observation in the ED. The patient reports several prior similar episodes. She has been managed on high-dose oral and inhaled corticosteroids, neither of which reduces the number or severity of these episodes.

Of the following, which diagnosis best describes her symptoms?

(A) Severe persistent asthma
(B) Allergic bronchopulmonary aspergillosis
(C) Exercise-induced asthma
(D) Vocal cord dysfunction (VCD)
(E) Laryngomalacia

The answer is D: **Vocal cord dysfunction (VCD).** The history and presentation for the patient in the vignette are most consistent with vocal cord paralysis or dysfunction. VCD is characterized by abnormal adduction of the vocal cords, especially during inspiration. This produces an obstruction to air flow at the level of the larynx. Patients with VCD typically present with sudden episodes of shortness of breath, hoarseness, wheezing, stridor, or inspiratory difficulty. The exact cause of VCD has not been determined, though there is an association with psychological illness. The acute episodes of VCD are typically self-limited and require minimal intervention, though heliox therapy has been shown to help. Often, VCD is confused with asthma and patients undergo treatment with corticosteroids and β_2-agonists without any improvement in their symptoms. Diagnosis is made through laryngoscopy and observation of the vocal cords during an inspiratory cycle. In the long term, techniques for prevention and management of future episodes can be learned though speech therapy and psychotherapy.

(A) Severe persistent asthma and exercise-induced asthma do improve with the use of corticosteroids and β_2-agonists. **(C)** Her symptoms are not reported to be exaggerated with exercise making exercise-induced asthma an unlikely diagnosis. **(B)** Allergic bronchopulmonary aspergillosis is caused by *Aspergillus* colonization of the lungs in a patient with a preexisting respiratory disease, such as asthma or cystic fibrosis. Patients typically have daily symptoms including chronic wheezing and cough. **(D)** Laryngomalacia is a condition that affects infants and is outgrown by 1 year of age.

49 A 14-year-old girl presents with malaise, fatigue, and throat pain. Her examination is significant for erythematous and enlarged tonsils as well as a palpable spleen tip. She was given amoxicillin for presumed bacterial pharyngitis, but subsequently was instructed to discontinue its use after she developed a diffuse maculopapular rash.

Of the following, which is the best test to confirm her most likely diagnosis?

(A) Liver function tests
(B) Complete blood count
(C) Heterophile antibody test
(D) Throat culture
(E) Clinical suspicion

The answer is C: **Heterophile antibody test.** A confirmatory test should be the test with the highest specificity. The higher a test's specificity, the lower its false positive rate. For example, a test with 100% specificity has a 0% false positive rate, so a positive test confirms the diagnosis with 100% accuracy.

The patient in the vignette has symptoms consistent with infectious mononucleosis. Infectious mononucleosis is caused by Epstein-Barr virus (EBV) and can be confirmed with the heterophile antibody test or EBV titers. The heterophile antibody test is highly specific for this disorder.

(A, B) Although liver function tests and complete blood counts may be abnormal in patients with infectious mononucleosis, they are not specific to this disease. **(D)** Throat culture is not useful in patients with viral infections, but would be specific for a patient with pharyngitis caused by bacterial organisms. **(E)** Clinical suspicion is useful in guiding a diagnostic and treatment plan, but is not as specific as the heterophile antibody test for mononucleosis.

50 During a routine health maintenance visit, the parents of a 2-year-old child state that they are moving to a house with a pool.

Of the following, what is the most appropriate anticipatory guidance that should be provided to this family regarding drowning prevention?

(A) Recommend installation of a fence around the yard with pool access only through the home
(B) Recommend installation of a fence around the pool with a self-closing and latching gate
(C) Do not allow children who cannot swim into the backyard
(D) Enroll children in swimming lessons
(E) Install an alarm on the pool gate

The answer is B: **Recommend installation of a fence around the pool with a self-closing and latching gate.** Drowning remains one of the major causes of death in children. The peak ages for drowning are the toddler years and adolescence. Younger children typically drown in the home. Infant drowning usually occur in bathtubs, either as a result of abuse or lapses in adult supervision. Toddlers often drown in swimming pools. Adolescent drowning often occurs in natural bodies of water and is associated with risk-taking behavior.

Submersion of a child leads to panic and aspiration of fluid. This in turn causes laryngospasm for protective measures, followed by relief of laryngospasm leading to flooding of the water into the lungs. Aspiration of large amounts of water into the lungs causes breakdown of surfactant and therefore inhibits alveolar capillary gas exchange resulting in hypoxemia and eventually cardiac arrest and hypoxic brain injury. Even if resuscitation occurs, the inhibition of alveolar capillary gas exchange leads to poor lung compliance and atelectasis, which, when severe enough, result in acute respiratory distress syndrome (ARDS). ARDS is an inflammatory process that leads to pulmonary edema due to leakage of proteinaceous fluid into the alveoli and interstitium and is associated with significant mortality.

(A, B) Enclosing pools with a four-sided, full perimeter fence with a self-closing, latching gate has been shown to reduce drowning rates in children. Adult supervision is recommended at all times. **(C, D, E)** Pool alarms, not allowing children in the pool area, or swimming lessons have not been shown to reduce drowning.

CHAPTER 8

Nephrology

RINKU PATEL

1 An 8-year-old boy with a history of minimal change disease presents to the emergency department with increasing facial edema. His mother states that these are similar symptoms to when he was first diagnosed, except this time he appears more ill, and he complains of abdominal pain and fever. He is currently on steroid treatment.

Of the following, which is the most common organism and condition responsible for this patient's presentation?

(A) *Escherichia coli*; spontaneous bacterial peritonitis (SBP)
(B) *Streptococcus pneumoniae*; SBP
(C) *Klebsiella pneumoniae*; appendicitis
(D) *Staphylococcus aureus*; appendicitis
(E) *Proteus mirabilis*; pyelonephritis

The answer is B: *Streptococcus pneumoniae*; SBP. A common complication for patients with nephrotic syndrome is an increased susceptibility to serious infections, such as bacteremia and SBP. Patients lose significant amounts of protein in the urine. This lost protein includes immunoglobulins, complement factors, and antibodies and can lead to immune compromise. Steroid dependency can also predispose these patients to an immunocompromised state. The most common microorganism seen in SBP in patients with nephrotic syndrome is *Streptococcus pneumoniae*, **(A)** followed by gram-negative bacteria such as *E. coli*. If there is a concern for SBP, appropriate antibiotic therapy should be initiated. **(D)** *Staphylococcus aureus* is a rare pathogen in the context of SBP.

(C, E) *Klebsiella pneumoniae* and *P. mirabilis* are generally not responsible for SBP. **(C, D, E)** Appendicitis and pyelonephritis are less likely given the patient in the vignette's presentation and history of nephrotic syndrome.

2 A 15-year-old boy presents to the clinic complaining of brown-colored urine for 1 day. He has recently started attending summer football camp. His daily activities include weightlifting, sprints, and push-ups.

He denies fevers, dysuria, or flank pain. He also denies any recent illness and does complain of muscle cramps following camp activities.

Of the following, which would most likely be found on this patient's urine studies?

(A) Dipstick: negative for blood; microscopy: 0 red blood cell and 0 white blood cell
(B) Dipstick: positive for blood; microscopy: 0 red blood cell and 0 white blood cell
(C) Dipstick: positive for blood; microscopy: 75 red blood cells and 0 white blood cell
(D) Dipstick: positive for blood; microscopy: 75 red blood cells and 75 white blood cells
(E) Dipstick: positive for leukocyte esterase; microscopy: 0 red blood cell and 75 white blood cells

The answer is B: **Dipstick: positive for blood; microscopy: 0 red blood cell and 0 white blood cell.** Rhabdomyolysis is the result of the breakdown products of large amounts of damaged skeletal muscle cells, such as myoglobin, phosphate, and creatinine kinase. This breakdown can be the result of many causes, including medications, drug abuse, infections, electrolyte abnormalities, or physical injury, including trauma and strenuous exercise. Symptoms of rhabdomyolysis include muscle pain, vomiting, fatigue, and confusion. These patients are also at risk for dysrhythmias and renal injury. Renal injury is generally due to an accumulation of myoglobin in the tubules leading to acute tubular necrosis. The urine color in rhabdomyolysis is typically brown due to the excreted myoglobin and can appear very similar to hematuria. **(A)** The dipstick test is positive for blood due to the test strip reagent's cross-reaction with myoglobin. **(C, D)** Unlike true hematuria, red blood cells are not seen on microscopy in patients with myoglobinuria. **(E)** Patients with urinary tract infections can have leukocyte esterase, nitrites, and/or blood in their dipstick, along with white and red blood cells visualized on microscopy.

3 A 2-month-old infant, new to the practice, presents for his immunizations. He has been in good health since birth and does not have any pertinent past medical history. On examination, a right flank mass is noted. On further questioning, his mother states that she has always felt that side to be fuller and it does not appear to bother him. She also states the infant has always had good wet diapers and describes a normal urinary stream.

Of the following, which is the most likely cause of his right flank mass?

(A) Posterior urethral valves (PUVs)
(B) Neuroblastoma
(C) Multicystic dysplastic kidney (MCDK)
(D) Bilateral renal agenesis
(E) Congenital pulmonary adenomatoid malformation

The answer is C: Multicystic dysplastic kidney (MCDK). MCDK is a common cause of an asymptomatic abdominal mass in the first few months of life. MCDKs are usually found incidentally during prenatal ultrasound evaluation. It is a condition where the kidney is replaced by cysts and does not retain any function. MCDK differs from polycystic kidney disease in that the latter condition retains some functioning kidney parenchyma. **(D)** Bilateral MCDK, similar to bilateral renal agenesis, is not compatible with life. The palpated mass is generally that of the enlarged cysts; however, over time the dysplastic kidney does involute. There is an association with vesicoureteral reflux in the normally functioning contralateral kidney.

(A) PUVs would be associated with bilateral hydronephrosis and manifest as bilateral flank masses on examination. The patient or parent also generally complains of other symptoms of urinary tract obstruction, such as a poor urinary stream. **(B)** Neuroblastoma may present as a flank mass but is less likely than cystic disease. **(E)** Congenital pulmonary adenomatoid malformation, previously called congenital cystic adenomatoid malformation, is a rare pulmonary malformation, which would not present as a flank mass.

During a delivery, the obstetrician is concerned about the significantly low level of amniotic volume for a baby that did not receive prenatal care. On delivery, the baby requires resuscitation immediately. Despite the effort from the team, the baby passes away. The neonatologist suggests the baby likely had pulmonary hypoplasia. On examination, the baby has a broad nose, compressed flat face, and significant limb contractures.

Of the following, which other finding is most likely to be found in this patient?

(A) Tetralogy of Fallot
(B) Single transverse palmar crease
(C) Bilateral renal agenesis
(D) Blueberry muffin rash
(E) Cataracts

The answer is C: Bilateral renal agenesis. The patient in the vignette with pulmonary hypoplasia likely has Potter sequence. The findings of this syndrome are due to bilateral renal agenesis or severe polycystic kidney disease. In utero, significant oligohydramnios occurs secondary to the poor production of urine. Pulmonary development is dependent upon appropriate volumes of amniotic fluid during the 16th to 24th week of gestation. As a result, the lungs do not fully develop, and the fetus is compressed, leading to significant contractures and typical Potter facies as described in the vignette. Often patients with Potter sequence are stillborn; those that do survive may eventually pass away from pulmonary insufficiency. **(A)** There is not an associated increased incidence of congenital heart disease.

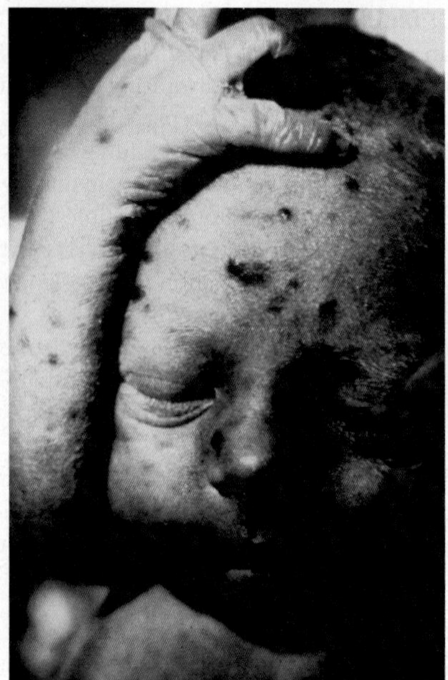

Figure 8-1

(B) A single transverse palmar crease is classically seen in trisomy 21. **(D)** A blueberry muffin rash (see *Figure 8-1*) is associated with TORCH infections, specifically cytomegalovirus and rubella, as a result of extramedullary hematopoiesis. **(E)** Cataracts may be found in metabolic syndromes, or with TORCH infections, specifically rubella.

---

5 A 4-month-old girl with no significant past medical history is hospitalized after 4 days of fever. The results of her partial septic workup reveal a urinary tract infection (UTI) with *Escherichia coli*. Antibiotics are initiated and her fevers have subsided. A renal ultrasound demonstrates that her right kidney is larger than her left.

Of the following tests, which is the next best step in evaluation of this patient?

(A) Voiding cystourethrogram
(B) Computed tomography scan of the abdomen and pelvis
(C) Cystoscopy
(D) 24-Hour urine collection
(E) Exploratory laparotomy

The answer is A: Voiding cystourethrogram. Based on the age and findings of a febrile UTI and abnormal renal ultrasound of the patient in the vignette, the patient warrants further evaluation for vesicoureteral reflux (VUR). VUR is an abnormal or retrograde movement of urine from the bladder into the ureters and/or kidneys. VUR can predispose patients to pyelonephritis, which can result in renal injury or scarring. The best test to evaluate VUR is a voiding cystourethrogram in which a catheter is placed through the urethra into the bladder, filled with contrast, and then monitored under fluoroscopy to look for abnormal retrograde flow from the bladder toward the kidneys. VUR is typically the result of abnormal valve insertion at the ureteral attachment to the bladder. There are five grades of reflux, and management can vary from supportive care to medical management to surgical intervention. Figure 8-2 illustrates the five grades of VUR.

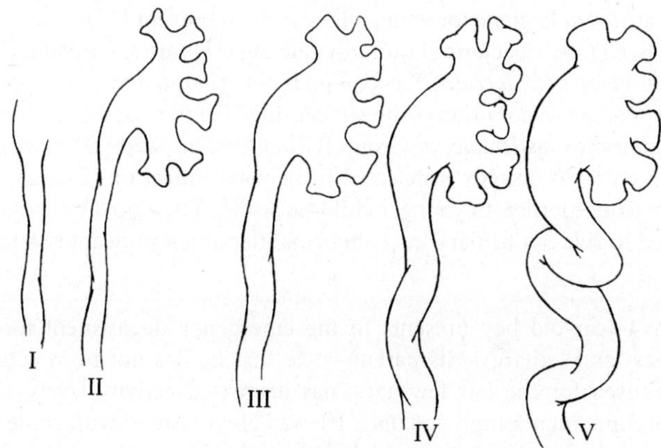

Figure 8-2

(B) A computed tomography scan would not provide superior information for the patient in the vignette and delivers a significant amount of radiation. **(D)** A 24-hour urine collection is not an appropriate test to evaluate for VUR. **(C, E)** Cystoscopy or exploratory laparotomy would be considered invasive tests and unnecessary.

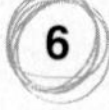

6 A 5-year-old girl is brought to the emergency department for abdominal pain and low-grade fever. She denies any nausea, vomiting, or diarrhea. She does report that she has been urinating more frequently and having discomfort with urination over the past 2 days. This is the first time she has experienced these types of symptoms. Urinalysis is positive for large bacteria, nitrites, and leukocyte esterase. A urine culture is pending.

Of the following, which is the most likely organism to grow on the urine culture?

(A) *Proteus mirabilis*
(B) *Staphylococcus saprophyticus*
(C) *Klebsiella pneumoniae*
(D) *Listeria monocytogenes*
(E) *Escherichia coli*

The answer is E: *Escherichia coli.* The most common pathogen to cause bacterial urinary tract infections (UTIs) is *E. coli*. In older children, UTIs generally result from an ascending infection of exterior fecal flora into the urinary tract. *E. coli* is unique from other microorganisms in the fecal flora because it has P-fimbriae, appendages on the bacterium that bacteria rely upon for adherence and attachment to uroepithelial cells. Given the risk of fecal flora, proper bathroom hygiene for young girls can help prevent UTIs.

(A, B, C) Other bacteria commonly causing UTIs are *P. mirabilis*, *K. pneumoniae*, *Enterococcus faecalis*, *Pseudomonas aeruginosa*, and *S. saprophyticus*. *S. saprophyticus* is a common pathogen causing UTI in sexually active teenagers. *Streptococcus agalactiae*, or Group B *Streptococcus*, and **(D)** *L. monocytogenes* are more commonly implicated in neonatal infections that are passed vertically from mother. In younger children with UTIs, a further workup may be needed to rule out urinary tract abnormalities as a significant risk factor.

7 A 4-year-old boy presents to the emergency department for weakness and lethargy. His parents state that he has not been acting like himself for the last few days, has decreased activity levels, and has become increasingly irritable. He was previously ill with some vomiting and diarrhea after a picnic last week. His parents are unclear the last time he urinated. His physical examination reveals pallor, edema, and a few scattered petechiae. His laboratory evaluation demonstrates a complete blood count and basic metabolic profile with the following results: white blood cell count of 10 × 10^3/μL, hemoglobin of 9.1 g/ dL and platelet count of 75 × 10^3/μL, sodium 136 mEq/L, potassium 4.0 mEq/L, chloride 100 mEq/L, carbon dioxide 24 mEq/L, blood urea nitrogen (BUN) 25 mg/dL, creatinine (Cr) 1.8 mg/dL, and glucose 108 mg/dL.

Of the following, what is this patient's most likely diagnosis?

(A) Hemolytic uremic syndrome (HUS)
(B) Sepsis
(C) Acute lymphoblastic leukemia
(D) Gastroenteritis due to rotavirus
(E) Systemic lupus erythematosus

The answer is A: Hemolytic uremic syndrome (HUS). The patient described in the vignette has findings of postinfectious HUS. The triad of microangiopathic hemolytic anemia, thrombocytopenia, and renal insufficiency classically characterizes HUS. The most common type is associated with a toxin-mediated response after an illness with bloody diarrhea. The two microorganisms most often associated with this condition are the verotoxin-producing *Escherichia coli* O157:H7 and the shiga toxin-producing *Shigella dysenteriae*. HUS can also be triggered by the neuraminidase-producing *Streptococcus pneumoniae* strain. The findings of HUS are the result of damaged endothelial cells that cause shearing of red blood cells, platelet aggregation and destruction, and decreased glomerular flow.

(B) Sepsis can present similarly, but the history of the recent diarrheal illness in the vignette makes HUS more likely. **(C, E)** The abrupt onset of symptoms following a diarrheal illness makes leukemia and systemic lupus erythematosus unlikely. **(D)** Complications from rotavirus are related to dehydration; abnormalities with red blood cells and platelets would not be expected.

8 An 11-year-old girl presents to the clinic with her concerned parents. She was recently at a school health fair where she was informed her blood pressure (BP) was elevated. Currently she is asymptomatic, and in the clinic has a normal BP and physical examination. She is significantly overweight, though her parents report they are working on her diet and activity level. All her previous BP readings in the office, including today, have been within normal limits.

Of the following, which is the most likely explanation for the high BP reading at the fair?

(A) White coat hypertension
(B) Coarctation of the aorta
(C) Inappropriate cuff size
(D) Acute glomerulonephritis
(E) Pheochromocytoma

The answer is C: Inappropriate cuff size. Hypertension in the asymptomatic pediatric patient is defined as BP measurements greater than the 95th percentile for age, gender, and height, on three separate occasions. Most children are asymptomatic, and therefore routine BP should be checked at every visit starting at the age of 3. The patient in the vignette is at risk for essential or primary hypertension based on her weight. However, if the BPs in the clinic have always been within normal limits, the most likely explanation for the high reading at the fair is an error in measurement.

BP in children should be measured in the sitting position after a period of being quiet. An appropriate cuff should cover at least two-thirds of the upper arm in width and the bladder should encircle 80% to 100% of the circumference of the upper arm. The patient in the vignette is overweight, and likely the cuff used at the fair was too small for her, therefore giving her a falsely elevated BP. **(A)** An elevated BP in the clinic and normal elsewhere would suggest white coat hypertension as the diagnosis. **(B, D, E)** Patients with secondary hypertension from underlying pathology such as coarctation of the aorta, acute glomerulonephritis, and pheochromocytoma would be expected to have persistently high BP measurements.

9 A 12-year-old boy complains of painless brown urine. He was seen recently for symptoms of upper respiratory illness, and discharged home with supportive care. He continues to have low-grade fevers controlled with antipyretics, along with a rhinorrhea, cough, and sore throat. On examination, he has inflamed turbinates and clear rhinorrhea. There is scant erythema without any exudates on his oropharynx. The rest of his examination is within normal limits. His BP is elevated compared with his last visit. His laboratory evaluation demonstrates a normal complete blood cell count, electrolytes and renal function, and complement levels. His urinalysis confirms hematuria.

Of the following, which condition is most likely responsible for this patient's presentation?

(A) Membranoproliferative glomerulonephritis (MPGN)
(B) Henoch-Schönlein purpura (HSP)
(C) Acute poststreptococcal glomerulonephritis (APSGN)
(D) Immunoglobulin A (IgA) nephropathy
(E) Lupus nephritis

The answer is D: Immunoglobulin A (IgA) nephropathy. The most likely cause for the findings of the patient in the vignette is IgA nephropathy. IgA nephropathy is one of the most common causes of chronic glomerular disease in children. Symptoms of gross hematuria occur concurrently with a viral infection such as an upper respiratory illness. **(C)** The hematuria of IgA nephropathy presents much earlier than that associated with APSGN. Patients with IgA nephropathy develop IgA deposits within the kidney that cause mesangial inflammation. The majority of the patients have a good prognosis, although rarely forms can progress to end-stage renal disease in adults. **(A)** Patients with MPGN do not have a prodrome such as a viral illness to cause hematuria and these patients have decreased complement levels. **(B)** Patients with HSP may go on to develop renal involvement identical to IgA nephropathy; however, the patient in the vignette does not have any of the other classic findings such as rash, arthritis, or abdominal pain. **(E)** Patients with lupus nephritis are expected to have decreased complement levels, along with other symptoms of systemic lupus erythematosus.

10 A 15-year-old boy presents to the clinic for a health maintenance visit. His mother is distraught over her father recently passing away from end-stage renal disease (ESRD). Upon further review of their family history, the patient reports his uncle also has problems with his kidneys. The patient states he does well in school but feels his hearing aid needs to be adjusted. Although he denies any urinary complaints, a urinalysis is positive for microscopic hematuria.

Of the following, which statement best describes the etiologic mechanism of his renal disease?

(A) IgA deposits causing mesangial inflammation
(B) Immune complex deposition in glomeruli after a recent illness
(C) Type IV collagen mutation affecting the basement membrane of glomeruli
(D) Antibodies to the basement membrane of glomeruli
(E) Chronic vesicoureteral reflux (VUR)

The answer is C: Type IV collagen mutation affecting the basement membrane of glomeruli. Alport syndrome, also known as hereditary nephritis, is a genetic disease caused by mutations in the genes coding for type IV collagen, a major component of the glomerular basement membrane. The majority of the mutations are passed along in an X-linked inheritance pattern; however, autosomal recessive and dominant mutations have also been described. Clinical findings of Alport syndrome include asymptomatic microscopic hematuria that can progress to ESRD, bilateral sensorineural hearing loss, and bowing of the lens capsule of the eye into the anterior chamber.

(A) IgA deposits are seen in both IgA nephropathy and Henoch-Schönlein purpura. **(B)** Immune complex deposition describes the mechanism of disease for postinfective glomerulonephritis. **(D)** Antibodies to the glomerular basement membrane describe the mechanism of disease for Goodpasture disease. **(E)** Chronic VUR is not associated with hearing loss.

11 A 7-year-old girl is admitted to the hospital after presenting to the emergency department with high fevers, chills, nausea, vomiting, and flank pain. She is diagnosed with pyelonephritis and gentamicin therapy is initiated secondary to a history of anaphylaxis to penicillin. Two days later, she no longer has fevers, vomiting, or flank pain, but is found to have a brown discoloration of her urine. Her BP on admission was 95/60 mmHg and now is 118/82 mmHg. Upon review of her records for the last 24 hours, her urine output has decreased significantly. Her urinalysis reveals red blood cells and granular casts and her complete blood cell count is within normal limits.

Of the following, which is the most likely cause for this patient's findings?

(A) Significant dehydration
(B) Ureteral obstruction
(C) Unresponsive pyelonephritis
(D) Acute tubular necrosis (ATN)
(E) Hemolytic uremic syndrome (HUS)

The answer is D: Acute tubular necrosis (ATN). The patient in the vignette is initially diagnosed with pyelonephritis, a bacterial infection of the upper urinary tract affecting the kidney, but has now developed signs of acute renal failure (ARF) with decreased urine output. The most likely cause for the patient in the vignette is ATN due to gentamicin therapy. ARF can be caused by pre-renal, intrinsic, or post-renal pathology. Significant dehydration and shock are examples of pre-renal causes of ARF. **(A)** Since the patient in the vignette was receiving intravenous fluids without further emesis, dehydration would be an unlikely cause of ARF. Nephrotoxic medications, such as aminoglycosides, can damage the tubules of the kidney and lead to ATN, an example of an intrinsic cause of renal failure.

(B, C) As the initial symptoms of the patient in the vignette have improved, it would be unlikely that she has a worsening infection or renal stone causing ureteral obstruction. **(E)** HUS can cause renal insufficiency and decreased urine output after an infection, most commonly a gastrointestinal illness. Without reports of abnormalities with red blood cells and platelets, this diagnosis is unlikely. Post-renal pathology includes obstructive conditions such as nephrolithiasis and ureteropelvic junction obstruction.

12 An 8-year-old boy with decreased urine output is diagnosed with acute renal failure (ARF). His blood urea nitrogen (BUN) and creatinine (Cr) are 28 and 1.2 mg/dL, respectively.

Of the following, which is the most likely cause for his ARF?

(A) Nephrotic syndrome
(B) Severe dehydration
(C) Acute poststreptococcal glomerulonephritis (APSGN)
(D) Acute tubular necrosis (ATN)
(E) Lupus nephritis

The answer is B: Severe dehydration. ARF is a clinical condition in which there is a sudden decrease in glomerular filtration rate and tubular function. This condition often manifests as a sudden decrease in urine output. Finding the cause of ARF relies upon history, physical examination, and blood work, such as urine electrolytes, fractional excretion of sodium (FE_{Na}), and BUN to serum Cr ratio. ARF is caused by etiologies that are pre-renal, intrinsic, or post-renal. In pre-renal causes, the FE_{Na} is typically found to be less than 1%

and the BUN to Cr ratio is greater than 20. The most common cause for this is dehydration. The patient in the vignette demonstrates laboratory results consistent with pre-renal failure, most likely from dehydration.

With intrinsic causes of ARF, the FE_{Na} is typically greater than 1% and the BUN to Cr ratio is less than 20. **(A, C, D, E)** Acute glomerulonephritis (such as poststreptococcal and lupus), nephrotic syndrome, and ATN are examples of intrinsic causes. Post-renal causes of ARF are secondary to obstruction of the urinary tract. Laboratory findings are variable in post-renal pathology; instead, imaging would be a more useful modality to establish diagnosis.

---

13 A 14-year-old boy with no significant past medical history presents to clinic for his yearly health maintenance visit. He states he has been in good health since his last visit, with no recent illnesses or hospitalizations. His vital signs and physical examination are within normal limits; however, his screening urinalysis is significant only for proteinuria. On further questioning, he denies any intense exercise, fevers, episodes of dehydration, or seizure-like activity in the last few weeks.

Of the following, which is the best next step in the workup of his proteinuria?

(A) Send urine culture and start antibiotics for possible urinary tract infection (UTI)
(B) Arrange for a renal biopsy
(C) Obtain serum electrolytes and renal ultrasound
(D) Refer to pediatric nephrology for consultation
(E) Repeat the urinalysis on a first morning void

The answer is E: Repeat the urinalysis on a first morning void. Asymptomatic proteinuria is a common finding on routine screening urinalysis. Proteinuria is usually the result of a benign condition, but can be a sign of serious renal disease. Transient causes of asymptomatic proteinuria include acute illness, fever, exercise, trauma, pregnancy, and seizures. The most common cause of persistent proteinuria in teenagers is orthostatic or postural proteinuria. In this type of proteinuria, there is normal protein excretion while laying supine, but significant proteinuria when standing. The exact mechanism for orthostatic proteinuria is unknown; however, it appears to be a benign process without the risk of long-term renal problems. The diagnosis is made based on the absence of proteinuria on urine collected immediately upon awakening. Repeating the urinalysis on the first morning void should be obtained prior to any additional workup.

(B, C, D) If there are abnormalities with the recumbent urine sample or any other abnormalities with the initial urine sample, such as hematuria, referral to a pediatric nephrologist for complete evaluation may be warranted. **(A)** Adolescents with UTIs typically have symptoms such as fever, dysuria, and frequency, along with other abnormalities on the urinalysis, for example, nitrites, leukocyte esterase, and bacteria.

14 A 15-year-old boy with spina bifida presents to clinic after a lapse of medical care. The patient was seen in the emergency department multiple times over the past 6 months for fevers and cloudy urine. Each time he was treated with antibiotics for urinary tract infections (UTIs) and remained asymptomatic for several weeks following. His medical records reveal a diagnosis of neurogenic bladder for which he was placed on antibiotic prophylaxis. He states he has been taking his antibiotics regularly. Currently, he is afebrile and does not report fever or cloudy urine.

Of the following, what is the next best step in the evaluation of this patient?

(A) Place the patient on a different antibiotic
(B) Send the patient for urology consultation
(C) Obtain urodynamic studies
(D) Order urinalysis and urine culture
(E) Review patient's intermittent catheterization regimen

The answer is E: Review patient's intermittent catheterization regimen. Patients with spina bifida can develop a neurogenic bladder secondary to poor or interrupted innervation of the bladder leading to urinary stasis and frequent UTIs. Neurogenic bladder can be a cause of incomplete emptying of the bladder and requires intermittent catheterization to mimic a normal voiding pattern. The next best step for the patient in the vignette is to make sure that he is still taking part in the intermittent catheterization regimen on a regular basis. Many adolescent patients have a difficult time continuing to provide daily self-medical care as they mature and become more independent. If patients with neurogenic bladder do not follow the intermittent catheterization regimen, there is an increase in urinary stasis in the bladder, leading to recurrent UTIs.

(A, B, C) After inquiring about this important historical point, it may be appropriate to refer him to a urologist to repeat urodynamic studies and consider altering his antibiotic prophylaxis. **(D)** If the patient in the vignette does not currently have symptoms, it is unlikely he has a UTI that would indicate starting a new antibiotic or obtaining urine studies at this time.

15 A 16-year-old girl presents to the office with the concern for a persistent cough. She has recently returned from Mexico, and now has a progressively worsening cough. She was seen in the office 2 days ago, where a tuberculin skin test was placed and is confirmed to be negative today. She now complains of headache, significant hemoptysis, and pink frothy urine. She is found to be afebrile and her BP is 155/95 mmHg. She also has mild edema to her face and extremities. A laboratory evaluation demonstrates decreased renal function, and a normal complete blood cell count. Her urinalysis is significant for hematuria and proteinuria. She is admitted to the pediatric intensive care unit for careful fluid and BP management. Her subsequent serum studies are

significant for normal complement levels, normal antistreptolysin O titers, negative antinuclear antibody, and positive antibodies against the glomerular basement membrane.

Of the following, which condition is most likely responsible for this patient's presentation?

(A) Wegener granulomatosis
(B) Lupus nephritis
(C) Henoch-Schönlein purpura (HSP)
(D) Goodpasture disease
(E) Tuberculosis

The answer is D: Goodpasture disease. The patient in the vignette presents with initial concern for cough and hemoptysis and is found to have symptoms of acute glomerulonephritis (hematuria, edema, hypertension, and renal insufficiency). The key to the diagnosis is the positive antibody to the glomerular basement membrane, which is seen in Goodpasture disease. The clinical manifestations of this disease are due to these antibodies that attack a specific type IV collagen found in the glomerular basement membrane (causing glomerulonephritis) and in the alveolar basement membrane (causing significant pulmonary hemorrhage).

(A) Wegener granulomatosis is an autoimmune vasculitis that can cause glomerulonephritis and upper or lower respiratory symptoms. These patients do not have antiglomerular basement membrane antibodies, but can have antibodies to neutrophil cytoplasmic components. **(B)** Patients with systemic lupus erythematosus can present with renal and pulmonary findings; however, these patients would not be expected to have a positive antibody test to the glomerular basement membrane. **(C)** Patients with HSP may progress to acute glomerulonephritis in the first few months after diagnosis, but generally do not have pulmonary findings. **(E)** Tuberculosis is not a common cause for acute glomerulonephritis.

A 5-year-old girl is brought to the clinic with complaints of dysuria and vague suprapubic abdominal pain. Her parents report they have been trying to teach the child the proper way to wipe after stooling. She also has a history of constipation, but reports no other complaints, and has been tolerating solids and liquids well. A urinalysis is obtained, which demonstrates nitrites, leukocyte esterase, and many bacteria. A urine culture is pending.

Of the following, which antibiotic is most appropriate to initiate for this patient?

(A) Ciprofloxacin
(B) Azithromycin
(C) Trimethoprim–sulfamethoxazole
(D) Gentamicin
(E) Piperacillin and tazobactam

The answer is C: Trimethoprim–sulfamethoxazole. The patient in the vignette presents with signs of acute cystitis, or lower urinary tract infection (UTI), limited to the bladder. Older children have symptoms similar to adults that include low-grade fever, frequency, urgency, dysuria, and hematuria. A common cause for girls to have UTIs is a result from ascending infection of exterior fecal flora into the urinary tract. Constipation is another common risk factor for UTIs as it can contribute to some voiding dysfunction. The organisms implicated in UTIs in this age group are those found in fecal flora, specifically *Escherichia coli*. Trimethoprim–sulfamethoxazole is the best choice for first-line uncomplicated acute cystitis. Nitrofurantoin, amoxicillin, and cephalosporins can also be used as outpatient treatment of UTIs based on the sensitivity reports of the microorganism involved. **(A)** Ciprofloxacin has appropriate coverage against most gram-negative organisms that cause UTIs; however, it is generally avoided in young children, secondary to concern for potential cartilage damage. **(B)** Azithromycin does not have activity against *E. coli*. **(D, E)** Gentamicin and piperacillin–tazobactam can be used for inpatient management of patients with pyelonephritis, who may not be responsive to third-generation cephalosporin therapy.

---

17 A 2-day-old neonate fails his newborn hearing screen. The infant was born full term by normal spontaneous vaginal delivery without any complications. His mother regularly visited her obstetrician and had an uncomplicated pregnancy. There is a family history of deafness. On physical examination, a small abnormality is noticed anterior to the right ear as seen in Figure 8-3.

Of the following which is the next best step for this patient?

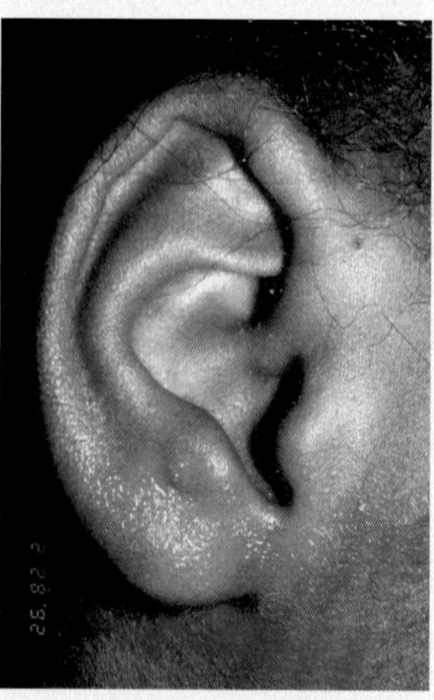

Figure 8-3

(A) Consult otolaryngology
(B) Karyotype assay
(C) Obtain computed tomography scan
(D) Obtain renal ultrasound
(E) Supportive care

The answer is D: **Obtain renal ultrasound.** The picture in the vignette demonstrates a preauricular pit. Preauricular pits are typically benign congenital malformations of the external ear; however, they are associated with an increased frequency of clinically significant structural renal anomalies. This is mainly due to the simultaneous embryologic development of the ears and kidneys. Auricular malformations often are associated with specific multiple congenital anomaly syndromes. **(D)** A renal ultrasound should be ordered in patients who fail the newborn hearing screen, have a family history of deafness, or present with other malformations or dysmorphic features. **(B)** Genetic testing for each syndrome varies; those identified in conjunction with preauricular pits have abnormalities at single gene loci, and thus, chromosome testing has limited value. **(A, C)** Typically, preauricular pits are benign; however, if they become infected, otolaryngology consultation may be warranted, in which case a computed tomography scan may provide additional anatomical information.

18 A 6-year-old boy without significant past medical history presents to the emergency department with a swollen face, hands, and feet for the last 2 days. His mother reports he has no other complaints. She denies any new food or environmental exposures. A laboratory workup reveals hypoalbuminemia and proteinuria.

Of the following, which is the next best step in the treatment of this patient?

(A) Prophylactic antibiotics
(B) Renal biopsy
(C) Epinephrine
(D) Fluid and salt restriction
(E) Steroid therapy

The answer is E: **Steroid therapy.** Nephrotic syndrome is a clinical condition caused by massive loss of protein in the urine due to glomerular pathology, specifically injury at the epithelial cells and basement membrane. The findings include proteinuria, edema, hypoalbuminemia, and hyperlipidemia. The most common cause for nephrotic syndrome is minimal change disease (MCD); therefore, any child presenting with primary nephrotic syndrome is considered to have MCD and should initially be treated with steroids.

(B) If the patient does not respond to steroid therapy, a renal biopsy may be warranted to assess for other potential causes of nephrotic syndrome. Patients with nephrotic syndrome are at risk for bacterial infections such as spontaneous bacterial peritonitis and bacteremia due to loss of significant amounts of immunoglobulin, complement factors, and antibodies in their urine. **(A)** However, without any symptoms of infection, prophylactic antibiotics are not routinely used.

(C) Patients with edema due to anaphylaxis require aggressive management with intramuscular or intravenous epinephrine and antihistamines. The patient in the vignette does not present with anaphylaxis. Patients with nephrotic syndrome have significant edema from loss of albumin, which leads to a decrease in oncotic pressure intravascularly. There is a subsequent fluid shift from the intravascular space to the interstitial space. Total body water may remain normal. The fluid management of patients with nephrotic syndrome can be difficult as initially the patients may be intravascularly depleted. Treatment includes replacement of albumin and the administration of diuretic medications, which result in fluid shift to the intravascular space. **(D)** Patients with nephritic syndrome often need fluid and salt restriction to regulate their fluid balance. The aggressive management of fluids is needed for all cases of nephrotic syndrome, but does not treat the underlying cause of the nephrotic syndrome itself.

---

19 An 8-week-old male infant is brought to the emergency department by his parents for inconsolable crying and irritability. On review of past charts, the patient was seen 3 weeks ago with the same complaint, and found to have hypernatremic dehydration. Currently, the parents deny fever or recent illness. The patient has been breastfeeding normally every 2 to 3 hours, and has heavy wet diapers every 30 minutes to 1 hour. Physical examination reveals a mild-to-moderately dehydrated patient. Blood and urine testing demonstrates hypernatremia, elevated serum osmolality, and a dilute urine sample with decreased urine osmolality. The patient is admitted for further workup and evaluation. He undergoes a vasopressin or antidiuretic hormone (ADH) test, which he fails.

Of the following, which medication is often used to treat this patient's underlying condition?

(A) Vasopressin
(B) Imipramine
(C) Oxybutynin
(D) Prednisone
(E) Hydrochlorothiazide

The answer is E: Hydrochlorothiazide. The patient in the vignette presents with symptoms and findings consistent with diabetes insipidus (DI). DI is a disorder of water and sodium metabolism that results in excessive thirst and excretion of large amounts of extremely dilute urine. Patients with DI are unable to reabsorb water and have increased serum sodium and serum osmolality, while having increased urine output with decreased urine sodium and urine osmolality.

DI is due to central or renal causes. In order to differentiate the etiology, the patient should be provided with vasopressin (ADH) and evaluated closely for improvement or change. **(A)** A positive response is consistent with central DI, in which the brain is producing insufficient amounts of ADH, but the kidneys are able to respond appropriately. With a male infant presenting with polyuria, hypernatremia, and diluted urine, hereditary nephrogenic DI should be considered as this condition is commonly an X-linked disorder and patients present with episodes of severe hypernatremic dehydration and failure to thrive. The etiology of nephrogenic DI is secondary to the inability of the kidneys to respond to ADH, thus, administering ADH does not have a therapeutic effect. Treatment of nephrogenic DI includes maintaining adequate fluid intake and minimizing urine output. Patients may need gastrostomy or nasogastric feedings to maintain caloric intake. To minimize urine output, some infants may benefit from a low-solute formula. In older patients, sodium intake should be limited. Thiazide diuretics are frequently used to induce sodium loss and reabsorption of water at the proximal tubule.

(B) Imipramine is a tricyclic antidepressant used to reduce bladder contractions in patients with nocturnal enuresis. **(C)** Oxybutynin is an anticholinergic agent also used for enuresis. Neither have a role in the treatment of nephrogenic DI. **(D)** Corticosteroids such as prednisone have not been proven to be beneficial in patients with nephrogenic DI.

---

20 A 9-year-old girl is admitted to the inpatient ward with intermittent flank pain. She complains of dysuria, urgency, and frequency. Her strained urine demonstrates small amounts of gravel-like material. Upon further analysis in the laboratory, the material is found to consist of struvite.

Of the following, which microorganism is most likely responsible for this patient's presentation?

(A) Adenovirus
(B) *Escherichia coli*
(C) *Streptococcus pyogenes*
(D) *Enterococcus faecalis*
(E) *Proteus mirabilis*

The answer is E: *Proteus mirabilis*. Primary urinary calculi in children can be due to recurrent urinary tract infections (UTIs), metabolic/dietary abnormalities, inadequate water intake, hypercalciuria, malabsorptive states, neuropathic bladder, and obstructive renal disease. The cause of the stones can be categorized by chemical composition, with most stones containing calcium. Struvite stones are caused by UTIs with a urea-splitting microorganism, most often *P. mirabilis*, and occasionally *Klebsiella pneumoniae* or *Pseudomonas aeruginosa*. These infections lead to alkalinization of the urine

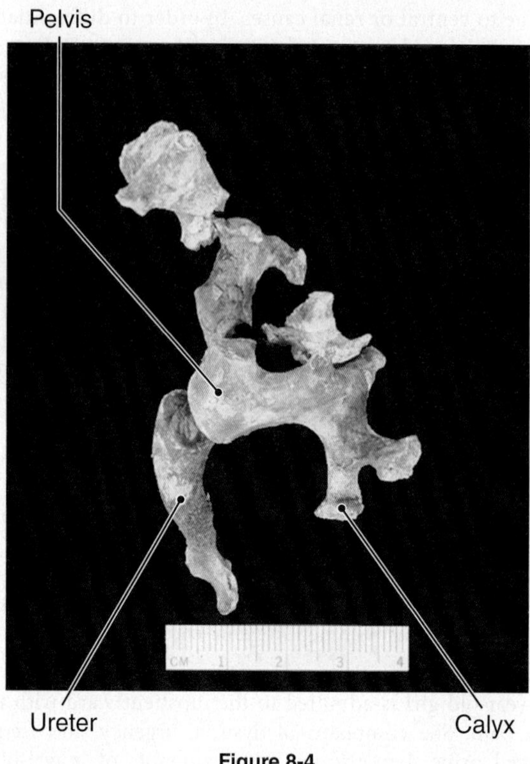

Figure 8-4

and high levels of urinary ammonia, which causes precipitation of magnesium ammonium phosphate. In the kidney, the calculi often have a "staghorn" appearance filling the calyces (see *Figure 8-4*). **(A, B, C, D)** The rest of the organisms listed are not associated with struvite stone formation.

---

21 A 3-week-old neonate is brought to the emergency department for evaluation of a rectal temperature of 40°C at home. His mother states that her son has been more sleepy than usual, but continues to feed, void, and stool appropriately. There are no sick contacts or significant past medical history. His physical examination is within normal limits. The infant has a temperature of 39.8°C in the emergency department. Prior to starting antibiotics, a full septic workup is initiated including cultures from blood, urine, and cerebrospinal fluid.

Of the following, which method of urine specimen collection would provide the most accurate results?

(A) Midstream clean catch
(B) Clean intermittent catheterization
(C) Sterile urine collection bag
(D) Urethral swab
(E) Directly from non-stool diaper

The answer is B: **Clean intermittent catheterization.** A fever in an infant less than 8 weeks old is concerning for a serious bacterial infection, including bacteremia, sepsis, pneumonia, urinary tract infection (UTI), and meningitis. Ideally, a culture from blood, urine, and cerebrospinal fluid should be obtained prior to initiating antibiotic therapy. For the patient in the vignette and any child who has not been toilet trained, there are two accepted methods for obtaining a urine sample to give reliable culture results: a catheterized sample or suprapubic needle aspiration. **(A)** In older children, a clean-catch midstream sample may be satisfactory. **(C)** A sterile urine collection bag should be avoided if treatment for UTI is planned, as there is a high rate of contamination with skin flora. **(D, E)** A urethral swab and any specimen collected directly from the diaper do not have a role in the evaluation for a UTI.

22 A 4-year-old boy who recently immigrated to the United States presents to the emergency department with evidence of end-stage renal disease (ESRD).

Of the following, which is the most likely etiology of his renal disease?

(A) Hypertension
(B) Diabetes mellitus
(C) Nephrotoxic drugs
(D) Chronic glomerulonephritis
(E) Posterior urethral valves (PUVs)

The answer is E: **Posterior urethral valves (PUVs).** In younger children, the most common cause for chronic kidney disease leading to ESRD is congenital and obstructive abnormalities, such as PUVs. PUVs are obstructive valve leaflets in the prostatic portion of the urethra, which can clinically manifest with a poor or absent urinary stream. PUVs are only found in men. The urinary tract obstruction at this level can lead to a dilated bladder with a dysfunctional detrusor muscle, vesicoureteral reflux, and bilateral hydronephrosis. Prompt surgical correction is indicated, although many patients may still develop ESRD.

(A, B) Hypertension and diabetes mellitus can lead to chronic kidney disease, but is the result of long-standing injury and more likely in an older patient. **(C)** Nephrotoxic medications are more likely to cause acute renal injury than ESRD. **(D)** The incidence of acquired diseases, such as chronic glomerulonephritis from systemic lupus erythematosus, or inherited diseases, such as Alport syndrome, is more likely to cause ESRD in older children.

23 The parents of a newborn baby girl present to the office for their first hospital follow-up visit. The baby was born 5 days prior without complications. She has been feeding, sleeping, voiding, and stooling appropriately. On examination, large, bilateral abdominal masses are palpated without any other significant findings.

Of the following, what is the most likely cause of the abdominal masses?

(A) Multicystic kidneys
(B) Wilms' tumor
(C) Posterior urethral valves (PUVs)
(D) Choledochal cyst
(E) Polycystic kidneys

The answer is E: **Polycystic kidneys.** The most common cause of an abdominal mass in the newborn period is of renal origin, usually cystic kidney disease (multicystic dysplastic or polycystic) or hydronephrosis from urinary tract obstruction (PUVs or ureteropelvic junction obstruction). The patient in the vignette has polycystic kidney disease, which generally presents with large, bilateral flank masses. She is more likely to have the autosomal recessive inheritance pattern, as these present earlier in life.

(A) A multicystic kidney consists of several irregular cysts within the kidney parenchyma leading to dysplasia and loss of function and is one of the most common causes of unilateral abdominal masses in the newborn. This kidney generally involutes over time and renders itself completely nonfunctional. Having bilateral, multicystic, dysplastic kidneys is incompatible with life. Tumors are rare in this age, but can present as painless abdominal masses in the newborn. **(B)** The more likely tumors are neuroblastoma and Wilms' tumor, as they can both present congenitally, but are far less likely than cystic renal disease. **(C)** PUVs are not seen in female patients. **(D)** Choledochal cysts are congenital cystic dilatations of the bile duct that can cause biliary obstruction leading to a direct hyperbilirubinemia. A choledochal cyst would present as a painless mass in the right upper quadrant, along with signs of jaundice.

24 A 15-year-old girl is found to be hypertensive on her routine school physical. Repeated BP readings confirm her diagnosis of hypertension. On further evaluation for the etiology of her hypertension, her primary care physician orders blood work, an echocardiogram, and abdominal ultrasound. The ultrasound displays multiple large dilated cysts throughout the renal parenchyma as well as a few hepatic cysts.

Of the following, what is the most likely inheritance pattern for her disease?

(A) Autosomal recessive
(B) Autosomal dominant
(C) X-linked recessive
(D) X-linked dominant
(E) Mitochondrial inheritance

The answer is B: **Autosomal dominant.** Cystic diseases of the kidney are a diverse group of disorders that include primary renal disease and many malformation syndromes. Of the primary renal diseases, polycystic kidney diseases can be inherited as autosomal dominant polycystic kidney disease (ADPKD) and autosomal recessive polycystic kidney disease (ARPKD). **(A, C, D, E)** ADPKD is the most common hereditary human kidney disease. The severity of renal disease and clinical manifestations are highly variable. Symptomatic patients with ADPKD usually present in the fourth decade of life but younger individuals can present with hematuria or hypertension, similar to the patient in the vignette. Family history may be helpful, but the spontaneous mutation rate is high. ADPKD is associated with extrarenal manifestations, particularly a high incidence of vascular aneurysms and cysts in other organs.

ARPKD is also referred to as infantile polycystic disease, as the time of presentation is seen much earlier. This form can be detected prenatally and may manifest with signs of oligohydramnios. Although ARPKD is much less common than ADPKD the prognosis is worse with a more rapid progression to end-stage renal disease. ARPKD is also associated with a wide range of extrarenal involvement, specifically congenital hepatic fibrosis, and pulmonary hypoplasia.

25 A 7-year-old girl presents to the emergency department with fevers and chills for the past 2 days. Her parents report she is also complaining of back pain and nausea. On examination, she has tenderness to her right flank area. Her laboratory workup reveals a leukocytosis with a left shift and elevated inflammatory markers. Her urinalysis reveals many bacteria, white blood cells, nitrites, and leukocyte esterase.

Of the following, which is her most likely diagnosis?

(A) Acute cystitis
(B) Acute pyelonephritis
(C) Vertebral osteomyelitis
(D) Pneumonia
(E) Acute appendicitis

The answer is B: **Acute pyelonephritis.** Acute pyelonephritis refers to a urinary tract infection (UTI) that involves the kidney. Pyelonephritis can clinically manifest with systemic signs of fever, nausea, vomiting, malaise, and focal signs of pain radiating to the back, abdomen, or flank region. In younger children, fever may be the only symptom. Most acute pyelonephritis infections occur from ascending UTIs; however, cases of hematogenous spread can be possible as well. The patient in the vignette has clinical symptoms, laboratory findings, and urine results consistent with acute pyelonephritis. Patients are typically hospitalized for initial treatment with intravenous antibiotics.

(A) The patient in the vignette unlikely has a simple acute cystitis with infection only limited to the bladder, given the pain, fever, and chills, indicative of a more systemic or involved process. **(C)** Vertebral osteomyelitis can present similar to pyelonephritis with fever and back pain; however, vertebral osteomyelitis should not present with urine findings consistent with an infection. **(D, E)** Patients with pneumonia and acute appendicitis will not have infectious urine findings, but both conditions can present with back pain, nausea, and fever. Acute appendicitis may cause a sterile pyuria, noted with white blood cells in the urinalysis with a negative urinary culture.

---

26 The parents of a 6-year-old boy bring him to the clinic for evaluation of cola-colored urine and mild swelling of his extremities. The symptoms started a few days prior, but have slowly increased in severity. He was sent home from school 3 weeks ago for having a fever and sore throat, which improved without intervention.

Of the following, which statement is true concerning this boy's condition?

(A) Acute poststreptococcal glomerulonephritis (APSGN) is the result of direct bacterial infection of the glomerular basement membrane
(B) APSGN is not seen following streptococcal skin infections
(C) Treatment of streptococcal pharyngitis with antibiotics would have prevented APSGN
(D) Only specific nephritogenic strains of *Streptococcus pyogenes* trigger the immune response that causes APSGN
(E) Urine cultures in patients with APSGN will be positive for *S. pyogenes*

The answer is D: **Only specific nephritogenic strains of *S. pyogenes* trigger the immune response that causes APSGN.** APSGN is one of the most common causes of acute nephritic syndrome in children and consists of hematuria, edema, hypertension, and renal insufficiency. **(A)** APSGN results from inflammation due to an immune-mediated response, specifically to a nephritogenic strain of *S. pyogenes*. This response is directed at the glomerular capillary wall leading to complement activation and eventual cell proliferation and injury. **(B)** APSGN occurs 5 to 21 days following the initial infection, usually of the pharynx or skin, such as impetigo. If the patient has an active infection at the time of diagnosis, antibiotics are needed; however, appropriate treatment does not prevent the immune response that leads to the development of APSGN. **(E)** APSGN is not the result of an active urinary infection. **(C)** Appropriate therapy of streptococcal pharyngitis does prevent rheumatic fever.

27 A 6-year-old boy who weighs 20 kg is admitted to the pediatric intensive care unit for severe dehydration due to acute gastroenteritis. He has received multiple intravenous fluid boluses, and now is on maintenance intravenous fluid therapy. He is noted to be in acute renal failure (ARF) with poor urine output.

Of the following what is the minimal acceptable goal urine output for this patient?

(A) 1 mL/h
(B) 5 mL/h
(C) 10 mL/h
(D) 25 mL/h
(E) 40 mL/h

The answer is C: 10 mL/h. The patient in the vignette is found to be in ARF due to a pre-renal etiology of severe dehydration. ARF is a clinical condition in which there is a sudden decrease in glomerular filtration rate and tubular function. This decrease causes the kidneys to be unable to properly maintain fluid and electrolyte balance. Oliguria, or decreased urine output, is one of the earliest signs of impaired renal function and is the result of the hypoperfusion of the kidneys. Oliguria is defined by urine output less than 1 mL/kg/h in infants, less than 0.5 mL/kg/h in children, and less than 400 mL/d in adults. The goal urine output for the patient in the vignette is greater than 10 mL/h (20 kg × 0.5 mL/h).

28 A 6-year-old boy presents with the rash seen in Figure 8-5, left knee pain, and crampy abdominal pain. He is admitted for observation and treated with supportive care. He continues to have normal BP readings, laboratory studies, and urinalysis. Over the next day, he quickly improves and is stable for discharge.

Of the following, which is the next best step for monitoring this patient upon discharge home?

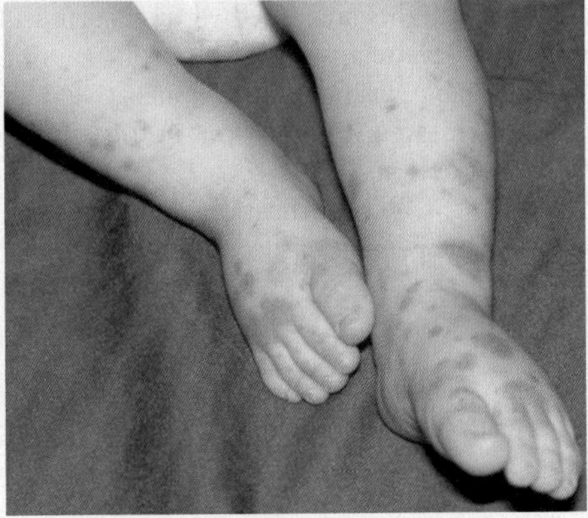

Figure 8-5

(A) Repeat a urinalysis weekly during active disease and then monthly for 6 months
(B) Obtain a renal biopsy
(C) Repeat the BP next month
(D) Refer patient to pediatric nephrology
(E) No further workup is needed unless patient develops clinical symptoms

The answer is A: **Repeat a urinalysis weekly during active disease and then monthly for 6 months.** The symptoms described in the vignette are consistent with a presentation of Henoch-Schönlein purpura (HSP). HSP is one of the most common systemic small vessel vasculitides of childhood. It is characterized by a palpable, purpuric rash, arthritis, and less frequently gastrointestinal pain or involvement. Children with HSP and renal involvement can have either acute or chronic conditions. **(C, E)** Most cases are mild and self-limited with isolated microscopic hematuria; however, patients can progress to severe glomerulonephritis with hematuria, edema, hypertension, and renal insufficiency within the first few months of presentation. Therefore, aggressive monitoring with urinalysis is recommended. **(D)** If a patient is found to have hematuria with proteinuria, renal insufficiency, or hypertension, consultation with pediatric nephrology may be warranted. **(B)** Although the patient in the vignette does not warrant a renal biopsy at this time, if a biopsy were to be performed, findings would appear similar to patients with immunoglobulin (IgA) nephropathy: increased mesangial cellularity and IgA deposition on immunofluorescence.

29 A frustrated mother brings her 8-year-old daughter to clinic for continued issues with nocturnal enuresis. She denies any daytime symptoms, polyuria, polydipsia, or dysuria. Her mother states she has eliminated extra sugar and caffeine from her diet. Her parents have also been limiting the child to 2 ounces of fluids after dinner and encourage her to void prior to bedtime. They have tried using motivational therapy with a star chart for dry nights and a bedwetting alarm in the past, but the child continues to have relapses. Her physical examination and urinalysis are unremarkable. Urine culture is negative. Her mother understands that most children will grow out of this condition, but inquires of other treatment options.

Of the following, which medication would be the most appropriate next step in the management of this patient?

(A) Doxazosin
(B) Desmopressin
(C) Cephalexin
(D) Trimethoprim–sulfamethoxazole
(E) Steroids

The answer is B: Desmopressin. Primary nocturnal enuresis is a condition in which a child continues to have nightly bedwetting despite proper potty training. Patients with diurnal enuresis are more likely to have a urinary tract abnormality, infection, or metabolic issues, such as diabetes. There is a strong association of family history in patients with primary nocturnal enuresis. Evaluation of primary nocturnal enuresis begins with history and physical examination to assess for potential etiologies of increased urinary output such as diabetes insipidus, diabetes mellitus, urinary tract infection (UTI), chronic renal disease, or inadequate bladder emptying as seen in neurologic or spinal abnormalities. Treatment should begin with behavioral changes such as limiting fluid intake at bedtime, limiting sugar and caffeine, and encouraging bedtime voiding. Conditioning therapy involves bedwetting alarms, which can be curative, however, are associated with a significant relapse rate.

Pharmacologic therapy in conjunction with conditioning therapy can increase the response rate to primary nocturnal enuresis. **(B)** Desmopressin is a synthetic analog of vasopressin, or antidiuretic hormone, which reduces the volume of urine made at night, and can be administered in the evening to reduce the occurrence of nocturnal enuresis. **(A)** Doxazosin is an α-antagonist that can be used in daytime enuresis by reducing bladder outlet resistance. **(C, D)** The patient in the vignette does not demonstrate any signs or symptoms consistent with a UTI and would not benefit from antibiotic therapy. **(E)** Steroids do not have a role in the treatment of enuresis.

CHAPTER

9

Fluids and Electrolytes

RINKU PATEL

1 A child protective services detective presents to the emergency department with a 7-year-old boy, a 4-year-old girl, and an 8-month-old infant after removal from their home. The detective states the neighbors were concerned about the children after having suspicions of parental abandonment. The 7-year-old boy is not sure how long the children have been alone without food, but does report they have had access to drinking water. On examination of the youngest infant, his weight is less than the 3rd percentile; he is pale, with decreased subcutaneous fat. The children are admitted to the hospital for nutritional rehabilitation.

Of the following, which is the most likely electrolyte abnormality to be seen once feedings are restarted?

(A) Hypermagnesemia
(B) Hyperkalemia
(C) Hypophosphatemia
(D) Hyponatremia
(E) Hypocalcemia

The answer is C: Hypophosphatemia. Worldwide, pediatric malnutrition is a leading cause of death in young children. Malnutrition can be seen in patients with increased caloric requirements, caloric malabsorption, or reduced caloric intake. When nutritional rehabilitation begins, the gastrointestinal tract may not tolerate a rapid increase in intake and the kidneys may not be able to tolerate the excess fluid and solute load; therefore, the initiation and advancement of feeds should be completed with caution and judicious monitoring. **(A, B)** Refeeding syndrome is a complication of advancing nutrition rapidly in a malnourished patient, which can be characterized by fluid retention, hypophosphatemia, hypomagnesemia, and hypokalemia. The serum phosphorus level specifically can fall significantly due to the shift from extracellular to intracellular compartments, as demands for synthesis of phosphorylated compounds, such as adenosine triphosphate, increase.

(D, E) Hyponatremia and hypocalcemia are generally not electrolyte abnormalities seen in refeeding syndrome.

A first time mother presents to the clinic with her newborn infant for a routine hospital follow-up visit. Both the mother and the baby are doing well. The mother's family has suggested giving the baby water when it is hot outdoors, however, the mother reports she read online to avoid water until 6 months of age.

Of the following, what is the most likely reason to avoid free water in the newborn age group?

(A) Increased risk of seizures
(B) Increased urine output
(C) Increased risk of sudden infant death syndrome
(D) Increased risk of urinary tract infections
(E) Increased risk of ear infections

The answer is A: Increased risk of seizures. A healthy newborn infant should be exclusively fed breast milk or formula for the first 6 months of life. Newborns have low glomerular filtration rates and are not able to produce dilute urine. This puts newborns at increased risk for water intoxication that can lead to hyponatremic seizures. The glomerular filtration rates of older children and adults are higher and allow their kidneys to be able to excrete free water in order to produce dilute urine in response to increased water consumption. **(C, D, E)** There is not a reported association with free water consumption and sudden infant death syndrome, urinary tract infections, or ear infections.

A 3-year-old boy arrives to the emergency department with his father after 3 days of vomiting and diarrhea. His father states that the symptoms have gradually worsened over the past 24 hours, and the child is unable to tolerate any oral intake. The patient has had three to four large watery bowel movements per day with fewer-than-normal wet diapers. On examination, he is restless and irritable, and only consolable in his father's arms. His vital signs are temperature 37.6°C, heart rate 140 beats/min, and blood pressure 90/60 mmHg. He is crying with few tears and he has dry mucous membranes. His pulses are 2+ throughout and his capillary refill less than 2 seconds with slightly decreased skin turgor.

Of the following, which percentage accurately depicts this patient's degree of dehydration?

(A) 1%
(B) 5%
(C) 10%
(D) 15%
(E) 20%

Table 9-1 Physical examination findings associated with mild, moderate, and severe dehydration.

	Mild	Moderate	Severe
Weight loss	<5%	10%	>10%
Vital signs			
Heart rate	Increased	Increased	Greatly increased
Respiratory rate	Normal	Normal	Increased
Blood pressure	Normal	Orthostasis	Decreased
Skin			
Capillary refill	<2 s	2–3 s	>3 s
Mucous membranes	Normal/dry	Dry	Dry
Anterior fontanelle	Normal	Sunken	Sunken
Eyes			
Tearing	Normal/absent	Absent	Absent
Mental status	Normal	Altered	Depressed
Stage of shock	Not in shock	Compensated shock	Uncompensated shock

The answer is C: 10%. Dehydration in children can often be due to gastroenteritis secondary to ongoing water losses. The assessment of degree of dehydration is important in determining the volume of fluid needed for rehydration. See *Table 9-1* for the clinical findings that are associated with the various degrees of dehydration.

(A, B, D, E) The patient in the vignette presents with signs and symptoms consistent with moderate dehydration, and thus, a loss of 10% total body weight.

4 An 8-year-old boy presents to the clinic after being recently diagnosed with new-onset diabetes mellitus. The patient is now doing well and has transitioned to a subcutaneous insulin regimen. The patient's initial laboratory results on presentation were as follows: pH 7.11, glucose 678 mg/dL,

sodium 130 mEq/L, potassium 4 mEq/L, chloride 102 mEq/L, bicarbonate 8 mEq/L, blood urea nitrogen 18 mg/dL, and creatinine 0.8 mg/dL.

Of the following options, which is consistent with the anion gap for the patient on his initial presentation?

(A) 8
(B) 10
(C) 20
(D) 28
(E) 30

The answer is C: **20.** An anion gap represents the unmeasured extracellular anions and is calculated by subtracting the major serum anions from the major serum cations. **(A, B, D, E)** The formula to calculate the patient in the vignette's anion gap is [sodium] – [chloride + bicarbonate] and his anion gap is 20. An elevated anion gap typically signifies an increase in organic acid production while a normal anion gap signifies increased excretion of bicarbonate or increased production of chloride. The differential diagnosis for a normal anion gap metabolic acidosis can include diarrhea, renal tubular acidosis, and iatrogenic causes such as hyperalimentation, ammonium chloride administration, and carbonic anhydrase inhibitors. The differential for increased anion gap metabolic acidosis can include conditions with elevated intrinsic organic acids such as lactic acidosis, ketoacidosis, and inborn errors of metabolism or conditions with elevated extrinsic organic acids including ingestions of salicylates, ethylene glycol, and methanol.

5 A 13-year-old boy presents to the emergency department with abdominal pain, emesis, and increased lethargy for the past 3 days. His parents report that he has been losing weight over the past 3 weeks despite an increased appetite and thirst. A bedside glucose reading is >500 mg/dL. Serum glucose level is 628 mg/dL, arterial pH is 7.20, serum carbon dioxide level is 12 mEq/L, and urinalysis is significant for ketones and glucose. The patient is given an intravenous (IV) bolus of normal saline and IV insulin prior to admission to the pediatric intensive care unit.

Of the following, which electrolyte abnormality is this patient at risk for as his acidotic state is corrected?

(A) Hyperkalemia
(B) Hypokalemia
(C) Hyponatremia
(D) Hypophosphatemia
(E) Hypomagnesemia

The answer is B: **Hypokalemia.** Diabetic ketoacidosis (DKA) occurs in patients with type 1 diabetes mellitus as a result of insulin deficiency and presents with dehydration, hyperglycemia, and ketone production secondary to fatty acid oxidation. Additional confirmatory laboratory workup for DKA includes decreased arterial pH, decreased serum carbon dioxide, and increased serum and urine ketones. **(A, C, D, E)** Electrolyte abnormalities occur as a result of three mechanisms: loss of electrolytes in the urine (hypophosphatemia and hypomagnesemia), intracellular transmembrane shifts from metabolic acidosis (hyperkalemia), and intracellular transmembrane shifts from hyperglycemia (hyponatremia). Once extracellular, potassium is also cleared by the kidneys, leading to a decrease in total body potassium. With insulin and appropriate fluid replacement therapy, the ketosis resolves, along with the acidotic state. **(B)** Potassium subsequently shifts back intracellularly, placing patients with resolving DKA at risk for hypokalemia.

6 A 12-year-old girl presents to the emergency department with lethargy and fatigue. Her mother states she has not been eating or drinking well the past few days and has had multiple episodes of vomiting and diarrhea. In the last 24 hours, the patient has not had any urine output. On examination, the patient's pulse is 164 beats/min and her blood pressure is 81/64 mmHg. She is anxious with cold sweaty skin. Her pulses are diminished and her mucous membranes are very dry.

Of the following, which is the next best step in the management of this patient?

(A) 20 mL/kg bolus of D5 half-normal saline over 20 minutes
(B) 20 mL/kg bolus of lactated Ringer's solution over 2 hours
(C) 20 mL/kg bolus of normal saline over 20 minutes
(D) D5 half-normal saline with 20 mEq/L of potassium chloride at maintenance rate
(E) Oral rehydration solution challenge

The answer is C: 20 mL/kg bolus of normal saline over 20 minutes. The patient in the vignette has symptoms consistent with severe dehydration and requires immediate intervention to restore adequate tissue perfusion. **(A, B, D, E)** The best initial option to restore intravascular volume is aggressive fluid therapy with a bolus of 20 mL/kg of an isotonic solution, either normal saline or lactated Ringer's solution. The bolus should be given quickly, ideally within 20 minutes. Once the initial fluid bolus is administered, the patient should be reassessed for clinical improvement and additional fluid boluses given as necessary. Once resuscitation is complete, an appropriate fluid plan can be determined to include maintenance fluid therapy needs and replacement of any ongoing losses. Severely dehydrated patients may have acute renal failure, thus, potassium is initially withheld from resuscitation fluids until adequate renal function is established.

7 An 8-month-old infant is brought to the emergency department with the complaint of diarrhea for the past 2 days. His parents report his stool output continues to remain unformed and watery and is now

increasing in frequency. The patient has been uninterested in eating since the onset of symptoms. On physical examination, the patient is moderately dehydrated. An arterial blood gas reveals a pH of 7.31, carbon dioxide partial pressure ($PaCO_2$) of 25 mmHg, and bicarbonate of 20 mEq/L.

Of the following, which acid–base state best explains this patient's findings?

(A) Metabolic acidosis without respiratory compensation
(B) Metabolic acidosis with respiratory compensation
(C) Respiratory acidosis with metabolic compensation
(D) Metabolic alkalosis without respiratory compensation
(E) Respiratory alkalosis with metabolic compensation

The answer is B: Metabolic acidosis with respiratory compensation. In order for cellular and metabolic processes to work optimally, the body maintains the acid–base balance to ensure homeostasis with the assistance of the kidneys, lungs, and cellular buffers. The patient described in the vignette has significant diarrhea, which is the most common cause of a normal anion gap metabolic acidosis in pediatric patients. **(D, E)** The pH is indicative of an acidosis. An abnormality in pH with any abnormal values of $PaCO_2$ (normally controlled by respiratory processes) or bicarbonate (normally controlled by metabolic processes) should help distinguish between respiratory and metabolic processes. Elevated $PaCO_2$ levels result in an acidotic state, while elevated bicarbonate levels result in an alkalotic state. **(B)** For the patient in the vignette, the decreased bicarbonate level, secondary to diarrhea, is causing a metabolic acidosis. **(A, C)** However, the $PaCO_2$ is also decreased, as a result of the respiratory system attempting to compensate for the acid–base disturbance by hyperventilation.

8 Paramedics bring in a 3-year-old boy after his parents discover him unresponsive on the kitchen floor. On examination, he is only responsive to painful stimuli, diaphoretic, febrile, and tachypneic. His Glasgow Coma Scale is 7 and he is intubated to protect his airway. His blood pressure and heart rate are within normal limits. His parents arrive immediately stating they found an empty bottle of aspirin near his playpen.

Of the following, which is the most likely arterial blood gas result for this patient?

	pH	$PaCO_2$	PaO_2	HCO_3^-
(A)	7.56	44	92	38
(B)	7.26	56	64	24
(C)	7.38	40	96	26
(D)	7.24	36	84	14
(E)	7.46	24	98	17

The answer is D: pH: 7.24, $PaCO_2$: 36, PaO_2: 84, HCO_3^-: 14. Aspirin is the most common over-the-counter salicylate medication. The incidence of salicylate poisoning in pediatrics has greatly declined over the years as acetaminophen and ibuprofen have replaced aspirin for analgesic and antipyretic purposes. Salicylate toxicity has multiple effects, including direct stimulation of the respiratory center, as well as modulation of multiple physiologic processes, including a number of metabolic pathways. Clinical manifestations of salicylate poisoning include tachypnea, diaphoresis, tinnitus, bleeding or easy bruising, fever, vomiting, lethargy, and coma. Laboratory findings include abnormal coagulation studies, hyperglycemia, and abnormal blood gas values. **(A, B, C, E)** The typical blood gas result found in salicylate poisoning reveals a mixed primary respiratory alkalosis and a primary metabolic acidosis. Therefore, the pH initially may be close to normal, but the $PaCO_2$ and HCO_3^- are both decreased.

9 A 3-year-old boy with hepatoblastoma presents to the pediatric oncology clinic for follow-up after a recent hospitalization for routine chemotherapy with cisplatin and doxorubicin. He did not have any complications during the hospitalization. His parents state he has had a normal activity level, a good appetite without any vomiting or diarrhea, and has remained afebrile. His vital signs and physical examination are within normal limits. Laboratory results drawn in the clinic demonstrate a complete blood count that is recovering well from the chemotherapy. His basic metabolic panel reveals a normal anion gap metabolic acidosis, which was not present previously.

Of the following, which is the most likely explanation for his acidosis?

(A) Severe dehydration
(B) Diarrhea
(C) Toxic ingestion
(D) Inborn error of metabolism
(E) Renal tubular acidosis (RTA)

The answer is E: Renal tubular acidosis (RTA). The most common cause for a normal anion gap metabolic acidosis in the pediatric population is secondary to significant bicarbonate loss in diarrhea. **(A, B)** The most likely explanation for the acid–base disturbance for the patient in the vignette, who denies any diarrhea, is from nephrotoxicity of his chemotherapy agents, specifically cisplatin causing an RTA. **(E)** RTA is characterized by a hyperchloremic, normal anion gap metabolic acidosis due to altered function of the renal tubules, leading to impaired urine acidification or bicarbonate wasting. Distal, or type 1, RTA results from impaired hydrogen ion secretion at the distal tubule. Causes of distal, or type 1, RTA include intrinsic renal pathology, urologic pathology, or from toxins such as cisplatin or amphotericin B. Patients with distal RTA cannot acidify their urine. These patients have a urine pH greater than 5.5 despite the significant metabolic acidosis.

Proximal, or type 2, RTA is seen secondary to wasting of bicarbonate from decreased reabsorption at the proximal tubule. These patients have a urine pH less than 5.5, which can increase with bicarbonate administration. Hyperkalemic RTA, or type 4 RTA, is unique as it is the only RTA with elevated potassium levels. The etiology of this condition is due to the inability of the kidney to respond to aldosterone.

(C, D) Toxic ingestions, such as salicylates, ethylene glycol, and methanol, and inborn errors of metabolism typically have an increased anion gap metabolic acidosis.

---

10 An 8-year-old boy presents to the clinic with symptoms of abdominal cramping and diarrhea for 2 days. His parents report that he did have a few episodes of vomiting during the onset of the illness, but is no longer having emesis. Currently, he is having four to five watery stools, without any blood. There have been other members of the family who have had similar symptoms. His parents deny any fevers or rashes. On examination, he is slightly tachycardic with a normal blood pressure. He has dry mucous membranes. Abdominal examination reveals hyperactive bowel sounds, without any tenderness, distension, or masses. His peripheral perfusion is normal.

Of the following, which treatment option is optimal for this patient?

(A) Intravenous (IV) bolus with isotonic solution, then oral rehydration
(B) IV bolus with isotonic solution, then maintenance fluids over 48 hours
(C) Oral rehydration only
(D) IV maintenance fluids over 24 hours
(E) IV bolus with isotonic solution only

The answer is C: Oral rehydration only. Symptoms of viral gastroenteritis typically begin with vomiting for 2 to 4 days followed by diarrhea that can last 7 to 10 days. The treatment for viral gastroenteritis is supportive care with adequate liquid intake, and resumption of a normal diet as soon as possible. Older children with mild-to-moderate dehydration from a diarrheal illness can be treated effectively with an oral rehydration solution containing glucose and electrolytes. Oral rehydration therapy has significantly reduced the morbidity and mortality from acute diarrhea worldwide. **(A, B, D, E)** For the patient in the vignette who is able to tolerate fluids, oral rehydration therapy alone is the best initial treatment choice. Treatment consists of an adequate volume of fluid administered gradually to treat the dehydration and then a smaller supplementary amount to replace ongoing losses.

11 A 7-year-old boy with a history of chronic renal failure presents to the emergency department with right elbow pain. His parents provide a detailed history of the patient playing outside and falling on his right arm. They provide a list of his renal medications and he currently undergoes nightly peritoneal dialysis awaiting a kidney transplant. Radiography of his extremity demonstrates a nondisplaced supracondylar fracture, along with subperiosteal resorption of the bone, and widening metaphyses. His parents report this is his seventh fractured bone.

Of the following, what is the most likely mechanism of this patient's recurring fractures?

(A) Non-accidental trauma
(B) Congenital defect in collagen production
(C) Primary hyperparathyroidism
(D) Increased phosphate retention and decreased production of activated vitamin D
(E) Infiltration of the bone marrow by leukemic cells

The answer is D: **Increased phosphate retention and decreased production of activated vitamin D.** Children with chronic renal failure are at risk for multiple medical problems, including growth failure, renal osteodystrophy, acidosis, anemia, and medication toxicity. **(D)** Renal osteodystrophy results from the long-standing combination of increased phosphate retention and decreased production of activated vitamin D (1,25-dihydroxycholecalciferol). Vitamin D deficiency results in hypocalcemia due to poor intestinal absorption of calcium. In response to hypocalcemia, there is an increase in parathyroid gland activity, also known as secondary hyperparathyroidism, which leads to an increase in bone resorption. This increase in bone turnover presents in patients as muscle weakness, bone pain, and/or fractures with minor trauma. Radiographic findings include osteopenia, subperiosteal demineralization, and widening of the metaphyses. Medical management for patients with renal osteodystrophy includes decreasing phosphorus consumption and administering phosphate-binding medications, vitamin D, and calcium.

(A) Child abuse should be considered in any patient with recurrent bone fractures. The patient in the vignette has other chronic medical conditions that make abuse less likely. **(B)** Osteogenesis imperfecta is a congenital disease affecting collagen production resulting in patients with extremely fragile bones and multiple fractures. **(C)** Given the renal disease for the patient in the vignette, secondary hyperparathyroidism is more likely than primary hyperparathyroidism. **(E)** Leukemia can present with bone pain secondary to bone marrow infiltration; however, given the renal failure described in the vignette, this option is less likely.

12 An 8-year-old boy with a past medical history of asthma presents to the emergency department (ED) with increased work of breathing. His mother reports that his symptoms began yesterday with a runny nose. She tells you his asthma has been difficult to control for the past 6 months, and he has been seen in the ED multiple times for breathing treatments. The only new change at home is that his mother's boyfriend has been around more frequently and is a smoker. On examination, his vital signs are significant for an elevated respiratory rate and a pulse oximetry reading of 92% on room air. He is in mild respiratory distress, with symmetrical wheezing auscultated throughout his lung fields. An albuterol nebulizer treatment is ordered for the patient.

Of the following, which arterial blood gas would most likely be found in this patient?

	pH	$PaCO_2$	PaO_2	HCO_3^-
(A)	7.26	56	72	24
(B)	7.58	45	90	44
(C)	7.40	42	88	26
(D)	7.36	64	82	35
(E)	7.22	35	80	12

The answer is D: pH: 7.36, $PaCO_2$: 64, PaO_2: 82, HCO_3^-: 35. Asthma is a chronic obstructive pulmonary disorder characterized by airway hyperresponsiveness, inflammation, bronchoconstriction, and increased mucus production. Patients with obstructive lung disease have difficulty removing carbon dioxide; therefore, these patients' carbon dioxide levels are higher than those with healthy pulmonary function. The increase in carbon dioxide leads to an acidotic pH value; however, patients with chronic respiratory conditions are able to compensate through metabolic pathways to maintain a normal pH level. The blood gas expected for the patient in the vignette is one with a normal pH, elevated $PaCO_2$, and elevated HCO_3^- (primary respiratory acidosis with chronic metabolic compensation). **(A)** If the patient in the vignette did not have a history of asthma and presented with respiratory distress leading to respiratory failure, one would expect a blood gas to reveal a low pH, elevated $PaCO_2$, and normal HCO_3^- (primary respiratory acidosis without metabolic compensation).

13 A 2-year-old boy has just returned from the operating room after open reduction and internal fixation of his right femur. The boy is still drowsy and will need to be placed on intravenous (IV) fluid therapy to maintain hydration. He weighs 14 kg (31 lb).

Of the following, which is the correct hourly rate to run his maintenance fluid therapy?

(A) 14 mL/h
(B) 28 mL/h
(C) 31 mL/h
(D) 50 mL/h
(E) 62 mL/h

The answer is D: 50 mL/h. Maintenance IV fluids are composed of a solution containing glucose, sodium, potassium, and chloride that replace electrolyte losses from urine, stool, lungs, and skin. The goal of maintenance IV fluids is to prevent dehydration, electrolyte abnormalities, and acidosis. The rate at which maintenance fluids run is based on the patient's weight. The gold standard method for calculating daily maintenance fluid rates is the Holliday-Segar method: 100 mL/kg/d for the first 10 kg of body weight + 50 mL/kg/d for the next 10 kg of body weight + 25 mL/kg/d for each additional kilogram of body weight thereafter. For example, the patient in the vignette weighs 14 kg (10 kg + 4 kg). The daily maintenance rate for the patient in the vignette is calculated as follows: (100 mL/kg/d × 10 kg) + (50 mL/kg/d × 4 kg) + (25 mL/ g/d × 0 kg) = 1,200 mL/d. The hourly maintenance rate is then calculated by dividing the daily rate by 24 hours. Therefore, the appropriate hourly rate for the patient in the vignette is 1,200 mL/d/24 hours/d = 50 mL/h.

14 A 3-year-old previously healthy boy arrives to the emergency department by ambulance after his parents found him unresponsive at home. He was intubated in the field. On examination, he is unresponsive, afebrile with a normal heart rate, blood pressure, and pulse oximetry saturations. A quick secondary survey is unremarkable without any signs of trauma or environmental exposures. Two large bore IV catheters are placed, along with a Foley catheter. Initial laboratory results reveal a normal complete blood count, sodium level of 136 mEq/L, potassium of 4.0 mEq/L, chloride of 99 mEq/L, bicarbonate of 6 mEq/L, calcium of 6.9 mEq/L, glucose of 103 mg/dL, blood urea nitrogen of 8 mg/dL, and creatinine of 0.4 mg/dL.

Of the following, which condition is most likely given this patient's presentation and laboratory findings?

(A) Septic shock
(B) Renal tubular acidosis (RTA)
(C) Epilepsy
(D) Ethylene glycol ingestion
(E) Severe dehydration

The answer is D: Ethylene glycol ingestion. The approach to an unresponsive pediatric patient first begins with taking measures to ensure the patient is hemodynamically stable. Once this has been established, the workup toward the cause can begin, which includes history and physical examination. A laboratory workup can also aid in diagnosis. The laboratory results documented in the vignette demonstrate an increased anion gap metabolic acidosis, with an anion gap of 31. The differential diagnosis for an increased anion gap metabolic acidosis can include conditions with elevated intrinsic organic acids or conditions with elevated extrinsic organic acids. Some causes of increased anion gap metabolic acidosis include uremia, diabetic ketoacidosis, inborn errors of metabolism, lactic acidosis, and ingestions of substances, such as methanol, paraldehyde, iron, salicylate, isoniazid, ethanol, and ethylene glycol. For the patient in the vignette, ethylene glycol, found in antifreeze, ingestion is the most likely explanation from the choices provided. These patients can also have hypocalcemia, as calcium precipitates to make calcium oxalate stones. **(B)** RTA causes a normal anion gap metabolic acidosis. **(A)** Sepsis is unlikely without any fevers, normal vital signs, and a normal complete blood cell count. **(E)** Severe dehydration is also unlikely with a normal heart rate and blood pressure. **(C)** Epilepsy is an unlikely cause of an increased anion gap metabolic acidosis, but can be a common cause of an unresponsive pediatric patient. Long-standing sepsis, severe dehydration, and recurrent seizures can all lead to increased lactic acid production, which is consistent with metabolic acidosis with an increased anion gap; however, this would not be expected in an acute setting.

15 A 6-year-old girl with a history of central diabetes insipidus presents to the emergency department for increasing urine output. Her mother states that the patient had been doing well for the last few years and she has not needed to refill her vasopressin since she ran out last month. Over the last 2 weeks, her mother has noticed that the patient has decreased energy levels and increased urine output. On examination, she is tachycardic, moderately dehydrated, and has decreased skin turgor. Her laboratory results reveal a sodium level of 168 mEq/L.

Of the following, what is the next best step in the management of this patient with regard to fluid resuscitation?

(A) Bolus with hypotonic fluid to replace intravascular volume
(B) Bolus with hypertonic fluid to replace intravascular volume
(C) Bolus with isotonic fluid to replace intravascular volume
(D) Administer maintenance fluid with isotonic fluid
(E) Administer maintenance fluid with hypotonic fluid

The answer is C: Bolus with isotonic fluid to replace intravascular volume. Children with central diabetes insipidus possess an inability to produce adequate amounts of antidiuretic hormone and are treated with exogenous administration of vasopressin, or antidiuretic hormone. Hypernatremic dehydration develops in the setting of inadequate vasopressin levels.

Rapid correction of hypernatremia, such as administering a large amount of hypotonic solution, can lead to intracellular fluid shifts in response to the decreasing serum osmolality. This intracellular fluid shift can lead to cerebral edema that can cause seizures, coma, or death. For the patient in the vignette, the first step is to replace the intravascular volume deficit with isotonic fluids, such as normal saline and lactated Ringer's solution (LR). **(A, B)** Normal saline or LR should be the initial fluid choice for replacing any fluid deficit in a moderately dehydrated patient requiring intravenous therapy. Following the initial fluid bolus, a slow correction of hypernatremia should take place, with close monitoring of serum sodium to make sure that the rate of sodium decline is not greater than 0.5 mEq/L/h, or 10 to 12 mEq/L/d. **(D, E)** As the patient in the vignette is clearly dehydrated, there is not a role at this time for maintenance fluid therapy until intravascular volume is replenished with a bolus of isotonic fluid therapy. **(B)** Hypertonic therapy is contraindicated for a patient with hypernatremia.

---

16 A 4-year-old girl presents to the clinic for a routine school physical. Her parents state she has been in good health, but are concerned that she is much shorter than her classmates. On physical examination, her vital signs are within normal limits. She is plotted below the 3rd percentile in height and the 10th percentile for weight. Upon standing upright, the patient has significant bowing of her lower extremities, a prominent forehead, and enlarged wrists. Her extremities do not demonstrate any clubbing or edema. A urine dipstick in the clinic reveals increased protein and glucose. Laboratory results demonstrate a metabolic acidosis with a normal anion gap, low phosphorus, and a normal albumin level.

Of the following, which is the most likely diagnosis for this patient?

(A) Nephrotic syndrome
(B) Fanconi syndrome
(C) Vitamin D deficiency
(D) Inflammatory bowel disease
(E) Cystic fibrosis

The answer is B: Fanconi syndrome. The patient in the vignette has clinical signs and symptoms consistent with rickets, a condition of inadequate bone mineralization in growing children. Clinical features include failure to thrive, craniotabes, frontal bossing, widened costochondral junctions, kyphoscoliosis, enlargement of wrist and ankles as seen in *Figure 9-1*, and valgus or varus deformities. Rickets can result from vitamin D disorders, calcium deficiency, phosphorus deficiency, or certain renal disorders. **(C)** The most common cause of rickets is vitamin D deficiency, but for the patient in the vignette that alone does not explain the patient's urine abnormalities and metabolic acidosis. The most likely diagnosis in this patient is Fanconi syndrome. Fanconi syndrome

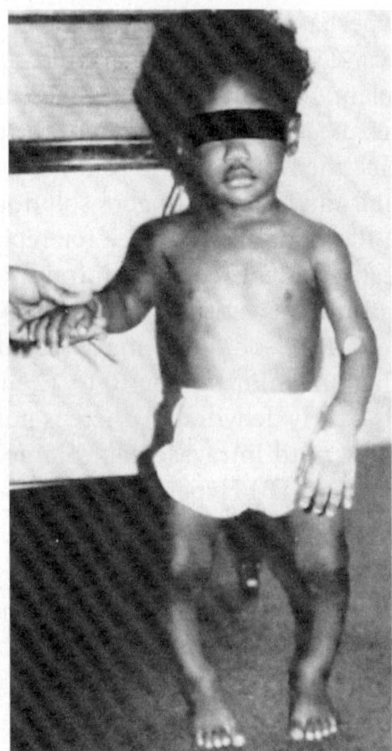

Figure 9-1

is a condition with generalized dysfunction of the proximal tubule leading to a proximal renal tubular acidosis and increased urinary losses of bicarbonate, protein, amino acids, glucose, uric acid, and phosphorus. The chronic hypophosphatemia leads to rickets.

(A) Patients with nephrotic syndrome do not typically present with rickets. Although patients with Fanconi syndrome may have mild proteinuria, it is generally not in the nephrotic range. **(D)** Patients with inflammatory bowel disease can have failure to thrive; however, this would be a less likely diagnosis given the lack of abdominal symptoms for the patient in the vignette. **(E)** Cystic fibrosis can lead to failure to thrive and malabsorption of fat-soluble vitamins, including vitamin D; however, the patient in the vignette does not have any respiratory or gastrointestinal symptoms that are associated with the disease.

17 A 15-year-old boy recently diagnosed with Burkitt lymphoma begins induction chemotherapy. He tolerates the first few hours of chemotherapy without any complaints; however, a couple hours later, his cardiac telemetry reading displays tall, peaked T waves. He is also complaining of diffuse muscle weakness. A basic metabolic profile is obtained, which reveals a potassium of 7.4 mEq/L.

Of the following treatment options, which intervention decreases total body potassium levels?

(A) Sodium bicarbonate
(B) Sodium polystyrene resin
(C) Insulin
(D) Albuterol nebulized treatment
(E) Calcium gluconate

The answer is B: Sodium polystyrene resin. The majority of total body potassium is found intracellularly. The kidneys regulate the serum level of potassium, and excretion is affected by acid–base balance, aldosterone, and renal function. Tumor lysis syndrome, as seen in the patient in the vignette, is one of the many conditions that can change the distribution of potassium between the intracellular and extracellular compartments. Tumor lysis syndrome is the result of the release of intracellular products from rapid cell turnover, generally seen at the initiation of chemotherapy for acute leukemia and high-grade lymphomas. The typical laboratory findings in tumor lysis syndrome include hyperkalemia, hyperphosphatemia, hyperuricemia, and hypocalcemia. The patient in the vignette is demonstrating clinical symptoms secondary to hyperkalemia, as the membranes of the cardiac and skeletal muscle are adversely affected. As hyperkalemia progresses, electrocardiography changes begin with peaking of the T waves and progress to an increased PR interval, flattening of P waves, widening of the QRS complex, and ultimately ventricular fibrillation and death. The goal of hyperkalemia treatment is to prevent life-threatening arrhythmias and to remove the potassium from the body. To prevent arrhythmias, interventions are needed to shift potassium intracellularly and stabilize the cardiac membrane. **(A, C, D)** Sodium bicarbonate, insulin, and β-agonists such as albuterol shift the potassium intracellularly while **(E)** calcium gluconate is used to stabilize the cardiac membrane. **(B)** To remove potassium from the body, sodium polystyrene or dialysis is used. Sodium polystyrene is an exchange resin given orally or rectally, in which sodium in the resin is exchanged for potassium. The potassium-containing resin is then excreted from the body.

CHAPTER 10

Endocrinology

PATRICIA M. NOTARIO

1 A 12-year-old boy is admitted from the emergency department with a 2-week history of diffuse headaches and worsening vision. He denies any history of trauma. He has a history of poor weight gain (see *Figure 10-1*). On examination, his extraocular movements are intact

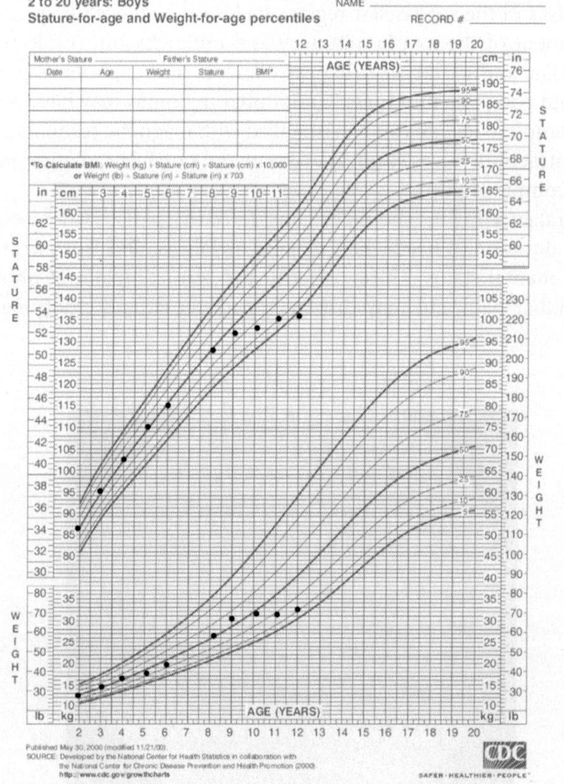

Figure 10-1

and his vision is 20/100 in both eyes. His funduscopic examination is shown in *Figure 10-2*. The patient's genital development is at sexual maturity rating (SMR) 2, but his pubic hair is at SMR 1. A magnetic resonance image of the brain confirms suspicions about the etiology of these findings.

Of the following, what is the most likely explanation for this patient's complaints?

(A) Craniopharyngioma
(B) Viral encephalitis
(C) Migraine headaches
(D) Pseudotumor cerebri
(E) Subarachnoid hemorrhage

The answer is A: Craniopharyngioma. The patient in the vignette presents with decreasing weight percentile, delayed sexual maturation, and evidence of increased intracranial pressure (i.e., papilledema) with poor visual acuity suggestive of a brain mass. These findings suggest a craniopharyngioma, which typically arises in the suprasellar region. Its location allows for spread toward and engulfment of the nearby pituitary and optic chiasm, resulting in both endocrinologic and visual disturbances. Patients may experience panhypopituitarism and complete blindness. Craniopharyngiomas may have both cystic and solid components that can be visualized with magnetic resonance imaging (MRI). Treatment involves surgical excision and possible radiation in the case of large or complex tumors.

(B) Viral encephalitis should be considered in a patient who presents with a few days' duration of headaches, malaise, myalgias, and fever with or without altered mental status. These patients may also complain of photophobia and retrobulbar pain and may display hyperesthesia and emotional lability.

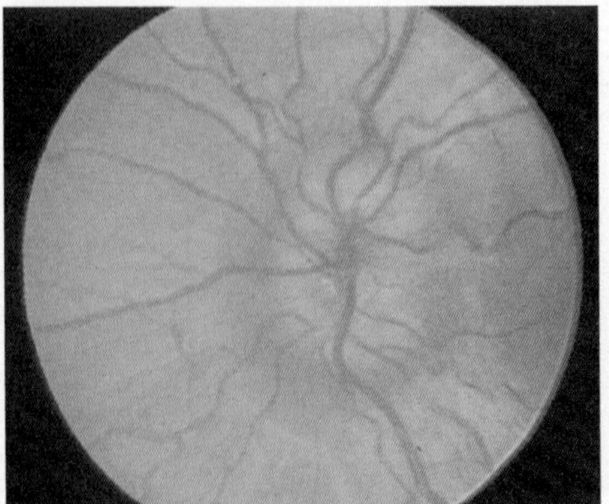

Figure 10-2

Common etiologic agents include echovirus, coxsackievirus, varicella zoster virus, and West Nile virus. Diagnosis is clinical but can be supported by mild mononuclear predominance on cerebrospinal fluid evaluation. Viral encephalitis is more acute in presentation than that described in the vignette and does not account for growth failure or delayed puberty described. **(C)** Similarly, although migraine without aura could explain the patient's headache and is often associated with vision changes, it does not account for his endocrinologic abnormalities. Neither disorder requires a brain MRI for diagnosis.

(D) The differential diagnosis of increased intracranial pressure should include idiopathic intracranial hypertension, also known as pseudotumor cerebri. Pseudotumor cerebri generally does not present with growth concerns. **(E)** Subarachnoid hemorrhage typically presents with acute onset of severe headache, focal neurologic deficits, and seizures. Underlying causes include arteriovenous malformations and aneurysms, the former of which is the most common cause in childhood. Diagnosis is made with angiography and patients require immediate attention. Subarachnoid hemorrhage does not have associated endocrinologic abnormalities.

A 3-week-old neonate presents to the emergency department with poor feeding and fussiness. The mother describes decreased urine output, but denies any fever. She reports the patient no longer wakes for feeds. On examination, the capillary refill is 3 seconds, the neonate's fontanelle is flat, and has tacky mucous membranes. Lungs are clear and there is no murmur appreciated or abdominal masses palpated. The neonate has normal male genitalia and both testes are descended. On initial laboratory evaluation, the sodium is noted to be 128 mEq/L, potassium 5.9 mEq/L, carbon dioxide 15 mEq/L, creatinine 0.8 mg/dL, and glucose 86 mg/dL.

Of the following, which is the ultimate treatment for this patient's underlying condition?

(A) Oral sodium supplements
(B) Insulin
(C) Ampicillin and cefotaxime
(D) Hydrocortisone and fludrocortisone
(E) Digoxin

The answer is D: Hydrocortisone and fludrocortisone. The patient in the vignette is demonstrating signs of altered mental status and dehydration, with concurrent hyponatremia and hyperkalemia. The most common cause of these findings is congenital adrenal hyperplasia (CAH), a disorder of cortisol synthesis that results in cortisol deficiency. The most common enzyme affected is 21-hydroxylase, seen in the majority of CAH cases. Without this enzyme, aldosterone and cortisol synthesis are halted, and the buildup of intermediate metabolites shunts the pathway to increased androgen secretion (see *Figure 10-3*). Men are more likely to present after a few weeks of life with severe salt wasting, as opposed to women who may be diagnosed earlier due to the appearance of virilized genitalia (see *Figure 10-4*). Patients with CAH require lifelong hormone replacement therapy. Hydrocortisone will replace cortisol and fludrocortisone will replace aldosterone. Treatment decreases the excessive secretion of androgens and prevents early-onset puberty and skeletal maturation.

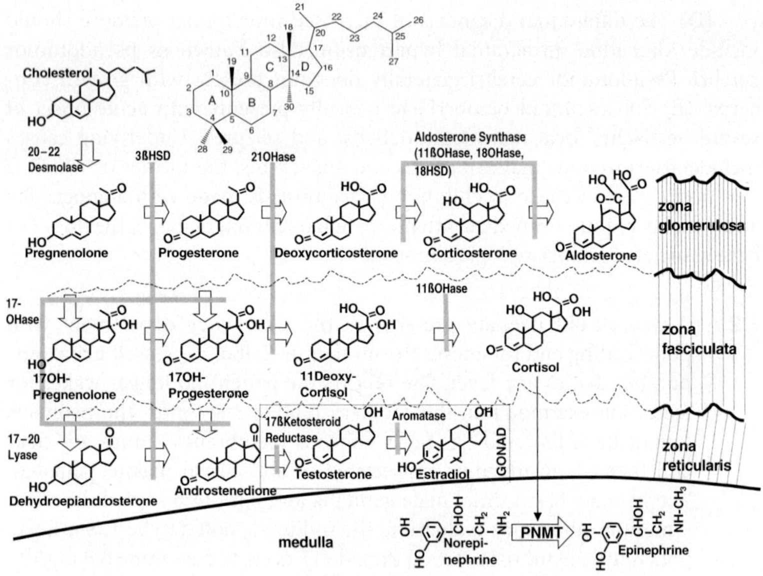

Figure 10-3

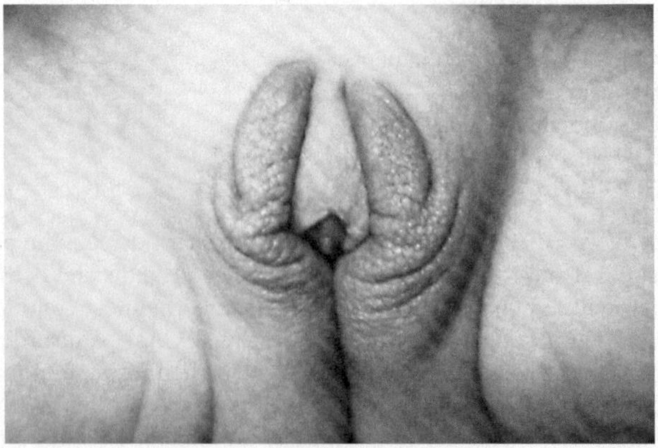

Figure 10-4

(A) Oral sodium supplementation does not address the patient's underlying diagnosis and will likely be renally excreted due to the absence of aldosterone. **(B)** Insulin is unnecessary as the patient in the vignette is normoglycemic and would result in hypoglycemia. **(C)** In a young patient with altered mental status, it is critical to consider sepsis and the need for antibiotic coverage with ampicillin and cefotaxime; however, neither would be as life saving as hydrocortisone and fludrocortisone in a patient with underlying CAH. **(E)** Digoxin, an antiarrhythmic, has no role in the case described in the vignette.

---

3 A 12-year-old girl comes to an outpatient clinic for the first time. Her father expresses concern about her weight and states that the patient has not seemed to have enough energy for daily exercise in the last few months. Her height is 145 cm and her weight is 60 kg. Although she denies fevers and dry skin, the patient states that she has infrequent bowel movements.

Of the following, what is the next best step in the evaluation of this patient?

(A) Obtain thyroid function tests
(B) Complete physical examination
(C) Abdominal radiograph
(D) Obtain urine sample for glucose
(E) Computed tomography (CT) of the head

The answer is B: Complete physical examination. The first step in evaluating a patient for potential pathologic conditions is a full history followed by a comprehensive physical examination. Often a detailed history and physical will help formulate a more appropriate differential diagnosis, and thus, a focused set of diagnostic evaluations. The patient in this vignette is experiencing symptoms consistent with hypothyroidism. This condition results from insufficient production or release of thyroid hormone. Primary hypothyroidism results from an intrinsic defect in the gland itself. Secondary hypothyroidism, also referred to as central or hypopituitary hypothyroidism, is typically the consequence of reduced or ineffective thyroid-stimulating hormone (TSH) activation of the thyroid follicles. Tertiary hypothyroidism results from deficient thyroid-releasing hormone production by the hypothalamus. Typical symptoms of hypothyroidism include fatigue, constipation, weight gain, depression, and muscle/joint pains. Less commonly, individuals may experience other effects such as bradycardia, menstrual irregularity, impaired cognitive function, and anemia.

(A) Ordering thyroid function testing, including a TSH level, free thyroxine, and triiodothyronine levels would be an appropriate next step for this patient after performing a complete history and physical examination. **(C)** An abdominal radiograph may help further investigate the patient's complaints of constipation, but is unlikely to help confirm the diagnosis. **(D)** A urine sample with urinalysis for glucose would help test for other potential causes for fatigue in the pediatric population such as diabetes but would be performed after a physical examination. **(E)** If a central pituitary or hypothalamic etiology for the patient's hypothyroidism is suspected, then CT scanning of the head may be warranted. However, this should not be performed until thyroid function testing has confirmed the presence of hypothyroidism.

4 A 16-year-old girl is brought in by her mother for evaluation of amenorrhea. The patient developed breasts at age 11 years but never developed pubic hair. Her mother experienced menarche at age 12 years. The patient is a long distance runner and does well in school. She is at the 90th percentile for height and 25th percentile for weight. On examination, she has sexual maturity rating (SMR) 3 breast development but SMR 1 pubic hair. She has no facial dysmorphism or cardiac murmur. She has no abdominal masses although there are 2 × 3 cm masses in the inguinal areas bilaterally. She has normal female external genitalia.

Of the following, what is the best explanation of this patient's amenorrhea?

(A) Hypothalamic amenorrhea
(B) Triple X syndrome
(C) Imperforate hymen
(D) Mayer-Rokitansky syndrome
(E) Complete androgen insensitivity

The answer is E: Complete androgen insensitivity. The patient in the vignette with evidence of thelarche has not yet achieved adrenarche or menarche, which is defined as primary amenorrhea. The differential diagnosis for primary amenorrhea includes gonadal dysgenesis, androgen insensitivity (also known as testicular feminization), triple X syndrome, true hermaphroditism, and all the causes of secondary amenorrhea such as hypothalamic amenorrhea, thyroid dysfunction, and pregnancy. Secondary amenorrhea is defined as the absence of menstruation for 6 months or more in a previously menstruating individual. This patient is tall for her age and is expected to have pubic hair as well as virilized external genitalia, neither of which is seen. In this case, the inguinal masses on examination are suspicious for testicles. This combination of findings strongly suggests complete androgen insensitivity, which is seen in patients whose chromosomes are 46,XY, but lack the ability to respond to testosterone. Although the external genitalia appear female, the vagina ends in a blind pouch and the uterus is absent. The gonads are testes, which are typically intra-abdominal but may descend to the inguinal canals.

(A) Hypothalamic amenorrhea is a common cause of secondary amenorrhea and is associated with high levels of stress, excessive exercise, and insufficient caloric intake; however, this condition does not explain her lack of pubic hair or the inguinal masses found on examination. **(B)** Females with triple XXX syndrome are much taller than their peers as is likely the case with this patient; however, most have normal pubertal development. **(C)** Anatomic reasons should be considered in a patient with amenorrhea, such as imperforate hymen. It may be diagnosed as early as infancy, when a bulging membrane may be seen in the vagina as stimulated by maternal estrogen levels during pregnancy. However, if asymptomatic, the bulging membrane regresses with time and may not present again until menarche when menstrual fluid collects. They typically present with primary amenorrhea and are found on examination to have a bluish, bulging membrane in the vagina. A pelvic mass may be palpable. **(D)** Another anatomic etiology is the congenital absence of the uterus and upper vagina. This can be seen if Müllerian duct development is prematurely arrested in the growing embryo. The most common cause is known as Mayer-Rokitansky syndrome. Patients are genotypically female and progress through puberty normally. They have a normal vulva but a dimpled or completely absent vagina. Internally, these patients have normal ovaries but hypoplastic fallopian tubes and an absent uterus.

5 A 3-year-old girl is brought to the office with the concern for breast development over the past 2 years. On examination, the girl's breasts are at sexual maturity rating (SMR) 3 and her external genitalia is at SMR 1. There is no clitoromegaly.

Of the following, what is the next best step toward establishing a diagnosis for this patient?

(A) Dehydroepiandrosterone sulfate (DHEA-S) level
(B) Pelvic ultrasound
(C) Magnetic resonance imaging of the brain
(D) Bone age radiography
(E) Reassure the mother that this level of development is normal and no further testing is needed

The answer is D: Bone age radiography. **(E)** Precocious puberty is defined by the onset of secondary sexual characteristics before 8 years of age in girls or 9 years of age in boys. It is important to perform a full physical examination and appropriately assign SMRs for breast and pubic hair development to ascertain which hormones may be involved as they may originate centrally or peripherally. The SMR or Tanner system assigns a number from 1 to 5 each for pubertal breast and pubic hair development, 1 being prepubertal and 5 being most mature. See *Figures 10-5* and *10-6* for illustrations of the SMR system in pubertal development.

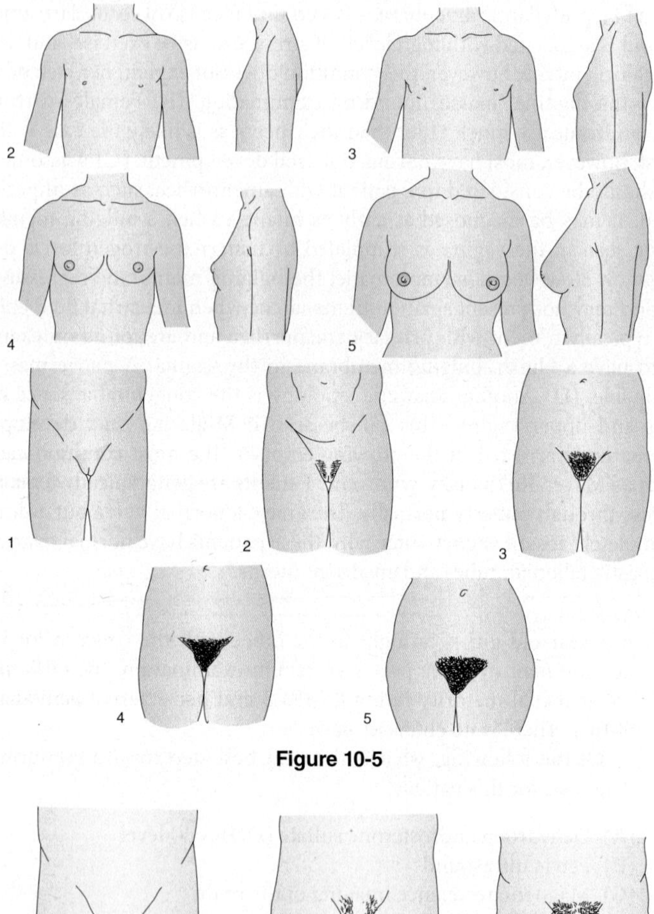

Figure 10-5

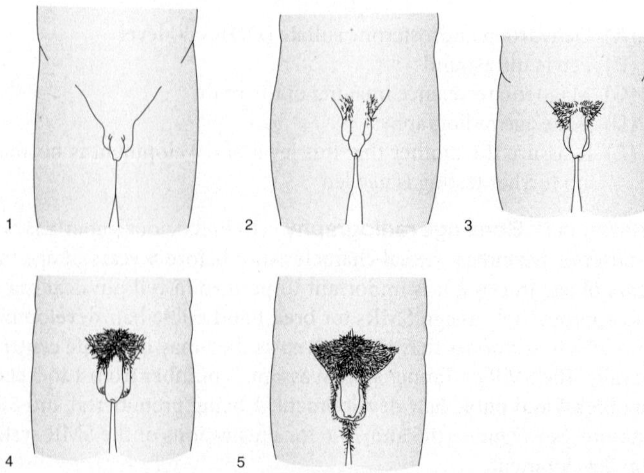

Figure 10-6

The main pubertal feature seen in the patient in the vignette is thelarche. Patients with isolated breast development typically do not progress further through puberty until an appropriate age. Thelarche can be seen shortly after birth and resolve by 2 years of age or persist to 5 years of age. **(B)** Genitalia and internal organ development is usually normal as is linear growth; thus, a pelvic ultrasound would likely not yield significant results. However, premature thelarche may be the first sign of true precocious puberty and these patients must be observed closely. Premature thelarche may also result from exogenous estrogen exposures necessitating a detailed history and physical examination. **(D)** A bone age radiograph should be obtained as the first step in the patient's workup in an attempt to identify signs of skeletal maturation, which would suggest progression in puberty and require a further workup.

In central precocious puberty, the patient develops through an expected progression (thelarche → adrenarche → growth spurt → menarche) via hypothalamic–pituitary–gonadal axis activation. **(A)** The patient in this vignette is displaying signs of central precocious puberty at a very young age, rendering a DHEA-S level unhelpful. DHEA-S is a helpful tool in the evaluation of premature pubarche. Causes of central precocious puberty include brain masses, head trauma, and hydrocephalus, all of which should be ruled out. **(C)** If this patient were to have an advanced bone age, brain imaging should be considered.

6 A 10-year-old girl presents for a well-child examination. She asks about puberty and when she can expect to experience menarche.

Of the following, which best describes normal female pubertal development?

(A) Peak height velocity → thelarche → adrenarche → menarche
(B) Thelarche → adrenarche → peak height velocity → menarche
(C) Adrenarche → thelarche → peak height velocity → menarche
(D) Thelarche → adrenarche → menarche → peak height velocity
(E) Adrenarche → thelarche → menarche → peak height velocity

The answer is B: Thelarche → adrenarche → peak height velocity → menarche. Pubertal changes in girls can be staged using the sexual maturity rating (SMR), also known as the Tanner staging system. These assign a rating or stage from 1 to 5 each for breast and pubic hair development. In both systems, 1 denotes prepubertal development and 5 denotes the most mature developmental stage. **(A, C, D, E)** The first sign of puberty in girls is thelarche, or breast bud development (SMR 2), which occurs on average at around 10 years of age. This is closely followed by adrenarche, or the appearance of pubic hair sparsely in the axillary and pubic regions. The breasts further develop at SMR 3 to a slightly fuller state with definition of the areola. Pubic hair becomes more abundant in its localized areas. As the breasts grow and pubic hair thickens, coils, and spreads to the inguinal area at SMR 4, the girl experiences a growth spurt followed by menarche. This is usually about 2 to 2½ years after the onset of thelarche. Other changes include enlargement of the ovaries, uterus, labia, and clitoris, and thickening of the endometrium and vaginal mucosa. At SMR 5, girls have well-defined breasts with darkened areolas and distinct nipples as well as thick, coiled pubic hair that extend to the medial thighs.

In contrast, boys experience testicular growth first, followed by elongation of the penis and development of pubic hair in the same progression as seen in girls. Boys reach peak height velocity as one of the final stages of pubertal development and thus continue linear growth longer than girls.

7 A 3-year-old patient in the pediatric intensive care unit was admitted for a closed head injury and renal laceration sustained after being thrown from her father's bicycle. She was intubated by the paramedics at the scene for altered mental status and airway protection and is postoperative day 2 for drainage of a subdural hematoma. The patient's urine output has increased from 3.4 to 6.7 mL/kg/h in the last 24 hours although there has been no change in the total amount and type of fluids she is receiving and her examination has remained stable. The following laboratory results have been obtained:

Serum: Sodium	159 mEq/L	Urine: Sodium	9 mEq/L
Potassium	4.4 mEq/L	Potassium	5 mEq/L
Urea nitrogen	24 mg/dL	Specific gravity	1.005
Creatinine	0.8 mg/dL	Osmolality	179 mOsm/kg
Glucose	89 mg/dL		
Osmolality	401 mOsm/kg		

Based on these laboratory results the patient received appropriate therapy and subsequent laboratory results are as follows:

Serum: Sodium	145 mEq/L	Urine: Sodium	28 mEq/L
Potassium	4.1 mEq/L	Potassium	15 mEq/L
Urea nitrogen	16 mg/dL	Specific gravity	1.015
Creatinine	0.7 mg/dL	Osmolality	283 mOsm/kg
Glucose	94 mg/dL		
Osmolality	351 mOsm/kg		

Based on these findings, of the following, which is the best treatment option for this patient?

(A) Replace all urinary losses with water
(B) Change intravenous fluids to hypotonic saline
(C) Routine desmopressin administration
(D) Thiazide diuretic
(E) Normal saline fluid bolus

The answer is C: Routine desmopressin administration. The patient in the vignette is demonstrating a sudden drastic increase in urine output with hypernatremia, increased serum osmolality, and dilute urine suggestive of diabetes insipidus (DI). DI can result from genetic anomalies or secondary to a variety of causes, including head trauma. Normally, antidiuretic hormone (ADH), also known as vasopressin, is released from the posterior pituitary in response to osmotic changes. Vasopressin acts via V2 receptors in the collecting tubules and thick ascending loop of Henle to insert aquaporin channels, allowing water to be reabsorbed and urine to be concentrated. In DI, the body cannot rely on ADH to appropriately balance sodium excretion and water retention, because of a central lack of ADH or a decreased renal responsiveness to the hormone.

DI must also be distinguished from other causes of polyuria such as postoperative fluid diuresis. Laboratory values can help to diagnose the underlying cause of polyuria. In DI, serum osmolality is >300 mOsm/kg while urine osmolality is <300 mOsm/kg, despite restriction of fluids. Patients with postsurgical diuresis should still be able to maintain normal serum osmolality as their body is appropriately diuresing excess fluid. In a post-neurosurgical setting with serum osmolality greater than urine osmolality, central DI would be the most likely cause. **(C)** Routine desmopressin administration is the mainstay therapy. **(A, B, E)** A normal saline bolus, hypotonic saline, or replacing urinary losses with water in the patient in the vignette would only result in further polyuria with hypernatremia. In nephrogenic DI, the issue is with the V2 receptor, and administration of desmopressin will not result in any change. **(D)** Patients with nephrogenic DI may respond to thiazide diuretics or amiloride, but these are not used in central DI.

A full-term newborn is seen in clinic for his 2-week visit. Prenatal maternal serologies were negative. Apgar scores were 9 and 9 at 1 and 5 minutes, respectively. The patient's mother denies any medication use during the pregnancy except a daily prenatal vitamin. She reports that the newborn was initially feeding well but has progressively seemed fussier and less interested in feeds. On examination, she has the findings shown in *Figure 10-7*. There is no evidence of a vagina. There are no abdominal or inguinal masses. Initial laboratory tests show a sodium level of 129 mEq/L, potassium of 6.1 mEq/L, and creatinine of 0.5 mg/dL.

Of the following, which best explains this newborn's examination and laboratory findings?

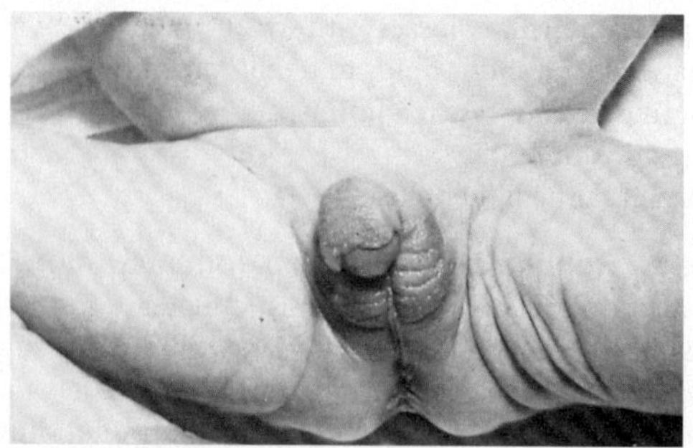

Figure 10-7

(A) 11β-Hydroxylase deficiency
(B) Complete androgen insensitivity
(C) Exogenous androgen exposure
(D) 21-Hydroxylase deficiency
(E) Autoimmune adrenal insufficiency

The answer is D: 21-Hydroxylase deficiency. The patient in the vignette demonstrates signs of virilization and altered mental status and presents with hyponatremia and hyperkalemia. The most common cause of these findings is congenital adrenal hyperplasia (CAH). In this autosomal recessive disorder of cortisol synthesis that results in cortisol deficiency, adrenocorticotropic hormone (ACTH) is increased via a feedback loop to hypersecrete intermediate metabolites depending on which enzymatic step is affected (see *Figure 10-8*). The adrenal cortex normally produces aldosterone, cortisol, and androgens. The vast majority of CAH cases involves a deficiency of 21-hydroxylase. Without this enzyme, aldosterone and cortisol synthesis is halted, leading to buildup of progesterone and 17-hydroxyprogesterone. The pathway is then shunted to increase

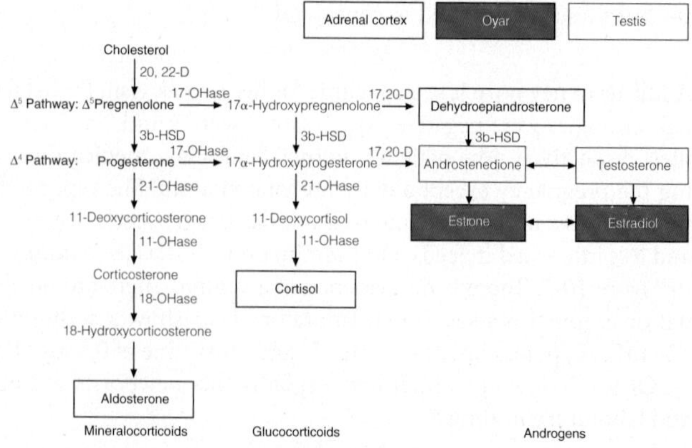

Figure 10-8

androgen secretion as the enzymes in those pathways are not affected. Thus, patients with 21-hydroxylase deficiency usually display evidence of salt wasting (hyponatremia with concurrent hyperkalemia), adrenal insufficiency (hypotension and hypoglycemia), and virilization. Females may present with clitoromegaly and ambiguous external genitalia, although their internal structures remain female. Males are more likely to demonstrate premature puberty and severe salt wasting.

(A) A small minority of patients with CAH have 11β-hydroxylase deficiency. In this case, the aldosterone pathway remains intact via buildup of a potent mineralocorticoid, deoxycorticosterone (DOC), from which some glucocorticoids can be formed. Thus, patients with this form of CAH do not usually display signs of adrenal insufficiency. In fact, the buildup of DOC leads to hypertension in many patients. However, these patients may still display virilization as intermediate metabolites continue to be shunted toward the androgen production pathway.

(B) Patients with complete androgen insensitivity, also known as testicular feminization syndrome, are genotypically male but phenotypically female as a result of a lack of recognition by androgen receptors to the present androgen hormones. These patients have testes and still produce high levels of luteinizing hormone and testosterone. These patients' vaginas end blindly in a pouch and they have no uterus because of the effect of anti-Müllerian hormone secreted by the testes. Frequently, these patients are raised as females from infancy but may present with an inguinal or labial masses, which are usually determined to be testicles. This disorder is not associated with any signs of adrenal insufficiency.

(C) Females exposed to excess androgen during intrauterine development are genotypically XX and have female internal organs including ovaries, uterus, and fallopian tubes; however, their external genitalia are virilized, showing clitoromegaly and labioscrotal fusion. This disorder is not associated with any signs of adrenal insufficiency (see *Table 10-1*).

Table 10-1 Disorders with genital abnormalities

	21-Hydroxylase Deficiency		**11β-Hydroxylase Deficiency**		**Complete Androgen Insensitivity**	**Excess Androgen Exposure**
Genotype	XY	XX	XY	XX	XY	XX
External Genitalia	Male	Virilized (clitoromegaly, labial fusion)	Male	Virilized (clitoromegaly, labial fusion)	Female (vaginal pouch)	Virilized (clitoromegaly, labial fusion)
Internal Genitalia	Male	Female	Male	Female	Male (testes, no uterus)	Female
Additional Findings	Hyponatremia, hyperkalemia, hypotension, hypoglycemia		Hypertension		Amenorrhea, thelarche w/o adrenarche	None

(E) The most common cause of primary adrenal insufficiency, or Addison disease, is autoimmune adrenal gland destruction resulting in glucocorticoid deficiency. Patients may also experience varying degrees of mineralocorticoid deficiency. Androgen production is not affected in this disease so the sexual genotype and phenotype correlate.

---

9 A previously healthy 10-year-old girl is brought to the office. Her mother expresses concern about her height, stating that the patient "has always been the shortest in her class." The mother is 5 feet tall and shares that the patient's father is 5 feet, 4 inches. The patient experienced menarche last month. On physical examination, the patient is well appearing, proportional, and has no facial dysmorphism. She has no cardiac murmurs or abdominal masses. Her radiographic bone age is within normal limits. Her growth chart is included in *Figure 10-9*.

Of the following, what is the best explanation of her findings?

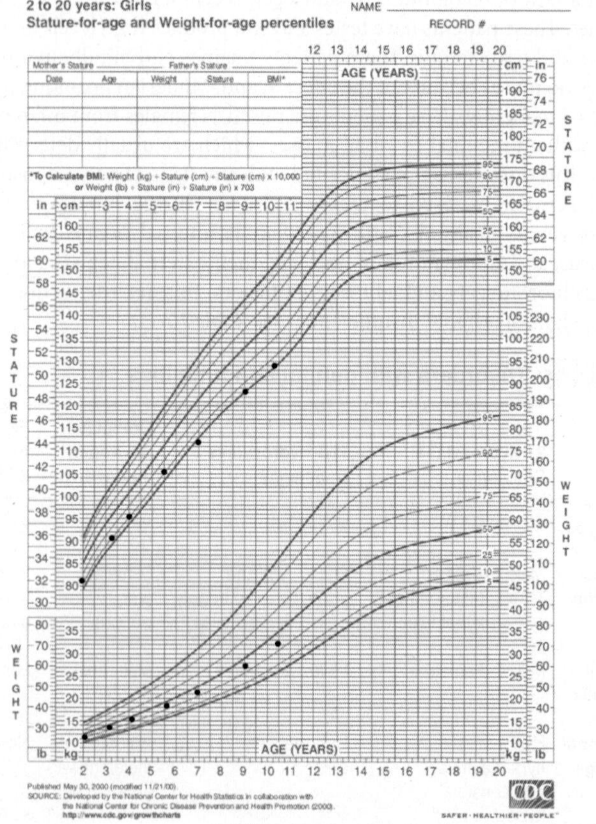

Figure 10-9

(A) Constitutional growth delay
(B) Familial short stature
(C) Turner syndrome
(D) Achondroplasia
(E) Congenital growth hormone deficiency

The answer is B: Familial short stature. The patient in the vignette demonstrates an expected pattern of growth based on the fact that her parents also have short stature. Height potential can be estimated by calculating the mid-parental height, which is slightly different given the gender of the patient.

For female patients: [Mother's height + Father's height − 5 inches (or 13 cm)] / 2
For male patients: [Mother's height + Father's height + 5 inches (or 13 cm)] / 2

The height potential for the girl in the vignette is 59.5 inches, or 4 feet 11.5 inches. It is also important to note that the patient's growth consistently has been between the 5th and 10th percentiles for height and near the 25th percentile for weight. Her examination is not suspicious for syndromic findings and she has achieved puberty at an appropriate age.

Patients with familial or genetic short stature are consistently small from birth, through childhood, and into adulthood. Growth pattern follows a normal curve although it typically runs just at or below the lower percentiles. Chronologic age and bone age are concordant. As with the patient in the vignette, these patients achieve puberty at an average age.

(A) In contrast with familial short stature, patients with constitutional growth delay have average height and weight for the first few years of life and then sustain lower height curves during childhood. These patients enter puberty later than average so their height remains lower than their age cohort. Even though these patients have a delayed beginning to puberty, they eventually attain their expected adult heights. This is not associated with any syndromic features or additional anomalies. Frequently, affected patients have other family members that describe short stature and delayed puberty with eventual attainment of height potential.

(C) Patients with Turner syndrome (monosomy of chromosome X, or XO) are usually small for gestational age as infants and display short stature as they grow. These patients can also have a variety of features, including webbing of the neck, renal anomalies, and congenital heart defects such as coarctation of aorta, mitral valve prolapse, and bicuspid aortic valve. These patients have gonadal dysgenesis with subsequent primary amenorrhea and lack of secondary sexual characteristics.

(D) Achondroplasia is a genetic dwarfism that involves shortened limbs, particularly of the proximal portions, a long narrow trunk, and a large head with a prominent forehead. Patients with achondroplasia are usually of low-normal size at birth but their growth parameters fall below the expected curve for both height and weight as they age.

(E) Most children with hypopituitarism are of normal weight and length at birth yet their heights fall below normal as they age at a rate dependent on the severity of their growth hormone deficiency. Infants with severe congenital pituitary hormone defects may present with apnea, hypoglycemia, or cyanosis. Boys have microphallus. These patients may also have hypothyroidism or hypoadrenalism.

---

10 A 17-year-old girl presents to the emergency department complaining of near-syncopal episodes associated with tachycardia that have occurred three times in the last week. She also complains of "feeling hot when everyone else feels cold." Her great aunt has a history of an unspecified thyroid disease. Her resting heart rate is 138 beats/min and her blood pressure is 130/80 mmHg. On examination, a mild protuberance of both eyes, a fine tremor, and anterior neck fullness are noted. She has brisk deep tendon reflexes. She has no murmur on cardiac auscultation, no abdominal masses, and no skin lesions.

Of the following, which explains the most likely etiology of her disease?

(A) Inhibitory thyroperoxidase enzyme antibody
(B) Iodide toxicity
(C) Excess catecholamine release
(D) Stimulatory thyroid hormone receptor antibody
(E) Hypoglycemia

The answer is D: Stimulatory thyroid hormone receptor antibody. The constellation of symptoms and findings of the patient in the vignette is most consistent with hyperthyroidism, particularly given the tachycardia, neck fullness, proptosis (see *Figure 10-10*), and fine tremor. This is further supported

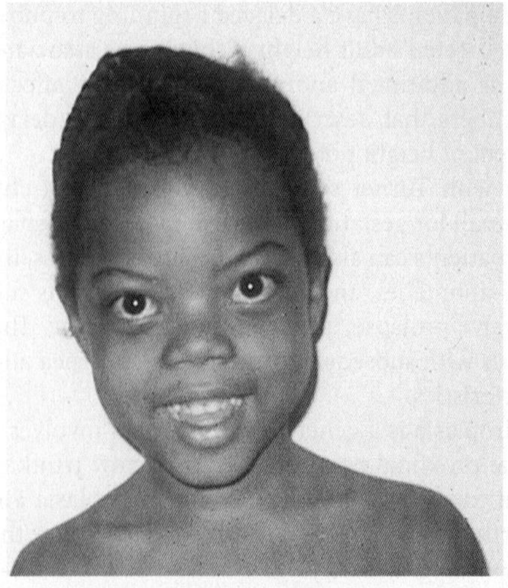

Figure 10-10

by the patient's family history of thyroid disease, the most common cause of which is autoimmune. Thyroid disease and autoimmune diseases can be seen with increased frequency among families with an affected member. In this case, the likely diagnosis is Graves disease which occurs via autoimmune thyroid hormone receptor stimulation. This stimulation causes increased cyclic adenosine monophosphate release that results in thyroid hyperplasia and unregulated overproduction of thyroid hormone.

(A) Autoimmune inhibition of thyroid peroxidase is seen in Hashimoto thyroiditis. This results in decreased thyroid hormone production as well as thyroid tissue destruction via natural killer cells. These autoantibodies can also stimulate natural killer cell cytotoxicity to destroy thyroid tissue. Patients with Hashimoto thyroiditis may also have anti-thyroglobulin antibodies as well as thyroid-stimulating hormone receptor-blocking antibodies.

(B) Chronic use of medications containing iodides, such as amiodarone, disrupts peripheral thyroxine to triiodothyronine conversion and results in hypothyroidism as opposed to hyperthyroidism. **(C)** Catecholamine excess is seen with pheochromocytomas, neuroendocrine tumors often located in the adrenal gland. Patients typically experience paroxysmal hypertension with tachycardia, flushing, dizziness, and abdominal pain. **(E)** Hypoglycemia can cause a large range of symptoms, including vision changes, palpitations, shakiness, anxiety, and sweating. Untreated hypoglycemia can result in altered mental status and seizures that require immediate attention.

---

11 A 7-year-old boy presents to the emergency department complaining of headaches, nausea, fatigue, and increased thirst. His mother states that his thirst seems to be insatiable and that he has been urinating much more frequently than usual. On examination, the patient is tired-appearing. His skin is dry and his mucus membranes are tacky. His lungs are clear and he has no murmur. His abdomen is soft with no abdominal masses. An initial bedside glucose level is 405 mg/dL. His sodium is 132 mEq/L, potassium 5.6 mEq/L, chloride 91 mEq/L, carbon dioxide 12 mEq/L, blood urea nitrogen 37 mg/dL, and creatinine 1.8 mg/dL.

Of the following, what is the next best step in management?

(A) Administer a 1 unit/kg bolus of insulin
(B) Administer a 20 mL/kg bolus of 0.45% saline
(C) Administer a 0.1 unit/kg continuous infusion of insulin
(D) Administer a 1 mEq/kg bolus of sodium bicarbonate
(E) Administer a 20 mL/kg bolus of 0.9% normal saline

The answer is E: Administer a 20 mL/kg bolus of normal saline. The patient in the vignette presents with polydipsia, polyuria, dehydration, hyperglycemia, and an anion gap acidemia. These are many of the features associated with diabetic ketoacidosis (DKA). DKA results from ineffective or severely inadequate circulating insulin. Hyperglycemia without an effective mechanism to deliver glucose to the tissues causes the cells to essentially function in starvation mode. Fats and proteins are broken down to produce ketones, or strong acids. Excess circulating glucose and ketone bodies cause osmotic diuresis that results in dehydration. **(C)** Thus, the first step in management is to address this patient's hydration status with isotonic fluid in the form of a 20 mL/kg bolus of normal (0.9%) saline bolus. This helps to improve renal excretion but care must be taken to avoid rapid rehydration as it can increase the risk of cerebral edema.

(B) Bolus therapy with hypotonic solutions such as 0.45% saline is not appropriate in this case, particularly in the face of hyponatremia. **(E)** Although a sodium bicarbonate bolus may provide a buffer for the patient's acidosis, it is not indicated, as it does not address the underlying problem of lipolysis and proteolysis. Insulin therapy is indicated after addressing hydration as it allows glucose to be utilized for metabolism and curbs ketone formation. **(A)** Insulin should be administered as a continuous infusion at a rate of 0.1 units/kg/h rather than as a bolus because the latter may result in hypokalemia and hypoglycemia due to rapid correction. Once glucose levels have fallen below 250 mg/dL, glucose is added to the patient's fluids while continuing to administer insulin, which continues to address ketone formation.

---

12 A 9-year-old obese male patient presents to the clinic with complaints of increased weight despite dietary changes and daily exercise. On examination, the boy is obese with a round face. Extraocular muscles are intact and his neck is supple. His cardiac and pulmonary examinations are unremarkable. His abdomen is obese, soft, and non-tender. He has several stretch marks along the sides of his abdomen. His blood pressure is 139/87 mmHg. His laboratory results reveal:

Fasting glucose	201 mg/dL	
Fasting triglycerides	142 mg/dL	
24 hours Urinary cortisol level	247 μg/dL	(Normal 10 to 100 μg/dL)
Morning cortisol level after midnight Dexamethasone administration	39 μg/dL	(Normal < 5 μg/dL)

Magnetic resonance imaging (MRI) of the brain with contrast is within normal limits. Of the following, what is the best explanation of the above findings?

(A) Hypothyroidism
(B) Prader-Willi syndrome
(C) Congenital adrenal hyperplasia (CAH)
(D) Cushing disease
(E) Cushing syndrome

The answer is E: Cushing syndrome. The most significant findings for the patient in the vignette are obesity, hyperglycemia, and elevated cortisol levels despite administration of dexamethasone (a positive dexamethasone suppression test). This is suggestive of cortisol hypersecretion, also known as Cushing syndrome. Patients with this disorder are usually obese, with moon facies, a buffalo hump, and abdominal striae. They may have thinned skin, poor wound healing, hyperglycemia, and hypertension. The most common cause of Cushing syndrome is prolonged exogenous high-dose administration of glucocorticoids. In these cases, patients may also develop osteoporosis, linear growth retardation, delayed pubertal onset, or secondary amenorrhea. Cushing syndrome may also be caused by endogenous hypersecretion of cortisol, which may result from an adrenal tumor that releases cortisol, a pituitary tumor-secreting adrenocorticotropic hormone (ACTH) that then raises cortisol levels, or by an ectopic tumor that secretes cortisol or ACTH.

Normally, cortisol levels are elevated in the morning and decrease overnight, except in infants and young children in whom this pattern is not yet established. Thus, an elevated midnight cortisol level is strongly suggestive of Cushing syndrome. Cortisol levels are also increased during a 24-hour urine collection. Finally, a one-step dexamethasone suppression test may also confirm this diagnosis. Dexamethasone acts via a negative feedback loop to decrease ACTH secretion, which in turn decreases cortisol levels. In patients with Cushing syndrome, where cortisol secretion is not regulated via this pathway, cortisol levels remain elevated despite dexamethasone administration.

Once the diagnosis is established, as is evident with the patient in the vignette, the underlying cause of the cortisol hypersecretion must be identified. Patients with cortisol-secreting tumors may have suppressed levels of ACTH due to the negative feedback loop, although this may not be the case in an ACTH-secreting pituitary adenoma. Adrenal tumors larger than 1.5 cm can be visualized by abdominal computed tomography while many pituitary tumors may be identified by a brain MRI with contrast. **(E)** The term Cushing disease is used to describe cortisol hypersecretion that results specifically from a pituitary source. In this patient, whose brain MRI with contrast is normal, Cushing disease is less likely.

(A, B) Cortisol levels are not expected to be starkly elevated in patients with hypothyroidism or Prader-Willi syndrome, although both may cause significant weight gain. Prader-Willi syndrome is a genetic condition acquired via paternal imprinting resulting in hypotonia, hyperphagia leading to obesity, short stature and extremities, developmental delay, and delayed pubertal development. **(C)** In patients with CAH, the defect is in cortisol biosynthesis leading to deficiency as opposed to excess of this hormone.

---

13 An 8-year-old patient presents to the urgent care clinic complaining of increasingly frequent episodes of headache, dizziness, flushing, and abdominal pain. Her blood pressure is 180/123 mmHg and her heart rate is 165 beats/min. Bedside blood glucose is 96 mg/dL. The remainder of her physical examination is otherwise normal.

Of the following, which test would confirm this patient's most likely diagnosis?

(A) Electrocardiogram
(B) Echocardiogram
(C) Venous Doppler study
(D) Urine metanephrines
(E) Thyroid function tests

The answer is D: Urine metanephrines. Hypertension in children may have a variety of causes including renal or renovascular disease, cardiac anomalies, hyperthyroid state, mineralocorticoid excess, adrenocortical tumors, essential hypertension, and anxiety. The most common cause of pathologic hypertension in children is associated with renal causes; however, as obesity is on the rise, the number of patients with essential hypertension continues to increase.

The patient in the vignette presents with episodic hypertension and tachycardia, which should prompt the provider to consider a pheochromocytoma, particularly in a previously healthy individual. Other causes of paroxysmal hypertension include porphyria, hyperthyroidism, familial dysautonomia, diabetes mellitus, and cerebral disorders. Pheochromocytomas are neuroendocrine-secreting tumors that release catecholamines. In children, this consists predominantly of norepinephrine, which can explain the presenting symptoms of headache, flushing, dizziness, palpitations, and abdominal pain. The hypertension is typically paroxysmal at first but evolves to become constant. Patients have elevated total urine catecholamine levels and metanephrines, a metabolite of norepinephrine. Computed tomography or magnetic resonance imaging can be used to detect these adrenal tumors, which may grow large enough to compress the renal vascular bed and account for the sustained hypertension.

(C) A venous Doppler study would diagnose a renal vein thrombosis, an uncommon disorder that may be caused by hypercoagulable disorders, dehydration, estrogen use, nephrotic syndrome, pregnancy, trauma to the back or abdomen, or a local tumor. In older children, the most common cause is nephrotic syndrome. In infants, the most likely cause is dehydration. It manifests as hypertension but it is not usually episodic or associated with tachycardia.

(A, B) Electrocardiogram and echocardiogram can give important diagnostic clues for left ventricular hypertrophy (LVH). The two most common and important pressure overload states are systemic hypertension and aortic stenosis. Hypertension secondary to LVH is sustained rather than episodic.

(E) Excess thyroxine release is seen in patients with hyperthyroidism. This condition shares many symptoms with pheochromocytoma such as flushing, palpitations, hypertension, and tachycardia although usually the symptoms are more constant as compared with the paroxysms experienced with a pheochromocytoma.

---

14 A 1-month-old neonate is following up in his pediatrician's clinic after being evaluated by an ophthalmologist for horizontal nystagmus. The ophthalmology report states that the patient has been diagnosed with optic nerve hypoplasia. On examination, the boy is a small-sized, sleeping baby with a wide, mildly sunken fontanelle and a micropenis. His testes are descended bilaterally. He has no murmur or abdominal masses.

Of the following, abnormality of which test is most consistent with this patient's diagnosis?

(A) Pituitary hormone levels
(B) Head ultrasound
(C) Urine toxicology screen
(D) Abdominal computed tomography (CT)
(E) Serum chemistries

The answer is A: Pituitary hormone levels. Optic nerve hypoplasia can be seen in patients with septo-optic dysplasia, a developmental disorder associated with midline brain structure defects including agenesis of the septum pellucidum, agenesis of the corpus callosum, and panhypopituitarism, although there can be a wide range in the severity of these malformations including hormone deficiencies. The most frequent hormone deficiency is that of growth hormone, which explains this patient's small size. If severe, patients may present with neonatal hypoglycemia, direct hyperbilirubinemia of unclear etiology, and micropenis in males. These patients may display horizontal nystagmus at 1 to 8 months of age and can display a range from normal vision to complete blindness. If septo-optic dysplasia is suspected, pituitary hormone levels should be obtained and replacement provided as indicated.

(B) A head ultrasound may reveal some abnormalities but a magnetic resonance imaging of the brain would be more specific, and indicated if ophthalmology examination reveals an abnormality. **(C)** A urine toxicology screen is an important part of the workup for neonatal nystagmus as nystagmus can result from in utero exposure to opiates and benzodiazepines. However, neither exposure is expected to cause optic nerve hypoplasia. **(D)** An abdominal CT scan is unlikely to be helpful in this case. **(E)** Serum chemistries might reveal hypoglycemia or signs of dehydration, but is not the best test to lead to the underlying diagnosis.

---

15 A previously healthy 14-year-old girl presents with a 3-week history of fatigue and infrequent stooling. She notes that she has also been "pulling out chunks of hair" whenever she washes it. She has gained 8 lb since her last visit 2 months ago. Her hemoglobin is 13.5 g/dL. Her thyroid-stimulating hormone (TSH) is 15.2 mIU/L and free thyroxine (fT4) is 0.4 ng/dL.

Of the following, what is the most likely underlying mechanism of this disease?

(A) Pituitary hormone deficiency
(B) Stimulatory thyroid hormone receptor antibody
(C) Thyroid enzyme inhibition by antibody formation
(D) Post-infectious enzyme deficiency
(E) Chronic amiodarone use

The answer is C: **Thyroid enzyme inhibition by antibody formation.** The patient in the vignette exhibits many symptoms that suggest hypothyroidism, confirmed by a low fT4 level along with an elevated TSH level. The primary problem is with the thyroid gland, such that the low fT4 levels stimulate the pituitary gland to secrete high levels of TSH in an attempt to produce more fT4 in a feedback loop. The most common cause of primary hypothyroidism is Hashimoto thyroiditis, which occurs through autoimmune inhibition of thyroid peroxidase to decrease hormone production. These autoantibodies can also stimulate natural killer cell cytotoxicity to destroy thyroid tissue. Patients with Hashimoto thyroiditis may also have anti-thyroglobulin antibodies as well as TSH receptor-blocking antibodies.

(A) Pituitary disease can cause acquired central hypothyroidism. TSH deficiency may be caused by a hypothalamic–pituitary tumor or as a result of treatment for the tumor. In this case, both TSH and fT4 levels are expected to be low. **(B)** Stimulatory thyroid hormone receptor antibodies are seen in Graves disease and typically are associated with hyperthyroidism. The antibody binds the TSH receptor and stimulates cyclic adenosine monophosphate to eventually cause thyroid hyperplasia and excess thyroid hormone release. Expected laboratory abnormalities are an elevated fT4 with decreased TSH because of the negative feedback loop to the pituitary. **(D)** Post-infectious enzyme deficiency can be seen with intestinal mucosal damage as with a viral gastroenteritis. This can cause a secondary lactase deficiency causing intolerance that typically improves as the mucosa heals. This process is not involved in the most common cause of hypothyroidism. **(E)** Amiodarone is an anti-arrhythmic medication that can cause thyroid dysfunction with chronic use. It can affect thyroid function via its high iodide content and by interfering with thyroxine to triiodothyronine conversion.

---

16 A 13-year-old girl who has been followed by her pediatrician for weight loss presents to the emergency department with a 3-day history of nonbloody, nonbilious emesis, generalized muscle weakness, and the feeling of lightheadedness when she sat up in bed. Her blood pressure is 91/56 mmHg while lying and 75/44 mmHg while sitting. She had upper respiratory symptoms 5 days prior. On examination, her mucus membranes are dry and her capillary refill is 3 seconds. She is thin-framed and ill-appearing although nontoxic. She is able to answer questions appropriately. Her mother states that the patient has had similar but

milder symptoms in the past whenever she experienced a viral upper respiratory infection. Her laboratory work reveals the following:

Serum: Sodium	121 mEq/L	Urine: Specific gravity	1.030
Potassium	6.1 mEq/L		
Chloride	97 mEq/L	Glucose	negative
Carbon dioxide	19 mEq/L	Ketones	positive
Urea nitrogen	34 mg/dL	Blood	negative
Creatinine	1.1 mg/dL	Urobilinogen	negative
Glucose	51 mg/dL	White blood cell	0–5 cells/hpf
Calcium	10.8 mg/dL	Red blood cell	0–5 cells/hpf

Of the following, which best explains this patient's findings?

(A) Gastroenteritis with dehydration
(B) Addison disease
(C) Bulimia nervosa
(D) Autoimmune polyglandular syndrome type 2 (APS-2)
(E) DiGeorge syndrome

The answer is B: Addison disease. The key point in the case described in the vignette is the recurrence of this patient's symptoms with viral illnesses as well as the history of weight loss. These factors, in combination with orthostasis, emesis, malaise, hypoglycemia, ketosis, hyponatremia, and hyperkalemia, suggest adrenal insufficiency, the most common cause of which is autoimmune destruction of the adrenal gland, Addison disease. This results in deficiencies of cortisol and aldosterone, which are particularly noticeable during periods of stress such as viral illnesses. Addison disease can have an insidious onset or could present acutely with severe hypotension, hypoglycemia, or even coma. Some patients may develop hyperpigmentation as a result of increased ACTH release in response to hypocortisolism via a feedback loop. This is because ACTH is formed from a pro-molecule that also produces melanocyte-stimulating hormone. Adrenal insufficiency can also be seen in patients who suddenly stop receiving exogenous steroids after having taken them chronically. The long-term administration of exogenous steroids suppresses adrenal production of glucocorticoids such that sudden removal causes adrenal insufficiency.

(A) Patients with gastroenteritis would be expected to have hypokalemia rather than hyperkalemia. **(C)** The history and physical examination of the patient in the vignette is not supportive of bulimia nervosa. Electrolyte abnormalities in bulimia are more common to include hypokalemia. **(E)** Hypoglycemia and emesis are not commonly associated with DiGeorge syndrome. In addition, the patient in the vignette has mild hypercalcemia and no evidence of cardiac disease.

(D) Autoimmune endocrinopathies can occur concurrently and are described in two main groups known as APS-1 and APS-2. APS-1 is caused by mutations in the autoimmune regulatory gene and is also known as APCED, or autoimmune polyendocrinopathy, candidiasis, and ectodermal dysplasia. It includes two of the following: hypoparathyroidism, Addison disease, or mucocutaneous candidiasis. APS-2 consists of Addison disease and either type 1 diabetes mellitus or autoimmune thyroid disease. Although the patient in this case may be at risk for developing either APS-1 or APS-2, she does not display any signs of other polyendocrinopathies at this time.

17 A 14-year-old boy with a history of recurrent renal calculi and behavioral problems is admitted from the emergency department to the general pediatrics ward with generalized abdominal pain. He also complains of several months' duration of constipation, generalized body aches, and frequent urination. His physical examination is normal except for mild diffuse abdominal tenderness to palpation without hepatosplenomegaly, masses, or hernias. His blood pressure is noted to be normal for height and age, and his blood glucose is within normal limits.

Of the following laboratory results, which best explains the underlying etiology of this patient's symptoms?

(A) Adrenal insufficiency
(B) Recurrent pancreatitis
(C) Hypothyroidism
(D) Primary hyperparathyroidism
(E) Secondary hyperparathyroidism

The answer is D: Primary hyperparathyroidism. Elevated parathyroid hormone (PTH) levels causing hypercalcemia are the likely cause of this patient's constellation of symptoms and result from unregulated production of PTH secondary to a parathyroid adenoma or gland hyperplasia. This is termed primary hyperparathyroidism. The patient in the vignette is likely suffering from a parathyroid adenoma. Although uncommon, this disease process typically manifests after the age of 10. Hyperparathyroidism is part of the multiple endocrine neoplasia syndrome types 1 and 2A; therefore, further screening for an autosomal dominant inherited syndrome is indicated if other family members have elevated PTH levels or endocrine neoplasms.

(E) A more common cause of an elevated PTH level in pediatric patients is secondary hypoparathyroidism, or increased PTH production as a result of compensatory mechanisms attempting to correct low systemic calcium levels. Low levels of body calcium can be due to vitamin D deficiency as in rickets, multiple malabsorption syndromes, or other causes of deficient calcium ingestion, absorption, and retention. This patient with likely elevated PTH levels is suffering from the effects of hypercalcemia, and therefore his elevation of PTH is not likely secondary to total body low calcium levels.

(B) If this patient's laboratory work had indicated an elevated lipase level, acute or acute-on-chronic pancreatitis may have been the cause of his abdominal pain. The pain of pancreatitis is typically epigastric to mid-abdominal in location, and often is described as radiating to the back. It is less likely that the constellation of symptoms the patient in the vignette is experiencing can be explained by pancreatitis alone; however, it may be a concomitant process in cases of acute hypercalcemia.

(C) Hypothyroidism can result in a broad range of symptoms including poorly localizable pain and neuropsychiatric symptoms; however, hypothyroidism is less likely to be related to this patient's recurrent renal calculi.

(A) Decreased cortisol secretion from the adrenal gland can result in renal dysfunction, weakness, vomiting, muscle cramping, and neuropsychiatric alterations. Although this patient is experiencing many of these symptoms, his blood glucose and blood pressure readings are normal for his age, which argues against low cortisol levels. Typically, low cortisol levels from adrenal insufficiency cause profound hypotension and hypoglycemia.

---

18 A full-term 9-month-old baby is brought to the office for the first time for a healthy checkup. Her mother states that the baby is exclusively breastfed and does not take any medications or supplements; however, the mother herself is still taking her prenatal vitamins. She has not yet started solid foods. She has one soft bowel movement every 2 days. Her family history is negative. She is at the 25th percentile for all growth parameters. Her radiograph is pictured in *Figure 10-11*.

Of the following, what is the most likely pathogenesis of these findings?

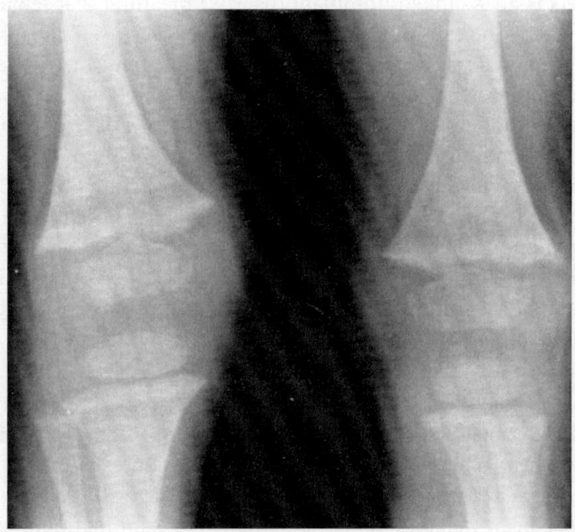

Figure 10-11

(A) Nutritional vitamin D deficiency
(B) Intestinal malabsorption
(C) Nutritional calcium deficiency
(D) Familial hypophosphatemia
(E) Decreased liver vitamin D 25-hydroxylase

The answer is A: Nutritional vitamin D deficiency. Based on the dietary history of exclusive breast milk without solid foods or vitamin supplementation, the child in the vignette is deficient in vitamin D as breast milk transmits an insufficient amount. The radiograph demonstrates rickets, a disorder of inadequate mineralization at sites of growing bone, particularly the growth plate. This causes a disproportionate widening that manifests as enlarged wrists and ankles. The demineralization leads to bone softening such that long bones may bow under the force of muscles or the weight of the body.

The most common cause of rickets is vitamin D deficiency. This can be seen through decreased intake as with the patient in the vignette or as a result of malabsorption. **(B)** There is no need to suspect intestinal malabsorption for the patient in the vignette as her stools are not greasy, foul-smelling, or bulky. Decreased serum levels of 25-hydroxyvitamin D confirm the diagnosis. Rickets can also be caused by hypocalcemia or hypophosphatemia from a variety of etiologies. Thus, additional laboratory testing should include serum calcium, phosphorus, alkaline phosphatase, parathyroid hormone (PTH), 25-hydroxyvitamin D, 1,25-dihydroxyvitamin D_3 (1,25-OH D_3), creatinine, and electrolytes.

(C) Another nutritional factor leading to rickets is inadequate calcium intake. It is usually seen once children are transitioned off of breast milk or formula, both of which contain sufficient calcium. **(D)** Familial hypophosphatemic rickets is an X-linked dominant disorder meaning that female carriers are also affected. The causative mutation results in increased phosphate excretion in the proximal tubule resulting in hypophosphatemia, increased alkaline phosphatase, but normal calcium and PTH. The 1,25-OH D_3 level is inappropriately low. Although this is the most common cause of hypophosphatemic rickets, it is less common than vitamin D deficiency.

(E) Patients with severe liver disease can have dysfunction of 25-hydroxylase, the enzyme that is responsible for the conversion of vitamin D to 25-hydroxyvitamin D so that it can then be converted to its active form, 1,25-dihydroxyvitamin D, in the kidney. However, this is not typically seen until a large majority of liver function has been compromised, and the patient in the vignette has no signs of liver failure.

---

19 A 6-year-old girl is being evaluated for body odor, breast development, and pubic hair growth over the last 3 months. She notes mild infrequent headaches and new onset blurred vision especially when she is tired. Her mother experienced menarche at age 10 years. She has otherwise been well and denies menarche. On examination, the patient is at the 25th percentile for height and the 50th percentile for weight. She has sexual maturity rating 3 breast and pubic hair development. She has no abdominal masses and has normal female genitalia without clitoromegaly. She has mild ataxia with finger-to-nose and 3+ patellar deep tendon reflexes.

Of the following, which would be the best treatment option for this patient based on the most likely cause of her symptoms?

(A) Referral to gynecologist for ovarian tumor removal
(B) Referral to general surgeon for adrenocortical tumor removal
(C) Close observation and reassurance
(D) Administration of an aromatase inhibitor
(E) Referral to neurosurgeon for brain tumor removal

The answer is E: Referral to neurosurgeon for brain tumor removal. The most concerning findings in the patient in the vignette are early-onset pubertal changes along with an abnormal neurologic examination making central precocious puberty the most likely etiology. Causes of central precocious puberty include brain masses, head trauma, and hydrocephalus. The complaint of vision changes in the vignette along with an abnormal neurologic examination requires immediate attention and evaluation with magnetic resonance imaging of the brain. Furthermore, the patient is displaying rapid-onset pubertal changes following the typical chronologic course, supporting a likely central cause. **(E)** A neurosurgery consult would then be appropriate management for a brain mass. **(A, B)** Neither a gynecologist or a general surgeon would be best to address this patient's brain mass; however, consultation might be helpful in the case of peripheral precocious puberty as it can be caused by ovarian tumors, adrenal gland tumors, and exogenous hormone administration. **(D)** For patients with persistent estradiol release, aromatase inhibitors may be helpful to lower levels. **(C)** Close observation and reassurance, while inappropriate in this case, can be an appropriate management for isolated premature thelarche, which tends to spontaneously regress.

at the 50th percentile for height and at the [illegible] percentile for weight. She [illegible] particular development, [illegible] [illegible] and [illegible] pubic [illegible] without [illegible]. She [illegible] [illegible] [illegible] [illegible] [illegible] [illegible].

Of the following, which would be the most appropriate initial management for this patient, based on the most likely cause of her [illegible]?

(A) Referral to gynecologist for [illegible] removal
(B) Referral to general surgeon for adrenocortical tumor removal
(C) Close observation and reassurance
(D) Administration of an aromatase inhibitor
(E) Referral to neurosurgeon for brain tumor removal

The answer is E: **Referral to neurosurgeon for brain tumor removal.** [illegible] the patient [illegible] [illegible] precocious puberty with abnormal neurologic examination findings [illegible] central precocious puberty. The most likely etiologies of central precocious puberty [illegible] brain tumor [illegible] and hydrocephalus. The complaint of vision changes [illegible] neurologic examination requires immediate attention and evaluation with magnetic resonance imaging of the brain [illegible] the patient's [illegible] [illegible] supporting a likely central cause [illegible] (A) [illegible] (B) [illegible] be appropriate in the case of peripheral precocious puberty, which can be caused by ovarian tumors, adrenal gland tumors, and exogenous hormone administration. (D) [illegible] may be [illegible] to lower [illegible]. (C) Close observation and reassurance [illegible] inappropriate [illegible] appropriate management [illegible] [illegible] to [illegible].

CHAPTER 11

Dermatology

KENT NELSON

1 A 16-year-old boy presents to the clinic with complaints of a persistent round, red lesion on his chest. He attempted to treat the lesion with an antifungal cream given to him by his wrestling coach, but the lesion remained and has now spread to his back. He denies pruritus. On examination, he is well-appearing and has a 3-cm oval lesion with a central clearing on his chest. There are several small scaly lesions spread on his upper back parallel to skin lines as pictured in *Figure 11-1*.

Of the following, what is this patient's most likely diagnosis?

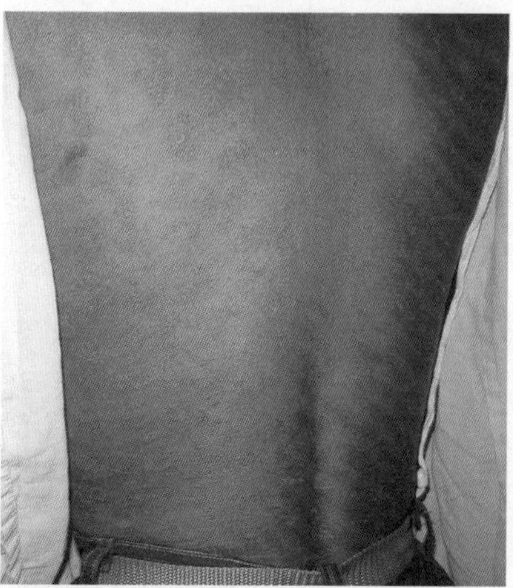

Figure 11-1

(A) Pityriasis alba
(B) Pityriasis rosea
(C) Guttate psoriasis
(D) Nummular eczema
(E) Tinea corporis

The answer is B: Pitryiasis rosea.

The boy in the vignette has pityriasis rosea, a dermatologic syndrome consisting of multiple erythematous macules that progress to small papular ovals on the back whose long axes parallel the lines of stress. Some papules may have a thin scale on the surface. A round lesion often precedes this eruption with a central clearing called a herald patch that resembles tinea corporis. The herald patch typically appears on the trunk and may precede the remainder of the rash by up to 1 month (see *Figure 11-2*). Pityriasis rosea is self-limited and resolves in 4 to 8 weeks without adverse sequelae. The pathogenesis is unknown, but infectious causes are suspected.

(A) Pityriasis alba is a common cutaneous condition among pediatric patients. Findings include hypopigmented patches on the face, trunk, and extensor surfaces without pruritus or discomfort. It is considered a form of atopic dermatitis. **(C)** Guttate psoriasis is characterized by multiple discrete thick, scaly plaques on the trunk and is associated with recent streptococcal pharyngitis. The plaques shown in *Figure 11-1* are not typical for guttate psoriasis. Nummular eczema and tinea corporis present with round, coin-like lesions and are difficult to distinguish from each other and from the herald patch of pityriasis rosea. **(D)** Nummular eczema usually involves round or oval erythematous and scaly lesions that present symmetrically on the extremities. The lesions are often intensely pruritic. **(E)** Tinea corporis is a

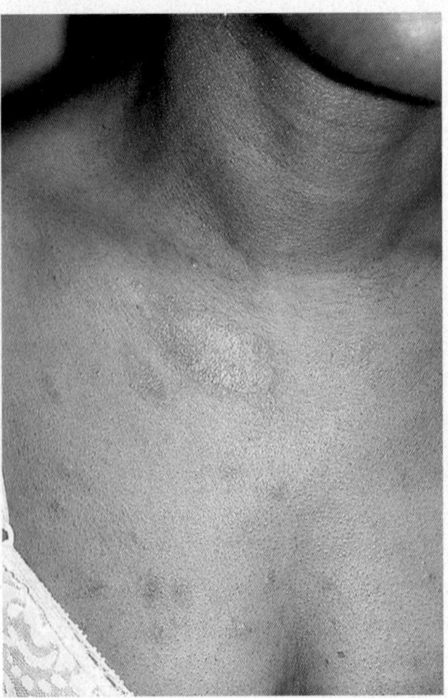

Figure 11-2

fungal infection that produces an annular lesion on the skin with a central clearing. It can be distinguished from a herald patch by the pattern of clearing. A herald patch is associated with central clearing of erythema with remaining central scale while the scaling of tinea corporis clears centrally but maintains scaling at the edge.

2 A mother brings her 15-month-old son to the pediatrician with complaints of dry skin. She reports that his skin has been dry and itchy since birth, but recently seems to have gotten worse. His older sister uses an albuterol inhaler twice weekly. On examination, the boy has dry, scaly skin on his face (see *Figure 11-3*) as well as his trunk. The skin is erythematous and flaky without severe thickening. The skin in the diaper area is soft and non-erythematous.

Of the following, what is the most appropriate recommendation for the treatment of this patient's rash?

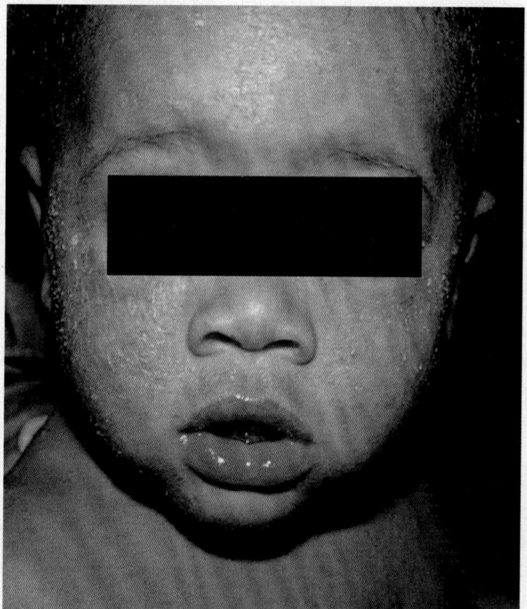

Figure 11-3

(A) Oral cephalexin
(B) Triamcinolone 0.1% ointment
(C) Mometasone 0.1% ointment
(D) Apply an emollient after bathing
(E) Pimecrolimus ointment

The answer is D: Apply an emollient after bathing. Atopic dermatitis, or eczema, is the most common dermatitis of childhood and is characterized by the following cardinal features: presence of dermatitis, dry skin, onset before the age of 2 years, and history of dermatitis in the flexural areas. Atopic dermatitis is a hereditary condition and is commonly associated with asthma or allergic rhinitis. The distribution of atopic dermatitis varies with age. Infants have involvement of the scalp, trunk, and extensor surfaces with relative sparing of the diaper area. Toddlers typically have involvement of the flexural areas as well as the hands, feet, and neck. Adolescents and adults have involvement that is concentrated to the hands, feet, and flexural areas. Itching is an important feature of atopic dermatitis and can be severe, leading to thickening and excoriations with an increased risk of bacterial superinfection. Diagnosis is clinical with the characteristic distribution of the dermatitis as well as family history.

The treatment of atopic dermatitis is chronic and involves baseline therapies with intermittent treatment of flares. There is no cure for atopic dermatitis although spontaneous remissions do occur. The mainstay of therapy is topical emollients and steroid creams or ointments. Adequate skin hydration and lubrication is the first-line therapy, often referred to as the soak and seal method. Frequent bathing and excess soaping or scrubbing of the skin should be limited. **(D)** Emollients should be applied liberally to gently dried skin immediately following baths. If the atopic dermatitis is mild to moderate as determined by erythema, scaling, or mild thickening, a low-potency steroid cream or ointment such as hydrocortisone may be applied prior to emollients. Apply the steroid cream only to the affected areas and use sparingly on the face and perineum to decrease the risk of skin thinning and hypopigmentation. **(B, C)** Moderate-to-severe flares require moderate potency steroid preparations such as mometasone 0.1% and triamcinolone 0.1%. **(E)** Topical calcineurin inhibitors, or pimecrolimus, may be effective in adolescents with chronic dermatitis limited to specific areas such as the face. Use of these medications is not recommended in children under the age of 2 years. **(A)** Systemic therapy with antistaphylococcal medications are recommended for children with signs of secondary bacterial infection.

---

3 A 15-month-old presents to the clinic the day after a visit to the emergency department for his first seizure. He had tactile fevers per his mother for each of the 3 days prior to presentation. She describes the seizure episode as shaking of his entire body and lasting approximately 4 minutes. It stopped without intervention before the ambulance arrived. He had returned to his baseline by the time they arrived at the emergency department. He was observed for several hours with no further adverse events and subsequently discharged home. In the clinic today, his mother reports he feels better than he had earlier this week except he has a rash on his body as shown in *Figure 11-4*. He has not felt warm since yesterday and his appetite has returned.

Of the following, what is the most likely etiologic agent causing this patient's rash?

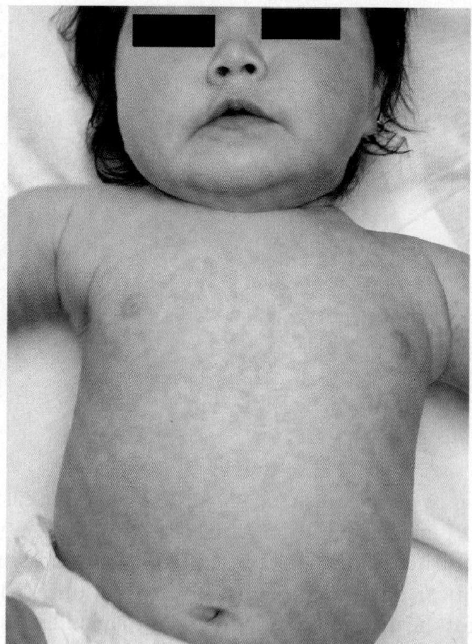

Figure 11-4

(A) Coxsackie virus
(B) Human parvovirus B19
(C) Human herpesvirus-6
(D) Varicella zoster virus (VZV)
(E) Rubeola virus

The answer is C: Human herpesvirus-6. The boy in the vignette has a viral exanthem caused by human hervpesvirus-6 or -7 known as roseola, or erythema subitum. This condition is a common exanthem seen most often in children younger than 2 years old. It is characterized by isolated and sustained high fevers for several days and followed by defervescence and eruption of a pink, morbilliform rash that fades within 24 hours. The rash appears similar to other exanthematous eruptions, but may be distinguished by the characteristic fever curve. Febrile seizures are associated with the high spiking fevers during the first few days of the illness.

The remaining options are associated with characteristic rashes as well, but unlikely to cause the presentation of the child in the vignette. **(A)** Coxsackie virus causes hand-foot-and-mouth disease and is characterized by the abrupt onset of papules and vesicles in the oral mucosa on the extremities including the palms and soles. **(B)** Human parvovirus B19 causes an exanthem called erythema infectiosum, or fifth disease. Patients present with the

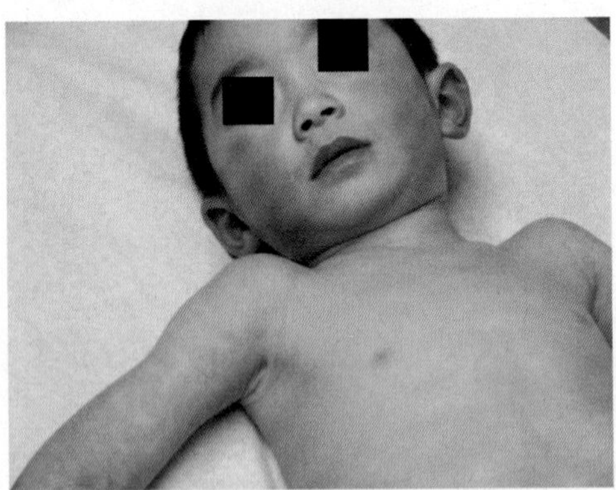

Figure 11-5

characteristic slapped cheek rash (see *Figure 11-5*) and occasionally progress to a widespread pink morbilliform rash. **(D)** VZV causes varicella (chickenpox) and zoster. Both infections present with crops of vesicular lesions in diffuse (varicella) or dermatomal (zoster) distributions. **(E)** Rubeola is the causative virus for the measles exanthem. Measles includes a severe prodrome lasting 3 to 5 days including fever, cough, and coryza that is followed by the typical exanthematous eruption that includes intense mucous membrane erythema, pinpoint white macules on the buccal surface called Koplik spots, and progression to a diffuse rash of discrete erythematous macules and papules on the face, trunk, and extremities.

4 A 10-year-old girl presented 3 days ago to an urgent care clinic at her local pharmacy with complaints of 4 days of fever, runny nose, sore throat with exudates, and fatigue. She was prescribed amoxicillin for presumed streptococcal pharyngitis and presents today to her pediatrician's clinic with a rash on her trunk and extremities. On examination, she is mildly ill-appearing and her temperature is 38.3°C. Her left tympanic membrane is dull and opaque without erythema. Her pharynx is erythematous and her tonsils have white exudates. Her abdomen is soft and a spleen tip is palpable. She has an erythematous maculopapular rash on her trunk and extremities that spares her palms and soles.

Of the following, what is the most likely cause of her presentation?

(A) *Streptococcus pyogenes*
(B) *Streptococcus pneumoniae*
(C) Influenza virus
(D) Epstein-Barr virus
(E) Anaphylactic reaction to amoxicillin

The answer is D: Epstein-Barr virus. Infectious mononucleosis is a viral syndrome characterized by fatigue, fever, lymphadenopathy, sore throat, exudative pharyngitis, headache, splenomegaly, and rarely a faint morbilliform rash. It is most often caused by infection with Epstein-Barr virus and affects children from school-age to adolescence. Because diagnosis is often made based on suggestive history and physical examinations, antibiotic therapy with penicillins or macrolides is often prescribed for concurrent diagnoses of otitis media or bacterial pharyngitis. The incidence and intensity of the viral rash is amplified with this antibiotic treatment. The presentation and rash in the vignette are typical for patients with clinically diagnosed infectious mononucleosis receiving amoxicillin therapy.

(A, B, C) Infections with influenza virus, *S. pyogenes*, and *S. pneumoniae* are not associated with rash eruption following antibiotic therapy. **(E)** The rash described is not characteristic of anaphylaxis or drug rash. These reactions are mediated by mast cell degranulation and more commonly lead to urticarial eruptions. Skin rash alone without involvement of other systems is not sufficient to diagnose anaphylaxis.

---

5 A 3-year-old boy presents to the emergency department because of an itchy rash that was present when he woke up this morning. The boy has been afebrile and has not had rhinorrhea or vomiting. On examination, he has several round and oval erythematous ringed lesions that are approximately 2 cm in diameter (see *Figure 11-6*). Many of the lesions have central clearings with dusky purple centers. His buccal mucosal surfaces are involved with shallow erosions. The remainder of his examination including conjunctivae, anus, and urethral surfaces is unremarkable.

Of the following, which statement regarding this patient's diagnosis is most accurate?

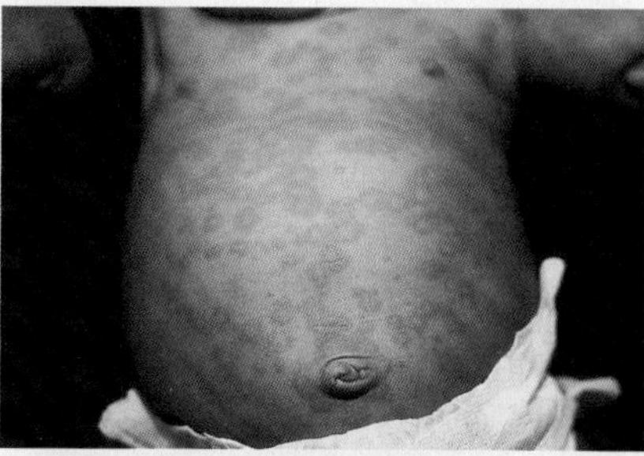

Figure 11-6

(A) Progression to Stevens-Johnson syndrome is likely
(B) Heart block is associated with this infection
(C) Episodes are associated with herpes simplex virus (HSV) infection
(D) Lesions typically resolve within 24 hours
(E) These lesions are caused by a rickettsial infection

The answer is C: **Episodes are associated with herpes simplex virus (HSV) infection.** The patient in the vignette is experiencing erythema multiforme (EM) as the lesions erupted acutely with absent prodromal complaints. The lesions may be numerous and progress to coalesce to concentric round areas of color change with dusky zones within. The rash often remains for up to 3 weeks and **(A)** may involve the buccal mucosa; however, EM does not progress in severity to Stevens-Johnsons syndrome or toxic epidermal necrolysis. **(E)** Several viral etiologies have been implicated in the pathogenesis of EM. **(C)** HSV, Epstein-Barr virus, cytomegalovirus, and other human herpes viruses have been reported to cause EM. **(D)** The EM rash is often confused with urticaria, but the EM eruption differs in that urticarial lesions change shape and location from day to day and any single lesion often does not last longer than 24 hours. **(B, E)** Lyme disease is associated with heart block. It is a rickettsial infection with *Borrelia burgdorferi* and may present with a characteristic target lesion at the site of a tick bite (see *Figure 11-7*). This rash is called erythema migrans.

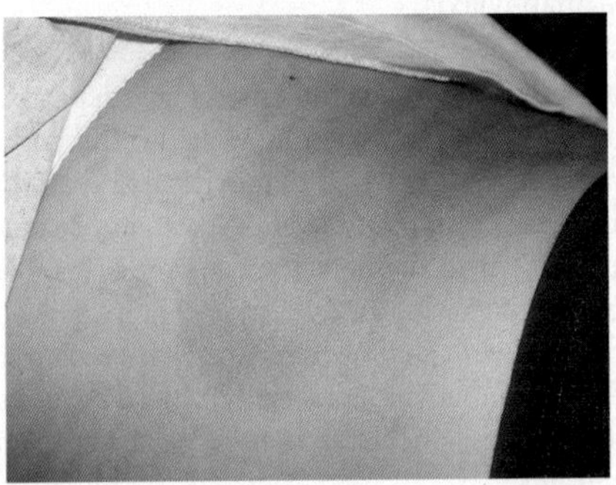

Figure 11-7

6 A 1-month-old infant has a birthmark on his eyelid as pictured in *Figure 11-8*.

Of the following complications, which is the patient at highest risk of developing?

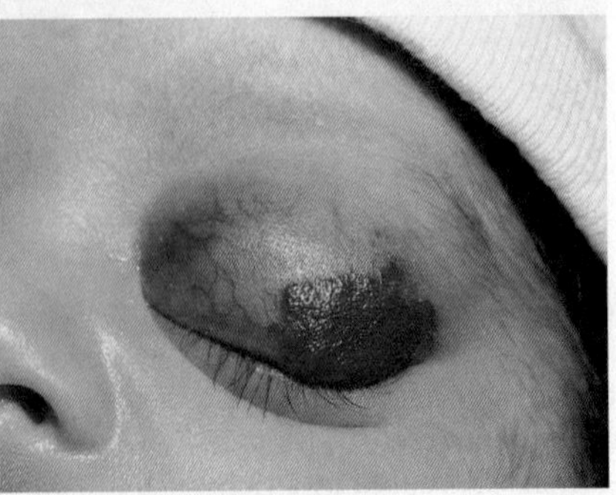

Figure 11-8

(A) Glaucoma
(B) Amblyopia
(C) Frontal lobe seizures
(D) Thrombocytopenia and hemolytic anemia
(E) Posterior fossa malformations–hemangiomas–arterial anomalies–cardiac defects–eye abnormalities–sternal cleft and supraumbilical raphe (PHACES) syndrome

The answer is B: Amblyopia. The patient in the vignette has a capillary hemangioma on his eyelid. Hemangiomas composed of proliferations of endothelial tissue are the most common benign tumor of infancy. Most simple hemangiomas have an excellent prognosis and involute without consequence within the first decade of life. Complications of hemangiomas include ulceration, pain, long-term deformity, and may threaten function or even life, depending on its location. The patient in the vignette is at increased risk for developing amblyopia (poor vision) because the hemangioma is located on his eyelid and obstructs his vision from the affected eye.

(A, C) Patients with Sturge-Weber syndrome present with a port wine stain (*Figure 11-9*) in the distribution of the first branch of the trigeminal nerve and are at increased risk for glaucoma and frontal lobe seizures secondary to associated leptomeningeal angiomatosis. **(D)** Kasabach-Merritt phenomenon is a life-threatening condition that is associated with coagulopathy, thrombocytopenia, and hemolytic anemia. It occurs in vascular tumors such as kaposiform hemangioendothelioma or tufted angioma. Kasabach-Merritt phenomenon is not associated with infantile hemangiomas such as the one described in the vignette. **(E)** PHACES syndrome is an

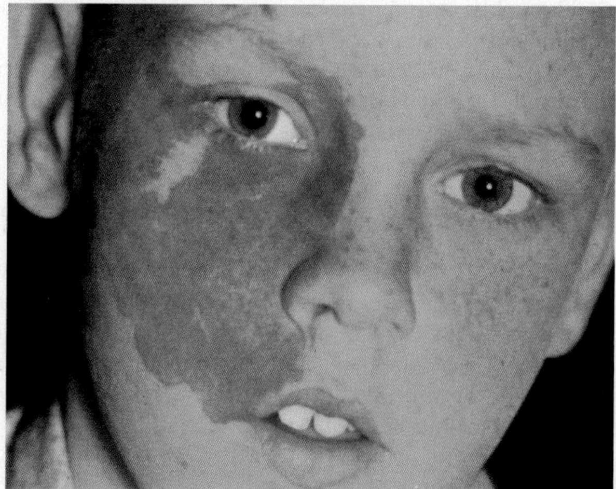

Figure 11-9

association of large facial hemangiomas with other systemic defects. The syndrome is characterized by posterior fossa defects, hemangioma, arterial anomalies, cardiac anomalies/aortic coarctation, eye abnormalities, and sternal clefting/supraumbilical abdominal raphe. The hemangioma of the patient in the vignette is small and is unlikely to be associated with PHACES syndrome.

The parents of a 5-month-old baby are planning a vacation to Hawaii. They come to clinic to ask about recommendations for sun protection.

Of the following, what is the best recommendation regarding sun protection for their child?

(A) Use a sunscreen with sun protection factor of at least 30
(B) Sunscreen should be applied to the entire body, including the face
(C) Limit sun exposure to the hours between 10 a.m. and 4 p.m.
(D) Sun exposure should be avoided as much as possible
(E) Apply sunscreen at least 15 minutes prior to sun exposure

The answer is D: Sun exposure should be avoided as much as possible. Solar radiation can have harmful effects with excessive exposure including sunburn, the development of nevi, and an increased risk of skin neoplasia. Infant skin is particularly sensitive to solar radiation and it is recommended to avoid sun exposure as much as possible before the age of 6 months. In addition to staying out of the sun, infants should wear large-brimmed hats and opaque clothing that covers their arms and legs. Sunscreen is not recommended for routine use in children younger than 6 months, but if applied, **(B)** it should be used sparingly and limited to the exposed areas of the body such as the face and hands.

(C) Children older than 6 months of age may have increased sun exposure, but should limit exposure between 10 a.m. and 4 p.m., the hours of most direct sunlight. **(A)** A sunscreen with a sun protection factor of at least 15 is recommended and **(E)** should be applied at least 30 minutes prior to sun exposure to allow adequate absorption into the epidermis.

The mother of a 6-year-old girl brings her to the pediatrician's office for evaluation of bumps on her face and chest that she noticed 2 weeks ago. She reports that her daughter has had no fevers and occasionally scratches her face. On examination, there are multiple round, pearly papules that measure 2 to 5 mm (see *Figure 11-10*) on her chest and face. The papules are arranged in a scattered pattern, but some appear to be along a linear arrangement and a few have a mildly erythematous base.

Of the following, what is the best recommendation to give this mother regarding her daughter's condition?

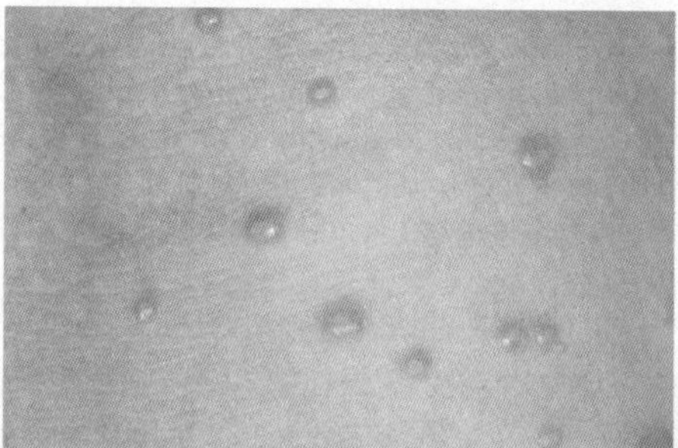

Figure 11-10

(A) Hydrocortisone ointment is an effective cure of this condition
(B) Removal by curettage is an effective cure of this condition
(C) These lesions will resolve spontaneously over several weeks
(D) Contact with pregnant women or immunocompromised contacts should be minimized
(E) She should receive a varicella vaccine booster at this visit

The answer is B: Removal by curettage is an effective cure of this condition. The patient in the vignette has molluscum contagiosum, an infection with a poxvirus that causes an eruption of discrete, pearly, small, 1- to 6-mm papules with a central umbilication. Some lesions may have an erythematous base. The typical distribution of lesions is on the face around the eyes, axillae, and proximal extremities, but lesions may be arranged on the trunk as well. The papules are often scattered, but may follow in a linear pattern secondary to autoinoculation from scratching. Children with atopic dermatitis may have extensive involvement with hundreds of lesions. **(D)** There is no vaccine for molluscum contagiosum and isolation from pregnant women or immunocompromised individuals is not indicated.

Removal of the papule is curative. There are several methods for removal including curettage or application irritants such as cantharidin or imiquimod 5% cream. While effective, these therapies can be painful and may leave scarring. **(C)** The lesions are self-limiting and may require months to years for resolution without treatment. **(A)** Treatment of concurrent atopic dermatitis with steroid creams may decrease the spread of molluscum contagiosum lesions, but this therapy is not considered curative.

Varicella is a vesicular eruption caused by the varicella zoster virus. The eruption occurs in crops and begins with vesicles that may evolve into pustules or papules and eventually crust over. **(D)** Contact with pregnant or immunocompromised individuals should be limited with active varicella infections. **(E)** Booster vaccination for varicella beyond the normal recommended schedule is not indicated.

9 A 15-month-old boy was seen in clinic 3 days ago for fever and tugging at his ear. His pediatrician prescribed amoxicillin for otitis media. The mother brings him back to the clinic today and reports that her son developed the rash pictured in *Figure 11-11* this morning. On examination, the boy is well-appearing and breathing comfortably. He scratches his skin often.

Of the following, what is the mechanism of this child's rash?

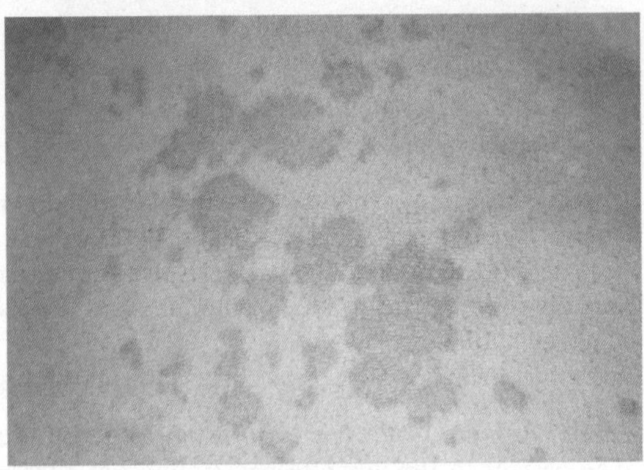

Figure 11-11

(A) Immunoglobulin (IgA) and immune complex deposition in arterioles
(B) Mast cell degranulation and secretion of histamine
(C) Exfoliative toxin release by *Staphylococcus aureus*
(D) Circulating toxin following *Streptococcus pyogenes* infection
(E) Infestation by *Sarcoptes scabiei* mite

The answer is B: Mast cell degranulation and secretion of histamine. The boy in the vignette is experiencing an urticarial drug reaction following administration of amoxicillin. These reactions are characterized by pruritic, edematous wheals of various shapes and sizes. The lesions typically erupt shortly following exposure to a drug and individual lesions resolve within 24 hours. The mechanism of urticarial drug reactions is IgE-mediated mast cell degranulation and histamine release. The reaction is halted by removal of the causative agent and symptomatic relief is obtained with oral antihistamines and topical antipruritic preparations.

(A) Henoch-Schönlein purpura (HSP), also known as anaphylactoid purpura, is a vasculitis that is mediated by IgA and immune complex deposition in arterioles. HSP can present with urticaria that progress to purpura. It is associated with abdominal pain, arthralgias, arthritis, and hematuria. Given the recent exposure to amoxicillin, the rash described in the vignette is unlikely to be secondary to HSP. **(C, D)** Toxins produced by *Staph. aureus* and *Strep. pyogenes* are associated with cutaneous findings, but not urticaria. **(E)** Infestation with *Sarc. scabiei* causes scabies, which presents with a pruritic eruption of papules, pustules, and burrows that are often located in the interdigital spaces. Scabies is not typically associated with urticaria.

---

10 A 5-year-old boy presents to the emergency department because of a severe headache and photophobia over the past 2 days. He had recently returned from a summer camping trip with his father. Cultures and analyses of blood and cerebrospinal fluid are drawn and he is admitted to the general pediatric floor to receive intravenous ceftriaxone therapy. Overnight he has a temperature of 39.2°C, is ill-appearing, and an erythematous, non-blanching rash similar to the one pictured in *Figure 11-12* develops on his wrists, soles, and extremities.

Of the following, what is the next best step in the treatment of this patient?

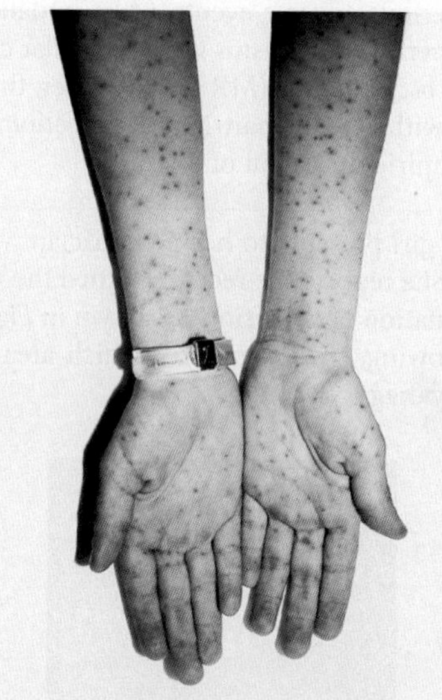

Figure 11-12

(A) Change the antibiotic to clindamycin
(B) Change the antibiotic to doxycycline
(C) Add chloramphenicol to his antibiotic regimen
(D) Continue ceftriaxone monotherapy
(E) Initiate corticosteroid therapy

The answer is B: Change the antibiotic to doxycycline. The patient in the vignette has Rocky Mountain spotted fever (RMSF) and is in the process of developing the typical rash associated with this rickettsial infection. RMSF is a small-vessel vasculitis that is characterized by fever, myalgias, severe headache, nausea, and vomiting. The characteristic rash that begins as erythematous macules or maculopapules on the wrists and ankles and spreads to the palms, soles, extremities, and trunk typically erupts within the first week of symptoms. Development of petechiae is an indicator of severe disease.

RMSF is caused by a gram-negative, obligate intracellular rickettsial organism called *Rickettsia rickettsii*. It is transmitted to humans via a tick vector, and exposure to ticks throughout the United States is a risk of contracting the infection. Diagnosis is by a fourfold or greater increase in IgG antibody titers.

(B, D) Doxycycline is the mainstay of treatment for all patients of all ages with suspected or confirmed RMSF. Risks of dental staining side effects associated with tetracyclines in children younger than 8 years of age are outweighed by the improved mortality achieved by early empiric coverage with doxycycline. **(C)** Chloramphenicol has activity against *R. rickettsii* but is not an ideal treatment option because its use is associated with a higher risk of fatal outcome and other serious adverse events. **(A)** Clindamycin is used to treat gram-positive and anaerobic organisms with particular coverage for methicillin-resistant *Staphylococcus aureus* (MRSA); however, the patient's symptoms are more consistent with RMSF than MRSA infection. **(E)** Corticosteroids have no role in the empiric treatment of RMSF.

11 A 12-year-old girl presents to her pediatrician with oval scaly lesions on her knees. She reports she recently joined the volleyball team at her school. Examination of the lesions is shown in *Figure 11-13*.

Of the following, involvement of which area or distribution supports her likely diagnosis?

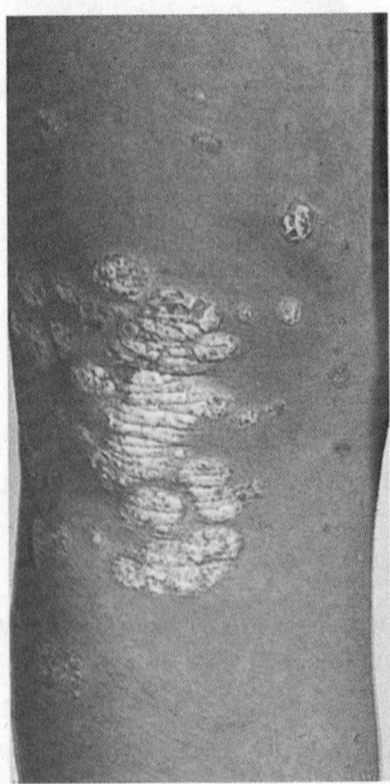

Figure 11-13

(A) Antecubital fossae
(B) Parallel to lines of skin stress on the back
(C) Circumferentially on the wrist
(D) Gluteal cleft
(E) Purple rash on the eyelids and face

The answer is D: Gluteal cleft. The patient in the vignette has lesions that are consistent with the diagnosis of psoriasis. Psoriasis is a dermatologic condition characterized by thick, scaly plaques that develop on the scalp, face, extensor surfaces, genital regions including the gluteal cleft, as well as at sites of skin trauma. The lesions begin as erythematous macular or papular lesions that progress to plaques with adherent silvery scales. The Koebner phenomenon describes the appearance of plaques at the sites of trauma and is consistent with the patient in the vignette developing new lesions shortly after starting volleyball practice. Psoriasis may also involve pitting of the nails and nail beds. Treatment is based on disease extent and severity and may require systemic retinoid therapy, but most pediatric psoriasis is well treated with topical corticosteroids and adjunctive therapies such as calcipotriene and anthralin.

The remaining distributions and descriptions of rashes are typical for other common pediatric dermatologic conditions. **(A)** Involvement of the antecubital fossa with scaly lesions suggests eczema. **(B)** A scaly, erythematous rash that is distributed to the back and is arranged parallel to lines of stress is consistent with pityriasis rosea. **(C)** A circumferential eruption of erythematous and scaly lesions on the wrist is suggestive of a contact dermatitis perhaps secondary to nickel in a metal watchband or jewelry bracelet. **(E)** A heliotrope rash, or purple coloration on the eyelids and face, is characteristic of dermatomyositis (see *Figure 11-14*).

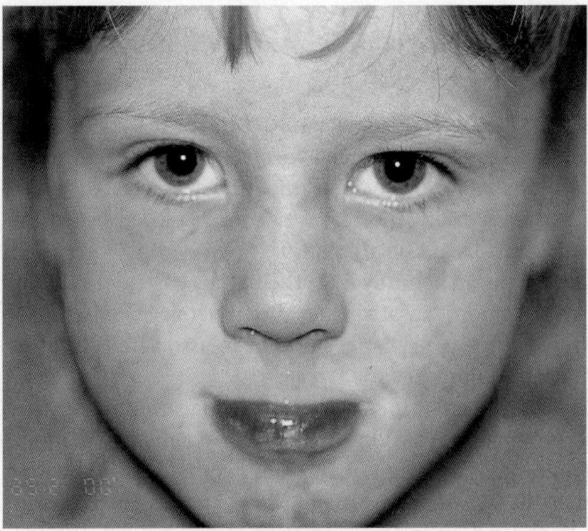

Figure 11-14

12 A 3-year-old boy presents to the clinic with complaints of a crusted and painful eruption around his mouth as shown in *Figure 11-15*. His mother reports that he attends daycare and his sister has a similar lesion on her hand.

Of the following, what is the most likely etiologic agent of this patient's rash?

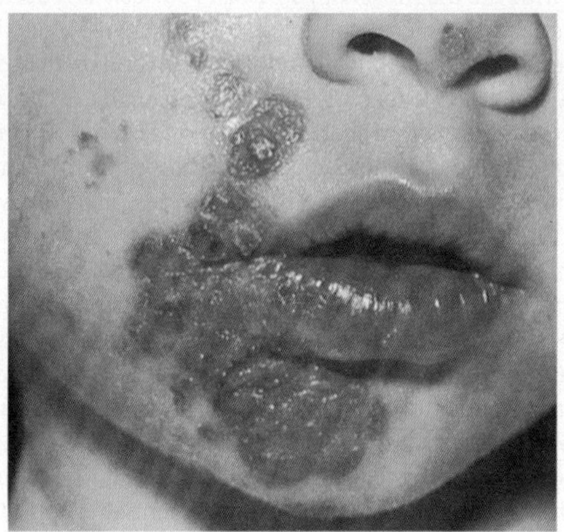

Figure 11-15

(A) *Streptococcus pyogenes*
(B) *Streptococcus pneumoniae*
(C) *Staphylococcus aureus*
(D) Herpes simplex virus (HSV)
(E) Varicella zoster virus (VZV)

The answer is C: *Staphylococcus aureus*. The patient in the vignette is suffering from impetigo, a superficial bacterial infection of the skin of the face or extremities. The common form of impetigo is associated with a superficial vesicle that ruptures easily and leaves a honey-colored crust. Bullous impetigo is characterized by the formation of fragile serous fluid-filled bullae that rupture easily and leave behind an erythematous base and surrounding collar. **(A)** The most common causative agent of impetigo is *Staphylococcus aureus*; however, *Streptococcus pyogenes* has also been associated. Treatment includes oral and topical antibiotic agents.

(D) HSV causes painful clusters of vesicular eruptions that rupture and leave deep erythematous erosions. HSV infection affects the mouth and other mucous membranes. The lesion pictured in *Figure 11-15* is affecting the skin of the face rather than the mucous membranes, and impetigo erosions are often not as deep as those seen in HSV infection (see *Figure 11-16*). **(E)** VZV is the causative agent of varicella and is associated with vesicular eruptions that begin

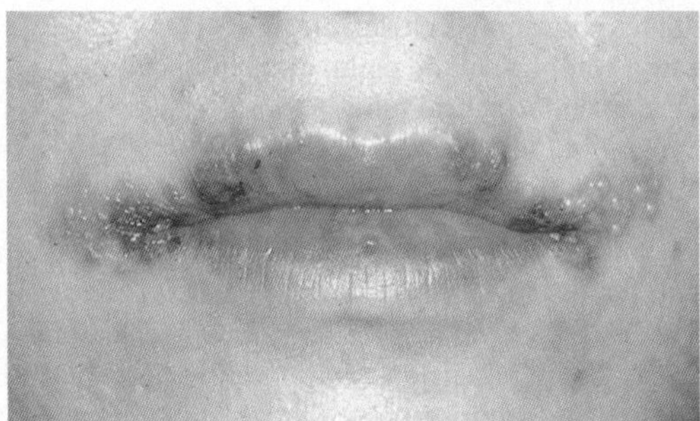

Figure 11-16

on the trunk and spread to the extremities. The mucous membranes are often involved. **(B)** *Streptococcus pneumoniae* is not associated with impetiginous eruptions.

---

13 A 16-year-old boy presents to the emergency department with fever, headache, malaise, and a rash that progressively worsened since yesterday. On examination, the boy is lethargic with shallow breaths, opens his eyes and withdraws from painful stimuli, and vocalizes with incomprehensible sounds. His trunk and extremities have blotchy, confluent areas of purple discoloration superimposed on gray, poorly perfused skin (see *Figure 11-17*).

Of the following, what is the next best step in the management of this patient?

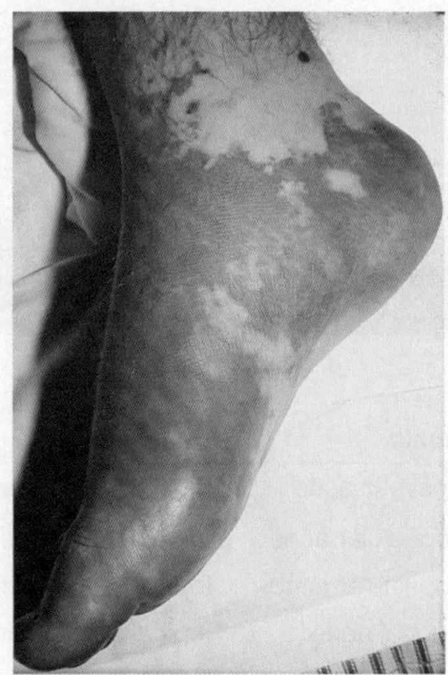

Figure 11-17

(A) Initiate intravenous ceftriaxone
(B) Draw a complete blood count and blood culture
(C) Insert an endotracheal tube
(D) Lumbar puncture
(E) Infuse fresh frozen plasma

The answer is C: **Insert an endotracheal tube.** The patient in the vignette has purpura fulminans secondary to bacteremia and sepsis with *Neisseria meningitidis*. His Glasgow Coma Scale score is 8 and his physical examination is showing signs of hypotension and poor peripheral perfusion. The next best step for this patient is to insert an endotracheal tube to secure his airway and ensure adequate aeration by mechanical ventilation. **(A, B, E)** Septicemia with *N. meningitidis* can be a fulminant process and should be diagnosed and managed aggressively with blood culture, complete blood count, intravenous ceftriaxone, fresh frozen plasma, and fluids; however, all of these events should take place after securing a reliable method of air exchange. **(D)** Most patients with *N. meningitidis* bacteremia do not have meningeal infiltration and only require lumbar puncture with cerebrospinal fluid analysis and culture if showing signs of meningeal inflammation.

14 A 14-year-old boy comes to his pediatrician's office with concerns about his acne. He reports that he is teased at school about his skin. An image of his skin is shown in *Figure 11-18*.

Of the following, which diagnosis and treatment pair is most appropriate for this patient?

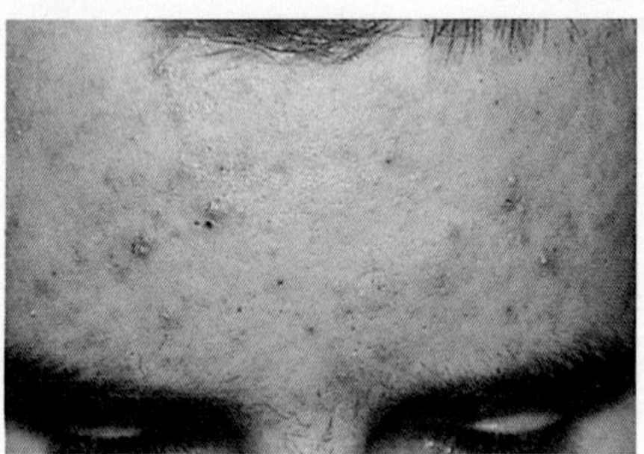

Figure 11-18

	Diagnosis	Treatment
(A)	Nodulocystic acne	Topical tretinoin and oral minocycline
(B)	Papulopustular acne	Topical tretinoin and benzoyl peroxide
(C)	Papulopustular acne	Topical tretinoin and oral minocycline
(D)	Comedonal acne	Topical tretinoin and oral minocycline
(E)	Comedonal acne	Topical tretinoin and benzoyl peroxide

The answer is B: Papulopustular acne; Topical tretinoin and benzoyl peroxide. The patient in the vignette has mild-to-moderate inflammatory papulopustular acne vulgaris. Acne vulgaris is the most prevalent skin condition affecting pediatric patients. It begins in preadolescence and affects the majority of patients older than 8 to 10 years. Acne occurs in sebaceous follicles that are located in abundance on the face and upper chest and back. There are several acne designations. Comedonal acne is defined as the presence of only open or closed comedones without inflammation. Comedones are dilated sebaceous follicles that are filled with keratinous material, lipids, and bacteria. Open comedones, or blackheads, are the most common lesions observed in early acne vulgaris and occur when the opening of a comedone is plugged by stratum corneum debris. Closed comedones, or white heads, are small papules without surrounding erythema and are the precursors to inflammatory acne. **(D, E)** Patients with a predominance of open or closed comedones without abundant erythematous papules or pustules are diagnosed with comedonal acne. **(B, C)** Patients are diagnosed with papulopustular acne when comedonal acne progresses to a mixture of open and closed comedones, superficial inflammatory and erythematous papules, and pustules. Inflammatory acne can be categorized into mild, moderate, or severe classification depending on the extent of erythema and nodularity of lesions. **(A)** Deep nodules and cysts characterize nodulocystic acne. Cystic acne may progress to permanent scarring and requires prompt medical attention.

The mainstay of treatment of acne vulgaris is topical retinoids, such as tretinoin, with the addition of other therapies, such as benzoyl peroxide or minocycline (see *Table 11-1* for a table of treatment options). Initial therapy for all categories of acne is daily topical retinoid application prior to going to bed. **(D, E)** Comedonal acne does not require additional therapies. **(C)** The treatment for papulopustular acne includes a topical retinoid with the addition of topical benzoyl peroxide. Oral minocycline is indicated if the inflammation is severe or if there are numerous pustules. **(B)** The patient in the vignette has

Table 11-1 Acne Treatment

Type of Acne	Treatment
Comedonal	Daily topical retinoid before bed
Papulopustular (few pustules)	Daily topical retinoid before bed + benzoyl peroxide every morning
Papulopustular (many pustules)	Daily topical retinoid before bed + benzoyl peroxide every morning + antibiotic (topical or oral) twice daily
Nodulocystic	Daily topical retinoid before bed + benzoyl peroxide every morning + oral antibiotic twice daily

mild inflammatory acne and few pustules. **(A)** Nodulocystic acne is treated with a daily topical retinoid, daily benzoyl peroxide, and twice-daily oral minocycline.

---

15 A 9-year-old boy presents to his pediatrician with the complaint of a circular area of hair loss. He denies fever. On examination, there is a 4-cm area of alopecia as pictured in *Figure 11-19* and he has a 2-cm nontender lymph node at his posterior hairline.

Of the following, what is his most likely diagnosis?

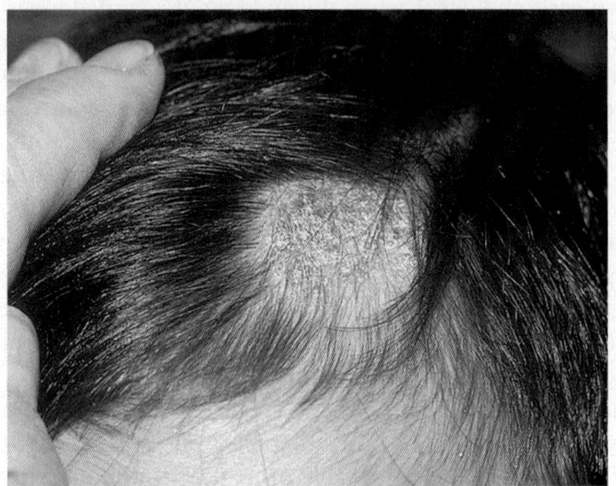

Figure 11-19

(A) Tinea capitis
(B) Kerion
(C) Alopecia areata
(D) Trichotillomania
(E) Tinea corporis

The answer is A: Tinea capitis. Tinea capitis is an infection of the scalp with dermatophytes, or fungi that invade and proliferate within the outer layer of the epidermis as well as the hair and nails. The most common dermatophytic cause of tinea capitis in North America is *Trichophyton tonsurans*. This condition typically begins as a noninflammatory stage that evolves over 2 to 8 weeks to an inflammatory stage, which is associated with hair loss and posterior cervical adenopathy. The patient in the vignette has a typical presentation for tinea capitis. Diagnosis of tinea capitis can be made with yellow-green fluorescence on Wood's lamp examination, microscopic examination with potassium hydroxide, and fungal culture.

(B) An exaggerated host response to the fungal infection can result in an erythematous, boggy, pustular eruption called a kerion (see *Figure 11-20*). This

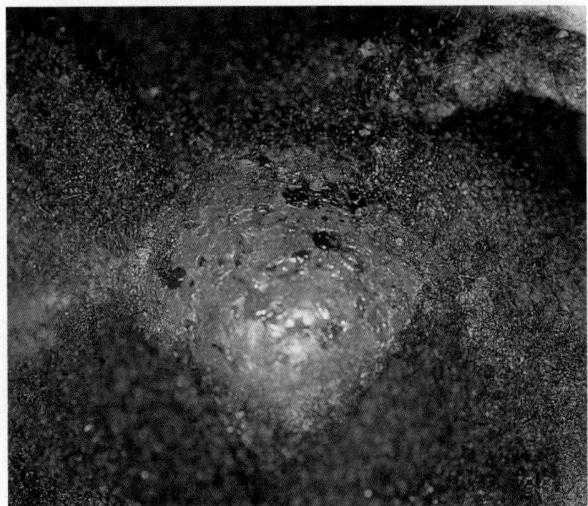

Figure 11-20

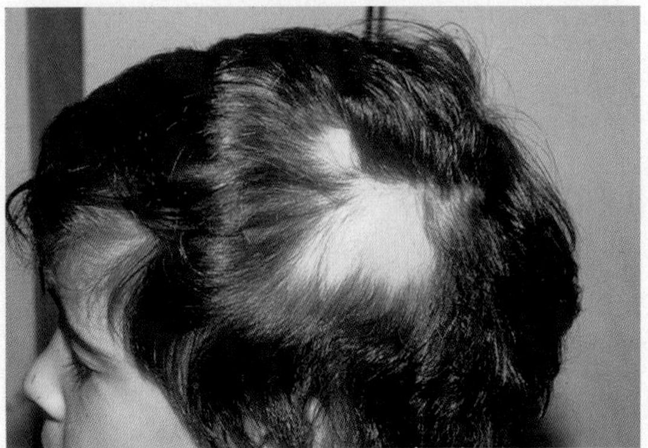

Figure 11-21

lesion appears up to 2 months following the original infection and can lead to scarring and permanent hair loss if left untreated. Both tinea capitis and kerion respond well to oral griseofulvin therapy. **(C)** Alopecia areata (see *Figure 11-21*) is a well-circumscribed area of complete hair loss involving the scalp hair, body hair, sexual hair, eyebrows, or eyelashes. It is an autoimmune-mediated process that often has a very good prognosis for future hair regrowth. **(D)** Trichotillomania is a disorder of hair pulling that is characterized by circumscribed areas of hair loss with irregular borders and varying lengths of broken hairs. The frontoparietal and frontotemporal scalp are the most common areas for hair loss from trichotillomania. **(E)** Tinea corporis consists of dermatophytic infection involving the skin of the body rather than the scalp.

Figure 11-[illegible]

Figure 11-[illegible]

lesion appears up to 2 months following the original irritation and can lead to scarring and permanent hair loss if left untreated. [illegible] respond well to oral griseofulvin therapy. (C) Alopecia areata (see Figure 11-30) is well circumscribed area of complete hair loss involving the scalp, face, body and [illegible] including eyebrows or eyelashes. It is an autoimmune mediated process that often has a very good prognosis for future hair regrowth. (D) Trichotillomania is a disorder of hair pulling that is characterized by irregular, patchy areas of hair loss with irregular borders and varying lengths of broken hairs. The contralateral parietal and frontotemporal scalp are the most common areas for hair loss from pulling. (E) Tinea corporis consists of dermatophyte infection involving the skin of the body rather than the scalp.

CHAPTER 12

Allergy and Immunology

CORRIE FLETCHER

1 A 16-year-old girl who has recently taken trimethoprim–sulfamethoxazole for a urinary tract infection presents to the emergency department in distress. She complains of cough, chest pain, and joint pain. Her conjunctivae are injected. She has sloughing of her oral mucosa, erythematous and edematous lips, and erythematous macules, vesicles, and bullae on her face, trunk, and hands. Notably she has no skin tenderness.

Of the following, what is her most likely diagnosis?

(A) Erythema multiforme
(B) Bullous pemphigoid
(C) Stevens-Johnson syndrome
(D) Toxic epidermal necrolysis
(E) Staphylococcal scalded skin syndrome

The answer is C: Stevens-Johnson syndrome. Stevens-Johnson syndrome is a bullous mucocutaneous disorder. Medications such as sulfonamides, nonsteroidal anti-inflammatory drugs, and anticonvulsants, as well as infections with *Mycoplasma pneumoniae* have been associated with developing Stevens-Johnson syndrome. Progression of the disease begins with cutaneous symptoms including erythematous macules that progress to bullae. Lesions occur in crops and may linger for more than 1 month following the removal of the offending agent. Additional criteria for Stevens-Johnson syndrome include the involvement of at least two mucosal surfaces such as eyes, oral mucosa, and gastrointestinal or genitourinary tracts. Ophthalmic involvement may be severe including corneal ulcers and anterior uveitis. Other systemic symptoms include pneumonitis, myocarditis, hepatitis, arthritis, and acute tubular necrosis with resultant renal failure. Treatment of Stevens-Johnson syndrome is supportive with intravenous fluids and nutrition, a burn unit, and special dressings and tension-relieving bedding.

(A) Erythema multiforme may be similar in presentation to Stevens-Johnson syndrome but involves only cutaneous symptoms. **(D, E)**

Toxic epidermal necrolysis and staphylococcal scalded skin syndrome are both characterized by skin tenderness while the skin of patients with Stevens-Johnson syndrome is distinctly nontender. **(B)** Bullous pemphigoid is a cutaneous disorder where blisters develop in crops and progress to tense bullae often filled with blood or turbid in appearance. Given the additional mucocutaneous findings described in the vignette, this disorder is less likely.

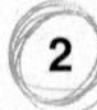

2 A 3-year-old boy presents to establish care at the pediatrician's office. His mother states that the patient has had multiple pneumonias, three of which required hospitalization for treatment. She also states he had tympanostomy tubes placed at 12 months of age following persistent otitis media and at birth he had to stay an additional day due to prolonged bleeding after his circumcision. On examination, he has severely dry, excoriated skin.

Of the following which is the most likely diagnosis of this 3-year-old boy?

(A) Ataxia-telangiectasia
(B) JAK3 deficiency
(C) DiGeorge syndrome
(D) Autoimmune polyendocrinopathy-candidiasis ectodermal dysplasia (APECED)
(E) Wiskott-Aldrich syndrome (WAS)

The answer is E: Wiskott-Aldrich syndrome (WAS). The patient described in the vignette has WAS. WAS is an X-linked recessive disease characterized by atopic dermatitis, thrombocytopenic purpura with small, ineffectual platelets, and T-cell deficiency. The mutated protein involved in this disorder is the Wiskott-Aldrich syndrome protein (WASP). It enables actin assembly for microvesicle formation with tyrosine kinase signaling. When the WASP mutation is present these T cells cannot signal antigen-presenting cells, B cells, or other T cells. Additionally, the cells have poor motility and cytoskeleton due to the disorganization of the actin filaments. In WAS, abnormally small platelets along with thrombocytopenia is frequently seen as well as decreased numbers of T cells and normal immunoglobulin G (IgG), decreased IgM, and normal to increased IgA and IgE. Patients with WAS are predisposed initially to multiple pneumococcal infections at younger ages and then later with *Pneumocystis jirovecii* and herpes virus. Treatment is with intravenous Ig, aggressive management of infections, and eventually bone marrow transplant. To manage the thrombocytopenia, patients may require a splenectomy, which can further increase their risk of infections from encapsulated organisms.

(A) Patients with ataxia-telangiectasia have mutations on chromosome 11 and have low CD3 and CD4 cell counts and decreased responsiveness of T and B cells to mitogens. The cells have defective DNA repair, poor cell cycle signaling, and an inability to control the cell cycle often leading to other chromosomal abnormalities. Patients present with progressive ataxia, oculomotor deterioration, nystagmus, and poor articulation. Telangiectasias of the skin and eyes typically appear around 3 to 6 years of age after the neurologic signs are present. Patients are at risk for multiple and concurrent sinopulmonary infections.

(B) The JAK3 mutation is an autosomal recessive form of severe combined immunodeficiency (SCID). Patients have elevated levels of B cells with few to no T and natural killer cells. There is a defect in the γ-chain on cytokine receptors leading to ineffective intracellular signaling. Patient with JAK3 mutation, like other SCID syndromes, present at a young age with recurrent or persistent diarrhea, pneumonia, sepsis, and cutaneous infections. Infections with opportunistic organisms are common, including *P. jirovecii*, cytomegalovirus, Epstein-Barr virus, and *Candida*. A patient with a JAK3 mutation would not present as late as 3 years nor would he have any risk factors for prolonged bleeding as described in the vignette.

(C) In DiGeorge syndrome, a mutation on chromosome 22q11.2 leads to varying degrees of thymic hypoplasia and low numbers of impaired T cells. Patients with complete thymic aplasia present similarly to SCID patients.

(E) APECED is a syndrome of chronic mucocutaneous candidal infections coupled with multiple endocrinopathies, usually hypoparathyroidism and primary adrenal dysfunction. Patients may also have alopecia, pernicious anemia, vitiligo, or other autoimmune conditions.

Of the following CD4 counts, what is the threshold for initiating *Pneumocystis jirovecii* prophylaxis in a teenager infected with human immunodeficiency virus (HIV)?

(A) 50 cells/μL
(B) 200 cells/μL
(C) 350 cells/μL
(D) 1,000 cells/μL
(E) 1,500 cells/μL

The answer is B: 200 cells/μL. The risk of various opportunistic infections in patients with HIV is based on the patient's CD4 levels. Infants born with vertically transmitted HIV are to start prophylaxis with trimethoprim–sulfamethoxazole (TMP–SMX) for *P. jirovecii* at 4 weeks and continue through 1 year of life. **(C, D, E)** Older children through adulthood should receive daily TMP–SMX prophylaxis against *P. jirovecii* starting at CD4 counts <200 cells/μL. **(A)** At CD4 counts <50 cells/μL, patients should be started on mycobacterium-avium complex (MAC) prophylaxis regardless of age. MAC prophylaxis includes daily clarithromycin and weekly azithromycin.

Children with HIV should continue to receive their routine immunizations, despite thoughts that their immune response may function suboptimally.

Children with CD4 counts >200 cells/μL should receive the 23-valent pneumococcal vaccine and the measles, mumps, and rubella vaccine. Patients with cell counts >1,000 cells/μL are safe to receive vaccination against varicella split into two doses and administered 3 months apart. All patients should receive yearly influenza vaccinations.

4 A 4-year-old girl presents with a history of recurrent infections with *Streptococcus pneumoniae*, *Streptococcus pyogenes*, and *Haemophilus influenzae* type b despite receiving appropriate vaccinations.

Of the following, which is most likely to confirm B-cell–specific immunodeficiency?

(A) Delayed hypersensitivity skin tests, immunophenotyping, and lymphocyte count
(B) Nitroblue tetrazolium dye test, chemotaxis assay, and a myeloperoxidase stain
(C) Quantitative immunoglobulin (Ig) levels, isohemagglutinin titers, and specific antibody levels
(D) CH50, C1-inhibitor level and function, and an AP50
(E) Computed tomography (CT) scan of the sinuses, urinalysis, and a blood culture

The answer is C: Quantitative immunoglobulin (Ig) levels, isohemagglutinin titers, and specific antibody levels. The workup for a potential B-cell deficiency includes a complete blood count, quantitative Ig levels, isohemagglutinin titers, and specific antibody levels. Quantitative Ig levels report serum IgG, IgM, IgA, and IgE levels. Antibody titers to vaccinations reflect the ability of the patient's immune system to react to antibody stimulation and create memory B cells. Checking isohemagglutinin titers such as anti-A and anti-B can help to measure the function of IgM. An abnormality in any of these tests is suggestive for a B-cell defect.

Immunophenotyping is the first step in the workup of a T-cell–mediated immunodeficiency. Immunophenotyping uses flow cytometry to count the percentages and absolute numbers of T cells, B cells, and natural killer cells as well as their subsets. **(A)** Delayed-type hypersensitivity tests help to determine the presence of antigen-specific memory T cells. Specific T-cell proliferation assays can assess the T cells' ability to respond and proliferate when exposed to antigens or mitogens.

(B) Nitroblue tetrazolium tests neutrophil function and is an appropriate workup for a defect in phagocytic cellular function. **(D)** CH50 assesses the components of the classical complement pathway and AP50 evaluates the alternative complement pathway. A C1-inhibitor level and function is a test for a specific complement defect leading to hereditary angioedema.

(E) While the patient in the vignette may need a CT scan of the sinuses to determine chronic damage, this will not confirm a B-cell immunodeficiency.

A 7-year-old boy is admitted to the general pediatric inpatient floor with a right lobar pneumonia. His medical history reveals multiple hospitalizations for recurrent pneumonias and several skin boils requiring incision and drainage. On physical examination, he is several inches shorter than the rest of his family and below his mean parental height.

Of the following, what is the most likely pathogenesis of his disease?

(A) Excessive accumulation of neutrophils at inflamed sites
(B) Decreased binding of neutrophils with impaired adhesion
(C) Impaired chemotaxis
(D) Inability of phagocytic cells to activate respiratory burst
(E) Absent or impaired function of splenic macrophages

The answer is D: Inability of phagocytic cells to activate respiratory burst. The boy described in the vignette has chronic granulomatous disease (CGD). Phagocytic function is crucial to the protection of deeper organs from microorganisms. The skin, mucus membranes, and linings of the respiratory and gastrointestinal tracts are susceptible to repeated infections when neutrophils do not function properly as phagocytes are the first line of defense. In CGD, neutrophils and macrophages are able to ingest the microorganism; however, due to a defect in initiating respiratory burst, they are unable to kill catalase-positive organisms. Respiratory burst is a process during which cells release reactive oxygen molecules such as superoxide and hydrogen peroxide to assist in killing bacteria. Nicotinamide adenine dinucleotide phosphate (NADPH) oxide is utilized by immune cells to reduce oxygen to free radical oxygen, a superoxide.

Myeloperoxidase then combines with free radical oxygen molecules to produce hydrogen peroxide and hypochlorite to destroy bacteria. In patients with CGD, phagocytic cells ingest the microorganism but then cannot produce the superoxide necessary to induce respiratory burst due to the lack of NADPH oxide.

This process is particularly important in catalase-producing organisms such as *Staphylococcus aureus*, *Aspergillus*, *Nocardia*, and *Salmonella* species. Catalase-positive organisms produce an enzyme that breaks down hydrogen peroxide in cells. In normal functioning phagocytes, the respiratory burst cycle can overwhelm the capacity of catalase; however, in CGD-affected individuals the catalase-positive organisms produce hydrogen peroxide resulting in a microbicidal effect on the hosts own cell. Accumulation of these cells leads to granuloma formation leading to the clinical presentation of multiple abscesses, recurrent pneumonias, lymphadenitis, and osteomyelitis.

(A) An excessive accumulation of neutrophils at inflamed sites is seen in phagocytic disorders of abnormal cell motility such as with familial Mediterranean fever (FMF). In FMF an autosomal recessive gene encodes for a protein that modifies neutrophil activation. This frequently leads to the clinical manifestation of recurrent fevers, peritonitis with abdominal pain, pleuritis, and arthritis.

(B) A decreased binding of neutrophils with impaired adhesion is seen in leukocyte adhesion deficiencies (LADs) and clinically presents as recurrent bacterial infections without pus formation. This can be associated with neutrophilia and is due to impaired adhesion to activated endothelium.

(C) Impaired chemotaxis can be seen with multiple phagocytic disorders including Chédiak-Higashi syndrome, neutrophil actin dysfunction, LAD, and hyper-IgE syndrome. Chemotaxis is the direct migration of cells into sites of infection as signaled through chemokines and inflammatory markers such as tumor necrosis factor and interleukin-1.

(E) Absent or impaired function of splenic macrophages as seen with congenital absence of the spleen, splenic removal, or auto-infarction with syndromes such as sickle cell anemia also predispose individuals to infections with encapsulated bacteria.

---

6 A 4-year-old previously healthy boy is admitted to the intensive care unit. He has required mechanical ventilation for encephalopathy secondary to acute hepatic failure and necrosis. Laboratory workup reveals an overwhelming sepsis syndrome secondary to Epstein-Barr virus (EBV). Immunophenotyping demonstrates elevated levels of CD8 T cells. Following his infection, significant hypogammaglobulinemia persists and later he develops aplastic anemia.

Of the following which family history is most compatible with his underlying immunodeficiency?

(A) The patient's twin sister is also affected
(B) The patient's father has human immunodeficiency virus (HIV)
(C) The patient's mother and father are first cousins
(D) The patient's paternal grandfather died suddenly at age 32
(E) The patient's maternal uncle died at a young age of an EBV

The answer is E: The patient's maternal uncle died at a young age of an EBV. The patient described in the vignette has X-linked lymphoproliferative disease. This is an X-linked recessive disease with symptomatic onset around 3 to 5 years of age. The mutation is at the SH2DIA gene on the X chromosome and leads to an inability to stop communication in proliferating T cells. Patients are usually unaffected until exposure to EBV, after which the mutation results in an expansion of CD8 cells leading to hepatic necrosis and often death. Patients who survive their first EBV infection have chronic hypogammaglobulinemia along with residual T- and NK cell dysfunction. These patients are at increased risk for developing acute aplastic anemia, leukemia, and lymphoma. The hypogammaglobulinemia is treated symptomatically with intravenous immunoglobulin; however, the only curative treatment is with a stem cell transplant.

In an X-linked recessive disorder inheritance is through the maternal affected X chromosome. The mother is not affected because her other X chromosome asserts dominance over the mutated one. In an X-linked inheritance pattern, the maternal uncles are at risk to have inherited and manifest symptoms from the affected X chromosome. Therefore, of the choices, the only choice consistent with an X-linked recessive pattern is choice E.

(A) The patient in the vignette's twin sister could not be affected, as she will inherit one healthy chromosome X from her father. She may, however, be an asymptomatic carrier. **(C)** Consanguinity is a risk for autosomal recessive diseases. **(B)** The patient's father's HIV status does not necessarily reflect the patient's status. However, if the patient in the vignette were infected with HIV, his CD8 levels would be expected to be low rather than elevated. **(D)** If the patient in the vignette's paternal grandfather died suddenly at the age of 32, suspicion could be higher for sudden cardiac death, however, not specifically relevant to his current presentation.

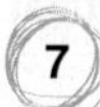

7 A 38-week gestational age neonate is born to a mother who had minimal prenatal care. Initially the baby was reported to do well, but after several hours he developed difficulty with feeding. He is brought to the nursery where a pulse oximeter shows a preductal saturation of 98% and a postductal saturation of 84%. An echocardiogram reveals an interrupted aortic arch, type B. On examination, the patient has low set ears, a short philtrum, and downward slanting eyes. Thirty minutes later the patient experiences a tonic–clonic seizure.

Of the following, which is the most likely genetic process involved in this neonate?

(A) JAK3 mutation
(B) Wiskott-Aldrich syndrome protein (WASP) mutation
(C) Nondisjunction of chromosome 21
(D) Substitution of glutamic acid for valine
(E) 22q11.2 mutation

The answer is E: 22q11.2 mutation. The patient in the vignette has DiGeorge syndrome. A microdeletion on chromosome 22 leading to a 22q11.2 mutation causes a spectrum of clinical manifestations. Patients with DiGeorge syndrome can have a variety of defects including anomalies of the heart such as conotruncal defects, septal defects, and interrupted aortic arch, type B. Typical facies of DiGeorge syndrome include short philtrum, hypertelorism, low set ears, mandibular hypoplasia, and downward slanted eyes. Patients may also have thymic and parathyroid hypoplasia. This leads to varying degrees of T-cell dysfunction and hypocalcemia. The seizures described in the vignette are most likely secondary to hypocalcemia.

(A) JAK3 mutations are seen in an autosomal recessive form of severe combined immunodeficiency. Patients with JAK3 mutations present with severe T-cell dysfunction and a predisposition to life-threatening infections. Differentiating features from the neonate described in the vignette include a lack of abnormal facies and normal calcium levels. **(B)** The WASP mutation is seen in association with Wiskott-Aldrich syndrome. Wiskott-Aldrich is an X-linked recessive syndrome composed of severe dermatitis, thrombocytopenia, and T-cell dysfunction.

(C) Trisomy 21 is most frequently caused by the nondisjunction in meiosis of the affected chromosome. While trisomy 21 is associated with cardiac anomalies and abnormal facies, interrupted aortic arch, type B is not associated with trisomy 21. **(D)** In patients with sickle cell disease, hemoglobin S is caused by an amino acid substitution of glutamic acid for valine in the β-globulin chain of hemoglobin. The result is the formation of abnormal hemoglobin that sickles when exposed to stress causing the clinical manifestations of sickle cell disease.

8 Of the following, which description is most characteristic of a patient with a T-cell defect?

(A) A patient aged less than 6 months at diagnosis, who is failing to thrive, has chronic diarrhea, and may have had fungal, parasitic, or viral infections
(B) A patient aged 6 months to a year or older with recurrent sinopulmonary infections, infections with *Streptococcus*, *Staphylococcus*, and *Haemophilus*
(C) A young childhood patient with a history of multiple boils and abscesses, poor dentition, staphylococcal infections, and poor wound healing
(D) A patient with recurrent sinopulmonary infections, more than one infection with *Neisseria meningitidis* or septicemia, and a history of angioedema
(E) A patient with fatigue, arthritis, thrombocytopenia and leukopenia, renal failure, and painless oral ulcers

The answer is A: **A patient aged less than 6 months at diagnosis, who is failing to thrive, has chronic diarrhea, and may have had fungal, parasitic, or viral infections.** While all the patients described in the answer set have immune system abnormalities, the one with classic T-cell dysfunction is the patient aged less than 6 months at diagnosis, with failure to thrive, chronic diarrhea, and infections with fungi, parasites, and viruses. Patients with T-cell defects are usually diagnosed within months of birth and are predisposed to infections with opportunistic organisms such as *Pneumocystis jirovecii* and mycobacteria along with fungal and severe viral infections.

(B) In contrast, patients who have recurrent sinopulmonary infections, severe bacterial infections, and a predisposition to autoimmunity often have B-cell dysfunction. Patients with B-cell dysfunction are usually diagnosed after 6 months of age when maternal antibodies are no longer circulating in the infant. However, many of these patients may not be diagnosed until older if the defect is minor such as in common variable immunodeficiency.

(C) In patients with recurrent boils and abscesses, especially those with internal organ involvement such as liver abscesses or osteomyelitis, a granulocyte defect such as chronic granulomatous disease should be considered. Patients with defects in granulocyte function are often diagnosed early in life following multiple skin infections with *Staphylococcus* sp.; however, these patients are also at risk for more unusual infections such as *Nocardia* and *Aspergillus*. Granulocyte defects should be considered in any patient with consistently poor wound healing as well as any patient with a prolonged attachment of the umbilical cord.

(D) Patients with recurrent sinopulmonary infections, more than one infection with *N. meningitidis* or septicemia, or a history of angioedema should be considered for a complement defect. Many autoimmune conditions such as systemic lupus erythematosus (SLE) or vasculitides also have complement defects and thus should be monitored secondary to an increased risk of severe, invasive infections.

(E) A patient with fatigue, arthritis, thrombocytopenia and leukopenia, renal failure, and painless oral ulcers should be investigated for having SLE, an autoimmune disease characterized by autoantibodies targeting specific organs causing inflammation and organ damage.

9 A 15-month-old child is brought in for her scheduled health maintenance visit. Her physical examination is significant for the findings in *Figure 12-1*. The family history is significant for her 6-year-old sister with a history of asthma and her mother reveals she has chronic seasonal allergies.

Of the following, what is the best recommendation for initial skin care?

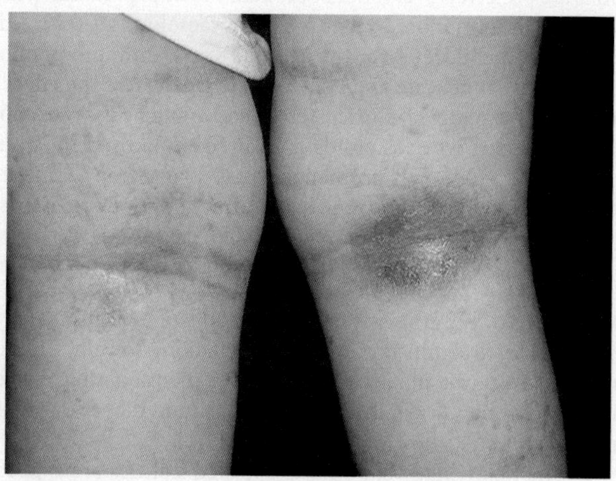

Figure 12-1

(A) Initiating a trial treatment with antihistamines
(B) Initiation of therapy with tacrolimus
(C) Lukewarm baths followed by application of emollients
(D) Every other day administration of a low-dose corticosteroid
(E) High-dose topical steroids on affected areas

The answer is C: **Lukewarm baths followed by application of emollients.** The patient described in the vignette has physical examination findings consistent with atopic dermatitis. Atopic dermatitis is a chronic, relapsing skin inflammation characterized by pruritus and hyperirritability of the skin. Nearly half of all infants with severe atopic dermatitis have food allergies as a contributing factor and allergies to egg and milk are common instigators. Additionally, the majority of infants with severe atopic dermatitis go on to develop other allergic conditions such as allergic rhinitis (AR) or asthma.

The diagnosis of atopic dermatitis requires pruritic skin irritation plus at least three of the following: history of involving skin creases, history of asthma or AR in a first-degree relative if the patient is less than 4 years old, history of generally dry skin within the last year, onset of age less than 2, and visible flexural dermatitis.

Initial skin care begins with attempting to restore the skin's natural barrier functions through the soak-and-seal method. The soak-and-seal method involves lukewarm baths, patting dry with a towel, and liberal application of emollients to seal in cutaneous moisture.

If the soak-and-seal method is not effective alone, the next-line therapy is topical corticosteroids to reduce inflammation and itching, especially during acute flares. **(E)** Patients with atopic dermatitis should be treated with the lowest effective dose of topical corticosteroid and titrated as indicated. Ointment preparations are preferred over lotions secondary to improved skin penetration.

(B) The use of immunomodulators such as tacrolimus is reserved for second-line therapy in children over the age of 2 years. Immunomodulators are particularly useful on delicate areas such as the face where the effect of striations or thinning from topical corticosteroid use would be the most noticeable. **(D)** Additionally, oral corticosteroids are infrequently used in severe flares. **(A)** Antihistamines, although not beneficial as sole therapy, can be used in conjunction with any of the above listed treatment options to assist with the pruritus and ideally stop the inflammatory cycle.

---

10 A 4-year-old girl presents with fever and pharyngitis. Her physical examination is significant for thrush extending from her mouth down into her posterior pharynx. Her mother mentions that her daughter has had chronic thrush infections and resistant diaper dermatitis since infancy.

Of the following, what other associated features are expected if she has an immunodeficiency?

(A) Autoimmune endocrinopathies
(B) Hypocalcemia
(C) Small platelets
(D) Failure to shed primary teeth
(E) Telangiectasias

The answer is A: Autoimmune endocrinopathies. The immunodeficiency most consistent with the patient in the vignette is chronic mucocutaneous candidiasis, also known as autoimmune polyendocrinopathy-candidiasis-ectodermal dystrophy (APECED). APECED is an autosomal recessive immunodeficiency that frequently is diagnosed between ages 3 and 5. It is due to a mutation in the autoimmune regulator gene, which when dysfunctional causes the thymus to fail to recognize normal host tissue antigens resulting in an autoimmunity. There is also decreased or absent response of lymphocyte proliferation secondary antigenic stimulation despite having antibodies that are produced normally.

As a result, patients with chronic mucocutaneous candidiasis have recurrent skin, mucosal, and nail infections with *Candida*. The infections are often resistant to topical antifungal therapy and require oral treatment. Many patients in late adolescence or early adulthood develop hypoparathyroidism and adrenal failure. Frequent surveillance for autoimmune conditions is a necessary part of their care.

The remaining choices are not associated with APECED. **(B)** Hypocalcemia is associated with DiGeorge syndrome. **(C)** Wiskott-Aldrich syndrome is associated with small platelets and thrombocytopenia. **(D)** A patient who fails to shed her primary teeth by the time she has her permanent teeth grow in should be considered for hyper-IgE syndrome. **(E)** Telangiectasias are associated with immunodeficiency in patients having ataxia-telangiectasia syndrome.

11 A 3-year-old girl presents because her mother states she has been called by the daycare to come pick her up early several days over the past month after she starts complaining of abdominal pain followed by diarrhea. The child has not had any new exposures to chemicals or toxins in the environment at daycare and attends a high-end daycare where only organic and healthy foods are served. She has noticed that on the days they serve edamame for the afternoon snack, she almost always gets called to pick her up. On examination, the girl has widespread eczema.

Of the following, what is the best advice to give this mother?

(A) Skin allergen testing for all legumes
(B) Avoid eating edamame
(C) Continue to eat edamame, but keep an epinephrine autoinjector for home
(D) Recommend 12.5 mg diphenhydramine prior to consumption of edamame
(E) Continue eating edamame, but gradually introduce larger amounts of it into her daughter's diet until her symptoms cease

The answer is B: Avoid eating edamame. Food allergies are increasingly prevalent in Western societies. The most common food allergy experienced by children is to cow milk protein. The development of specific food hypersensitivity is typically complex ranging from immunoglobulin E (IgE)-mediated mast cell activation to cytokine secretion from allergen-sensitized T lymphocytes.

The clinical manifestations of food hypersensitivities are broad and include classic anaphylaxis symptoms such as wheezing, shortness of breath, hypotension, flushing, and edema, and frequently involve multiple organ systems. Gastrointestinal manifestations include irritability or spitting up in younger infants, diarrhea, poor weight gain, hypoproteinemia, malabsorption, and flatulence in toddlers to adults. Atopic dermatitis and allergic rhinitis often accompany chronic allergen exposure.

Identifying specific reactive food allergens is complex and often difficult. **(A)** Skin prick tests can rule out IgE-mediated reactions to specific antigens, but often are hindered by false-positive reactions in that a child has skin-mediated reaction without any clinical reaction to the ingested food. Additionally, serum IgE testing for suspected foods is highly specific but limited in scope beyond a few foods. There is no testing that identifies cell-mediated food hypersensitivities. The process of an elimination diet followed by food challenge is the only validated method to establish a true diagnosis. For IgE-mediated food responses, avoidance of the suspected allergen for 10 to 14 days is recommended prior to oral food challenges within a controlled setting such as a pediatrician's office. For cell-mediated responses, avoidance for up to 8 weeks might be necessary prior to reintroduction. Once the food has been avoided for the recommended allotment of time, a food is reintroduced. If the challenge has a positive reaction, continued allergen avoidance is the key treatment.

Thus, initial treatment for food hypersensitivities is strict avoidance of the suspected agent. **(C, D, E)** Treatments with diphenhydramine or continued exposure to the allergen, even with the backup of an epinephrine autoinjector, are not safe options for handling food allergies.

12 A 9-month-old infant presents to the clinic following his second infection with *Neisseria meningitidis*.

Of the following, what is the most likely deficiency to be found in this patient?

(A) Deficiency of C1 inhibitor
(B) Deficiency of C3
(C) Deficiency C3b receptor
(D) Deficiency C5a inhibitor
(E) Deficiency of C8

The answer is E: Deficiency of C8. The complement cascade is a complex system that aids in the innate immune response as well as antibody-mediated immunity. The complement system can be activated through three pathways. The classic pathway is activated through antigen–antibody complexes or inflammatory markers such as C-reactive protein. The alternative pathway is activated through endotoxins, fungal antigens, or C3b generated via the classical pathway. Lastly, the lectin pathway is activated by the interaction of microbes with mannose-binding lectin.

All three of the above pathways culminate with the formation of C3. C3 initiates the common pathway and the membrane attack complex (MAC) is formed. The MAC, composed of C5 to C9, results in the lysis of pathogens and target cells. See *Figure 12-2* for an illustration of the complement pathways.

Deficiencies of complement early in the cascade have minimal immunologic effects although are often associated with rheumatologic conditions. **(B, C)** Deficiencies of C1, C2, C3, and C3b are all associated with systemic lupus erythematosus. Patients with C2 defects may have mild recurrent infections.

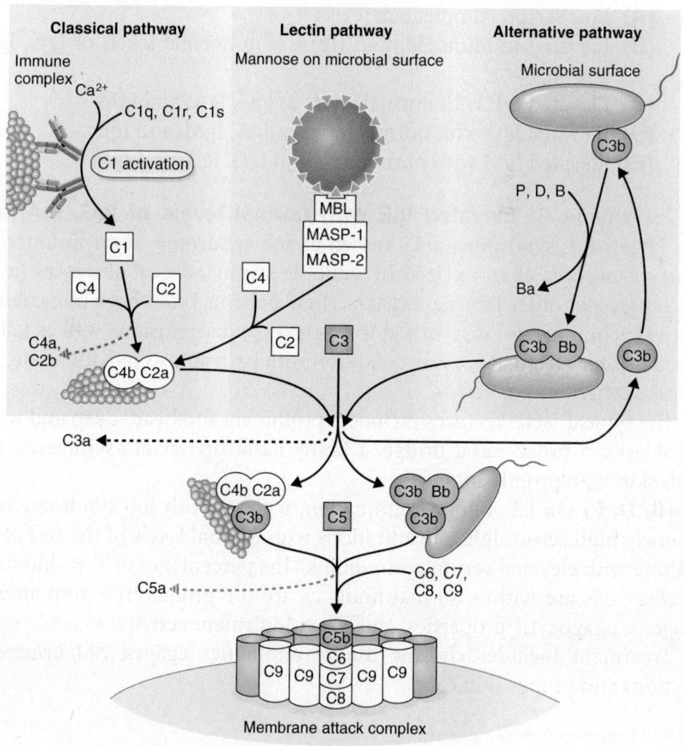

Figure 12-2

(D) A deficiency in the C5a inhibitor is associated with the development of FMF, a periodic fever syndrome inherited through families of Mediterranean descent that results in autoinflammation of serosal surfaces.

(A) Deficiency in C1 inhibitor leads to hereditary angioedema.

The patient in the vignette has a deficiency of C8, a component the MAC, as evidenced by recurrent *N. meningitidis* infections.

---

13 An 8-year-old boy presents following a dentist visit in which he was told several of his permanent teeth are coming in and yet he has not lost any of his primary teeth. On examination, both the patient and his mother have a broad forehead, widely spaced eyes, a protruding mandible, and rough, excoriated skin. On further history, his mother states he has been hospitalized on several occasions for multiple skin boils, septic arthritis, and several pneumonias.

Of the following, which set of laboratory results is most likely for this patient?

(A) Low serum complement levels
(B) Elevated immunoglobulin (Ig)A with normal levels of IgG, IgM, and IgE
(C) Elevated IgE with normal levels of IgG, IgA, and IgM
(D) Elevated IgG with normal levels of IgA, IgM, and IgE
(E) Elevated IgM with normal levels of IgG, IgA, and IgM

The answer is C: **Elevated IgE with normal levels of IgG, IgA, and IgM.** Hyper-IgE syndrome, also known as Job syndrome, is an immunodeficiency syndrome characterized by multiple staphylococcal abscesses in the skin, lungs, and other internal organs. These patients often have bony abnormalities including a predisposition to fractures and scoliosis as well as failure to shed primary teeth. It is a rare condition with both autosomal dominant and recessive inheritance patterns.

The typical facial features include a prominent forehead, deep and wide-spaced eyes, a broad nasal bridge, a fleshy nasal tip, facial asymmetry, and rough skin with prominent pores.

(B, D, E) On laboratory examination, patients with Job syndrome have extremely high serum IgE concentrations with normal levels of the rest of the Igs along with elevated serum eosinophilia. The percentages of T, B, and natural killer cells are within normal limits as are the proliferative responses to mitogens, phagocytic properties, and **(A)** complement activity.

Treatment includes chronic use of antibiotics against *Staphylococcus* infections and proper skin care.

14 A 6-month-old infant diagnosed with severe combined immunodeficiency as a newborn presents 1-month post-hematopoietic stem cell

transplant. He has an erythematous, maculopapular rash on 25% of his body, has difficulty with feedings due to persistent diarrhea, and scleral icterus. A complete metabolic panel reveals bilirubin and liver enzymes that are moderately elevated.

Of the following, what is the most likely pathogenesis behind his current presentation?

(A) Host lymphocytes rejecting donor stem cells
(B) An infection with an opportunistic microorganism
(C) Medication side effect due to immunosuppression
(D) Donor lymphocytes activating against the patient's own antigens
(E) Underproduction of host cytokines leading to an ineffectual uptake of the transplant cells

The answer is D: Donor lymphocytes activating against the patient's own antigens. The patient described in the vignette is experiencing graft-versus-host disease (GVHD), which occurs following an allogeneic hematopoietic stem cell transplant. **(A)** The donor T cells from the transplant attack the recipient's antigens on target tissues. This mechanism occurs in two phases. First, the patient's own tissue is damaged through preparation for stem cell transplant, which activates the patient's own antigen-presenting cells and brings the patient's antigens to the newly acquired donor T cells. Second, the donor T cells, in response to these antigens, activate CD4 and CD8 cells that then produce cytokines including tumor necrosis factor, interleukin 2, and interferon gamma causing tissue damage.

Acute GVHD develops within 2 to 6 weeks post-transplantation and involves primarily endothelial damage and lymphocytic infiltration. Primarily skin, liver, and intestinal endothelium is damaged leading to the symptoms of rash, vomiting or diarrhea, jaundice, and anorexia. Treatment includes steroids, monoclonal antibody targeting, and extracorporeal photophoresis to attempt to induce cytotoxic effects on the activated donor T cells.

Patients who receive hematopoietic stem cell transplant are in a state of immunodeficiency post-transplant and are at risk for severe bacterial and fungal infections. Infections with *Candida* or *Aspergillus* can be devastating for the patients. **(B)** While these patients are at risk due to absent neutrophils following transplant, GVHD is not an infectious process; however, it can increase the risk of a severe infection.

(C) Patients post-transplantation are treated with immunosuppressive medications such as cyclosporine, tacrolimus, and methotrexate in order to help prevent GVHD. These medications are used to suppress the immune system from activating, rather than causing the immune system to activate.

A 9-year-old girl with severe food allergies is diagnosed with celiac disease. Quantitative immunoglobulin (Ig) levels are drawn in the workup of her celiac disease and the results demonstrate absent serum IgA levels.

Of the following, what is the most likely inheritance pattern for selective IgA deficiency?

(A) X-linked dominant
(B) Autosomal
(C) Mitochondrial
(D) Imprinting
(E) Spontaneous mutation

The answer is B: **Autosomal.** Selective IgA deficiency is defined as isolated serum IgA levels < 10 mg/dL. Prior to 4 years of age, serum IgA levels are not accurate, as IgA levels do not fully reach adult levels until then. Often patients with IgA deficiency are asymptomatic; however, in patients who are symptomatic, selective IgA deficiency can be associated with sinopulmonary infections, allergies, autoimmunity, and celiac disease. **(A, C, D, E)** Selective IgA deficiency has been shown to run in families and its inheritance is thought to be autosomal in nature. A patient with a family history of selective IgA deficiency is at an increased risk of developing common variable immunodeficiency.

16 Stem cell transplantation is often the only curative treatment for many immunodeficiencies.

Of the following, which immunodeficiency can be successfully treated without stem cell transplantation?

(A) Severe combined immunodeficiency (SCID)
(B) Hyper-immunoglobulin (Ig)M/CD40 ligand deficiency
(C) X-linked lymphoproliferative disease
(D) Complete DiGeorge syndrome with thymic aplasia
(E) Selective IgA deficiency

The answer is E: **Selective IgA deficiency.** Stem cells reside in the patient's bone marrow and cord blood. While stem cells are found in peripheral blood, they usually are not in high enough quantities to be harvested for transplant. When picking a stem cell donor, the major histocompatibility complex of a donor's stem cells is carefully analyzed to provide the best match for the recipient in order to reduce the receiving patient's risk of graft-versus-host disease.

(A, B, C, D) Most severe T-cell defects are curable by stem cell transplantations, including all forms of SCID, hyper-IgM/CD40 ligand deficiency, X-linked lymphoproliferative disease, and complete DiGeorge syndrome. Additionally, patients with Wiskott-Aldrich syndrome, autoimmune lymphoproliferative syndrome, Chédiak-Higashi syndrome, familial hemophagocytic lymphohistiocytosis, and leukocyte adhesion deficiency type 1 also are candidates for cure by stem cell transplant.

Fortunately, for most patients with selective IgA deficiency, their course is often mild and often asymptomatic. The most common symptoms include sinopulmonary infections, chronic gastrointestinal giardiasis, and a predisposition to allergies and celiac disease. Patients with selective IgA deficiency are not candidates for stem cell transplantation and should not be treated with intravenous immunoglobulin (IVIG) as most IVIG preparations contain levels of IgA and can lead to anaphylactic reactions.

17 A 7-year-old boy presents to the emergency department with fevers, fatigue, severe exudative tonsillitis, posterior cervical lymphadenopathy, and splenomegaly.

Of the following, which set of symptoms is most consistent with a reactive hemophagocytic lymphohistiocytosis (HLH) process?

(A) History of recent treatment of the patient's sore throat with amoxicillin followed by a generalized maculopapular rash after initiating the antibiotic
(B) Fever for 5 days consecutively, erythematous lips and a fissured tongue, cracked peeling skin on the patient's palms and soles
(C) Generalized maculopapular rash, hepatomegaly, headache, neutropenia, thrombocytopenia, and hyperlipidemia
(D) Severe headache, photophobia, and stiff neck
(E) Generalized lymphadenopathy, pancytopenia, and persistent fevers

The answer is C: **Generalized maculopapular rash, hepatomegaly, headache, neutropenia, thrombocytopenia, and hyperlipidemia.** Histiocytosis is a group of individual disorders that share a common thread. There is a proliferation and accumulation of monocytes or macrophages that lead to organ damage and neoplasia. There are three main types of histiocytosis. Langerhans cell histiocytosis (LCH) is considered class I. Langerhans cells are antigen-presenting cells of the skin and bone. LCH is defined by proliferation of these cells within the skin leading to severe petechial or seborrheic rashes and lytic bone lesions in the skull, femur, or vertebrae, as well as bone marrow infiltration causing cytopenias. Other organs can also be involved leading to hepatomegaly, lymphadenopathy, and diabetes insipidus with pituitary involvement.

HLH is class II. HLH class II is a familial form in which patients present younger than 4 years of age with severe immunodeficiency. Symptoms include prolonged fevers, splenomegaly, a generalized maculopapular rash, respiratory, and/or central nervous system involvement. Diagnosis is made with cytopenia of at least two cell lines, hyperlipidemia or hypofibrinogenemia, and elevated ferritin levels.

Class III histiocytosis is a malignant form leading to cancers of the myeloid cell line and is rarely seen in pediatric patients.

(A) The development of a generalized maculopapular rash following treatment with amoxicillin for a sore throat is consistent with an infection with Epstein-Barr virus. **(B)** A patient with fever for 5 days consecutively, erythematous lips, a fissured tongue, and cracked peeling skin on the palms and soles should be considered for Kawasaki disease. **(D)** A patient with a fever, severe headache, photophobia, and stiff neck is consistent with meningitis.

(E) A patient with generalized lymphadenopathy, pancytopenia, and persistent fevers should be evaluated for an oncologic process.

18 An 18-year-old adolescent presents to the emergency department following a week of severe coughing. He states he has been fatigued for several months and has lost 15 pounds. On examination, he appears ill and gaunt and his pulse oximeter is reading 88% on room air. He has erythematous scars and open healing wounds on his bilateral forearms and antecubital spaces. His chest radiograph is shown in *Figure 12-3*.

Of the following, what is the best initial screening test to perform on this patient?

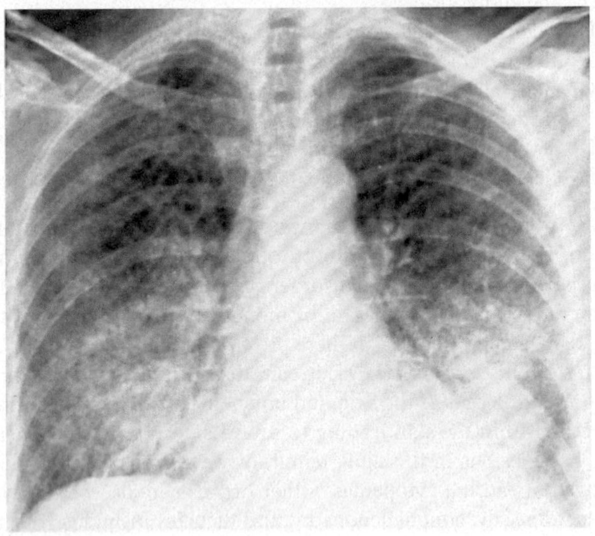

Figure 12-3

(A) Western blot
(B) Human immunodeficiency virus (HIV) culture
(C) Enzyme-linked immunosorbent assay (ELISA)
(D) HIV DNA or RNA polymerase chain reaction (PCR)
(E) CD4 cell count

The answer is C: Enzyme-linked immunosorbent assay (ELISA). The boy in the vignette engages in high-risk behaviors and has a chest radiograph consistent with *Pneumocystic jirovecii* pneumonia, making a diagnosis of HIV likely. HIV is an RNA virus that infects CD4 cells and causes dysgammaglobulinemia. Once infected, the virus replicates within the cells causing lysis, inducing increased speed of apoptosis, and leading to an increased activation of the CD8 cells. This leads to a declining number of CD4 cells, eventually causing the loss of cell-mediated immunity and increased risk of opportunistic infections and cancers.

ELISA is the standard initial screening test for HIV diagnosis. The test is an immunoglobulin G-based antibody with a high sensitivity but lower specificity. In other words, the ELISA test correctly identifies a high percentage of those patients with HIV infection, or true positives, while identifying an acceptable number of patients without HIV as infected with HIV, or false positives. **(A)** The confirmatory test to the ELISA for HIV diagnosis in patients older than 2 years is the Western blot. The Western blot has a higher specificity, thus, of the patients that tested positive on the ELISA, it eliminates the false positives leaving only the true positives.

(D) HIV, DNA, or RNA PCR can identify viral load. DNA PCR is the preferred test to diagnose HIV infections in children younger than 18 months. **(B)** HIV culture also has a high level of sensitivity; however, it is costly and requires up to a month for final results. Thus, it is not practical for clinical use.

(E) CD4 counts are measured once the diagnosis of HIV is confirmed. It is neither sensitive nor specific for HIV diagnosis.

---

19 A 14-year-old girl with large tonsils, splenomegaly, and pernicious anemia is seen for follow-up in clinic. She reports a recent history of several pneumonias with *Streptococcus pneumoniae*. Quantitative immunoglobulins (Igs) reveal pan-hypogammaglobulinemia.

Of the following, what is the best treatment option for this patient?

(A) Stem cell transplant
(B) Intravenous immunoglobulin (IVIG)
(C) Chronic prophylaxis with trimethoprim–sulfamethoxazole (TMP–SMX)
(D) Bi-weekly infusions with infliximab
(E) Social services care

The answer is B: Intravenous immunoglobulin (IVIG). The patient described in the vignette has common variable immunodeficiency (CVID) with hypogammaglobulinemia of IgG, IgM, IgA, and IgE. As is the case with most B-cell disorders, the first-line therapy is to replace the Igs through infusions with IVIG. The infusion of IVIG helps to provide passive immunity for patients with CVID. This allows their bodies to respond to microorganisms and reduce the severity and frequency of infections. Igs are administered intravenously every 3 to 4 weeks or subcutaneously every 1 to 2 weeks. Levels are measured frequently to maintain therapeutic levels of IgG. Complications of IVIG include the risk of anaphylaxis, especially in patients with absent IgA, and headache associated with chemical meningitis.

Antibiotic prophylaxis is often used in concurrence with IVIG therapy for B-cell disorders. Frequently, TMP–SMX or amoxicillin is used for prophylaxis and often on alternating days to help combat resistance in susceptible patients. **(C)** While TMP–SMX is used in B-cell disorders for prophylaxis, it alone is not the best treatment option.

(A) Stem cell transplantation is the treatment of choice for patients with T-cell deficiencies. Often these patients continue to have poor B-cell function and later require Ig replacement as well, but primary approach is through stem cell transplantation with an human leukocyte antigen–matched sibling.

(D) Infliximab is a chimeric monoclonal antibody that binds to tumor necrosis factor-α and is therefore beneficial in several autoimmune conditions including inflammatory bowel disease and rheumatoid arthritis. It is not beneficial in use for patients with CVID.

(E) Supportive care may be appropriate for any child with a chronic disease, including additional emotional and psychological care. While considering these aspects is important to provide holistic care to a child, it alone will not treat the underlying condition of the patient in the vignette.

20 A 14-year-old girl is seeing a pediatrician for the first time since relocating from another state. She is fair skinned with very blond hair. She reports the sun bothers her eyes and she always wears sunglasses. She has a history of multiple pneumonias, recurrent gingivitis, and poorly healing skin ulcers. She underwent menarche at age 12 and describes heavy menses. She states on occasion she notices she is bleeding without realizing she had cut herself. At the time of her visit she complains of feeling off balance. Her examination is significant for a wobbly gait and a slapping motion of her feet when she walks.

Of the following, what is the mechanism of this patient's most likely diagnosis?

(A) Decreased complement levels
(B) Low levels of immunoglobulin (Ig)G, IgM, and IgA
(C) Impaired neutrophil chemotaxis and degranulation
(D) Microdeletion on chromosome 22q11.2 leading to thymic aplasia
(E) Inappropriate Ig class-switching

The answer is C: **Impaired neutrophil chemotaxis and degranulation.** The patient described in the vignette has Chédiak-Higashi syndrome (CHS). Patients with CHS have a constellation of symptoms secondary to defective degranulation of neutrophils, ineffective neutrophil chemotaxis, impaired platelet aggregation, and development of giant melanocytes due to the formation of giant cytoplasmic granules with unregulated fusion of lysosomes. The symptoms of CHS include light skin and hair, photophobia, a mild bleeding diathesis, progressive peripheral neuropathy, frequent mucus membrane and skin infections, and most concerning the predisposition for an accelerated lymphoma-like syndrome.

(A) Decreased complement levels are seen in complement-deficiency syndromes including congenital deficiencies of C1 to C9 or secondary disorders of complement, as seen with membranoproliferative glomerulonephritis, sickle cell disease, or premature infants.

(B) Hypogammaglobulinemia characterized by low levels of all the Igs is seen with common variable immunodeficiency. Most cases are sporadic or autosomal dominant in inheritance. Clinically, these patients often have enlarged lymphoid tissue such as lymph nodes, tonsils, and spleen, and are predisposed to multiple infections, celiac-like disease, and other diseases of autoantibody formation.

(D) A microdeletion on chromosome 22q11.2 leading to thymic aplasia is classically seen with DiGeorge and velocardiofacial syndromes. The clinical spectrum of these patients includes cardiac anomalies that are typically conotruncal, abnormal facies, thymic hypoplasia, cleft palate, and hypocalcemia. The severity of the immunodeficiency associated with 22q11.2 deletions is related to the degree of thymic hypoplasia. Patients with mild hypoplasia grow at normal rates with minimal impact from opportunistic infections. Patients with complete thymic aplasia, however, resemble patients with severe combined immunodeficiency and require a bone marrow transplant.

(E) The inability to class switch from IgM to IgG, IgA, or IgE is consistent with hyper-IgM syndrome. Normal-to-elevated IgM levels with absent levels of the other Igs characterize this disease: The clinical syndrome of small tonsils, no palpable lymph nodes on examination, and neutropenia leading to recurrent infections with *Staphylococcus* sp., *Pneumocystis jirovecii*, and *Cryptosporidium*.

21 A 5-year-old girl is hospitalized with temperature to 39.8°C and found to have her fourth urinary tract infection. Her most recent urine culture was positive for *Escherichia coli* that was resistant to amoxicillin. She is reported to have an allergy to amoxicillin for which her reaction was a rash.

Of the following what is the best advice regarding the use of cephalosporins in this patient?

(A) Before administering the antibiotic, skin testing should be performed
(B) The risk of cephalosporin anaphylaxis is high
(C) The cephalosporin should be run over a slower rate to decrease the risk of reaction
(D) Patients with late-onset rashes to penicillins are not at risk to cross-react with anaphylaxis
(E) A lower dosage of cephalosporin should be prescribed in order to decrease the risk of reaction

The answer is D: Patients with late-onset rashes to penicillins are not at risk to cross-react with anaphylaxis. Penicillin is the most frequently reacted to antibiotic, often causing an immunoglobulin (Ig)E-mediated reaction. β-Lactam hypersensitivity is the cause of the majority of anaphylaxis to medications and anaphylactic drug-related mortality. Skin testing is available to determine the presence of penicillin-specific IgE for patients with an allergy to penicillin. Beyond penicillin, other antibiotics including synthetic penicillins such as amoxicillin, cephalosporins, and carbapenems also share a β-lactam ring.

In patients with a possible penicillin allergy, the degree of reaction can help to determine the risk of cross-reactivity with a cephalosporin. **(B)** Patients who have had an anaphylactic reaction to penicillin have a risk of cross-reactions, including anaphylaxis, to cephalosporins. **(A)** If a patient with a history of penicillin anaphylaxis requires a cephalosporin, skin testing for antigens should be performed prior to administration. If the skin tests are negative, the cephalosporin can be safely administered without any additional risk of anaphylaxis. **(D)** However, in patients with non-anaphylactic reactions to penicillin involving late-onset rashes, there is no increased risk of anaphylaxis with either synthetic penicillins or cephalosporins. **(C, E)** In general, slowing the infusion rate or decreasing to a subtherapeutic dose will not influence the risk of anaphylaxis to a medication.

22 A 14-year-old boy was bitten by a black widow spider while hiking through a forest 2 weeks ago. He was urgently treated with antivenom. He had been back to baseline until 2 days ago when he began to have temperatures to 102°F, feelings of fatigue and myalgias, and developed a pruritic rash. He has been taking ibuprofen for his achiness and diphenhydramine for his pruritus. This was initially effective until he began to also experience nausea, diarrhea, and chest pain.

Of the following, what is the most appropriate workup to establish his diagnosis?

(A) Complete metabolic panel and complete blood count
(B) Complete blood count and electrocardiogram
(C) Erythrocyte sedimentation rate (ESR), serum complement levels, and complete blood count
(D) Urinalysis, skin biopsy, and complete metabolic panel
(E) ESR, chest radiograph, and allergy testing

The answer is C: ESR, serum complement levels, and complete blood count. The boy in the vignette has findings consistent with serum sickness, an immune-complex–mediated reaction that is an example of a type III hypersensitivity reaction. This can occur following an exposure to serum, for example, the antivenom to the black widow spider as described in the vignette; but more frequently occurs in response to antibiotics such as penicillin or cefaclor and occasionally to human intravenous immunoglobulin.

The symptoms of a type III hypersensitivity reaction occur after antigen exposure within the blood stimulates antibody production. As the antigen concentration decreases due to clearance from antibodies, immune complexes form. The small complexes circulate freely and the larger ones are cleared by the reticuloendothelial system. The circulating intermediate-sized complexes deposit within walls of smaller blood vessels and cause a vasculitis.

The damage to the walls induces complement activation promoting chemotaxis and neutrophil adherence to the site. Activation of mast cells then occurs and further promotes tissue injury resulting in the symptoms described in the vignette. Patients with serum sickness often have a stereotypical rash described as a serpiginous band of erythema starting peripherally.

(A, B, D, E) While all of the tests named in the answer choices potentially could be useful in fully understanding the extent of the pathophysiology of the boy in the vignette, the best option to establish the diagnosis of serum sickness is to check the ESR, complement levels, and a complete blood count. With the activation of complement, C3 and C4 levels are typically at their lowest when circulating immune complexes are at their highest. The ESR is typically elevated and a thrombocytopenia, proteinuria, hemoglobinuria, or hematuria may be seen as well.

23 Of the following which infant is most at risk for transmission of human immunodeficiency virus (HIV)?

(A) The infant of a mother who acquired HIV prenatally and is formula feeding
(B) The infant of a mother who acquired HIV postnatally and is formula feeding
(C) The infant of a mother who acquired HIV prenatally and is breastfeeding
(D) The infant of a mother who acquired HIV postnatally and is breastfeeding
(E) The infant of a mother who acquired HIV prenatally, is receiving treatment with highly active anti-retroviral therapy (HAART), and is breastfeeding

The answer is D: The infant of a mother who acquired HIV postnatally and is breastfeeding. While a relatively uncommon mode of transmission in developed nations, maternal transmission through breastfeeding is significant in developing nations. **(C)** HIV has been identified as both free-floating and attached to human cells within breast milk, passing easily from the mother to the infant during breastfeeding. There is additional risk to breastfeeding infants whose mothers acquire primary HIV infection postnatally. Initial viremia in HIV infection often leads to >100,000 copies/mL of the virus, thus potentially exposing neonates to large burdens of viral copies. Therefore, the risk of transmission to the infant through breastfeeding doubles compared with those who acquired the infection prenatally.

(A, B) Due to the risk of transmission, it is recommended that HIV-infected mothers or mothers who have known ongoing exposure to HIV substitute formula for breastfeeding. However, adequate clean water and safe infant formula is not readily available in many developing countries. Given the high prevalence of severe diseases including diarrheal illnesses, dehydration, and malnutrition in these countries, the World Health Organization recommends that breastfeeding continues even in endemic areas as the nutritional benefits outweigh the risk of vertical transmission.

(E) Since the advent of HAART, mothers on proper HIV treatment can have essentially negligible viral levels. There have been established cases of vertical transmission of HIV despite viral copies <1,000/mL and formula feeding is recommended for women in developed nations even when receiving HAART.

24 A 7-year-old girl with a known peanut allergy exchanges lunch with a friend at the school cafeteria. Within minutes she feels tightness in her throat, abdominal pain, and shortness of breath. She goes to the school nurse with complaints of a rash and her vital signs are heart rate of 110 beats/min, respiratory rate of 24 breaths/min, and blood pressure of 70/40 mmHg.

Of the following, what is the best initial step in the management for this patient?

(A) Administration of 25 mg of diphenhydramine
(B) Administration of 75 mg of ranitidine
(C) Immediate intravenous injection of diphenhydramine
(D) Immediate intramuscular (IM) injection of 1:1,000 epinephrine
(E) Immediate IM injection of 1:10,000 epinephrine

The answer is D: Immediate IM injection of 1:1,000 epinephrine. The patient in the vignette is having classic symptoms of anaphylaxis. Anaphylaxis is the activation of mast cells and basophils as the result of IgE-mediated release. Patients with anaphylaxis have to be exposed to the allergen previously in order to develop allergen-specific antibodies. Once exposed, additional exposures lead to the release of histamine and cytokines causing allergic response.

While food allergy is the most common cause of anaphylaxis, multiple other exposures can also cause anaphylaxis including, but not limited to, insect stings, medications, and latex. Reactions can occur immediately to 48 hours after exposure. In order to classify the reaction as anaphylaxis at least three organ systems must be involved. Symptoms include cutaneous involvement, such as generalized pruritus, flushing, and rash; respiratory, including tightness of the throat, dyspnea, chest pain, and wheezing; and gastrointestinal symptoms, such as nausea, abdominal cramping, and vomiting. Systemic involvement includes hypotension with or without shock.

(E) Anaphylaxis is a medical emergency and should be treated promptly with IM epinephrine of 1:1,000 strength initially. **(A, B, C)** Additional therapy includes antihistamines, H1 and H2 blockers, oxygen, fluids, inhaled β-agonists, and corticosteroids based on the severity of the reaction and organ involvement. Patients with known anaphylactic reactions should be educated on strict avoidance of allergens, given an autoinjectable epinephrine device, and have a written emergency action plan if allergen exposure occurs.

25 The mother of a 4-week-old newborn makes an appointment with her pediatrician because she is concerned that the umbilical stump of her newborn has not yet fallen off. She is more anxious now because the area surrounding the umbilicus has changed color and appears dusky gray. She has not noticed any pus. A complete blood count reveals a white cell count of $28 \times 10^3/\mu L$ with a predominance of neutrophils.

Of the following, which complication is this patient most at risk for developing in the future?

(A) Progression to obstructive sleep apnea
(B) An anaphylactic reaction to penicillin
(C) Development of pancytopenia
(D) Recurrent bacterial and fungal infections
(E) Severe, recurrent croup infections

The answer is D: Recurrent bacterial and fungal infections. The concern with the infant in the vignette is the delayed separation of the umbilical cord along with clinical signs of infection without pus formation. Normal umbilical cord separation should occur by approximately 10 days of life. This clinical scenario suggests an abnormality of phagocyte adhesion as seen in leukocyte adhesion deficiency (LAD). LAD is an autosomal recessive disorder characterized by a deficiency in β_2-integrin leading to failure of activated neutrophils to bind to intercellular adhesion molecules (ICAM-1 and ICAM-2) on inflamed endothelial cells. Secondary to their inability to bind, the neutrophils cannot migrate out of the circulation and into the area of inflammation. The neutrophils that are able to migrate out of the blood vessel often have decreased function including decreased degranulation and oxidative metabolism. Patients with LAD may present with delayed umbilical stump separation secondary to poor wound healing or infection.

Consequently, patients with LAD are at risk for high levels of neutrophilia, as the activated neutrophils cannot move outside of the blood vessel into the areas of damage. These patients present similarly to those with neutropenia, with severe and recurrent bacterial and fungal infections. The skin and areas of mucosa are particularly affected including the lining of the lungs, the gastrointestinal tract, and the genitourinary tract. With the development of these infections the typical signs of inflammation such as erythema, warmth, swelling, and pus formation are often not seen.

The diagnosis can be undertaken with assessment of neutrophil and monocyte function. Specific flow cytometry measurements can also be taken. Once identified, patients with LAD often require early stem cell transplantations. Infections are aggressively managed with broad-spectrum antibiotics and prophylaxis with trimethoprim–sulfamethoxazole is appropriate.

(A, B, C, E) There is no association in patients with LAD with the development of obstructive sleep apnea, pancytopenia, an increased risk of anaphylaxis to penicillin, or recurrent croup infections.

---

26 A 2-year-old boy is seen in clinic for concerns of failure to thrive, chronic eczema, and a history of multiple skin infections. On further review of systems, his mother reveals a history of five incision and drainages for skin abscesses found to be positive for *Staphylococcus aureus*. In addition, he has been hospitalized for an empyema and has received multiple courses of antibiotics for acute otitis media. A nitroblue tetrazolium dye test and flow cytometry using dihydrorhodamine 123 are ordered and both return with positive results. The workup for stem cell transplantation is initiated.

Of the following, what is the best additional therapy available while he awaits a stem cell transplant?

(A) Intravenous immunoglobulin (IVIG)
(B) A 4-week course of intranasal administration of mupirocin
(C) Administration of granulocyte colony stimulating factor (G-CSF)
(D) Recombinant interferon gamma (INF-γ)
(E) Therapeutic isolation within a negative pressure room

The answer is D: Recombinant interferon gamma (INF-γ). Positive nitroblue tetrazolium dye tests and flow cytometry using dihydrorhodamine 123 are diagnostic for chronic granulomatous disease (CGD). While the only cure for CGD is a hematopoietic stem cell transplant, aggressive care can be undertaken in the time prior to transplantation. Specifically for CGD, recombinant therapy with INF-γ is beneficial. Intravenous therapy three times per week reduces the number of serious infections in patients with CGD. Additionally to INF-γ, patients with CGD should receive antibiotic therapy for developing infections as well as prophylaxis with trimethoprim–sulfamethoxazole. There is an increased risk of fungal infections with *Aspergillus*. If a diagnosed infection with *Aspergillus* occurs, treatment with amphotericin should be promptly initiated. Prophylaxis with itraconazole may be considered in certain high-risk patients with CGD. **(B)** Patients with infections with *S. aureus* should be tested for nasal carriage and treated appropriately with twice a day mupirocin for 5 days. Any extended treatment has not been shown to be effective.

(A) IVIG is the treatment of choice for patients with B-cell and severe T-cell disorders, including common variable immunodeficiency and severe combined immunodeficiency. **(C)** G-CSF is useful in treating patients who have neutropenia. Daily intravenous or subcutaneous administration can help quicken the bone marrow production of neutrophils. Patients on G-CSF therapy should be monitored closely for the development of splenomegaly, thrombocytopenia, and vasculitis. **(E)** Isolation within a negative pressure room while waiting for a stem cell transplant would be over-excessive and unnecessary for this patient at this time.

27 A first-time expectant mother comes to establish care with her pediatrician 4 weeks before her baby is due.

Of the following, which statement regarding the benefits of breastfeeding is most accurate?

(A) Breastfed infants have a higher stool pH that contributes to establishing healthy intestinal flora
(B) Breastfed infants gain weight faster than their formula-fed counterparts
(C) Breastfed infants have a lower mortality rate than formula-fed infants
(D) Breastfed infants receive immunoglobulin (Ig)A through breast milk
(E) Breastfed infants receive adequate vitamin D

The answer is D: Breastfed infants receive immunoglobulin (Ig)A through breast milk. The immunologic protective effects of breast milk are well documented. Breast milk contains bacterial and viral antibodies including the transfer of IgA. IgA binds to the intestinal mucosa and prevents microorganisms from attaching. This helps to decrease the prevalence of serious bacterial infections such as those causing diarrhea, otitis media, and pneumonia in exclusively breastfed babies during the first year of life. Additionally, human milk contains macrophages that produce complement, lysozymes, and lactoferrin that bind a high percentage of iron. This prevents the overgrowth of *Escherichia coli* and other harmful bacteria in the intestine. **(A)** Infants fed with breast milk have a lower stool pH that promotes establishment of healthy intestinal flora including lactobacilli and bifidobacteria.

(C) Breastfeeding, while associated with lower rates of morbidity as described above, has little overall effect on mortality for infants receiving adequate care. **(B)** There is no difference in the rate of weight gain in breastfed infants once mothers have established adequate milk supply. The average weight gain for an infant, breastfed or formula-fed, is 20 to 30 g/d within the first several weeks, although breastfed infants may initially have a slower weight gain until adequate milk supply develops.

(E) A healthy mother eating a well-balanced diet can produce milk that provides most of the essential nutrients her infant needs, but breast milk does not contain sufficient amounts of fluoride or vitamins D and K.

28 A 14-year-old boy presents to his pediatrician with complaints of chronic cough. He complains of nasal congestion, runny nose, and frequent sneezing. His family has a cat. His physical examination reveals a distinct nasal crease with boggy nasal mucosa.

Of the following, which is the most appropriate initial management for this patient?

(A) Daily antihistamine therapy
(B) Prescription for epinephrine autoinjector
(C) Avoidance of allergen
(D) Trial of albuterol therapy
(E) Intranasal corticosteroids

The answer is C: Avoidance of allergen. The boy in the vignette has symptoms consistent with allergic rhinitis (AR). AR is an IgE-mediated inflammation of the nasal mucosa. Symptoms can either be intermittent or persistent. Intermittent AR is usually seasonally based and persistent AR is year round. Seasonal symptoms are frequently associated with outdoor allergens, including pollen, ragweed, grasses, and trees. Accordingly, persistent symptoms are usually due to indoor allergens including animal dander, dust mites, and mold.

Treatment for AR begins with avoidance of the allergen. In persistent AR due to animal dander, it may be necessary to get rid of the pet. Similarly, avoiding outdoor exposure as much as possible during ragweed season also would be advised. **(E)** The most appropriate next therapy option for the patient in the vignette is treatment with intranasal corticosteroids, such as fluticasone, beclomethasone, and mometasone. **(A)** Oral antihistamines, such as loratadine and diphenhydramine, are appropriate adjunctive therapy. **(B)** Epinephrine autoinjectors should be prescribed for patients with concern of anaphylaxis. AR symptoms alone do not lead to anaphylaxis. **(D)** Prophylactic use of albuterol therapy for AR is not indicated without a diagnosis of asthma.

29 A 14-year-old boy presents with progressive debilitating unbalanced gait, making ambulation extremely difficult. He is noted to have a proliferation of blood vessels on his skin and eyes, and his past medical history reveals frequent antibiotic use for recurrent sinus infections.

Of the following, which is the inheritance pattern for this patient's most likely diagnosis?

(A) X-linked recessive
(B) X-linked dominant
(C) Autosomal recessive
(D) Autosomal dominant
(E) Mitochondrial

The answer is C: Autosomal recessive. The boy described in the vignette has ataxia-telangiectasia. Ataxia-telangiectasia is a syndrome composed of immunologic, neurologic, and cutaneous manifestations and **(A, B, D, E)** is inherited in an autosomal recessive pattern. A mutation in the ataxia-telangiectasia gene on chromosome 11 leads to defective DNA repair. Consequently, patients develop decreased proliferative response of T and B cells to antigenic stimulation leading to both T- and B-cell deficits.

Clinically, patients with ataxia-telangiectasia present with progressive ataxia beginning as young as their first steps and eventually leading to incapacitation and wheelchair dependence. In addition, ocular and skin telangiectasias are seen as early as 3 years of age. Neurologically, patients often have cognitive difficulties leading to varying degrees of intellectual disability. The majority of patients with ataxia-telangiectasia also develop chronic sinopulmonary infections secondary to B-cell deficits. There is an increased risk of leukemia and lymphoma. Diagnosis is made through detection of the genetic mutation and supported by low immunoglobulin (Ig)A and IgE levels with normal levels of IgM. IgG may be low or normal. Treatment is largely supportive with infusions of intravenous IG pending severity of immunodeficiency and avoidance of live vaccines.

30 A 3-year-old boy with known hemoglobin SS sickle cell disease presents to the emergency department with 1 day of fever to 104°F, lethargy, and abdominal pain. He quickly deteriorates with a blood pressure of 70/30 mmHg, capillary refill in his lower extremities of 4 seconds, and a white blood cell count of $30 \times 10^3/\mu L$. On further history, his mother states that he does take a medication daily, but he ran out a month ago and she has not had a chance to refill it.

Of the following, what is the most likely organism to grow from his blood culture?

(A) *Aspergillus fumigatus*
(B) *Candida albicans*
(C) *Streptococcus pneumoniae*
(D) *Escherichia coli*
(E) *Listeria monocytogenes*

The answer is C: *Streptococcus pneumoniae*. Children with sickle cell anemia have known immunologic dysfunction. Occasionally, as young as 6 months but almost universally by 5 years old, patients have functional asplenia. Functional asplenia implies patients have a spleen but its reticuloendothelial function is limited or absent. In healthy individuals, the spleen works to filter and trap bacteria, particularly encapsulated bacteria such as *S. pneumoniae*, *Haemophilus influenza* type B (Hib), and *Neisseria meningitidis*.

Due to the inability to filter out encapsulated bacteria, children with sickle cell anemia are at increased risk for bacterial sepsis, leading to significant increases in morbidity and mortality. Patients with sickle cell anemia should receive prophylaxis with penicillin V potassium. Additionally patients should receive routine childhood immunizations, including those against *S. pneumoniae*, Hib, and *N. meningitidis*.

(A, B, D, E) Of the choices listed, a sickle cell anemia patient is most at risk for bacteremia from *S. pneumoniae* rather than aspergillosis, candidiasis, *E. coli*, or *Listeria*.

CHAPTER 13

Gastroenterology

TARA ALTEPETER

1 A 2-year-old girl is brought to the emergency department by her frantic mother. She reports that she had stepped out of her house to retrieve the mail, and when she returned, she found her daughter sitting on the bathroom floor with an open bottle of drain cleaner. The product had spilled on the floor and was on the child's hands and face. She is not sure if the child ingested it.

Of the following, what is the mechanism of potential damage caused by ingestion of drain cleaner?

(A) Direct burn from the chemical
(B) Inhalation damage to the lungs
(C) Dermatitis from direct contact
(D) Liquefaction necrosis
(E) Coagulation necrosis

The answer is D: Liquefaction necrosis. Accidental poisoning with household cleaning products remains an important cause of morbidity and mortality in young children. It is most likely to occur in children between the ages of 1 and 6 years. A detailed history regarding potential exposures is of utmost importance. Acidic agents constitute a minority of household ingestions as these agents are sour or bitter and a child is likely to spit out at the first taste. **(E)** If ingested, acidic agents cause coagulation necrosis on contact with mucosal surfaces. Often a thick eschar forms, which prevents further tissue damage. In contrast, alkaline products, such as toilet and drain cleaners, are tasteless, allowing children to ingest a significant quantity. **(D)** Alkaline products cause deep liquefaction necrosis, which can be full thickness and may result in severe damage, esophageal perforation, and eventual stricture formation. Symptoms of caustic ingestions may include oropharyngeal burns, drooling, dysphagia, inability to swallow saliva, refusal to drink, vomiting, crying, coughing, and stridor. It is important to note that a significant esophageal injury can exist in the absence of visible oropharyngeal burns. Any symptomatic child with the history of a possible ingestion should be considered for upper endoscopy within 6 to 24 hours to assess the esophageal integrity.

(B) The mechanism of action for hydrocarbon (such as lamp oils) ingestion may include damage to the lungs and pulmonary system. **(A, C)** Skin and mucosa dermatitis is generally minor with alkaline products, such as drain cleaner, although these products should always be handled with care.

A 12-year-old boy is brought to the emergency department with complaints of the acute onset of abdominal pain and vomiting. He describes the pain as sharp and located in his mid-upper abdomen which spreads to the middle of his back. He has had multiple episodes of non-bilious vomiting today. His physical examination is unremarkable except for a mild purple discoloration around his umbilicus. His initial evaluation included a complete blood cell count which was notable for a mildly elevated white blood cell count, basic metabolic profile which included a serum glucose of 97 mg/dL, and evidence of mild dehydration.

Of the following tests, which would best aid in making the diagnosis for this patient?

(A) *Helicobacter pylori* stool test
(B) Liver function tests
(C) Amylase and lipase
(D) Blood culture
(E) Stool culture for bacteria

The answer is C: Amylase and lipase. Acute onset vomiting has a broad differential diagnosis. While viral gastroenteritis is the most common etiology of pediatric vomiting, it is typically accompanied by diarrhea. When vomiting is an isolated symptom, it should prompt further evaluation. Other causes to consider include pancreatitis, diabetic ketoacidosis, pneumonia, increased intracranial pressure, and urinary tract infection.

Pancreatitis in children is caused by viral infection, drug reaction, gallstones, cystic fibrosis, and inheritable or autoimmune pathology. As described in the vignette, patients with pancreatitis present with emesis and abdominal pain, often radiating to the back. **(C)** Diagnosis is made with elevated amylase and lipase levels. Physical examination findings can include a discoloration around the umbilicus, called the Cullen sign, or bruising to the flank areas, otherwise known as the Grey Turner sign (see *Figure 13-1*). Both of these rare findings are consistent with more severe, necrotic cases, or suggest retroperitoneal involvement of pancreatitis. Treatment of pancreatitis in children is mostly supportive. Aggressive intravenous hydration, bowel rest, and pain control constitute the pillars of treatment. Evaluation for genetic causes is generally not recommended for the first episode of pancreatitis.

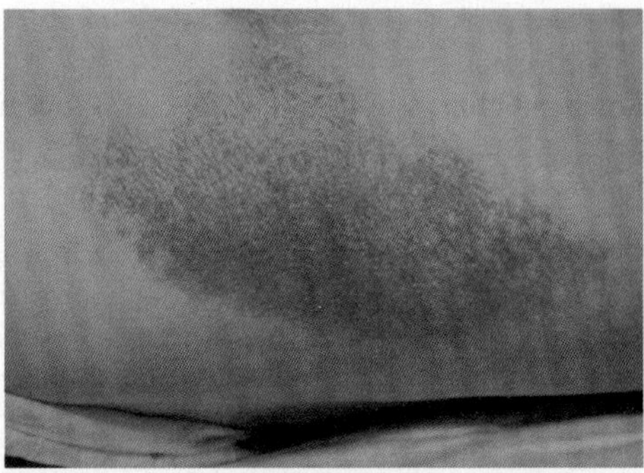

Figure 13-1

(A) Peptic ulcer disease (PUD) generally presents with a more subacute presentation than that described in the vignette. Patients would be expected to have epigastric pain, vomiting, and weight loss. Diagnosis of PUD can be made with evidence of *H. pylori* in the stool. **(B)** Liver function tests would be beneficial with regard to evaluation for possible hepatitis; however, some degree of jaundice on examination would be expected. The description of pain radiating to the back is not consistent with hepatitis. **(D, E)** Blood and stool cultures are less likely to be of assistance in diagnosis for the patient in the vignette who does not present with any signs of enteral infection.

---

3 A 6-year-old girl is brought to the emergency department with complaints of abdominal pain and rash. The abdominal pain has been ongoing for about 1 week. The family initially attributed her pain to a viral infection, but today she developed a purplish raised rash on her legs and buttocks (see *Figure 13-2*), which prompted her visit to the emergency department.

Of the following, which is the most worrisome complication related to her pain that could develop overnight for this patient?

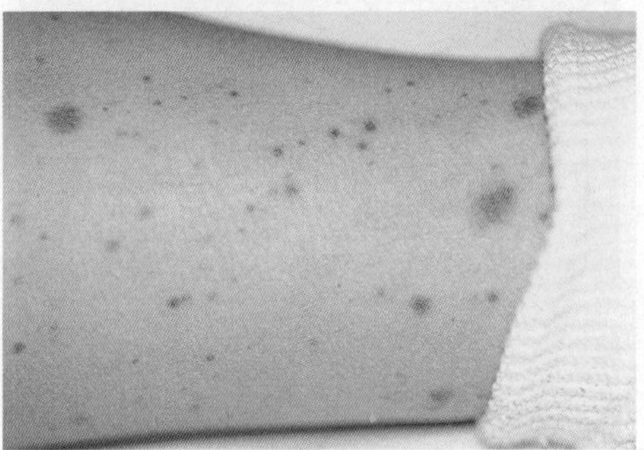

Figure 13-2

(A) Ileo-ileal intussusception
(B) Ileo-colic intussusception
(C) Progression of the rash to Stevens-Johnson syndrome
(D) Bacteremia progressing to sepsis
(E) Symptomatic anemia due to hematuria

The answer is A: Ileo-ileal intussusception. Henoch-Schönlein purpura (HSP) is a small-vessel vasculitis and is the most common vasculitic syndrome of childhood. Many common childhood infections have been implicated as an inciting cause. The presentation of HSP includes abdominal pain, joint pain, and a palpable, purpuric rash located on the lower extremities.

The rash in HSP can at first be worrisome, as the differential for purpuric rash includes life-threatening infections such as **(C)** meningococcal disease and Rocky Mountain spotted fever. However, patients with those conditions are generally toxic appearing, and often the rash is not localized only to the lower extremities. **(B)** The rash in HSP does not involve mucosal surfaces as seen in Stevens-Johnson syndrome (see *Figure 13-3*). The abdominal symptomatology associated with HSP can range from mild abdominal pain due to mucosal inflammation, to intussusception, which occurs in a small number of cases. **(A, D)** Of note, the intussusception in HSP is more likely to be ileo-ileal, as opposed to ileo-colic, as seen in typical intussusception.

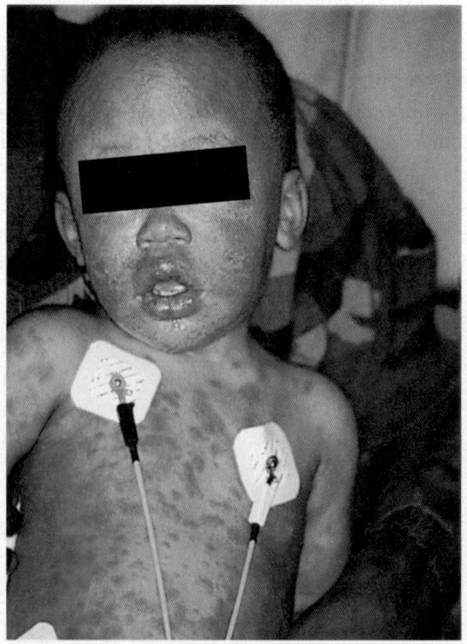

Figure 13-3

Many children will have some degree of renal involvement. The spectrum of renal disease is wide, ranging from asymptomatic hematuria/proteinuria, to frank nephritic disease, and progression to chronic renal disease. **(E)** Symptomatic anemia is not a typical consequence of hematuria. Children are at risk for developing renal disease anytime within 4 months of diagnosis; thus, even those with normal findings at the time of diagnosis require close follow-up with frequent blood pressure and urinalysis screenings.

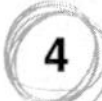
4 An 8-year-old boy is brought to the office with complaints of bleeding while stooling. He was seen for this same complaint about 2 months ago. At that time, he was placed on stool-softening medications for constipation. His mother reports that he is taking the medication every day. He stools daily and denies any hard stools or pain with stooling. However, he has had three more episodes of bleeding. The patient reports a significant amount of bright red blood in the toilet following defecation. He denies any abdominal pain associated with these episodes.

Of the following options, which is the most likely cause of this patient's bleeding?

(A) Juvenile polyps
(B) Familial adenomatous polyposis (FAP) syndrome
(C) Constipation
(D) Intussusception
(E) Peutz-Jeghers syndrome

The answer is A: Juvenile polyps. Intermittent painless bleeding associated with defecation should raise the suspicion for colonic polyps. Juvenile polyps typically present in children aged 2 to 10 years old. The diagnosis is made by colonoscopy. Treatment of a juvenile polyp is removal at the time of colonoscopy.

(B, E) There are several inherited polyposis syndromes, which can also present similarly but are much less likely than juvenile polyps. These include FAP, which is an autosomal dominant condition caused by a mutation in the APC gene. Typically 5 or more polyps are seen at the time of diagnosis and will progress to 100 or more by early adulthood. Patients will ultimately require surgical colectomy, as the risk of colon cancer is extremely high if left untreated. Peutz-Jeghers syndrome is another autosomal dominant polyposis syndrome, which can present with rectal bleeding. Children with Peutz-Jeghers typically have freckling of the lips and gingiva. These patients have polyps that are benign hamartomas. Patients with Peutz-Jeghers syndrome have an increased risk of breast, colon, and gynecologic cancers. **(C)** Constipation is unlikely for the patient in the vignette given his current stooling pattern and medication compliance. **(D)** Intussusception generally presents with intermittent episodes of colicky abdominal pain and eventually bloody stools.

5 The parents of a 3-week-old neonate bring him to the pediatrician and they report that he has been vomiting after each feeding for the past day. He always spits up a little, but they now report that the vomiting is becoming more forceful. It appears white-colored like his formula. They are confused because he appears happy and hungry in between episodes, and actually wants to feed again immediately after vomiting.

Of the following options, which diagnostic test is most useful for diagnosis?

(A) Computed tomography scan of the abdomen
(B) Plain radiograph of the abdomen
(C) Upper gastrointestinal (GI) series with contrast
(D) Abdominal ultrasound
(E) Barium enema

The answer is D: **Abdominal ultrasound.** Hypertrophic pyloric stenosis is a condition that occurs due to hypertrophy of the pylorus muscle. It is more common in Caucasian men and in firstborn children. Presentation is most common between 2 weeks and 2 months of age. Persistent vomiting typically leads to hypochloremic metabolic alkalosis in these infants. The diagnostic test of choice is abdominal ultrasound. Children with pyloric stenosis typically have a pylorus measuring >4 mm in thickness. Treatment of this condition is surgical. A pyloromyotomy is performed in order to relieve the obstruction. It is imperative that electrolyte abnormalities be corrected prior to surgery to reduce the risk of complications from anesthesia.

(A) A computed tomography scan is inappropriate to evaluate the pylorus and exposes the patient to unnecessary radiation. **(B)** Plain abdominal radiography does not visualize the pylorus. **(C)** Though a barium swallow, or upper GI series, may suggest some obstruction, this is not the optimal test of choice as it is not as sensitive as an abdominal ultrasound. **(E)** A barium enema, or lower GI series, is inappropriate to evaluate the pylorus.

6 A 14-year-old boy presents to the emergency department with complaints of maroon-colored stools. His parents report he has been complaining of abdominal pain on and off for the past few days. They did not think much of it until today, when he called them to the bathroom, because he passed a large, maroon-colored stool with streaks of mucous. He has passed three more similar stools in the past 4 hours. On further history he admits that his stools have been black-colored for the past several days. He is complaining of feeling dizzy and lightheaded. Laboratory evaluation is notable for hemoglobin of 7.6 g/dL. A normal saline fluid bolus is initiated.

Of the following, which is the next best step in evaluating the cause of bleeding for this patient?

(A) Nasogastric tube with gastric lavage
(B) Plain radiograph of the abdomen
(C) Emergent colonoscopy
(D) Ultrasound of the abdomen
(E) Meckel scan

The answer is A: **Nasogastric tube with gastric lavage.** There are many causes of gastrointestinal (GI) bleeding. In a child who is having profuse bleeding, it is first imperative to determine if the bleeding is from an upper or lower GI source. A brisk upper GI bleed, such as that from an ulcer or severe gastritis, can cause severe bleeding and rapid transit time, resulting in passage of maroon to bright red blood per rectum. Generally, darker stools are indicative of an upper GI bleed, and bright red stools are indicative of a lower GI bleed. The quickest way to evaluate for an upper GI source of bleeding is to place a nasogastric tube and lavage or wash out the stomach to evaluate for the presence of blood. The history of ongoing abdominal pain and black stools followed by progression to frank bleeding and anemia is suspicious for a bleeding peptic or duodenal ulcer of the patient in the vignette. Initial care should focus on achieving hemodynamic stability and includes fluid resuscitation or blood transfusions. An urgent upper endoscopy is indicated as soon as the patient is stable for anesthesia. It is important to ask about the chronic use of nonsteroidal anti-inflammatory medications, as these medications may increase the chances of an upper GI bleed secondary to mucosal irritation.

(B) Abdominal radiography is not likely to be helpful for the patient in the vignette to elucidate a cause to the GI bleed. **(C)** While colonoscopy may identify a cause of bleeding, it should not be considered until the patient is stabilized. **(D)** Ultrasound may be helpful in evaluating for conditions such as intussusception, but the age and history of the patient in the vignette are not suggestive of intussusception. **(E)** A Meckel scan can be helpful in searching for the cause of bright red painless bleeding per rectum. However, a Meckel diverticulum is likely to present at a younger age with acute painless bright red blood per rectum as opposed to the progression of symptoms for the patient in the vignette.

A 12-year-old boy is referred to the gastrointestinal (GI) clinic by his pediatrician. The boy has had vague intermittent complaints of abdominal pain for the past year. Recently, he has complained of pain in his knee, although evaluation did not uncover any injury or infectious cause. In the past week, he has experienced loose stools, fecal urgency, and one episode of bloody diarrhea. His complete blood cell count notes a white blood cell count of 8 × 10^3/μL, hemoglobin of 11.5 g/dL, and a platelet count of 615 × 10^3/μL. His erythrocyte sedimentation rate is 56 mm/hour and C-reactive protein is 4 mg/L. Pathologic reports of an esophagogastroduodenoscopy and colonoscopy note chronic, active gastritis in the stomach, lymphocytic infiltration and destruction of crypt architecture in the duodenum, and areas of focal granuloma formation within the ascending colon, with normal biopsies noted in the descending and transverse colon.

Of the following, which is the most likely etiology of this patient's presentation?

(A) Ulcerative colitis (UC)
(B) Infectious colitis
(C) Crohn disease
(D) Systemic-onset juvenile idiopathic arthritis
(E) Celiac disease

The answer is C: Crohn disease. The clinical vignette is consistent with Crohn disease. Crohn disease is a form of inflammatory bowel disease, which can affect any portion of the GI tract, from the mouth to the anus. Presenting symptoms vary, but can include upper GI symptoms such as abdominal pain, nausea, and vomiting, as well as lower GI symptoms such as diarrhea, hematochezia, and fecal urgency. Extraintestinal manifestations vary and can include eye pain or vision changes from uveitis, joint pain and swelling, skin rashes such as pyoderma gangrenosum (see *Figure 13-4*) and erythema nodosum (see *Figure 13-5*), weight loss, decreased height velocity, fatigue, and depression.

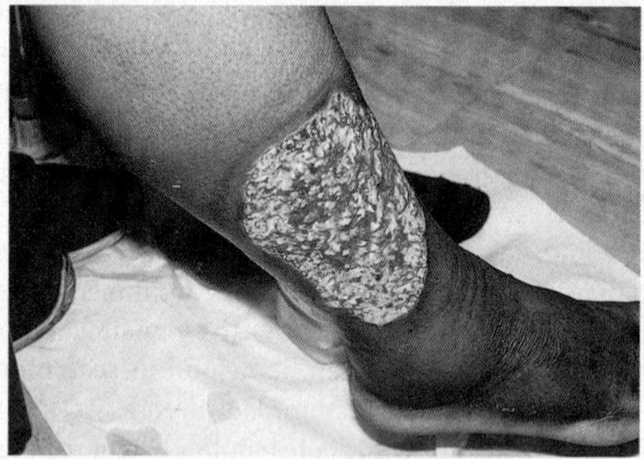

Figure 13-4

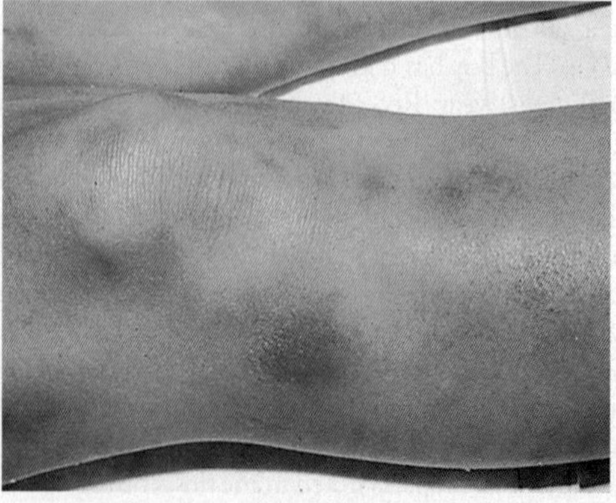

Figure 13-5

Evaluation of a pediatric patient with suspected inflammatory bowel disease should include review of the growth chart, complete blood cell count, inflammatory markers, and an albumin level. Other causes of weight loss and growth failure should be considered, such as celiac disease. Ultimately, both Crohn disease and UC require pathologic examination to confirm a diagnosis, thus endoscopy is required. Granulomas seen on microscopic examination are characteristic of Crohn disease.

(A) UC is characterized by a continuous segment of involvement in the colon. The patchy nature of the disease with areas of normal mucosa in between described in the vignette is more suggestive of Crohn disease. **(B)** Infectious colitis in children is generally characterized by an abrupt onset of severe diarrhea, which may progress to bloody diarrhea. **(D)** Systemic-onset juvenile idiopathic arthritis, otherwise known as Still disease, can also present with joint involvement, fatigue, weight loss, and elevated inflammatory markers; however, diarrhea or blood in the stool would not be expected. **(E)** Celiac disease is a gluten-mediated enteropathy, characterized by destruction of the villi in the duodenum. Normal biopsies from the duodenum exclude this diagnosis.

8 A patient recently had blood work completed for a pre-college physical. He received a letter in the mail stating that his test for hepatitis B surface antibody was positive. The mother is very concerned about how her son could possibly have hepatitis.

Of the following statements, which should be included in the discussion with this mother?

(A) Hepatitis B is a common infection, but if he does not feel sick, there is nothing to worry about
(B) He has chronic hepatitis B infection, which puts him at high risk of liver cancer
(C) Hepatitis B early antigen is a marker for resolved infection
(D) Antibody to hepatitis B surface antigen indicates immunity rather than infection
(E) This test was done erroneously, and should be repeated

The answer is D: Antibody to hepatitis B surface antigen indicates immunity rather than infection. Hepatitis B is a DNA virus that causes infectious hepatitis. It can be transmitted via blood products or sexual contact. In the United States, the most important risk factor for the development of hepatitis B infection is to be born to a mother who is hepatitis B positive. Routine perinatal testing of mothers and vaccination of newborns have dramatically reduced the number of new cases each year in the United States. Many patients are asymptomatic from their primary infection. When symptoms do occur, they typically start around 6 weeks after exposure and may include jaundice, malaise, and anorexia. The majority of patients clear the primary infection, with a small minority becoming chronic carriers. Patients with chronic

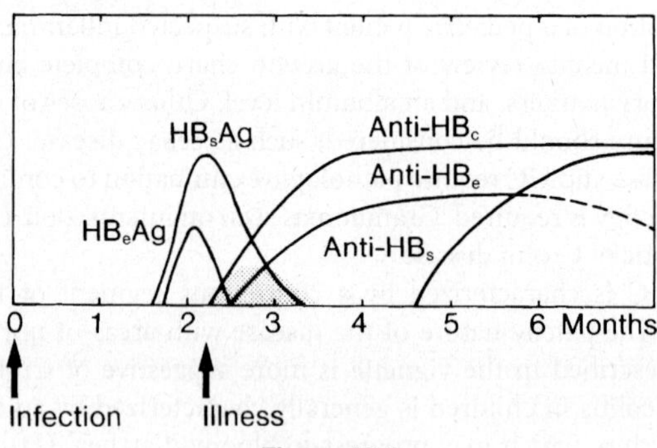

Figure 13-6

hepatitis B are at increased risk for cirrhosis and hepatocellular carcinoma. Blood testing for hepatitis B includes several tests. Hepatitis B surface antigen is the first serologic marker to develop after acute infection (see *Figure 13-6* for the serologic changes in hepatitis B infection). Antibodies to the core antigen (anti-HB_c) develop next. Hepatitis B core antigen immunoglobulinM is a marker for acute infection and may persist for months. Antibody to surface antigen (anti-HB_s) indicates protective immunity. This can develop either after a person has cleared a primary hepatitis B infection, or in response to the hepatitis B vaccine. **(C)** Early antigen (HB_eAg) is a marker of infectivity. Testing for anti-HB_s is commonly used to verify that someone has been appropriately vaccinated. **(A, B)** Presence of this antibody indicates immunity, which is likely the case for the patient in the vignette.

9 A 12-year-old boy is being followed in the outpatient clinic for short stature. His tissue transglutaminase antibodies are found to be elevated. An esophagogastroduodenoscopy confirms his diagnosis. The mother has a lot of questions regarding his diagnosis.

Of the following, which recommendation should be included in discussion with this mother?

(A) Keep epinephrine autoinjector at all times
(B) There is no need for an epinephrine autoinjector
(C) Replace wheat products with those made with rye
(D) Hives will occur with wheat exposure
(E) Occasional wheat intake is permitted

The answer is B: There is no need for an epinephrine autoinjector. Celiac disease is an immune-mediated enteropathy caused by gluten, a specific protein found in wheat, **(C)** rye, and barley. The screening test of choice is a blood test, looking for tissue transglutaminase immunoglobulin (Ig)A antibody. It is important to check the total IgA level at the same time, as patients with selective IgA deficiency cannot be reliably screened this way. The gold standard for diagnosis of celiac disease is tissue biopsy. Under the microscope, duodenal biopsies demonstrate blunting of the villi, and chronic lymphocytic infiltration. **(E)** Treatment for celiac disease entails strict avoidance of all gluten-containing products. Even small amounts of gluten can cause continued inflammation and may not allow the mucosa to heal. Celiac disease is a T-cell–mediated phenomenon triggered by a response to gluten peptides in a genetically susceptible individual. Although celiac disease is a reaction to wheat, it is not mediated by IgE hypersensitivity. **(A, D)** Accordingly, patients with celiac disease do not develop hives or anaphylaxis with exposure to wheat.

10 The mother of a 5-week-old baby calls the office at 5:00 p.m. to report that her infant is becoming more "yellow." She was told at the 1-week checkup that this problem should get better with time, but she feels it is worsening. The infant has been eating well, is formula-fed, and stools daily. The mother is instructed to report to the emergency department for further evaluation. Laboratory tests in the emergency department are notable for a total bilirubin of 15 mg/dL, with a direct component of 13.6 mg/dL. On examination, the infant appears well hydrated and nontoxic with jaundice and scleral icterus.

Of the following, which is the most appropriate next step in the diagnostic evaluation of this patient?

(A) Change to soy formula
(B) Discontinue oral feedings and start intravenous fluid therapy
(C) Inpatient abdominal ultrasound and cholescintigraphy scan
(D) Refer for urgent liver transplantation
(E) Reassure the mother that jaundice is a benign finding at this age

Answer C: Inpatient abdominal ultrasound and cholescintigraphy scan. The differential diagnosis for conjugated, or direct, hyperbilirubinemia in the neonate is vast. *Table 13-1* shows a few basic categories of the etiology of direct hyperbilirubinemia.

The table is not all-inclusive, but covers some of the more common causes of conjugated hyperbilirubinemia.

Biliary atresia is secondary to embryonal or neonatal destruction of the extrahepatic biliary duct system. Clinical symptoms of biliary atresia include prolonged jaundice with direct hyperbilirubinemia and acholic stools. Evaluation of neonates with prolonged conjugated hyperbilirubinemia should include an abdominal ultrasound, looking for obstructive processes such as choledochal cysts and the presence or absence of the gallbladder. **(C)** The next best step in the diagnosis of the patient in the vignette would be to obtain a nuclear medicine cholescintigraphy scan, to evaluate the uptake of dye by the liver, and its excretion through the biliary system. A patient with biliary atresia has normal hepatic uptake of the tracer molecule, but fails to excrete

Table 13-1 Several common causes of direct hyperbilirubinemia in the neonatal period

Systemic Illness/ Metabolic	Hepatic Outflow Obstruction	Intrahepatic Cholestasis
Galactosemia	Biliary atresia	α1-Antitrypsin deficiency
Hypothyroidism	Choledochal cyst	Transport defects
Sepsis	Neonatal sclerosis cholangitis	Cystic fibrosis
Hypopituitarism		Defects in bile acid synthesis

it into the intestine. Ultimately, all patients with suspected biliary atresia require laparotomy with an intraoperative cholangiogram, and a portohepatoenterostomy procedure when indicated. The success of the portohepatoenterostomy procedure is dramatically improved when performed prior to 60 days of life, thus, diagnosing biliary atresia is time-sensitive. The goal of the procedure is to provide an alternate drainage pathway for bile to be excreted from the liver and reach the intestine, minimizing the hepatotoxic effects of retained bile, and allowing the patient to grow. **(D)** Patients with biliary atresia will eventually require a liver transplant. However, this is generally not completed urgently as an improved nutritive state and growth assist in better tolerance of the overall transplant procedure.

(E) Direct hyperbilirubinemia is never a normal finding, and always warrants further evaluation.

(A) Changing to soy formula would be an appropriate next step for a patient with galactosemia, but as the patient in the vignette is nontoxic and feeding well, evaluating for biliary atresia is the more pressing concern. **(B)** Bowel rest would not assist in making a diagnosis for the patient in the vignette.

11 A 3-year-old girl is referred to the gastrointestinal (GI) clinic for complaints of chronic diarrhea. She has four to five loose stools each day, which occasionally contain pieces of undigested food. There is no blood or mucous in the stool. She is growing well and denies abdominal pain, nausea, or other complaints. Her diet consists of a variety of table foods. Her mother reports that the girl does not like milk and drinks mostly apple juice instead. Her pediatrician has sent two sets of stool cultures for bacteria, viruses, and parasites, which have yielded negative results.

Of the following, which is the most appropriate next step in the management of this patient?

(A) Schedule a colonoscopy and endoscopy to look for underlying inflammation
(B) Prescribe a course of antibiotics for empiric treatment of bacterial overgrowth syndrome
(C) Instruct the mother to limit fruit juice to 4 oz or less per day
(D) Order testing for *Clostridium difficile* infection
(E) Reassure the mother that 4 to 5 stools per day is normal for some children

The answer is C: **Instruct the mother to limit fruit juice to 4 oz or less per day.** The patient in the vignette has symptoms consistent with toddler's diarrhea, an osmotic diarrhea caused by excessive intake of fruit juices. The child will have multiple watery stools per day, and the parents often describe that there are chunks of undigested food in the stools. Toddler's diarrhea occurs in an otherwise healthy child, who is growing and gaining weight normally. There is no blood or inflammatory cells in the stool and this condition can be resolved by changes in the diet. The treatment involves removing fruit juice from the diet and increasing the fat and fiber content.

(A) Esophagogastroduodenoscopy and colonoscopy are invasive procedures requiring the child to undergo anesthesia. Although these tests are invaluable in the evaluation of some serious conditions such as inflammatory bowel disease and celiac disease, this procedure is not indicated in an otherwise healthy child with isolated diarrhea. **(B)** Bacterial overgrowth can cause malabsorptive diarrhea. However, the patient in the vignette does not have any risk factors, such as a chronic condition or prematurity. *C. difficile* is becoming an increasingly important cause of disease in childhood. **(D)** *C. difficile* infection typically causes bloody, foul-smelling diarrhea and is often associated with other symptoms such as fever, abdominal pain, and cramping. **(E)** Normal stooling patterns can vary greatly from one child to the next with stooling every other day to two to three times per day as normal.

A 4-year-old girl presents to the emergency department with jaundice and fever. The parents report that she was previously healthy, and developed a fever 3 days ago. She has been complaining of abdominal pain and has had a decreased appetite. Today the parents noticed that she appears yellow, and brought her in for further evaluation. Her laboratory results demonstrate an aspartate aminotransferase of 700 IU/L and an alanine aminotransferase of 986 IU/L. Her bilirubin is 2.8 mg/dL, with a direct component of 1.2 mg/dL.

Of the following tests, which would most aid in establishing a cause of this patient's condition?

(A) Blood tests for common viral pathogens
(B) Plain abdominal radiography
(C) Magnetic resonance imaging of the abdomen
(D) Amylase and lipase
(E) Renal ultrasound

The answer is A: **Blood tests for common viral pathogens.** Acute hepatitis can be from many different causes. Viruses such as hepatitis A, B, and C, as well as Epstein-Barr virus, cytomegalovirus, and adenovirus could be responsible for causing an acute hepatitis. There are many other noninfectious causes of hepatitis including autoimmune hepatitis, metabolic disease of the liver, inherited disease such as α1-antitrypsin deficiency, and hemochromatosis. A complete workup should be initiated including an ultrasound of the abdomen to asses for tumors and hepatic echotexture. It is also important to check γ-glutamyl transpeptidase levels to assess for damage to the biliary tree, which can be seen in diseases such as primary sclerosing cholangitis.

(B) Plain abdominal radiography is not helpful in evaluating the cause of acute hepatitis. **(C)** Magnetic resonance imaging of the abdomen is nonspecific and should not be the next step in establishing a likely cause. **(D)** Screening for pancreatic enzymes is not unreasonable, although there is generally the presence of significant vomiting and pain in patients with pancreatitis. Gallstone pancreatitis could cause mildly increased liver enzymes, but not typically to this level. **(E)** A renal ultrasound would be helpful in establishing a diagnosis of renal origin, such as a pyelonephritis, or hydronephrosis, neither of which is expected to cause jaundice.

13 A 2-year-old child is brought to the emergency department by his father. He reports that while changing his son's diaper, he found it full of maroon blood. His son did not seem to be in acute pain or distress. He is now sitting in the examination room, smiling and playing. He is afebrile, with a heart rate of 90 beats/min, respiratory rate of 20 breaths/min, and blood pressure of 90/50 mmHg. His abdomen is soft, non-tender, non-distended, without any palpable masses. There are no fissures detected in the perirectal area. A complete blood count is obtained and is within normal limits.

Of the following, what is the next best step in the evaluation of this patient?

(A) Nuclear medicine technetium-99m scan
(B) Plain radiograph of the abdomen
(C) Colonoscopy
(D) Barium enema
(E) Upper gastrointestinal (GI) series

The answer is A: Nuclear medicine technetium-99m scan. Painless significant bleeding per rectum in a toddler should raise suspicion for a Meckel diverticulum. A Meckel diverticulum is an outpouching of the ileum, which may contain ectopic gastric mucosa. If present, the ectopic acid-secreting mucosa will cause damage to the surrounding tissue and bleeding that is typically painless, brisk, and described as maroon. A Meckel diverticulum can also act as a lead point for intussusception. The diagnostic test of choice is a technetium scan. The technetium is absorbed by gastric mucosal cells, but not ileal cells. Treatment of a patient with a symptomatic Meckel diverticulum is surgical resection.

(B) Plain abdominal radiography is typically not helpful in the evaluation of lower GI bleeding, especially if there is a concern for a Meckel diverticulum. **(C)** A colonoscopy should be reserved for a child with a negative technetium scan who continues to have significant bleeding. **(D)** A barium enema frequently misses a Meckel diverticulum, based on location. **(E)** An upper GI series is helpful for evaluating for malrotation, but not for a Meckel diverticulum.

14 A 2-month-old infant is brought to the emergency department with inconsolable crying. His mother reports that he was in his normal state of health until a few hours ago. She was changing his diaper and noticed a bulge in his groin. The bulge did not seem to bother him at first, but with the next diaper change he was crying more, and she believes that the bulge is tender. He had one episode of non-bloody, non-bilious emesis. On examination, the infant is crying vigorously. His genitourinary examination is notable for a soft bulge in the right groin that is purplish-blue in color and does appear to be tender. Gentle but firm pressure does not appear to reduce the bulge.

Of the following, which is the most appropriate next step in the management of this patient?

(A) Obtain an ultrasound of the area with Doppler evaluation
(B) Schedule elective repair once the child is 12 months old
(C) Immediate call to a pediatric surgeon
(D) Perform a needle aspiration of the mass
(E) Reassure the family that most hernias resolve on their own

The answer is C: Immediate call to a pediatric surgeon. The clinical presentation of the patient in the vignette is consistent with an incarcerated inguinal hernia. This is a surgical emergency. Within hours, a tightly strangulated hernia can become ischemic and result in bowel infarction. **(A)** An ultrasound can help differentiate between a hydrocele, hernia, or testicular torsion if the presentation is unclear; however, the description in the vignette is clear and sufficient to make the diagnosis without imaging. **(B)** Once an inguinal hernia is identified in a young infant, surgical repair should be scheduled promptly. An easily reducible hernia may be repaired electively, but should be completed by 1-year age, because of the risk of incarceration. The incidence of incarceration is greatest in infants less than 6 months age. **(E)** Repair of the hernia in the vignette should not be delayed as it is currently incarcerated. The hernia usually contains a bowel loop. **(D)** It is not an abscess or fluid collection; thus, needle drainage is not appropriate.

---

15 A 5-year-old boy is brought to the emergency department with complaints of fever, anorexia, and right lower quadrant abdominal pain over the past 12 hours. His parents state that he complained of pain around his belly button yesterday.

Of the following, what is the most likely cause of this patient's complaints?

(A) Food poisoning
(B) Genetic predisposition
(C) Fecalith
(D) Viral infection
(E) Incomplete rotation of the foregut during embryogenesis

The answer is C: Fecalith. The history in the vignette is most consistent with a diagnosis of acute appendicitis. The pathophysiology of appendicitis is well described. The inciting event is generally obstruction of the tubular appendix with a fecalith. The obstructed appendix results in increased pressure and eventually reaches a point where the blood supply to the wall of the appendix is affected. The appendix can become necrotic, and if not removed promptly, perforation and intra-abdominal infection can occur. Acute appendicitis is considered a surgical emergency. Appropriate treatment involves surgical appendectomy as soon as possible. Antibiotic therapy may be given as adjunctive therapy or for treatment of a perforation. **(B)** Appendicitis is not contagious and there is no genetic predisposition.

(A, D) The history and pattern of symptoms described in the vignette is inconsistent with either bacterial or viral enteral infections. **(E)** Problems with gut rotation during embryogenesis may result in malrotation, which presents with bilious emesis, most commonly in the first month of life.

---

16 A 5-year-old girl is brought to the emergency department with abdominal distention, vomiting, and pain. Plain abdominal radiography demonstrates a large number of small, radiopaque densities in the stomach. On further discussion with the mother, she reports she was recently diagnosed with anemia and did have a bottle of iron tablets on her dresser. She is not sure if her child had access to them.

Of the following, what is the next best step in the management of this patient?

(A) Placement of a nasogastric tube and initiation of whole bowel irrigation
(B) Administration of syrup of ipecac to induce vomiting
(C) Initiate chelation therapy
(D) Admit for observation with serial abdominal radiographs
(E) Observe for 6 hours and discharge home if stable

The answer is A: Placement of a nasogastric tube and initiation of whole bowel irrigation. Iron is one of the leading causes of poisoning-related death in the United States. Iron overdose causes gastrointestinal toxicity and can lead to bleeding and bowel perforation. Systemic absorption leads to hypotension and shock. Liver damage can result, resulting in hepatic necrosis and coagulopathy. Direct central nervous system effects include lethargy and eventual progression to coma. Emergent management of iron ingestion should begin with attempts to remove the remaining tablets visible on radiography as soon as possible to prevent further iron absorption. This should be attempted by whole bowel irrigation. **(A)** Syrup of ipecac is never recommended secondary to a risk of aspiration. Activated charcoal is not useful in iron overdose. **(C)** A serum iron level should be obtained, and the child should be considered for chelation therapy with deferoxamine, depending on the level and clinical symptomatology. **(D, E)** Observation alone is not adequate treatment in a situation with a high index of suspicion for iron overdose.

17 A 9-month-old infant was recently hospitalized for dehydration secondary to a rotavirus diarrheal illness. He was discharged home once rehydrated and demonstrating adequate oral intake. However, 1 day after discharge, the mother reports that since he started drinking normal amounts of his formula, she is seeing a dramatic increase in the amount of diarrhea. He had five loose stools today and she is worried that he is going to end up back in the hospital. A temporary switch to a soy-based formula is suggested.

Of the following, which is the underlying mechanism for this patient's current diarrhea?

(A) Recurrence of his infectious diarrhea
(B) Hospital-acquired infection from *Clostridium difficile*
(C) Allergy to milk-based formula
(D) Transient lactase deficiency
(E) Inadequate bowel rest duration

The answer is D: Transient lactase deficiency. Postinfectious transient lactase deficiency is common among pediatric patients. The inflammation caused by the infection of the gut lumen causes damage to the brush border, and subsequent decreased enzyme production, such as lactase. As the child improves after a diarrheal illness and resumes intake of lactose-containing products, such as milk or formula, malabsorption occurs secondary to a temporary inability to break down the sugars. This will result in watery diarrhea and increased gas. If the symptoms are mild and the child is maintaining adequate hydration, with time, this condition is self-limited and will resolve. If the diarrhea is profuse, a reasonable alternative is to switch to a soy-based formula for a few weeks, as all commercially available soy formulas are lactose free.

True congenital lactase deficiency is extremely rare at infancy.

(B) A secondary infection such as *C. difficile* should be considered, but patients with this infection typically have bloody diarrhea. **(C)** Allergy to milk protein generally presents earlier than 9 months of age, usually within the first 3 months of life. **(E)** There is not an indication for bowel rest in a stable child with uncomplicated viral-induced infectious diarrhea. **(A)** Rather than a recurrence of his infectious diarrhea or infection with a new virus, it is more likely the patient in the vignette has developed a known complication of gastroenteritis.

18 A 4-year-old girl is brought to the office with complaints of high fever, cough, congestion, and fatigue. Her rapid influenza test is positive.

Of the following statements, which is accurate while providing anticipatory guidance to this family?

(A) Antiviral treatment is not prescribed to children less than 7 years old
(B) Antibiotics will prevent development of secondary pneumonia
(C) Urinary tract infection is a common coinfection
(D) She will not need an influenza vaccine next year
(E) Symptomatic treatment of her fever with acetaminophen is appropriate, but aspirin should be avoided

The answer is E: Symptomatic treatment of her fever with acetaminophen is appropriate, but aspirin should be avoided. A feared complication of the use of salicylates is the development of Reye syndrome. Reye syndrome occurs in genetically susceptible individuals and seems to be triggered by a viral illness with concurrent salicylate usage. This combination results in severe liver dysfunction and can progress rapidly to coma and death. Although rare, it is prudent to remind parents not to treat their children with aspirin-based products.

(A) Antiviral treatment is available and useful in certain clinical situations. Patients can be offered antiviral treatment for an influenza infection in certain situations. The medication has the greatest effect when given within 48 hours of symptoms. Children <5 years old, and particularly those <2 years old, are among those at greatest risk for complications and should be given treatment. **(C)** Secondary pneumonia can be associated with influenza. **(B)** Early use of antiviral therapy may reduce the risk of pneumonia. Most pneumonias are due to the influenza virus itself, although secondary bacterial pneumonia can develop as well. **(D)** As the strains of influenza change yearly, the child should still receive the vaccination next year.

19 A 9-year-old boy is brought to the pediatrician's office by his parents because of diarrhea. He first started having loose stools 3 days ago, which were watery and green. This continued until this morning, when he noticed that there was blood in his stool. He is having four to five episodes of diarrhea daily with some cramping abdominal pain. He is afebrile and has been eating and drinking enough to stay adequately hydrated.

Of the following, which test is most likely to help identify the cause of his illness?

(A) Stool test for ova and parasites
(B) Stool test for *Clostridium difficile* toxin
(C) Stool cultures for bacterial pathogens
(D) Stool viral culture
(E) Complete blood cell count

The answer is C: Stool cultures for bacterial pathogens. Bloody diarrhea in a previously healthy child is most commonly secondary to an infectious cause. It is important to obtain stool cultures early in the course of the illness. Many bacterial pathogens can cause bloody diarrhea, including enterohemorrhagic *Escherichia coli*, *Shigella sonnei*, *Salmonella enteritidis*, *Campylobacter jejuni*, and *Yersinia enterocolitica*. Identification of the specific pathogen is important, as treatment varies. It is critically important to identify those who may have disease caused by the *E. coli* O157:H7 strain, as these patients are at risk for developing hemolytic uremic syndrome.

(A) Testing for ova and parasites in those with prolonged diarrhea may be helpful in certain circumstances, particularly if there are other factors in the history that suggest a parasite infection, such as recent camping, swimming in fresh water, and an immunocompromised status. However, most diarrhea caused by parasites is non-bloody. **(B)** Infection caused by *C. difficile* is becoming more prevalent. Exposure to antibiotics in the past 6 months or recent hospitalization are important risk factors. **(E)** A complete blood cell count should be considered for any child with protracted bloody diarrhea. Although this is an important part of the evaluation, it does not help to determine which infectious agent is the cause. **(D)** Viral agents frequently cause diarrheal illnesses. However, most virus-mediated diarrhea is non-bloody. Common viral causes of diarrhea include rotavirus, norovirus, and adenovirus.

20 A 1-hour-old newborn in the nursery is in respiratory distress. He was born full term to a 24-year-old woman without any known risk factors. He did well initially, but he coughed and choked immediately with the initiation of the first feeding. The nurses had difficulty passing a nasogastric tube to suction his oropharynx. The nasogastric tube was reinserted and an urgent plain radiograph of the chest and abdomen was obtained. On review of the film, the nasogastric tube is coiled up within the upper chest.

Of the following, which is the most likely condition consistent with this clinical presentation?

(A) Diaphragmatic hernia
(B) Hyaline membrane disease
(C) Transient tachypnea of the newborn
(D) H-type tracheoesophageal fistula (TEF)
(E) Esophageal atresia with distal TEF

The answer is E: **Esophageal atresia with distal TEF.** The presence of cyanosis, coughing, gagging, and pooling of oral secretions with initiation of feedings is highly suggestive of esophageal atresia, which is generally associated with a distal TEF. **(D)** H-type TEFs are much less common and generally present later with difficulty feeding, coughing, and growth issues. Patients with H-type TEFs have a patent esophagus and are able to ingest milk or formula. Initial management of this condition includes securing the airway, control of oropharyngeal secretions in order to prevent aspiration, and prompt surgical repair. **(A, B, C)** Though diaphragmatic hernia, hyaline membrane disease, transient tachypnea of the newborn, and congenital heart disease all may present with respiratory distress in the newborn, none are associated with coiling of the nasogastric tube in the esophagus, which is only found in cases of esophageal atresia.

21 A 12-month-old infant is brought to the emergency department by his mother. She states that he had several episodes of green-colored vomiting earlier in the day and has become progressively more tired and less interactive. On initial assessment, the patient is a lethargic child and minimally responsive to stimuli. The physical examination is notable for a tense, distended, and tender abdomen, which has hypoactive bowel sounds. A plain abdominal radiograph demonstrates free air in the abdomen. The child is taken to the operating room, where an exploratory laparotomy is performed. The surgeons note a duodenal hematoma as well as perforation.

Of the following, which is the most likely cause of this patient's condition?

(A) Non-accidental blunt trauma
(B) Motor vehicle accident
(C) Falling down a flight of stairs
(D) Intussusception
(E) Henoch-Schönlein purpura (HSP)

The answer is A: **Non-accidental blunt trauma.** A duodenal hematoma is an uncommon finding in pediatric patients, but can be a complication of blunt trauma to the abdomen, such as a handlebar injury or seatbelt injury in an older child. Duodenal hematomas may present as obstruction with bilious vomiting. In an infant, the presence of a duodenal hematoma should raise immediate suspicion and evaluation for possible child abuse. After stabilization, complete evaluation for the patient in the vignette should include a skeletal radiographic survey looking for evidence of other fractures including posterior rib fractures, skull fractures, and extremity fractures, a computed tomography scan of the head to look for evidence of a new or previous intracranial bleed, and a social work evaluation.

Certain fractures increase the suspicion for non-accidental trauma, including posterior rib fractures, multiple fractures in different stages of healing, and bucket handle fractures. Bucket handle fractures are metaphyseal fractures that form an arc along the proximal margin of the metaphysis on radiograph, mimicking a handle. These fractures are caused by excessive torsion. An example of this type of fracture can be seen at the distal end of the tibia pictured in Figure 13-7. A subdural hemorrhage may be seen on head imaging as a result of a shaking injury. This injury occurs when the bridging veins, which extend from the cortex to the dural sinuses, experience shear stress and bleed.

(B) Though a motor vehicle accident could cause a duodenal hematoma, it is not expected for a patient of this age, who should still be placed in a rear-facing car seat. **(C, D, E)** Falls down a flight of stairs, intussusception, and HSP have not been specifically associated with a duodenal hematoma.

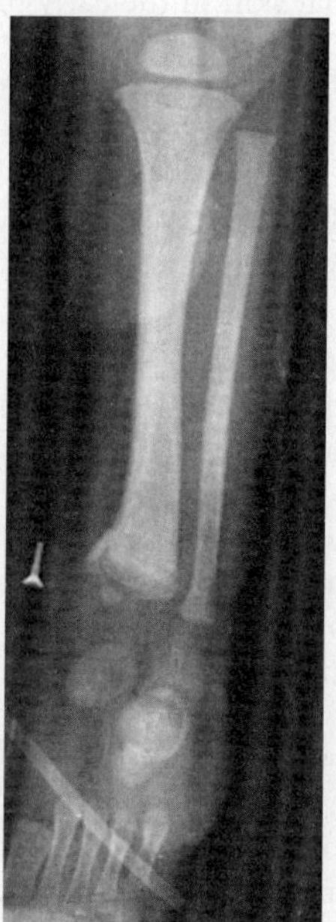

Figure 13-7

22 A mother brings her 6-year-old daughter into the pediatrician's office. The child has been scratching her buttocks to the point of causing excoriations. Her mother notes that the itching seems to be the worst at night and that the child has not been sleeping well. She is worried that her daughter may have a yeast infection. She has been applying diaper rash cream to the area, with no improvement. On examination, the child has normal-appearing external genitalia, and no evidence of candidal infection.

Of the following, which treatment is most appropriate for this patient's likely condition?

(A) Mebendazole
(B) Amoxicillin
(C) Clarithromycin
(D) Topical nystatin
(E) Topical hydrocortisone

The answer is A: Mebendazole. The history and physical examination of the patient in the vignette is most consistent with a diagnosis of pinworms, or *Enterobius vermicularis*. This helminth causes perianal itching, especially at night because of migration of the parasite to the perianal area. The best way to diagnose this condition is to have the parent place a piece of cellophane tape on the perianal skin in the early morning, and then examine the specimen microscopically. The presence of ova is strongly suggestive of pinworm infection. Treatment is with an antihelminthic drug, such as mebendazole. The whole family should be treated as well, as pinworms are easily spread.

(B, C, D, E) Amoxicillin, clarithromycin, nystatin, and hydrocortisone therapies do not eradicate pinworms.

23 A new mother brings her daughter in for the 2-month health maintenance visit. She reports that her baby cries all the time and that she does not know what to do. Her relatives do not enjoy helping out because the child is always fussy. She has tried all the techniques she was taught in the nursery, such as swaddling or swaying, with little to no relief. She has an appropriate affect, states that she loves her baby, but fears that she is a failure as a mother or that there is something seriously wrong with her baby. The mother reports the baby has six wet diapers per day, stools daily, and tolerates breast and bottle feeds well. Her vital signs are temperature 37.5°C, heart rate 130 beats/min, respiratory rate 38 breaths/min, and blood pressure 70/50 mmHg. Pulse oximetry is noted to be 100% on room air. On examination, the baby appears well cared for, is thriving, and there are no abnormalities appreciated.

Of the following, which is the most likely diagnosis for this clinical scenario?

(A) Colic
(B) Milk protein allergy
(C) Cardiac anomaly
(D) Postpartum depression
(E) Child abuse

The answer is A: Colic. Colic is diagnosed in infants who seem to cry and experience more pain than the average infant. An infant who cries for more than 3 hours each day, more than 3 days/wk, for more than 3 consecutive weeks is generally considered to have colic. Colic is a diagnosis of exclusion, and it is important for the pediatrician to rule out other common causes of crying, such as an anal fissure, hair tourniquet, supraventricular tachycardia, corneal abrasion, constipation, gastroesophageal reflux disease, and sepsis. An infant with colic generally feeds adequately, gains weight appropriately, and lacks other evidence of organic disease. Colic usually begins around 3 weeks of age, and the crying peaks around 6 weeks of age. The condition improves with time, and many infants show resolution around 12 weeks, and almost all by 16 weeks. It is crucial to provide reassurance and support to parents of an infant with colic. They may feel overwhelmed or as though they are failing as parents. **(D)** Mothers should be carefully screened for postpartum depression and provided with appropriate support and resources. The mother in the vignette is unlikely to be depressed as she has an appropriate affect and a genuine concern for her child.

(B) The patient in the vignette has no signs to suggest milk protein allergy such as diarrhea, mucous or blood in stool, or poor weight gain. **(E)** Infants with colic are at increased risk for non-accidental trauma and it is important to discuss with parents about their support system including a plan to implement when they feel overwhelmed. However, the patient in the vignette appears well cared for without any signs of trauma or abuse. **(C)** A cardiac anomaly is unlikely given a normal blood pressure, heart rate, and pulse oximetry, and physical examination.

24 A worried mother brings her 1-year-old child to the office for a health supervision visit. She has been reading online regarding the recommended vaccinations for this visit, and although she understands the importance of the measles/mumps/rubella and varicella vaccines, she is questioning the need for the hepatitis A vaccine. She reports her family lives in a nice suburb, is not planning to take the child to any developing nations, and inquires if this vaccine is needed for her child.

Of the following statements, which is accurate regarding hepatitis A and vaccination?

(A) The vaccine is not recommended as long as the family does not plan to travel to an endemic area
(B) Hepatitis A is rare in the United States compared with other causes of viral hepatitis
(C) Hepatitis A infection is highly contagious and daycares are a common place that children are exposed
(D) Hepatitis A causes a lifelong, chronic hepatitis in those infected
(E) It is safer to administer the hepatitis A vaccine on a separate day from the varicella vaccine to reduce the chances of an adverse reaction

The answer is C: **Hepatitis A infection is highly contagious and daycares are a common place that children are exposed.** **(A, B)** Contrary to popular belief, hepatitis A is a common infection in the United States. The hepatitis A virus is highly contagious and can be spread easily among children in a daycare or school setting via the fecal–oral route. The clinical presentation varies, especially by age. Very young children are likely to have a nonspecific viral syndrome, often with diarrhea and vomiting. Older patients are more likely to have symptomatic acute hepatitis, with abdominal pain, jaundice, vomiting, and malaise that can last for 7 to 14 days. Patients who are older or immunosuppressed are at highest risk for serious complications, which include acute liver failure. **(D)** Hepatitis A virus does not cause chronic hepatitis, in contrast with hepatitis B and hepatitis C. **(E)** Safety is not compromised by administering the hepatitis A vaccine at the same time as other recommended childhood vaccinations.

25 A young mother brings her 4-week-old son to the office for his 1-month health maintenance visit. She reports that he spits up constantly and is worried that he might be allergic to her breast milk. She describes the vomit as appearing like milk. The infant does not cry or fuss with these episodes. The mother notices the vomiting more after feedings. On examination, he is alert, interactive, and well hydrated. He is gaining weight appropriately along the 50th percentile. The remainder of the physical examination is unremarkable.

Of the following, which best describes the mechanism of action for this patient's condition?

(A) Failure of recanalization of the duodenum
(B) Hypersensitivity reaction
(C) Relaxation of the lower esophageal sphincter
(D) Incomplete rotation of the foregut during embryogenesis
(E) Hypertrophy of the gastric outlet

The answer is C: **Relaxation of the lower esophageal sphincter.** The description provided by the mother in the vignette is consistent with infantile gastroesophageal reflux (GER). **(C)** Most infants have GER due to transient relaxations in the lower esophageal sphincter. It is important to take a complete history to determine if the reflux falls into the spectrum of normal physiologic reflux or has characteristics of gastroesophageal reflux disease (GERD). Historical points that would increase the concern for GERD requiring treatment would be posturing or back arching, excessive crying or fussing around feedings, and failure to gain weight. If one or more of these symptoms is present, then a diagnosis of GERD should be considered, and the infant may be a candidate for acid suppression therapy.

(B) Although vomiting may be a sign of milk protein allergy, there would generally be other signs of systemic illness such as diarrhea or poor weight gain. **(E)** Hypertrophic pyloric stenosis is another diagnosis that must be considered in this age group with repetitive non-bilious emesis. Children with pyloric stenosis present with progressive emesis, which becomes forceful or projectile and occurs with every feed. Characteristically, these patients are hungry after an episode of emesis. Untreated, infants with pyloric stenosis eventually develop hypochloremic, hypokalemic metabolic alkalosis. **(D)** Malrotation, or incomplete rotation of the midgut during embryogenesis, is associated with a risk of volvulus and would present with bilious emesis. **(A)** Failure of recanalization of the duodenum, or duodenal atresia, would present with emesis within the first few hours of life and requires neonatal surgical intervention.

---

26 A 24-month-old child is brought to the emergency department with complaints of lethargy. The parents report he appears pale and has been sleepy all day. He has not improved despite acetaminophen therapy at home and has not been interested in eating anything. A plain radiograph of the abdomen is obtained and suggests the likely diagnosis (see *Figure 13-8*).

Of the following, what is the most appropriate next step for this patient?

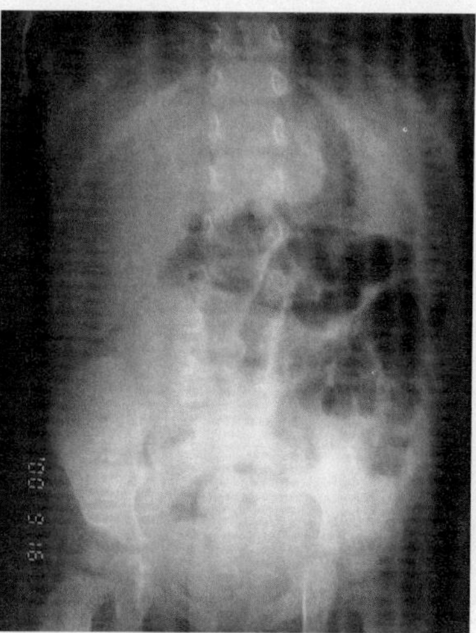

Figure 13-8

(A) Endotracheal intubation
(B) Intravenous antibiotic therapy
(C) Computed tomography of the head
(D) Emergent surgical intervention
(E) Contrast enema

The answer is E: Contrast enema. The clinical scenario and plain abdominal radiograph in the vignette is consistent with intussusception. Intussusception is the most common cause of intestinal obstruction in young children. The majority of cases occurs in children 6 months to 24 months old, but can occur in children up to 6 years of age. The classic triad of symptoms includes episodic severe abdominal pain, a palpable mass in the right upper quadrant, and bloody mucous on rectal examination. Most patients do not present with all three components of the triad; thus, a high index of suspicion is required for diagnosis. Some patients may present with unexplained pallor or lethargy as the only complaint. Evaluation of intussusception is best completed with an abdominal ultrasound. Although abdominal radiography may demonstrate a paucity of gas in the right upper and lower quadrants, an ultrasound is still the more sensitive and specific test. The treatment of choice in most situations is an air or contrast enema. The enema is considered ultimately both diagnostic and therapeutic (see *Figure 13-9*). **(D)** Surgical intervention may be necessary if air or contrast enema therapy is unsuccessful at reduction.

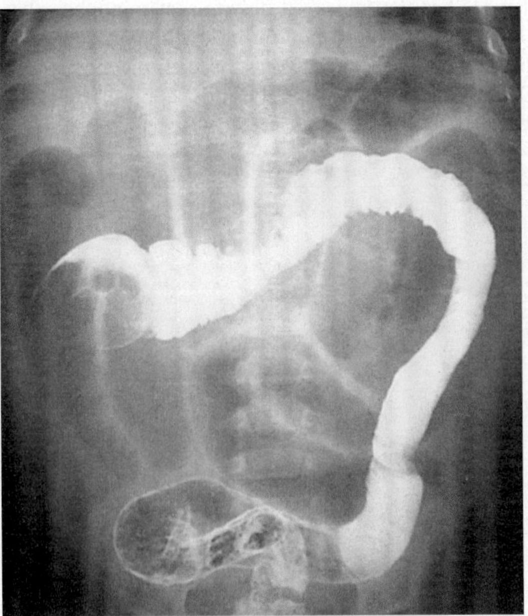

Figure 13-9

(A) Based on the information presented, the patient does not require mechanical ventilation. **(B, C)** Although lethargy may be a presenting sign of sepsis or meningitis, the abdominal radiograph suggests intussusception as the most likely diagnosis.

27 A 4-year-old boy with a past medical history of constipation is brought to the outpatient clinic with complaints of diarrhea. His parents report for the past week he has been having daily accidents. When he comes home from school, they note small marks or larger volumes of loose stool in his underpants. A rectal examination demonstrates mildly lax anal tone with a normal anal wink and palpable soft stool in the vault.

Of the following, which is the best explanation for this patient's condition?

(A) Improper hygiene
(B) Spinal cord mass
(C) Medication side effect
(D) Enteritis
(E) Overflow incontinence

The answer is E: Overflow incontinence. Encopresis refers to fecal incontinence and is frequently associated with chronic constipation in children. Long periods of constipation, or long-standing fecal withholding behaviors, cause the rectum to become stretched, making it more difficult for the child to sense the need to defecate. Additionally, with fecal impaction, the child may have loose stools that leak around the impacted stool. This can easily be misconstrued as diarrhea and cause families to discontinue medications for constipation.

The treatment for chronic constipation with encopresis includes removal of any impaction with a bowel cleanout. This can be accomplished with rectal enemas, manual disimpaction, oral laxatives, and stool softeners. Once the impacted stool is removed, the long-term management focuses on maintaining soft stools and allowing the child to defecate one to two times per day every day. Consistent treatment with a stool softener allows the rectum to eventually regain its normal caliber and tone. It is important to make parents aware that this type of problem often requires months of medical therapy and that consistency at home is crucial.

(A) Although the boy in the vignette may have improper hygiene, it does not explain his incontinence. **(B)** A spinal cord tumor should be considered if a true loss of continence is noted. Physical examination would demonstrate poor rectal tone, lack of an anal wink, and diminished lower deep tendon reflexes. Any neurologic deficit warrants emergent imaging of the spine for possible compressive lesions. **(C)** Excessive use of stool softeners can result in watery stools and stool incontinence. Given the history of the patient in the vignette, overflow incontinence is more likely. **(D)** Acute infectious enteritis as a cause of diarrhea is common in children; however, this is often associated with vomiting, abdominal pain, or fever.

28 A 12-year-old girl was recently discharged from the hospital after a 1-week stay for bacterial pneumonia. She received antibiotic therapy with a third-generation cephalosporin for a total of 10 days. For the past 2 days, she has been experiencing profuse, foul-smelling diarrhea. Today her mother reports she has been to the bathroom 10 times and noted streaks of blood in the stool.

Of the following options, which is the most appropriate initial therapy for this patient?

(A) Oral amoxicillin
(B) Oral vancomycin
(C) Oral ciprofloxacin
(D) Oral metronidazole
(E) Intravenous metronidazole

The answer is D: Oral metronidazole. Given the history and clinical presentation, *Clostridium difficile* infection is the most likely cause of this patient's diarrhea. Although classically considered a hospital-acquired infection, there are now increasing numbers of patients experiencing community-acquired infection as well. Antibiotic treatment within the last 6 months places a patient at increased risk for developing *C. difficile* colitis.

First-line treatment is oral metronidazole for 10 to 14 days. **(B)** Oral vancomycin should be reserved for those who fail or cannot tolerate metronidazole or have recurrent disease. **(E)** The preferred treatment route is oral, and intravenous treatment should be reserved only for those who are unable to tolerate enteral medication. **(A, C)** Ciprofloxacin and amoxicillin are not appropriate choices to treat a *C. difficile* infection.

29 A 7-day-old neonate is brought to the emergency department by his parents. He was born full term to a mother without any known risk factors. He was discharged home at 48 hours of life and was breastfeeding well until this morning when he started vomiting. They describe the vomit as bright green in color. He has vomited many times today with each feeding and now is disinterested in feeding. On examination, the patient is lethargic and difficult to arouse. His vital signs are temperature 36.9°C, heart rate 165 beats/min, respiratory rate 45 breaths/min, and blood pressure 60/30 mmHg. His abdomen is distended and he cries with palpation. He appears poorly perfused with mottled extremities. Blood and urine cultures are obtained and broad-spectrum antibiotic and fluid therapy is initiated.

Of the following, which is the most important next step in the evaluation of this patient?

(A) Computed tomography scan of the head
(B) Lumbar puncture
(C) Urgent surgical consultation
(D) Renal ultrasound
(E) Chest radiography

The answer is C: Urgent surgical consultation. The green emesis described in the vignette is consistent with bile. The abrupt onset of bilious emesis, especially in a young infant, should always raise the possibility of volvulus secondary to malrotation. Malrotation of the midgut occurs early in gestation. The failure of rotation results in the majority of the small bowel being located in the right side of the abdomen, with the colon located to the left. The mesentery is not adequately anchored to the abdominal wall and predisposes the patient to a potential midgut volvulus. The mesentery twists, cutting off blood supply through the superior mesenteric artery, and causes acute obstruction (see *Figure 13-10*).

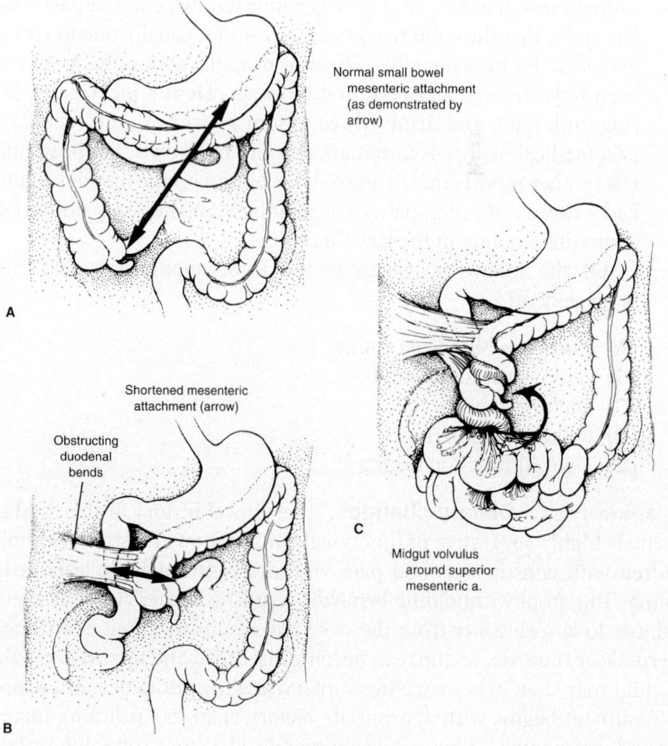

Figure 13-10

Malrotation with midgut volvulus is a surgical emergency as ischemic damage to the bowel can occur within hours. The patient in the vignette is severely ill and in shock. **(C)** Urgent surgical correction of a volvulus is needed to prevent loss of the majority of the small bowel. Malrotation is best diagnosed with an upper gastrointestinal (GI) contrast study.

A full septic evaluation should be considered on a young infant presenting with shock. **(B)** However, it would be reasonable to delay the lumbar puncture for the patient in the vignette, until a surgical evaluation has been completed, and until the patient is fluid resuscitated and hemodynamically stable. **(A)** A computed tomography scan of the head should be considered in a lethargic infant to evaluate for an intracranial bleed; however, the presence of bilious emesis is more suggestive of a GI catastrophe rather than an intracranial process. **(E)** A chest radiograph can be included in the septic evaluation when respiratory symptoms are present, but the most important priority for the patient in the vignette is urgent surgical evaluation. **(D)** A renal ultrasound would not be helpful in this situation.

30 A mother brings her 4-year-old child to the office because he has started soiling himself at school. This has happened twice in the past 3 weeks. She states that the child has small hard stools, usually one to two times per week. He occasionally complains of vague abdominal pain but has been toilet trained since 30 months of age. He is a picky eater, preferring junk food, and drinks three to four glasses of milk each day. His past medical history is unremarkable and his growth has been normal. His mother reports that he passed meconium on the first day of life and had a normal stooling pattern as an infant. She has only noticed problems with stooling in the last 3 months.

Of the following, which is the most appropriate next step in management?

(A) Complete blood cell count
(B) Abdominal ultrasound
(C) Dietary changes
(D) Rectal manometry
(E) Thyroid function testing

The answer is C: Dietary changes. The clinical history of the child in the vignette is highly suggestive of functional constipation and stool withholding. Children with constipation and pain with defecation quickly learn to avoid stooling. This stool withholding behavior results in firmer stools as the colon continues to absorb water from the stool and results in a vicious withholding pattern. Over time, the rectum can become distended and lose its normal tone. The child may then experience involuntary fecal incontinence, or encopresis. **(C)** Treatment begins with appropriate dietary changes, including increasing fiber and water intake. Many children may need a stool-softening or laxative medication as well. A rectal examination is an important portion of the physical examination for a child with constipation. Findings of significant stool in the rectal vault support the diagnosis of stool withholding. The finding of normal rectal tone is reassuring that an underlying spinal cord lesion is not to blame.

The diagnosis of functional constipation can be made with a detailed history and physical examination. It is first important to establish that the child did have a period of normal stooling in infancy and early childhood. A history of significant constipation in infancy is a concern for organic disease such as Hirschsprung disease or allergic enteropathy. **(D)** The diagnosis of Hirschsprung disease is supported by abnormal rectal pressure on manometry. **(A)** Fecal occult blood testing is more cost effective and timely in excluding GI blood loss than obtaining a complete blood cell count. **(E)** Although hypothyroidism can cause constipation, the history of normal weight gain and normal linear growth makes this diagnosis less likely. **(B)** Although an obstruction or mass could cause constipation, routine screening with an ultrasound is not appropriate in the absence of suspicious findings on examination.

A 7-year-old girl comes to the office with complaints of abdominal pain and nausea. The mother describes that the girl has been complaining of epigastric abdominal pain intermittently for the past month, but has increased recently. She has noticed that her daughter has a poor appetite although she seems to have some relief of the pain after eating.

Of the following, what is the mechanism regarding this patient's most likely diagnosis?

(A) Ulceration in the third portion of the duodenum
(B) Increased stress
(C) Nonsteroidal anti-inflammatory medication use
(D) Oversecretion of acid
(E) *Helicobacter pylori* infection

The answer is E: *Helicobacter pylori* infection. The signs and symptoms of the patient in the vignette are consistent with peptic ulcer disease. **(A)** Primary ulcers are most commonly located in the first portion of the duodenum, or duodenal bulb. **(D)** They are associated with *H. pylori* infection for the majority of cases. Effective treatment requires eradication of the *H. pylori* infection, as well as acid suppression therapy. The first line of treatment consists of a 14-day course of triple therapy, including amoxicillin, clarithromycin, and a proton pump inhibitor.

Secondary ulcers may be due to excessive nonsteroidal anti-inflammatory drug (NSAID) use, or stress. Chronic use of NSAIDs causes an inhibition of prostaglandins, which impairs the ability of the stomach mucosa to protect itself from acid. **(C)** There is no suggestion that the patient in the vignette is using NSAIDs. **(B)** A stress ulcer refers to erosion or ulceration of the gastric mucosa that occurs secondary to physiologic stress. This generally occurs in critically ill patients, usually within the first 24 hours of illness. Many pediatric intensive care units have protocols to initiate acid suppression therapy in all critically ill patients, in an attempt to avoid this condition. Secondary ulcers are usually located in the gastric antrum. A secondary ulcer in a patient who does not have *H. pylori* infection can be treated with acid suppression alone.

32 A 17-year-old girl is brought to the office by her mother. The girl has been complaining of abdominal pain intermittently for the past 2 months, particularly after eating. Today she complains of worsening abdominal pain, which is mostly in the right upper quadrant. In the office, her temperature is 39.0°C and she has a positive Murphy sign.

Of the following, which diagnosis is most likely for this patient?

(A) Acute cholecystitis
(B) Cholelithiasis
(C) Acute viral hepatitis
(D) Pelvic inflammatory disease
(E) Acute appendicitis

The answer is A: Acute cholecystitis. Right upper quadrant pain that is worsened with eating is indicative of gallbladder disease. Cholelithiasis refers to the presence of stones in the gallbladder. **(B)** Although cholelithiasis can cause intermittent pain as small stones pass, the presence of stones does not explain the fever, tenderness, vomiting, and persistent pain presented in the vignette. **(A)** The patient has acute cholecystitis, or inflammation and/or infection of the gallbladder. Diagnosis is suggested with fever, cessation of inspiration with right upper quadrant palpation (Murphy sign), and abdominal pain that is worsened with eating. Ultrasound is the confirmatory test of choice. The most common cause of cholecystitis is calculus cholecystitis, or a stone obstructing the cystic duct. However, it is possible to develop acalculous cholecystitis. Treatment for cholecystitis involves broad-spectrum antibiotic therapy, intravenous fluid therapy, bowel rest, and pain control. If a cholecystectomy is needed, it is typically completed 6 to 8 weeks after the acute episode of cholecystitis has resolved.

(C) The presentation of viral hepatitis can include right upper quadrant pain; however, hepatitis presents more insidiously and is frequently associated with jaundice. **(D)** A complication of pelvic inflammatory disease is seeding of the liver with bacteria, a condition known as Fitz-Hugh and Curtis syndrome, which can present with right upper quadrant pain and fever. Given the relationship between the food intake and pain for the patient in the vignette, gallbladder disease is more likely. **(E)** Appendicitis may present with fever and abdominal pain, but the pain is typically in the right lower quadrant and would not be intermittently present for 2 months.

---

33 A 15-year-old girl with a history of ulcerative colitis is brought to the emergency department by her parents. She has been experiencing a

flare of her colitis over the past week, with increased stooling, abdominal pain, and hematochezia. Today, she has had a high fever, increased abdominal pain, abdominal distention, and vomiting. On physical examination, she is ill-appearing with dry mucus membranes. Her vital signs are temperature 40°C, heart rate 140 beats/min, and blood pressure is 85/40 mmHg. Her abdomen is firm and moderately distended. Plain radiography films demonstrate air fluid levels and massive dilation of the colon with loss of haustral markings.

Of the following, which is this patient's most likely diagnosis?

(A) Hirschsprung colitis
(B) *Escherichia coli* infection
(C) Appendicitis
(D) Toxic megacolon
(E) Abdominal abscess

The answer is D: Toxic megacolon. Toxic megacolon is one of the most serious complications of inflammatory bowel disease. It can occur anytime, but is more common at the time of initial diagnosis or after a rapid taper or discontinuation of therapy. The patient in the vignette demonstrates the typical constellation of findings including signs of systemic illness such as fever, tachycardia, abdominal distention, and radiographic evidence of colonic distention. Toxic megacolon is a life-threatening emergency. Treatment should be initiated promptly and includes decompression of the colon with a rectal tube, fluid resuscitation, electrolyte replacement, intravenous corticosteroids, and empiric antibiotic therapy.

(A) Hirschsprung disease can present as toxic megacolon, but is most likely to occur in a young infant prior to surgical repair. **(B)** *E. coli* infection has not been associated with toxic megacolon. **(C)** Appendicitis presents with right lower quadrant pain, fevers, abdominal tenderness, but does not demonstrate colonic distention on radiography. **(E)** Though abdominal abscesses are possible in patients with inflammatory bowel disease, the clinical presentation and radiography of the patient in the vignette are more indicative of toxic megacolon rather than abscess formation.

A 4-year-old girl is brought to the emergency department with complaints of bright green vomiting. Her parents report that she was adopted 1 month ago from Guatemala. Per history, she was previously healthy. Plain abdominal radiography is obtained which suggests obstruction. An upper gastrointestinal (GI) study does not demonstrate evidence of a malrotation. She is managed conservatively with bowel rest and nasogastric tube decompression, but fails to improve. Ultimately she is taken to surgery, where a definitive diagnosis is made.

Of the following etiologies, which is most likely to cause her obstruction?

(A) *Entamoeba histolytica*
(B) *Ascaris lumbricoides*
(C) *Cryptococcus neoformans*
(D) *Salmonella typhi*
(E) *Trichinella spiralis*

The answer is B: *Ascaris lumbricoides.* *A. lumbricoides* is a nematode that causes infection worldwide. The infection is transmitted via the fecal–oral route or by contact with contaminated fruits and vegetables. The ova are ingested and hatch in the small intestine, releasing the larvae. Larvae can travel to the lungs and cause pulmonary ascariasis. From the lungs, the larvae are coughed up and swallowed, and then mature into adult worms in the intestine (see *Figure 13-11*). The presentation is varied, but can involve cough, shortness of breath, and hemoptysis. The GI manifestations can include abdominal pain, vomiting, and distention. In a patient with a large worm burden, acute obstruction can occur. The worms can also travel up the biliary tree, resulting in jaundice, cholecystitis, and pancreatitis. Antiparasitic medications such as mebendazole and albendazole can provide effective treatment.

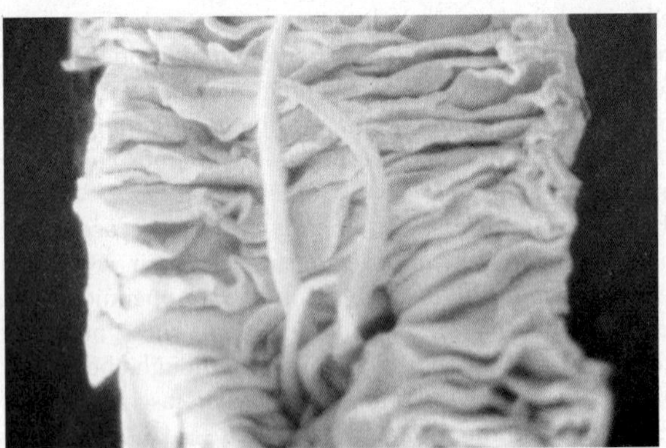

Figure 13-11

(A) *E. histolytica* is a parasitic infection common in developing countries. Infection is transmitted via ingestion of the cystic form. Most cases are asymptomatic, however, severe invasive disease is more common in children. Children between 1 and 5 years are particularly at risk for developing infectious colitis from the organism and can have bloody diarrhea, fever, chills, and severe electrolyte imbalance. A rare complication of infection is liver abscess. Liver abscesses can develop months to years after the initial infection, and symptoms may be vague with abdominal pain, distention, and tenderness in the right upper quadrant. Treatment is with metronidazole or tinidazole.

(C) *C. neoformans* is a fungal infection that is transmitted via inhalation of fungal spores. It causes pulmonary disease, meningitis, and ocular infection in immunosuppressed patients.

(D) *Salmonella* sp. are gram-negative enteric bacteria. *S. enteritidis* causes gastroenteritis, marked by cramping and profuse watery diarrhea that progresses to bloody diarrhea. The disease is generally self-limited, and antibiotic treatment is not recommended because it prolongs excretion and increases the risk of chronic carrier state. Infants less than 3 months of age, immunocompromised patients, or patients with invasive complications such as bacteremia and joint involvement require antibiotic therapy. *S. typhi* is a distinct serotype, which causes typhoid fever. The clinical disease is marked by high fever, myalgia, hepatosplenomegaly, abdominal pain, and anorexia. Typhoid fever should be treated promptly with antibiotics.

(E) *T. spiralis* is a parasite transmitted via ingestion of undercooked meat, most often pork, contaminated with larvae. The clinical presentation is nonspecific and includes diarrhea, abdominal pain, and vomiting. With progression of disease, the parasite invades the muscle, and symptoms can include cough, dyspnea, periorbital edema, myalgia, and a macular or petechial rash. Patients often have markedly elevated eosinophilia in the blood. Treatment is with mebendazole.

---

35 A healthy infant presents to the outpatient clinic for her 4-month health maintenance visit. Her mother is concerned because she has a bulge at her umbilicus that appears when she cries. She wants to know if her child will need surgery to correct this problem. A picture of this infant's examination finding is shown in Figure 13-12.

Of the following, what is the next best step in management?

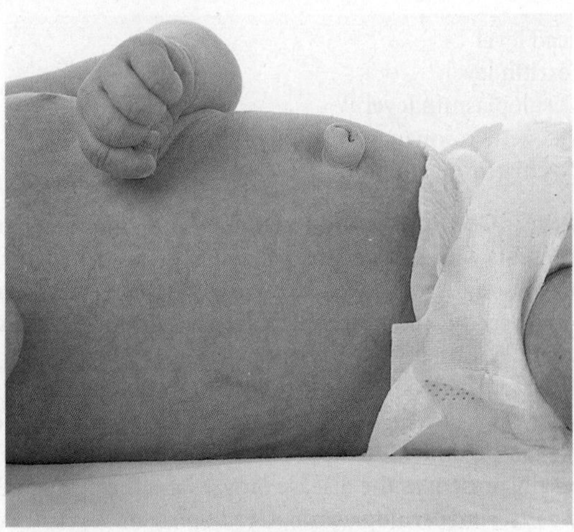

Figure 13-12

(A) Immediate surgical correction
(B) Abdominal ultrasound
(C) Surgical referral at 1 year of age
(D) Apply a compression dressing to the area
(E) Reassurance

The answer is E: Reassurance. The patient in the vignette has an umbilical hernia due to weakness or failure of complete closure of the umbilical ring. Physical examination demonstrates a bulge or outpouching at the umbilicus that is exacerbated when the child cries or strains and then reduces spontaneously. **(A)** Strangulation of this type of hernia is extremely rare, and if present requires emergent surgical correction. **(E)** The majority of umbilical hernias resolve without intervention by 2 years of age. **(C)** Those with a large defect greater than 2 cm are less likely to close without intervention and surgical correction in these patients can be considered electively if it persists remains beyond the age of 4 years. **(D)** A compression dressing is not indicated and does not change the natural course of an umbilical hernia. **(B)** There is no indication for any abdominal imaging to evaluate an uncomplicated umbilical hernia.

36 A 12-year-old boy is brought into the outpatient clinic by his mother because his school performance has been declining over the past year. The boy states he is having difficulty concentrating and completing assignments. A set of questionnaires is distributed to assess for attention deficit disorder, but the results are inconclusive. A screening laboratory evaluation notes an elevated aspartate aminotransferase and alanine aminotransferase.

Of the following, which would be the most appropriate next step in establishing the diagnosis?

(A) Lead level
(B) Ferritin level
(C) Ceruloplasmin level
(D) Magnetic resonance imaging of the brain
(E) Psychiatric consultation

The answer is C: Ceruloplasmin level. The combination of an adolescent patient who presents with elevated liver enzymes and psychiatric complaints is suspicious for Wilson disease. Wilson disease is an autosomal recessive disorder caused by a defect in the gene which encodes for a copper transport protein. Patients with Wilson disease present insidiously with deteriorating school performance, dysarthria, poor motor coordination, and hepatic inflammation. Kayser-Fleischer rings (see *Figure 13-13*) are discolorations around the border of the iris that can be difficult to appreciate without a slit lamp examination, but are universally present as the disease progresses. The best screening test for Wilson disease is serum ceruloplasmin. Ceruloplasmin levels are decreased in Wilson disease. Serum and urine copper levels may be increased.

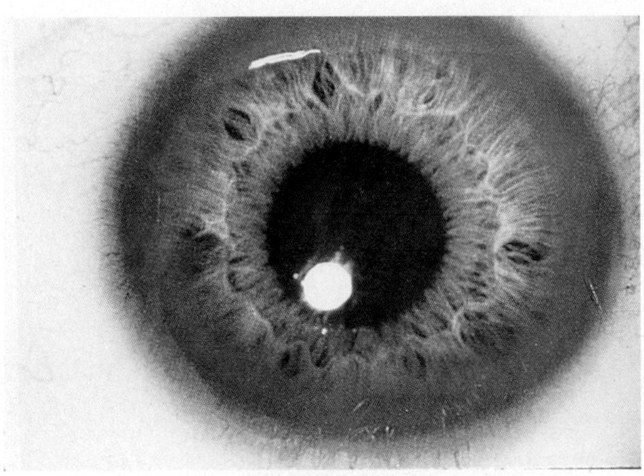

Figure 13-13

(A) Lead poisoning can cause neurologic symptoms at very high doses; it is less likely to occur in an older child. **(B)** Ferritin levels can be helpful in diagnosing hemochromatosis presenting with abnormal liver enzymes; however, hemochromatosis would not explain the patient's declining school performance. **(D, E)** Magnetic resonance imaging of the brain and psychiatric consultation may also be useful to assist with the neurologic complaints described in the vignette, but do not address the elevated liver enzymes.

CHAPTER

14

Hematology and Oncology

CAITLIN KELLY

1 The results of a newborn screen hemoglobin test show FSA.
Of the following, what is the next best step?

(A) Do not refer to a pediatric hematologist due to the diagnosis of sickle cell trait
(B) Do not refer to a pediatric hematologist due to the diagnosis of sickle cell disease
(C) Do not refer to a pediatric hematologist. Repeat a hemoglobin electrophoresis in 6 months
(D) Refer to a pediatric hematologist due to the diagnosis of sickle cell trait
(E) Refer to a pediatric hematologist due to the diagnosis of sickle cell disease

The answer is E: **Refer to a pediatric hematologist due to the diagnosis of sickle cell disease.** Newborn screening for various metabolic, endocrinologic, and hematologic disorders is mandatory in all 50 states and each state is responsible for determining which disorders to screen. Screening for sickle cell disease is performed universally. Diagnosis in the neonatal period is critical for the sickle cell population since prophylactic penicillin should be given by 2 months of age.

The newborn screen uses thin-layer isoelectric focusing and high-performance liquid chromatography to determine which types of hemoglobin are present. The hemoglobin fraction that is present in the largest quantity is listed first, followed by the other hemoglobin fractions in decreasing order. Therefore, the newborn screen described in the vignette shows the largest percentage of hemoglobin is F (fetal), followed by S (sickle), and lastly A (adult). It is normal for fetal hemoglobin to have the highest percentage on a newborn screen. Having the second highest quantity as hemoglobin S indicates sickle cell disease. **(D)** Sickle cell trait would have a newborn screen result of FSA indicating that the fraction of hemoglobin A is more prevalent than hemoglobin S.

(A, B, C) Any infant with an abnormal newborn screen suggestive of either sickle cell disease or trait should be referred immediately to a hematologist for genetic counseling and medical management.

2 A patient with newly diagnosed acute lymphoblastic leukemia (ALL) with an initial white blood cell count of 100 × $10^3/\mu L$ is given induction chemotherapy.

Of the following, which electrolyte abnormalities are most consistent with tumor lysis syndrome?

	Potassium	Phosphate	Uric acid	Sodium
(A)	↓	↓	↑	↑
(B)	↑	↓	↓	Normal
(C)	↑	↓	↑	↑
(D)	↑	↑	↑	Normal
(E)	↓	↑	↑	Normal

The answer is D: Hyperkalemia, hyperphosphatemia, high uric acid, normal sodium. Tumor lysis occurs due to the rapid breakdown of tumor cells. It occurs more frequently in those malignancies characterized by very high white blood cell counts such as acute leukemias, Burkitt lymphoma, and T-cell lymphomas. Acute renal failure occurs secondary to the high uric acid concentrations and leads to a worsening of the electrolyte abnormalities. The elevated electrolytes are those that are primarily intracellular, for example, potassium and phosphate, and are released into the serum when the cells lyse. The kidneys cannot excrete these electrolytes quickly enough so they accumulate within the body. Sodium concentrations are not affected by cell lysis because it exists mostly in the extracellular space. Tumor lysis syndrome is treated with hyperhydration and a xanthine oxidase inhibitor called allopurinol.

3 A 6-year-old boy is admitted to the pediatric ward for evaluation of complaints of increasing clumsiness over the past 2 months. His mother states that she has noticed him tilting his head to the right over the past 2 weeks. He complains of headaches when he first wakes up in the morning and has vomited several mornings this week. His midnight vital signs are as follows: temperature, 37.5°C; heart rate, 78 beats/minute; respiratory rate, 22 breaths/minute; blood pressure, 96/76 mmHg.

Of the following, which is most likely to establish a diagnosis for this patient?

(A) Computed tomography (CT) of the head without contrast
(B) Electroencephalogram
(C) Magnetic resonance imaging (MRI) of the brain with contrast
(D) Dilated funduscopic examination
(E) Lumbar puncture

The answer is C: Magnetic resonance imaging (MRI) of the brain with contrast. The boy described in the vignette presents with signs consistent with medulloblastoma. Medulloblastoma has a peak incidence between the ages of 5 and 7 years and is the most common malignant brain tumor of childhood. The majority arise in the cerebellum and present with ataxia. Ataxia can be reported as clumsiness by parents. Head tilt or neck stiffness may be seen due to meningeal irritation or trochlear nerve compression by the tumor. Children can have increased intracranial pressure with resulting nausea, vomiting that is worse in the morning, headache, and papilledema. Symptoms generally are present 2 to 3 months prior to diagnosis. Severely increased intracranial pressure can result in herniation of the brain through the foramen magnum. This herniation presses on the brain stem and results in Cushing triad: bradycardia, hypertension, and irregular breathing.

The optimal test to evaluate the posterior fossa is an MRI scan. **(A)** A CT scan without contrast is useful in evaluating an acute hemorrhage and does not adequately visualize the brain stem. **(B)** The patient in the vignette does not present with symptoms suggestive of seizure activity and his clumsiness is best attributed to cerebellar involvement. Therefore, an electroencephalogram is not a useful diagnostic test in this case. **(D)** Papilledema found on a dilated funduscopic examination suggests increased intracranial pressure, but is not diagnostic of an intracranial mass. **(E)** Lumbar puncture is not recommended in a 6-year-old patient with concerns for an intracranial mass because of the possibility of cerebellar herniation.

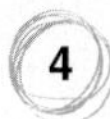

4 A 3-day-old infant born at home presents to the emergency department with a chief complaint of prolonged bleeding from her umbilical stump and bloody stools.

Of the following, which clotting factor is most likely to be deficient?

(A) Factor III
(B) Factor IV
(C) Factor VI
(D) Factor VII
(E) Factor XIII

The answer is D: Factor VII. (A, B, C, E) Vitamin K is necessary for the production of factors II, VII, IX, and X. A deficiency in vitamin K also leads to a decrease in proteins C and S, which plays a role in coagulation. The lack of any of these clotting factors and coagulation factors predisposes patients to bleeding. Newborn infants are born with a transient deficiency in vitamin K and thus are routinely given an injection of vitamin K at birth. Infants born outside of a hospital setting may not receive this injection. Infants with bleeding secondary to vitamin K deficiency present within the first 2 weeks following birth with bleeding of the mucosa, gastrointestinal tract, umbilical stump, or less commonly, intracranial bleeding. Breastfed infants of vitamin K–deficient mothers can experience late complications of vitamin K deficiency with bleeding occurring between 2 and 12 weeks of age.

Vitamin K is found in green leafy vegetables, legumes, plant oils, and liver. The normal flora of the intestinal tract also produces vitamin K naturally.

Vitamin K is a fat-soluble vitamin and requires bile salts for adequate absorption. Conditions characterized by exocrine pancreatic insufficiency or intestinal malabsorptive disorders require vitamin K supplementation. Medications such as warfarin, phenobarbital, and phenytoin interfere with vitamin K function. Vitamin K deficiency is associated with prolonged prothrombin time and partial thromboplastin time (PTT); however, these values may be normal in early deficiency.

5 A 15-year-old girl is seen in clinic for a school physical. She reports no issues and mentions that her last menstrual period was 2 weeks ago. Her examination is unremarkable except for a 3-cm rubbery nodule palpated in her anterior neck that elevates when she is asked to swallow.

Of the following, what is the next best step in establishing a diagnosis?

(A) Thyroid function testing
(B) Thyroid ultrasound
(C) Thyroid biopsy
(D) Fine needle aspiration
(E) Nuclear scintigraphy with technetium-99m pertechnetate

The answer is D: Fine needle aspiration. Although the majority of thyroid nodules detected in the pediatric population are benign, further investigation is indicated. Risk factors for potential malignancy include female gender and nodules greater than 1 cm in size. Fine needle aspiration is the diagnostic test of choice as it is **(C)** less invasive than a biopsy and provides the tissue sample necessary to confirm a diagnosis.

(A) Thyroid function testing is used to evaluate for abnormalities in circulating thyroid hormone but does not determine whether a nodule is benign or malignant. **(B)** An ultrasound of the thyroid gland should be performed to help with placement of the fine needle aspiration and helps to classify the nodule as cystic or solid but it does not give a definitive diagnosis. **(E)** Nuclear scintigraphy with technetium-99m pertechnetate is not useful in the diagnostic evaluation of thyroid nodules, but rather parathyroid disease.

6 What is the mechanism of action for methotrexate?

(A) Methotrexate is a prodrug that is converted intracellularly into a thioguanine nucleotide that has a cytotoxic effect.
(B) Methotrexate has a heavy metal component that has a cytotoxic effect due to platination of the DNA.
(C) Methotrexate binds to tubulin, which prevents the formation of microtubules, which interferes with mitosis.
(D) Methotrexate induces topoisomerase II, which leads to DNA strand breaks.
(E) Methotrexate is a structural analog of folic acid and is an inhibitor of folate metabolism.

The answer is E: **Methotrexate is a structural analog of folic acid and is an inhibitor of folate metabolism.** Methotrexate belongs to the antimetabolite class of chemotherapeutic agents. Antimetabolites are structural analogs of vital cofactors involved in the synthesis of DNA or RNA. Methotrexate is a structural analog of folic acid, which is vital for the synthesis of purines and thymidine. Methotrexate inhibits dihydrofolate reductase (DHFR) by binding to it and prevents the conversion of several folates to their active forms, which inhibits the synthesis of DNA. Methotrexate shares membrane-transport processes and intracellular metabolic pathways with the naturally occurring folates. It rapidly binds to DHFR and continues to be metabolized until all the receptors are bound. Methotrexate can be given orally, intravenously, and intrathecally. High doses can be given intravenously with leucovorin rescue. Leucovorin is a folic acid analog that does not require DHFR for metabolism. It allows for some purine/pyrimidine synthesis to occur in the presence of methotrexate.

(A) Mercaptopurine is a prodrug that is converted intracellularly into a thioguanine nucleotide, which has a cytotoxic effect. It is an example of another group of antimetabolite agents called thiopurines and is used in the maintenance phase of acute lymphoblastic leukemia therapy. Mercaptopurine is given orally.

(B) Platinum compounds are considered to be nonclassical alkylating agents. They have cytotoxic effects due to their heavy metal component, which results in the platination of DNA.

(C) Vinca alkaloids, a plant derivative, bind to tubulin, which prevents the formation of microtubules and interferes with mitosis. The most well-known agent from this group is vincristine. Vinca alkaloids work as mitotic inhibitors due to the binding of tubulin.

(D) Anthracyclines induce topoisomerase II, which leads to DNA strand breaks. These agents work multifactorially, but the induction of topoisomerase-II-mediated DNA breakage is the most important mechanism of action.

7 The circumcision of a 2-day-old full-term newborn is cancelled because his external urethral meatus exits on the ventral side of his penis. The remainder of his physical examination is unremarkable except for a lack of pigmentation of his eyes.

Of the following, which malignancy is this patient at increased risk for developing?

(A) Hepatoblastoma
(B) Acute lymphoblastic leukemia
(C) Wilms tumor
(D) Medulloblastoma
(E) Osteosarcoma

The answer is C: **Wilms tumor.** The patient in the vignette has aniridia, defined as the absence of the iris, and hypospadias, a genital anomaly. These are components of Wilms tumor-aniridia-genitourinary anomalies-mental retardation (WAGR) syndrome, which stands for Wilms tumor, aniridia, genital anomalies, and mental retardation. It is associated with mutations on chromosome 11. Wilms tumor usually develops by the age of 2 and requires routine screening abdominal ultrasounds for early detection. **(A, B, D, E)** The other tumors listed are not associated with aniridia, hypospadias, or WAGR syndrome. However, Wilms tumor is associated with other syndromes such as Beckwith-Wiedemann or Denys-Drash syndrome. These syndromes are collectively associated with hemihypertrophy of the body.

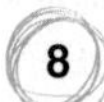

8 A 15-month-old boy comes to the outpatient clinic for a routine health maintenance visit. His mother reports that the family recently moved from another state and that her son has been a healthy boy with no complaints. During the examination, only one testicle is palpated in the scrotum. An ultrasound reveals the unpalpated testicle within the abdomen.

Of the following, what recommendation is most appropriate to give to this mother?

(A) Orchiopexy is recommended to eliminate his chances for future germ cell malignancy.
(B) Orchiopexy is recommended but his risk for germ cell malignancy will still be above the general public.
(C) Orchiopexy is not recommended, as his fertility will be maintained with only one testicle involved.
(D) Orchiopexy is not recommended, as it is normal for testes to be undescended by 15 months of age.
(E) Orchiopexy is not recommended given the undescended testicle is not at risk for torsion.

The answer is B: **Orchiopexy is recommended but his risk for germ cell malignancy will still be above the general public.** Cryptorchidism is a failure of descent of the testis. If the testis has not descended by 4 months of age, it will often remain undescended. Consequences include increased risk of germ cell tumors, as well as infertility, torsion, and associated hernias. Germ cell tumors are the most likely malignancy associated with cryptorchidism and the risk is two to four times higher than in normal testis. The risk is even higher if both testes are undescended. **(A, C, D, E)** Orchiopexy does not eliminate the risk of malignant transformation, however, placing the testicle in the scrotum allows for earlier detection of a testicular mass. Fertility is impacted by having an undescended testis but is usually preserved if corrected.

9 A 2-month-old infant with sickle cell anemia is evaluated in clinic. The infant will be starting a daily antibiotic.

Of the following, which is the best choice for a prophylactic antibiotic paired with the most likely organism to cause bacteremia in this patient?

(A) Azithromycin to prevent *Streptococcus pneumoniae*
(B) Clindamycin to prevent *Staphylococcus aureus*
(C) Penicillin VK to prevent *Staphylococcus aureus*
(D) Penicillin VK to prevent *Streptococcus pneumoniae*
(E) Penicillin VK to prevent *Salmonella* sp.

The answer is D: Penicillin VK to prevent *Streptococcus pneumoniae*. Infants with sickle cell anemia can become functionally asplenic as early as 6 months of age, and most are functionally asplenic by 5 years of age. The asplenia occurs because of repeated autoinfarction by sickled cells in the spleen. Asplenia leads to a risk of bacteremia caused by encapsulated organisms such as *Streptococcus pneumoniae* and *Haemophilus influenzae* type B. It is recommended that infants are started on daily prophylactic penicillin VK by 2 months of age to prevent potentially life-threatening bacteremia and sepsis. It is critical that children with sickle cell disease also receive all regular vaccines as well as the 23-valent pneumococcal polysaccharide vaccine after the age of 2.

(B, C, E) *Streptococcus pneumoniae* remains the more likely cause of bacteremia and sepsis over either *Staphylococcus aureus* or *Salmonella* sp. **(A, B)** Neither azithromycin nor clindamycin are appropriate choices for bacteremia prophylaxis in patients with sickle cell disease.

10 A mother brings her 6-year-old boy to clinic for his routine health maintenance visit. She reports she often finds him eating dirt and small toys and reports he has been complaining of abdominal pain and “not acting like himself” over the past month. A complete blood count reveals a hemoglobin concentration of 9.8 g/dL with a mean corpuscular volume (MCV) of 65 fL.

Of the following, which is the most likely cause of this patient’s anemia?

(A) Iron deficiency anemia
(B) Folic acid deficiency
(C) Vitamin B_{12} deficiency
(D) Lead poisoning
(E) Sideroblastic anemia

The answer is D: Lead poisoning. The combination of a microcytic anemia along with a history of pica, abdominal pain, and neurologic changes points to a diagnosis of lead poisoning with resulting anemia. Common sources of ingested lead particles include soil as well as paint used in older home construction and on imported toys or ceramics. Lead circulates through the body bound to the red blood cells. Lead binds to the enzymes that are involved in making heme, which results in decreased heme production. There is a concurrent increase in measurable erythrocyte protoporphyrin as a result of the decreased production of heme. Lead also decreases the red blood survival time, which leads to anemia. A screening value ≥2 μg/dL of lead is consistent with exposure and requires further testing. Chelation therapy is indicated for blood lead levels ≥45 μg/dL.

(A) Iron deficiency anemia causes a microcytic anemia but is less likely given the constellation of symptoms in the vignette. **(B, C)** Folic acid and B_{12} deficiency both cause megaloblastic anemia and increased MCV. **(E)** Sideroblastic anemia is a microcytic anemia that is very rare in children and is a result of acquired or hereditary disorders of heme synthesis. Peripheral blood smear reveals ringed sideroblasts.

A 6-month-old boy presents to his primary pediatrician for a well-child examination. His parents state they have no concerns regarding his growth and development. His ocular examination is as pictured in Figure 14-1.

Of the following, what is the next best step for this patient?

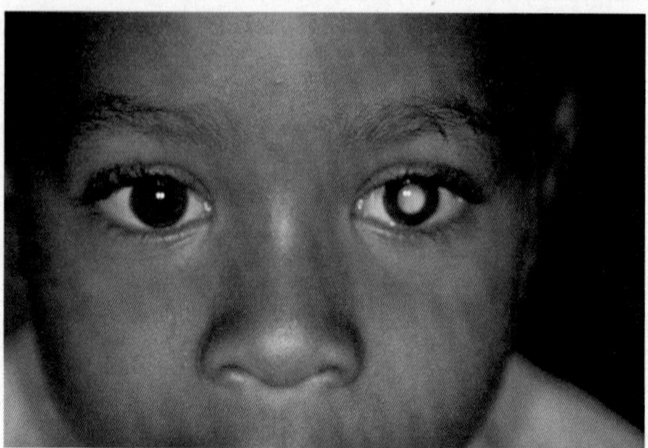

Figure 14-1

(A) Refer urgently to a pediatric ophthalmologist
(B) Refer to a pediatric ophthalmologist at the next available scheduled visit
(C) Repeat an ocular examination in 1 month
(D) Obtain a magnetic resonance imaging (MRI) scan of the orbits
(E) Provide reassurance and guidance in anticipation for his 9-month visit

The answer is A: Refer urgently to a pediatric ophthalmologist. Leukocoria, or a white pupillary reflex, is never a normal examination finding. In this age group, the diagnosis of retinoblastoma should be suspected and treated as an ophthalmologic urgency with **(B)** a rapid referral to a pediatric ophthalmologist. Retinoblastoma can be hereditary or sporadic. The hereditary type presents at a younger age and is often bilateral at diagnosis. Hereditary retinoblastoma is due to a loss of function of the retinoblastoma gene either through gene mutation or deletion. This gene is an example of a tumor suppressor protein. Retinoblastoma follows the "two-hit" model of tumor formation. In the hereditary form, the first mutation of the retinoblastoma gene is passed on to the child and the second mutation occurs sporadically in the somatic cells. Treatment for retinoblastoma is dependent on the extent of involvement of the tumor. If the tumor is localized and unilateral, enucleation may be performed. If the disease is bilateral, chemotherapy is indicated prior to enucleation in an attempt to salvage vision in at least one eye.

(C, E) Reassurance or repeating the ocular examination are both inappropriate next steps as the patient in the vignette has leukocoria and treatment delays for retinoblastoma will lead to disease progression and decrease the chances of vision salvage. **(D)** Although MRI of the orbits is indicated to determine the extent of the retinoblastoma, this should be done after urgent evaluation by an ophthalmologist.

A 14-year-old boy with Ewing sarcoma is being treated with chemotherapy. He is transfused packed red blood cells because his hemoglobin is found to be decreased on routine laboratory surveillance. Twenty minutes after starting the transfusion, he complains of chills and his temperature is 39.4°C.

Of the following, which is the next best step in the management of this patient?

(A) Slow the blood transfusion
(B) Stop the blood transfusion
(C) Give intravenous cefepime
(D) Give acetaminophen
(E) Continue to observe

The answer is B: Stop the blood transfusion. The patient in the vignette is having a transfusion reaction. The most important step is to stop the transfusion immediately. Transfusion reactions occur within 24 hours of a transfusion and can include fever, chills, pruritus, and urticaria. Transfusion-related reactions typically resolve without intervention. Other possible signs of a more severe transfusion reaction include hematuria, acute shortness of breath, and/or loss of consciousness. There should be a high index of suspicion of a transfusion reaction in any patient receiving blood products or with a recent history of transfusions that develops any of these symptoms. Once the transfusion has been stopped, the blood product should be rechecked to ensure it was given to the proper patient and it was properly cross-matched.

(A, E) Slowing the transfusion or observing the patient would not stop the transfusion reaction. **(C)** While fever and chills could indicate an infection and antibiotic therapy may be started, based on the timing of the symptoms in the vignette, a transfusion reaction is more likely than infection. **(D)** Acetaminophen can be given if the fever is causing the patient discomfort but if the fever is due to a transfusion reaction it is likely to resolve with cessation of the transfusion.

---

13 A newborn hemoglobin electrophoresis shows the following:

Hemoglobin A:	91%
Hemoglobin A_2:	2%
Hemoglobin F:	1%
Hemoglobin Barts:	6%

Of the following disorders, which condition is most consistent with this hemoglobin electrophoresis?

(A) Iron deficiency anemia
(B) β-Thalassemia trait
(C) Transient erythroblastopenia of childhood (TEC)
(D) Sickle cell trait
(E) α-Thalassemia trait

The answer is E: α-Thalassemia trait. Hemoglobin is made up of a heme group and a tetramer of four chains of globin isotypes—α, β, δ, or γ. Each of the three common types of nonpathologic hemoglobin consists of two α-globin chains and two chains of each of the remaining globin isotypes: hemoglobin A ($\alpha_2\beta_2$), hemoglobin A_2 ($\alpha_2\delta_2$), and hemoglobin F ($\alpha_2\gamma_2$). A group of disorders called thalassemias are characterized by mutations in one or more of the above globin chains.

The presence of hemoglobin Barts during infancy points to the diagnosis of α-thalassemia. Hemoglobin Barts consists of four γ-chains and is only found during the newborn period in patients with α-thalassemia trait. The percentage of hemoglobin Barts in the newborn period is typically between 3% and 8%. α-Thalassemia trait results from a deletion on two α-globin genes and causes a microcytic anemia outside the newborn period. The loss of only one α-globin gene does not produce any microcytosis or anemia. The loss of three α-globin genes results in the diagnosis of hemoglobin H. Patients with hemoglobin H have hemoglobin Barts as infants as well, but in larger quantities, often >25%. The deletion of all four α-globins leads to severe anemia and hydrops fetalis in utero.

(A, B, C, D) Hemoglobin Barts is not found with iron deficiency anemia, β-thalassemia trait, TEC, and sickle cell trait.

14 An infant in the special care nursery develops small, pinpoint, nonblanching erythematous lesions. On examination, the forearms appear deformed and the thumbs are present.

Of the following, which is his most likely diagnosis?

(A) Thrombocytopenia-absent radius (TAR) syndrome
(B) Wiskott-Aldrich syndrome
(C) Congenital amegakaryocytic thrombocytopenia
(D) Fanconi anemia
(E) Diamond-Blackfan anemia

The answer is A: **Thrombocytopenia-absent radius (TAR) syndrome.** The name of this disorder describes the most notable clinical aspects of this syndrome, thrombocytopenia and bilateral radial anomalies. Thrombocytopenia is due to the absence or hypoplasia of megakaryocytes, and the platelet count may normalize after the first year of life. The radial anomalies can range from minor to severe but the thumbs are present and normal in appearance. Other skeletal anomalies can be present in the ulnae and lower extremities.

(B) Wiskott-Aldrich syndrome in an X-linked disorder characterized by a triad of thrombocytopenia, eczema, and recurrent infections. The platelets in this disorder are small. Splenectomy will often cure the thrombocytopenia but will increase the risk of infections even further. Bony abnormalities are usually not present.

(C) Congenital amegakaryocytic thrombocytopenia becomes apparent within the first week of life with the presence of petechiae and/or purpura and no other physical examination abnormalities. It is due to a defect in the platelet hematopoiesis, which results in the complete absence of megakaryocytes. Bone marrow transplant is curative.

(D) Fanconi anemia is a primarily autosomal recessive disorder and presents with pancytopenia and bony abnormalities due to increased chromosomal fragility. Patients typically have hyperpigmentation of the skin and/or café-au-lait spots. Short stature and abnormal facies are also common. Patients can have bony abnormalities including thumb abnormalities. Treatment is bone marrow transplant.

(E) Diamond-Blackfan anemia is a pure red blood cell aplasia and does not affect the platelet cell line. Bony abnormalities including triphalangeal thumbs are characteristic.

15 A 2-year-old patient with Down syndrome is seen in clinic for the first time. Her parents mention that when she was a newborn she had abnormal blood work including blasts in her blood that resolved without any treatment beyond a few transfusions of packed red blood cells and platelets.

Of the following, which statement is the most likely explanation for her abnormal blood work?

(A) Neuroblastoma
(B) Lymphoma
(C) Acute lymphoblastic leukemia (ALL)
(D) Acute myeloblastic leukemia
(E) Transient myeloproliferative disorder

The answer is E: **Transient myeloproliferative disorder.** Transient myeloproliferative disorder occurs in Down syndrome and is identified by the presence of leukocytosis with peripheral blastocytes, anemia, and thrombocytopenia which resolve within the first 3 months of life without any chemotherapy; however, these patients are at higher risk for developing acute leukemias later in life. **(C, D)** Blastocytes are not expected to resolve without treatment in acute leukemias.

Children with Down syndrome are at increased risk for acute leukemia over the general population. In the first 3 years of life, acute myeloid leukemia (AML) is more common than ALL in these children, but children with Down syndrome tend to have a better prognosis with AML and a worse prognosis with ALL. It is important that every child with Down syndrome has routine surveillance of complete blood counts to monitor for acute leukemia. **(A, B)** There is not an increased incidence of neonatal blastocyte formation with neuroblastoma or lymphoma.

16 A 3-year-old girl presents to the emergency department with a chief complaint of fever, bruising, and progressive left knee pain with a limp that progressed over the past several days. Her skin examination reveals pallor with a non-blanching, erythematous macular rash and extensive bruising on her upper and lower extremities. She also has a 2/6 systolic ejection murmur at the left lower sternal border.

Of the following, which test is most likely to reveal this patient's diagnosis?

(A) Prothrombin time
(B) Complete blood count
(C) Echocardiogram
(D) Radiograph of the left knee
(E) Radiograph of the lumbar spine

The answer is B: **Complete blood count.** The combination of low-grade fever, limp, petechiae, bruising, and pallor is most consistent with the diagnosis of acute lymphoblastic leukemia. The bruising and petechial rash are due to thrombocytopenia, and pallor is caused by anemia. Infiltration of the bone marrow by leukemic cells causes bone pain and leads to limp. The bone pain can be severe enough to wake the patient at night. Other malignancies can present with bony pain including primary bone tumors such as osteosarcoma and Ewing sarcoma, which typically are not associated with thrombocytopenia or anemia.

Bone pain can also be a presentation of histiocytosis and in severe cases can cause anemia and thrombocytopenia, but acute leukemia is more likely. Histiocytosis commonly presents with a rash described as a scaly, papular, seborrheic dermatitis of the scalp, diaper, axillary, or posterior auricular regions that is often refractory to treatment. Lytic lesions on radiograph are characteristic of histiocytosis. Neuroblastoma can also present with bony pain secondary to metastasis but typically an abdominal mass is palpated with this diagnosis.

(D) Radiographs would be indicated if fractures or bone tumors were the cause of the pain but this is less likely for the patient in the vignette. **(E)** It is important to remember that spinal pathology can present as a limp in the pediatric population. However, orthopedic injuries do not impact the bone marrow and circulating blood cells as suggested by the patient in the vignette. **(C)** There is no role for an echocardiogram in this patient. The murmur is likely secondary to an anemic state. **(A)** Although prolongation of prothrombin time could explain the bleeding symptoms seen, it does not explain the limp or fevers.

17 A 3-year-old boy is evaluated in hematology clinic for pancytopenia. His physical examination is significant for a hyperpigmented patch on his posterior neck, several café-au-lait spots on his trunk, and absent thumbs. His height is below the 5th percentile for his age.

Of this following, which disorder is the best explanation for this patient's symptoms?

(A) TAR syndrome
(B) Shwachman-Diamond syndrome
(C) Diamond-Blackfan anemia
(D) Fanconi anemia
(E) Aplastic anemia

The answer is D: **Fanconi anemia.** The combination of pancytopenia and the physical anomalies mentioned in the vignette suggests a diagnosis of

Fanconi anemia. This disorder is associated with several cutaneous findings, including hyperpigmentation of the neck, trunk, and intertriginous areas, café-au-lait spots (see *Figure 14-2*), and vitiligo (see *Figure 14-3*). Patients with Fanconi anemia may also have short stature and abnormal facies. Bony abnormalities can involve the upper and lower extremities, and in particular, the thumbs may be hypoplastic, supernumerary, bifid, or absent. These patients have chromosomal fragility leading to genomic instability and are at increased risk for malignancies, including squamous cell carcinomas, liver tumors, and

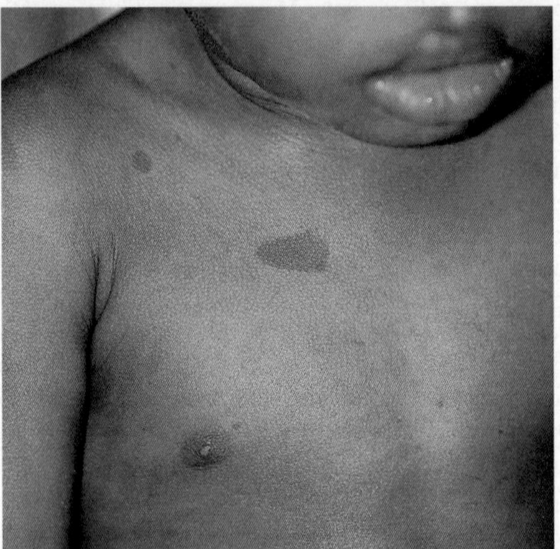

Figure 14-2

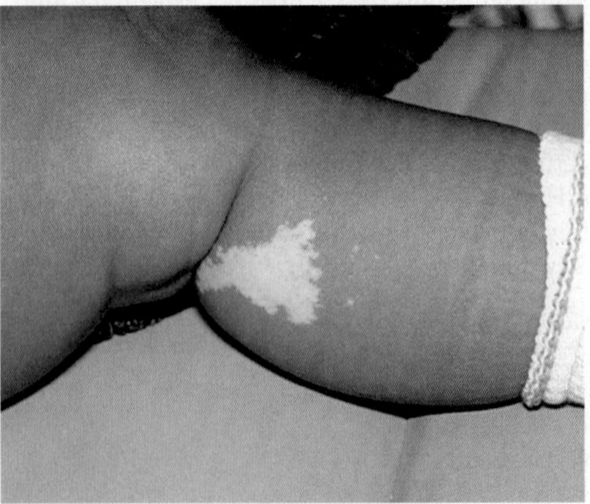

Figure 14-3

acute leukemia. Diagnosis is made with a lymphocyte chromosomal breakage study. It is inherited mainly as an autosomal recessive disorder but uncommonly can be X-linked. Treatment is a stem cell transplant, which can cure the hematologic changes only.

(A) TAR syndrome does not cause pancytopenia or the physical examination findings listed in the vignette. The radius is absent leading to forearm deformities, but the thumb anatomy remains normal. **(B)** Shwachman-Diamond syndrome is associated with pancytopenia and characterized by short stature and skeletal abnormalities, including metaphyseal dysplasia, short or flared ribs, thoracic dystrophy, and bifid thumbs. This disorder is also associated with fat malabsorption due to exocrine pancreatic insufficiency. Patients often suffer bacterial infections due to neutropenia. **(C)** Diamond-Blackfan anemia is a pure red cell aplasia and does not affect other cell lines. These patients can have craniofacial abnormalities, and thumb abnormalities including triphalangeal thumbs (see *Figure 14-4*). **(E)** Aplastic anemia can be acquired or congenital. It causes pancytopenia but the bony and skin changes described in the vignette would not be expected.

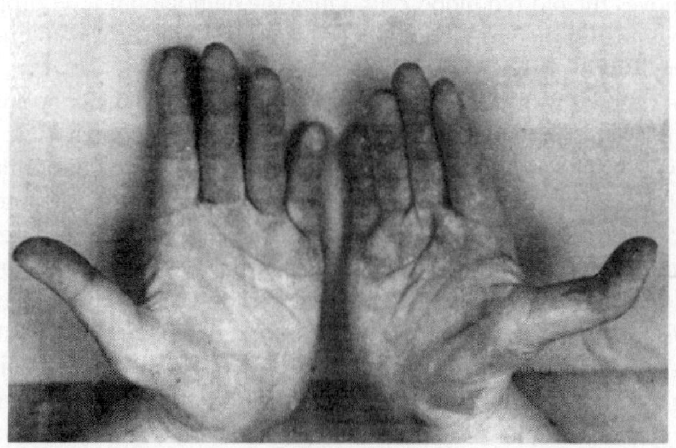

Figure 14-4

---

18 A 9-week-old, full-term infant comes to clinic. The infant is primarily breastfed, growing normally, and clinically doing well. Physical examination, including vital signs, is within normal limits. The complete blood count is remarkable for a hemoglobin concentration of 9 g/dL with a mean corpuscular volume (MCV) of 90 fL.

Of the following, what is the next best step with regard to this patient's care?

(A) Begin iron supplementation
(B) Transfuse the infant with 10 mL/kg of packed red blood cells
(C) Obtain a bone marrow aspirate
(D) Provide reassurance to the mother that the anemia will improve spontaneously
(E) Encourage the mother to transition to formula

The answer is D: Provide reassurance to the mother that the anemia will improve spontaneously. Reassurance is the next best step as this infant has physiologic anemia of infancy. This occurs normally in full-term infants between the ages of 8 and 12 weeks and, on average, the hemoglobin decreases to 9 to 11 g/dL. Infants are born with a higher hemoglobin concentration (16 to 18 g/dL) and their red blood cells are larger in size (MCV 95 to 105 fL). The hemoglobin decreases after birth due to the normal switch from fetal to adult hemoglobin. Adult hemoglobin has lower oxygen affinity than fetal hemoglobin, and thus, more oxygen is able to be delivered to the tissues. As the tissues are supplied with a high oxygen level, there is a decrease in erythropoietin production, and thus a decrease in erythropoiesis. Without new red blood cells being produced, the hemoglobin concentration decreases as the spleen naturally removes the old red blood cells. Once the hemoglobin level drops to the physiologic nadir, the production of erythropoietin is triggered and hemoglobin normalizes over the course of the next 1 to 2 months.

(A) The infant in the vignette does not have iron deficiency anemia, as the anemia is normocytic while iron deficiency causes a microcytic anemia. Typically, iron deficiency anemia does not occur until 9 to 12 months of age as infants have high iron stores even with an iron-poor diet. **(B)** There is no indication to transfuse this infant, as he is clinically stable. If the anemia was severe and causing symptoms such as tachycardia, lethargy, and cardiopulmonary instability, a 10 to 15 mL/kg transfusion of packed red blood cells would be appropriate. **(C)** There is no need for a bone marrow aspirate at this point as the infant's macrocytic anemia is physiologic. If the anemia did not improve over the expected time course, evaluation of the cellular components of the bone marrow may be appropriate. **(E)** There is no reason to recommend changing to formula since breast milk provides all the necessary nutrients for proper erythropoiesis.

A 2-year-old girl is newly diagnosed with acute myeloblastic leukemia. Which chromosomal anomaly is associated with the most favorable prognosis for this disorder?

(A) Translocation of (8;21)
(B) Deletion of chromosome 7
(C) Monosomy of chromosome 5
(D) Translocation of (9;22)(q34;q11)
(E) Philadelphia chromosome

The answer is A: Translocation of (8;21). AML in general has a worse prognosis than acute lymphoblastic leukemia. However, certain chromosomal abnormalities have been associated with an improved prognosis. A favorable prognosis has been associated with translocation (8;21), translocation (15;17), and inversion of chromosome 16. Acute promyelocytic leukemia, which is FAB-M3, is characterized by the translocation of 15;17 which involves the rearrangement of the gene involving the retinoic acid receptor. This rearrangement makes this subtype of AML very responsive to all-*trans*-retinoic acid. The introduction of this agent has greatly increased survival for acute promyelocytic leukemia. Obtaining remission after induction chemotherapy is a favorable prognostic indicator in AML.

(B) Deletion of chromosome 7, also called monosomy 7, **(C)** deletion of chromosome 5, also called monosomy 5, 5q-, and 11q23 abnormalities have all been associated with an unfavorable prognosis. Patients with these abnormalities should proceed to either a matched sibling or an unrelated donor bone marrow transplant instead of receiving standard chemotherapeutic regimens. **(D, E)** Presence of Philadelphia chromosome, or translocation of (9;22) (q34;q11), indicates an unfavorable diagnosis and is associated more often with chronic myeloid leukemia rather than AML.

---

20 A 2-year-old boy presents to the emergency department with diffuse bruising. His examination is remarkable for ecchymoses on the extremities as well as a diffuse petechial rash on the trunk as seen in Figure 14-5. He otherwise appears well and his vital signs are within normal limits. His mother reports he had congestion approximately 10 days prior.

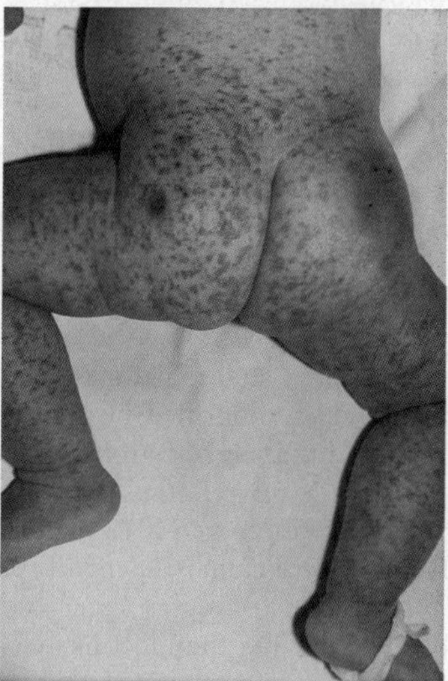

Figure 14-5

Of the following, which is the most likely cause for his presentation?

(A) Thrombotic thrombocytopenic purpura (TTP)
(B) Idiopathic thrombocytopenic purpura (ITP)
(C) Acute lymphoblastic leukemia (ALL)
(D) Acute myeloblastic leukemia
(E) Neuroblastoma

The answer is B: Idiopathic thrombocytopenic purpura (ITP). The most common cause for the acute onset of thrombocytopenia in children is ITP. The peak age at diagnosis is 1 to 4 years, and there is often a history of a preceding viral illness. This diagnosis should only be considered in those patients with isolated thrombocytopenia and who otherwise appear well with no abnormalities on physical examination, excluding the presence of ecchymoses or petechiae. Treatment options for ITP include observation, intravenous immunoglobulin administration, intravenous anti-D therapy, and steroids. Treatment is indicated in the setting of active bleeding and is generally given prophylactically if platelet counts are $\leq 20 \times 10^3/\mu L$. The most feared, but fortunately very rare complication of ITP is intracranial hemorrhage. Platelet transfusion is generally not indicated unless there is serious acute bleeding since the autoimmune destruction affects the transfused platelets as well.

The patient described in the vignette appears to have isolated thrombocytopenia based on examination findings and is well appearing. **(C, D)** These findings argue against an acute leukemia as these children typically have more than one cell line impacted and do not appear well. They also tend to have lymphadenopathy, hepatosplenomegaly, and/or fever. ALL is more common than AML. **(A)** TTP is rare in young children and typically presents in adolescents or adults. It consists of a pentad of fever, microangiopathic hemolytic anemia, thrombocytopenia, abnormal renal function, and central nervous system changes. **(E)** Neuroblastoma is a rare solid tumor that typically presents in children less than 2 years of age and often as an abdominal mass. The most common bruises seen with this tumor are periorbital due to tumor infiltration.

---

21 A 10-year-old boy with an abdominal mass is started on chemotherapy after his diagnosis is confirmed by pathology. After the initiation of chemotherapy, his serum electrolytes are as follows: sodium is 138 mEq/L, potassium is 6.5 mEq/L, chloride is 104 mEq/L, carbon dioxide is 26 mEq/L, urea nitrogen is 12 mg/dL, creatinine is 1.5 mg/dL, glucose is 113 mg/dL, calcium is 7.8 mg/dL, phosphorus is 7 mg/dL, and uric acid is 10 mg/dL.

Of the following, which is the most likely cause for this patient's abdominal mass?

(A) Burkitt lymphoma
(B) Wilms tumor
(C) Neuroblastoma
(D) Acute lymphoblastic leukemia
(E) Germ cell tumor

The answer is A: Burkitt lymphoma. The laboratory results in the vignette of hyperkalemia, hyperphosphatemia, hyperuricemia, and hypocalcemia are consistent with tumor lysis syndrome. Tumor lysis syndrome can result in acute renal failure, which is suggested by the elevated creatinine. The most common malignancies to cause tumor lysis syndrome are Burkitt lymphoma, T-cell lymphomas, and **(D)** acute leukemia presenting with significant leukocytosis. Of these, Burkitt lymphoma is most likely to present with an abdominal mass. T-cell lymphoma tends to present as a mediastinal mass. **(E)** Germ cell tumors can present as an abdominal mass in this age group but is not likely to cause tumor lysis syndrome. **(B, C)** Although Wilms tumor and neuroblastoma can present as abdominal masses, both are less likely in a 10-year-old patient and neither is characterized by a high risk for tumor lysis syndrome.

22 A 3-year-old girl with standard-risk precursor B-cell acute lymphoblastic leukemia presents to the emergency department with fever. The physical examination reveals a well-appearing child with mild rhinorrhea as her only symptom. The area surrounding an indwelling central venous catheter is clean, dry, and intact. A complete blood count is obtained which reveals a white blood cell count of $1.0 \times 10^3/\mu L$ with a differential of 35% neutrophils, 5% bands, 50% lymphocytes, and 10% monocytes.

Of the following, what is this patient's absolute neutrophil count (ANC)?

(A) 50 cells/μL
(B) 400 cells/μL
(C) 500 cells/μL
(D) 900 cells/μL
(E) 1,000 cells/μL

The answer is B: 400 cells/μL. The ANC for the patient in the vignette is 400 cells/μL. This is calculated with the following formula: ANC = (white blood cell count) × (neutrophils (%) + bands (%)). For example, the ANC of the patient in the vignette is calculated as follows: ANC = 1,000 × (0.35 + 0.05) = 400 cells/μL. An ANC greater than 1,500 cells/μL is considered normal.

23 Of the following, what is the next best step in management of the patient in the previous vignette?

(A) Obtain a blood culture from the patient's central venous line and begin cefepime immediately
(B) Obtain a blood culture from the patient's central venous line and wait to begin antibiotics if the culture is positive
(C) Obtain a blood culture from patient's central venous line and begin vancomycin immediately
(D) Obtain a blood culture from patient's central venous line and begin fluconazole immediately
(E) Reassure the family that her symptoms are likely caused by a viral illness and there is no need to begin antibiotics

The answer is A: Obtain a blood culture from patient's central venous line and begin cefepime immediately. Fever in the setting of neutropenia is considered a medical emergency. Patients being treated for leukemia are at increased risk for bacteremia due to their immunosuppression and presence of a central venous line. A complete physical examination should be done to search for a localizing source. Blood cultures should be obtained from all lumens of any central venous lines in place. **(B)** Even in the absence of a localizing source, broad-spectrum intravenous antibiotics should be started in those patients with fever and severe neutropenia, or absolute neutrophil count (ANC) of less than 500 cells/μL. Patients are at increased risk for both gram-positive organisms such as *Staphylococcus aureus* and *Staphylococcus epidermidis* and gram-negative organisms such as *Pseudomonas aeruginosa* and *Escherichia coli* and need coverage for both. Cefepime is a fourth-generation cephalosporin with good activity against both gram-negative and gram-positive organisms. It is generally well tolerated and makes an ideal choice for empiric coverage in febrile neutropenic patients.

(C) Vancomycin is used to treat gram-positive organisms. Its widespread use has led to the development of vancomycin-resistant *Enterococcus* and its use should be reserved for those patients with specific clinical indications. Vancomycin also has the potential for nephrotoxicity necessitating close monitoring of peak and trough serum levels. **(D)** Fluconazole can be used empirically when fungal infections are suspected in febrile neutropenic patients. Fungal infections are more likely in severely neutropenic patients who have had persistent fevers for longer than 3 to 5 days in the setting of appropriate antimicrobial coverage. **(E)** Although the patient in the vignette may indeed have a viral illness, she needs broad-spectrum antibiotic coverage until bacteremia can be safely ruled out. Generally, antibiotic coverage is continued until the patient becomes afebrile, has negative blood cultures for a minimum of 48 hours, and begins to have some recovery in the ANC.

24 A 5-year-old patient recently diagnosed with acute lymphoblastic leukemia is being discharged from the hospital.

Of the following, which medication should be included on his discharge medication list?

(A) Fluconazole
(B) Azithromycin
(C) Penicillin
(D) Trimethoprim–sulfamethoxazole
(E) Amoxicillin

The answer is D: **Trimethoprim–sulfamethoxazole.** Trimethoprim–sulfamethoxazole is given prophylactically to prevent pneumonia caused by *Pneumocystis jiroveci* in immunocompromised individuals. It is usually given 2 to 3 days/week and it should be started at the diagnosis of a malignancy and continued until the patient has been off of all therapy for 6 months. If a patient is allergic, alternatives include pentamidine and dapsone.

(A) Fluconazole is used as prophylaxis against fungal infections in certain high-risk malignancies, for example, AML. **(B)** Azithromycin is used as treatment against atypical bacterial infections. **(C)** Penicillin is used as prophylaxis in the sickle cell population against *Streptococcus pneumoniae* infections. **(E)** Amoxicillin is not typically used for prophylaxis in an immunocompromised patient.

25 A 15-year-old Caucasian boy presents to the emergency department with the chief complaint of leg pain. The review of systems is positive for fever, weight loss, and painful swelling noted in his lower leg. A radiograph is obtained, which demonstrates a lytic lesion with a significant multilaminar periosteal reaction (see *Figure 14-6*).

Of the following, which is this patient's most likely diagnosis?

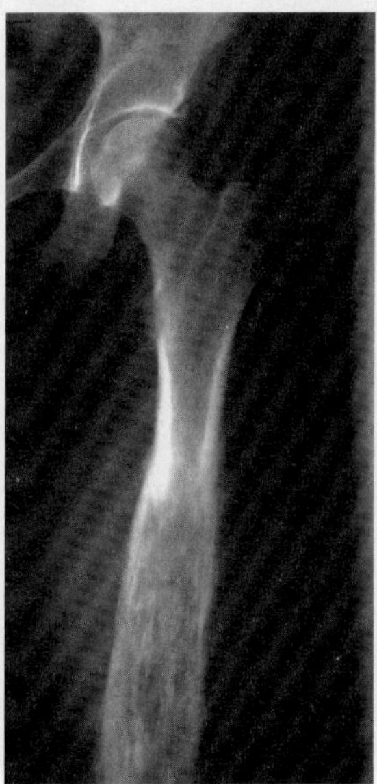

Figure 14-6

(A) Osteosarcoma
(B) Chondroblastoma
(C) Osteochondroma
(D) Osteoid osteoma
(E) Ewing sarcoma

The answer is E: Ewing sarcoma. The patient in the vignette has an examination that is consistent with a malignant bone tumor. Malignant bone tumors are most common in the second decade of life during the adolescent growth spurt and are more common in Caucasians. The most common bone tumors are Ewing sarcoma and osteosarcoma. Presence of systemic symptoms such as weight loss and fevers is more common with Ewing sarcoma. The radiographic finding in Figure 14-7 shows multilaminar periosteal reaction, otherwise known as onion skinning, and is consistent with Ewing sarcoma. Primary Ewing sarcomas can present either in the diaphyses of long bones or the axial skeleton, and metastasize most commonly to the lungs.

(A) Osteosarcoma can present with bony pain but usually does not present with systemic symptoms. The radiographic finding is described as sclerotic destruction in a sunburst pattern (see *Figure 14-8*). Osteosarcoma commonly affects the metaphyses of long bones with the lungs as the most common site of metastasis. Patients with familial retinoblastoma, Li-Fraumeni syndrome, and Paget disease are associated with a higher predisposition to develop osteosarcoma.

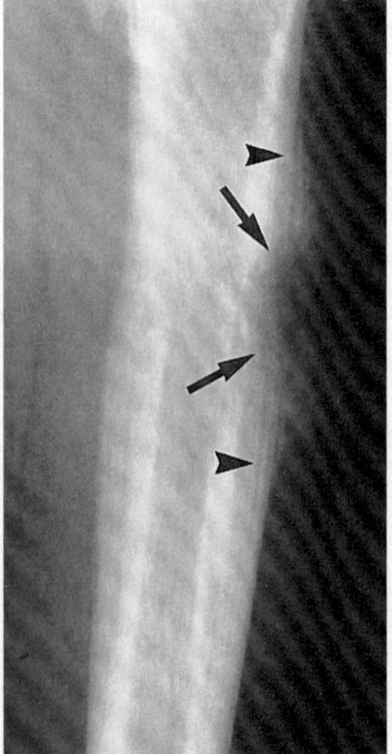

Figure 14-7

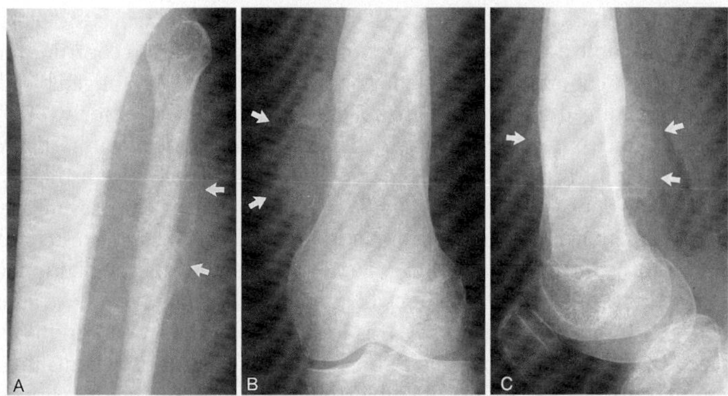

Figure 14-8

(B, C, D) Chondroblastoma, osteochondroma, and osteoid osteoma are all benign bone lesions that do not present with systemic symptoms. Chondroblastoma is a rare lesion found in the epiphyses of long bones and presents with joint pain. Osteochondroma is one of the most common benign bone tumors of childhood. Many lesions are completely asymptomatic and may go undetected. Osteoid osteoma is a small benign bone tumor that causes pain that is progressive and awakens the patient at night but is relieved by nonsteroidal anti-inflammatory drugs while pain caused from malignant bone tumors is not. Treatment of osteoid osteoma is removal of the lesion.

26 An 8-year-old boy has prolonged pharyngeal bleeding the evening following a tonsillectomy and adenoidectomy. Review of systems is positive for a history of occasional nosebleeds and his mother thinks he is an "easy bruiser." Family history reveals a maternal history of menorrhagia.

Of the following, which is the most likely cause of this patient's prolonged postoperative bleeding?

(A) Hemophilia A
(B) Hemophilia B
(C) Factor XIII deficiency
(D) Inadequate surgical cauterization
(E) von Willebrand disease (vWD)

The answer is E: von Willebrand disease (vWD). vWD is the most common hereditary bleeding disorder. It presents primarily with mucocutaneous bleeding episodes such as epistaxis, excessive bruising, menorrhagia, and postoperative bleeding. Von Willebrand factor is a large multimeric glycoprotein produced in megakaryocytes and endothelial cells and participates in normal coagulation by binding to exposed endothelium. Platelets then bind to von

Willebrand protein through the glycoprotein 1B receptor. Once the platelets bind, they become activated and cause more platelets to bind, contributing to clot formation. Laboratory testing may or may not reveal a prolonged bleeding time and prolonged PTT. There are specific diagnostic assays for vWD. The therapy of choice is desmopressin, which induces the release of von Willebrand factor from endothelial cells and is used as needed for bleeding episodes.

(A, B) Patients with hemophilia A or B may present with severe bleeding such as hemarthrosis and intraoperative bleeding. These disorders most often present prior to 8 years of age. Factor XIII is a fibrin-stabilizing factor in the clotting cascade that is responsible for stabilizing clots that have already formed. **(C)** Deficiency of factor XIII is less common than vWD and is characterized by delayed bleeding due to unstable clot formation. Patients present with mild bruising, poor wound healing, and recurrent spontaneous abortions. Neonates with this deficiency can have a delay in umbilical stump separation beyond 4 weeks. **(D)** Although inadequate surgical cauterization is a possible cause of postoperative bleeding, the constellation of personal and family histories for the patient in the vignette suggests a clotting disorder.

27 A 1-year-old boy comes to clinic for a routine health maintenance visit. The mother states that the family has recently moved from a livestock farm and that her son is a picky eater and drinks milk exclusively from the family's farm. She also states that she found him with a paint chip in his mouth last week. A screening complete blood count is drawn and shows the following results:

White blood cell count:	$7.2 \times 10^3/\mu L$
Hemoglobin:	8.1 g/dL
Hematocrit:	25%
Mean corpuscular volume:	105 fL
Platelets:	$350 \times 10^3/\mu L$

Of the following, which is the most likely explanation for this patient's blood work?

(A) Vitamin B_{12} deficiency
(B) Iron deficiency
(C) Folic acid deficiency
(D) Lead ingestion
(E) Copper deficiency

The answer is C: Folic acid deficiency. The complete blood count of the patient in the vignette shows a macrocytic, or megaloblastic, anemia and of the choices listed, only folic acid deficiency and vitamin B_{12} deficiency cause a megaloblastic anemia. Goat's milk does not contain folate. Humans are unable to make folate and thus depend on their diet to obtain the necessary amounts. Folate can be found in green vegetables, fruits, and animal organs; however, folate is heat labile so cooking foods will decrease the amount of the vitamin present. Infants have limited stores of folate, and if not provided in their diet, develop anemia within 2 to 3 months.

(A) Vitamin B_{12}, or cobalamin, deficiency also causes a megaloblastic anemia. Infants/children have a greater ability to store vitamin B_{12}; thus, anemia from deficiency generally does not present before the age of 3 to 5 years. Those adhering to a vegan diet are at increased risk for vitamin B_{12} deficiency since animal protein is a good source of vitamin B_{12}. **(B, D, E)** Iron deficiency, lead poisoning, and copper deficiency are all associated with microcytic rather than megaloblastic anemia. While eating paint chips of lead-based paints is a risk factor for anemia, the patient in the vignette's anemia is macrocytic rather than microcytic.

28 A 2-year-old boy is being evaluated in clinic for the first time after recently moving to the area. He has been taking 5 mg/kg/day of elemental iron over the past 2 months as prescribed by his previous pediatrician as treatment for iron deficiency anemia. A complete blood count drawn today shows the following:

Hemoglobin concentration:	9.8 g/dL
Mean corpuscular volume:	62 fL
Red cell distribution width (RDW):	12%

Of the following, which is the most likely reason for this patient's persistent anemia?

(A) β-Thalassemia major
(B) β-Thalassemia trait
(C) Transient erythroblastopenia of childhood (TEC)
(D) Nonadherence with iron therapy at home
(E) Inadequate prescribed iron therapy dosing

The answer is B: β-Thalassemia trait. Iron deficiency anemia and β-thalassemia trait commonly have similar presentations. They both cause a microcytic anemia but a key difference is the RDW. The RDW describes the variation of sizes among a population of red blood cells. Iron deficiency causes an increased RDW while β-thalassemia trait does not change the RDW from the normal range. One should suspect β-thalassemia trait when a microcytic anemia fails to improve with appropriate iron therapy. β-Thalassemia is caused by a mutation in the gene responsible for the β-subunit of hemoglobin.

(D) Nonadherence with prescribed therapy should be considered in any treatment failure, but the RDW in the vignette does not support iron deficiency as the underlying cause of the anemia. **(E)** The recommended dosage of iron therapy for iron deficiency anemia is 3 to 6 mg/kg of elemental iron per day. The patient in the vignette was prescribed an appropriate dose. **(A)** β-Thalassemia major is a more severe disorder that presents in the first few months of life with severe anemia. If untreated, infants can have cardiac decompensation and death by 6 months of age. Patients can develop massive hepatosplenomegaly, pathologic bone fractures, and have atypical facies such as maxilla hyperplasia, flat nasal bridge, frontal bossing (see *Figure 14-9*). These patients become transfusion-dependent and as a result, often have iron overload requiring iron chelation therapy. A hemoglobin electrophoresis done at birth reveals only fetal hemoglobin. Cure can be obtained with bone marrow transplantation. **(C)** TEC causes a normocytic anemia and commonly resolves over a period of 1 to 2 months and is inconsistent with the patient in the vignette.

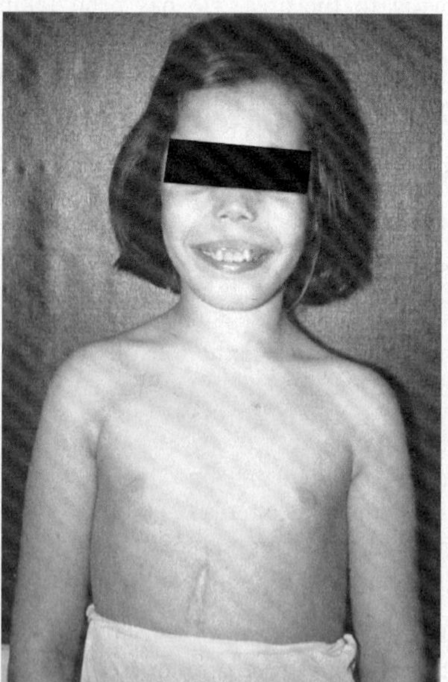

Figure 14-9

29 Which of the following laboratory patterns is most consistent with iron deficiency anemia?

(A) Decreased mean corpuscular volume (MCV), decreased serum ferritin, decreased total iron binding capacity
(B) Decreased MCV, increased RDW, increased ferritin
(C) Decreased MCV, decreased serum ferritin, increased total iron binding capacity
(D) Decreased serum ferritin, increased RDW, decreased total iron binding capacity
(E) Increased MCV, increased RDW, increased total iron binding capacity

The answer is C: Decreased MCV, decreased serum ferritin, increased total iron binding capacity. Iron deficiency anemia is the most common nutritional cause of anemia found worldwide; it is commonly caused by excess milk ingestion in children 9 months to 2 years of age. Bovine milk has low iron content and can cause chronic blood loss from milk protein colitis.

Iron deficiency causes a microcytic anemia with an increase in red blood cell distribution width and increase in total iron binding capacity. Ferritin is an excellent indicator of iron storage and a reliable indicator of iron deficiency. Iron levels are not always helpful as they are influenced by recent dietary consumption of iron but in general, they are decreased in iron deficiency anemia. Ferritin levels drop before iron levels as iron deficiency anemia develops and ferritin levels take longer to normalize than iron levels once treatment is initiated.

Recommended treatment is 3 to 6 mg/kg of elemental iron. Hemoglobin concentrations should normalize within approximately 1 month but treatment should continue until ferritin levels normalize which may take 2 to 3 months. If hemoglobin concentrations do not rise as expected, another diagnosis such as thalassemia should be considered.

30 A 7-year-old boy with sickle cell disease presents to the emergency department with fever. Physical examination is unremarkable except for an elevated temperature and slightly erythematous cheeks. A complete blood count is obtained which reveals a white blood cell count of $3.4 \times 10^3/\mu L$, hemoglobin concentration of 4.3 g/dL, and platelet count of $45 \times 10^3/\mu L$. A reticulocyte count is 0.1%.

Of the following, which is the most likely diagnosis?

(A) Splenic sequestration
(B) Acute chest syndrome
(C) acute lymphoblastic leukemia (ALL)
(D) Aplastic crisis
(E) Sickle cell pain crisis

The answer is D: Aplastic crisis. The combination of pancytopenia with a decreased reticulocyte count in a patient with sickle cell disease is consistent with an aplastic crisis. In sickle cell disease, this can often be brought on following an infection with parvovirus B19 but other viruses can also cause an aplastic crisis. Treatment is supportive with blood products only if the patient becomes symptomatic.

(A) Splenic sequestration can result in a decreased hemoglobin concentration and platelet count but should not impact the white blood cell count or reduce the reticulocyte count. This condition can also be preceded by a viral illness. Treatment is supportive and blood transfusions may be needed. Splenectomy may be indicated if a patient has recurrent splenic sequestrations. **(E)** Sickle cell pain crises occur when red blood cells deform to a sickle shape and become caught in the capillary circulation. **(B)** Acute chest syndrome occurs when this deformity takes places within the lung and presents with fever, cough, and hypoxia. It is associated with a new infiltrate on chest radiograph. Leukocytosis may be present as the etiology is often infectious, but pancytopenia and a depressed reticulocyte count are not routinely expected. Treatment is a combination of supportive care including oxygen and incentive spirometry along with antibiotics such as a cephalosporin and a macrolide. Simple transfusions of packed red blood cells can be used to increase a low hemoglobin concentration, but exchange transfusions may be necessary. **(C)** ALL may present with pancytopenia, but both of these diagnoses are less likely than aplastic crisis in a patient with known sickle cell disease.

---

31 A 14-year-old boy is diagnosed with Hodgkin lymphoma.

Of the following, which group of symptoms is associated with the worst prognosis?

(A) Fever >39°C, pruritus, weight loss of >10% body weight
(B) Weight loss of >10% body weight, drenching night sweats, pruritus
(C) Fever >39°C, painful adenopathy, weight loss of >10% body weight
(D) Fever >39°C, weight loss of >10% body weight, drenching night sweats
(E) Fever >39°C, weight loss of >10% body weight, anorexia

The answer is D: Fever >39°C, weight loss of >10% body weight, drenching night sweats. The prognosis of Hodgkin disease is impacted by the presence or absence of B symptoms. Presence of these is associated with poorer prognosis. The B symptoms are fever >39°C for at least 3 days, weight loss of 10% of the patient's body weight within the previous 6 months, and drenching night sweats. Other symptoms that can be present with Hodgkin disease but are not related to prognosis include pruritus, lethargy, anorexia, and pain that may worsen after the ingestion of alcohol.

32 A 14-month-old boy with a new diagnosis of neuroblastoma is being treated with chemotherapy. The nurse calls report that he has gross hematuria and is passing clots of blood from his urethra.

Of the following, which chemotherapeutic agent is most likely the cause of this side effect?

(A) Methotrexate
(B) Vincristine
(C) Cisplatin
(D) Cyclophosphamide
(E) Bleomycin

The answer is D: Cyclophosphamide. The patient in the vignette is experiencing hemorrhagic cystitis. This is characterized by dysuria and gross hematuria, often with the passage of clots. Both cyclophosphamide and ifosfamide are associated with this side effect. Patients receiving either of these chemotherapeutic agents receive aggressive hydration both before and after administration as well as mesna disulfide to avoid this complication. Mesna disulfide inactivates cyclophosphamide metabolites and helps protect the bladder.

(A) Some common side effects of methotrexate include mucositis and bone marrow suppression. **(B)** Vincristine is associated with jaw pain, constipation, and peripheral neuropathy. **(C)** Side effects of cisplatin include ototoxicity and nephrotoxicity. **(E)** Pulmonary fibrosis is a potential side effect of bleomycin.

CHAPTER

15

Rheumatology

DIANA C. BOTTARI

1 A 10-year-old girl with a past medical history of oligoarticular juvenile idiopathic arthritis (JIA) presents for a follow-up visit. She has been on naproxen 275 mg twice daily for the past 6 weeks with some improvement in her pain. Her physical examination is significant for an edematous, tender left knee with decreased range of motion.

Of the following, which is the most effective adjunctive therapy for this patient?

(A) Glucocorticoids
(B) Antitumor necrosis factor
(C) Methotrexate
(D) Intravenous immunoglobulin
(E) Cyclosporin

The answer is C: Methotrexate. The patient in the vignette has oligoarticular JIA and has been managed with nonsteroidal anti-inflammatory drugs (NSAIDs). NSAIDs are the first-line treatment agent for oligoarticular, polyarticular, or systemic-onset JIA. If improvement is absent or minimal with NSAID therapy, a second-line agent is added. The safest and most efficacious second-line medication to start for either oligoarticular or polyarticular JIA is methotrexate. **(A)** Second-line therapy for systemic-onset JIA is glucocorticoids. Steroids are used as a third-line treatment in polyarticular JIA and during a severe flare and are usually not indicated for oligoarticular JIA. **(B)** The third-line treatment of oligoarticular JIA is antitumor necrosis factor medications.

(D, E) Intravenous immunoglobulin and cyclosporine are steroid-sparing agents and can be used as third-line medications for systemic JIA and refractory cases of polyarticular JIA.

2 A 16-year-old girl presents to her pediatrician's office with complaints of facial redness. She states she is getting teased at school and is self-conscious about the redness. Her review of systems is positive for

morning stiffness that is not related to activity. Her physical examination notes the findings pictured in Figure 15-1 as well as bilateral edema of her knees and ankles. Her complete blood cell count is significant for hemoglobin of 10.1 g/dL with a mean corpuscular volume of 70 fL and mean corpuscular hemoglobin concentration of 33 pg per cell.

Of the following, which would best help establish her diagnosis?

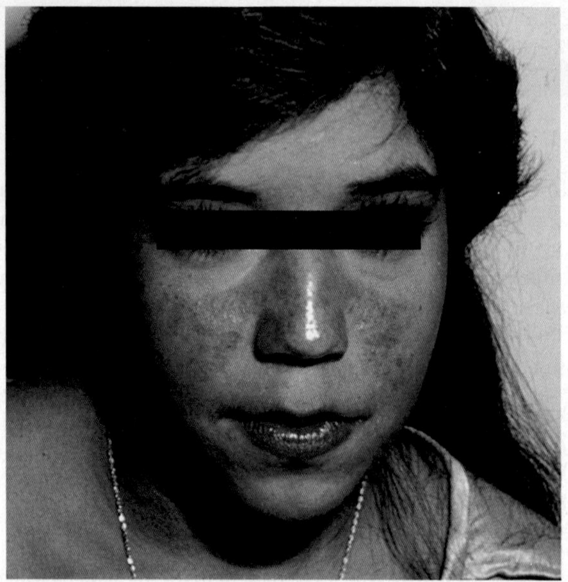

Figure 15-1

(A) Lymphopenia
(B) Elevated C-reactive protein
(C) Nasal ulcers
(D) Elevated erythrocyte sedimentation rate
(E) Fever

The answer is C: Nasal ulcers. The patient in the vignette has findings characteristic of systemic lupus erythematosus (SLE). SLE is a chronic inflammatory condition characterized by autoantibodies directed at self-antigens, immune complexes, and immune dysregulation. There is a female predominance. SLE can affect any organ system; however, it mainly affects the skin, kidney, joints, blood cells, and the nervous system.

Patients with SLE will have increased production of certain antibodies including anti-double-stranded DNA (anti-dsDNA), anti-Ro, anti-La, anti-Smith, anti-ribonucleoprotein (anti-RNP), and antiphospholipid antibodies. These antibodies can cause tissue damage by directly binding to the tissue or by forming immune complexes that are deposited into the tissues. The clinical manifestations of SLE are varied and include fever, fatigue, abnormalities seen on complete blood cell count, arthritis, rash, and renal disease.

To establish the diagnosis of SLE, patients require 4 of 11 criteria set forth by the American Academy of Rheumatology as follows:

- Malar rash: fixed erythema over the malar eminence with sparing of the nasal labial fold
- Discoid rash: erythematous raised patches with keratotic scaling, follicular plugging possibly leading to scarring
- Photosensitivity
- Oral or nasal ulcers
- Serositis: pleuritis or pericarditis
- Renal disease
- Neurologic disorder
- Immunologic disorder: anti-dsDNA, anti-Smith, antiphospholipid antibodies
- Antinuclear antibody (ANA)
- Hematologic disorder: anemia, leukopenia, lymphopenia, thrombocytopenia
- Arthritis: affecting two or more joints

The patient described in the vignette has a malar rash, arthritis, and microcytic anemia. Of the choices provided, only nasal ulcers are a diagnostic criterion for SLE for this patient. **(A)** Lymphopenia, anemia, and thrombocytopenia are all hematologic disorders and count as only one criterion in the same patient. **(B, D, E)** While most patients with SLE do have elevated C-reactive protein and erythrocyte sedimentation rates as well as fever, these findings are not diagnostic.

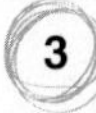

3 A 17-year-old young woman presents to clinic with complaints of dry mouth for the last 3 months. She continually has to drink while eating or the food feels like it gets stuck in her throat. She is unable to wear her contacts secondary to irritation. On physical examination, she has edema of her parotid glands bilaterally.

Of the following, what is her most likely diagnosis?

(A) Mumps
(B) Sjogren syndrome
(C) Gastroesophageal reflux (GER)
(D) Achalasia
(E) Scleroderma

The answer is B: Sjogren syndrome. The patient in the vignette has Sjogren syndrome, a chronic inflammatory disease characterized by lymphocytic infiltration of the salivary and lacrimal glands. Sjogren syndrome is most frequently seen in the third to fourth decades of life with the majority of those afflicted being women. Clinical manifestations of Sjogren syndrome include symptoms related to exocrine dysfunction of the epithelial surface of mucus membranes including the eye, mouth, nose, trachea, vagina, and skin. Symptoms include blurred vision, photophobia, dry eye, dry mouth, frequent dental caries, halitosis, hoarse voice, and angular cheilitis. In the pediatric population, the most common complaint is recurrent unilateral or bilateral parotid gland swelling or parotitis.

(A) Mumps is unlikely for the patient in the vignette based on her age, lack of fever, as well as the likelihood she received the mumps vaccination. **(C)** GER usually causes a bad taste in the mouth, burning in the chest, and may cause a feeling of having something lodged in the esophagus. GER is not associated with dry eyes or edema of the parotid glands. **(D)** Achalasia is a primary esophageal dysmotility. Patients with achalasia can present with complaints of feeling as if food is stuck in their throat; however, the dry mucus membranes and parotid edema described in the vignette are not found in achalasia. **(E)** Scleroderma is a connective tissue disorder which is characterized by fibrosis affecting the skin, arteries, gastrointestinal tract, and kidneys.

4 A 10-year-old girl presents to clinic for a follow-up visit for a 2-month history of recurrent left knee pain. She noticed that the pain first began following a hospitalization for dehydration and acute gastroenteritis. She has been to the clinic and multiple emergency departments for complaints of pain worse in the morning and evening. Radiography of her knee is within normal limits. She reports that her pain is gone today and she wants to return to gym at school. On examination, she is well appearing and has full range of motion of her joints with no evidence of edema or erythema.

Of the following, what is the most likely diagnosis for her resolved knee pain?

(A) juvenile idiopathic arthritis (JIA)
(B) Osteomyelitis
(C) Reactive arthritis
(D) Inflammatory bowel disease
(E) Primary gout

The answer is C: Reactive arthritis. Reactive arthritis is a postinfectious arthritis that occurs following an enteric infection or genitourinary tract infection. The most common organisms associated with reactive arthritis are *Salmonella* sp., *Shigella* sp., *Yersinia enterocolitica*, *Campylobacter jejuni*, *Cryptosporidium parvum*, *Giardia intestinalis*, *Chlamydia trachomatis*, and *Ureaplasma* sp. Arthritis may become apparent 1 to 2 months after the inciting infection. Large joints are typically affected asymmetrically and can remain affected up to 6 months or longer. Treatment is aimed at pain management with the first-line treatment being nonsteroidal anti-inflammatory drugs. Reactive arthritis is a diagnosis of exclusion and usually made once the arthritis has resolved. The patient in the vignette has a known history of acute gastroenteritis and developed asymmetric arthritis lasting less than 6 months; therefore reactive arthritis is the most likely diagnosis.

(A) JIA is unlikely, as the symptoms described in the vignette have completely resolved. **(B)** Osteomyelitis is associated with fever and does not resolve without treatment. **(D)** Inflammatory bowel disease is a possibility; however, there is no indication in the vignette that the patient has any continued gastrointestinal symptomatology. **(E)** Primary gout is a condition where hyperuricemia leads to deposition of urate crystals in the joints and surrounding tissue leading to joint pain and swelling, most commonly seen in middle-aged men.

5 An 18-year-old young man with ankylosing spondylitis presents for a follow-up appointment. His genetic testing notes human leukocyte antigen (HLA) B-27 positive.

Of the following, which is he at greatest risk for developing?

(A) Osteomyelitis
(B) Rheumatoid arthritis
(C) Long bone fractures
(D) Renal failure
(E) Uveitis

The answer is E: Uveitis. The HLA system is genetically encoded on chromosome 6 by the major histocompatibility complex (MHC). MHC plays a vital role in immunity and self-recognition in the body. MHC Class I includes HLA-A, HLA-B, and HLA-C which present antigens to CD8 or T-suppressor cells. MHC Class II, the HLA-D, presents antigens to CD4 or T-helper cells. HLA-B27 has the strongest correlation with ankylosing spondylitis. It has also been associated with many other diseases including reactive arthritis, psoriatic arthritis, and inflammatory bowel disease. Having HLA-B 27 increases the risk for patients with ankylosing spondylitis to develop anterior uveitis. The mechanism behind HLA-B27's involvement with disease is unknown; however, the current theory on the mechanism is molecular mimicry. Molecular mimicry describes an antigen from an infectious agent that closely resembles HLA-B27 and therefore results in an immune response to HLA-B27 rather than the original antigen.

(A, B, C, D) Patients who are HLA-B27 positive are not at increased risk for osteomyelitis, rheumatoid arthritis, long bone fractures, or renal failure.

6 A 7-year-old girl is admitted to the pediatric ward with complaints of abdominal and ankle pain. A photograph of her lower extremity is seen in Figure 15-2.

Of the following, what is the most likely mechanism for these findings?

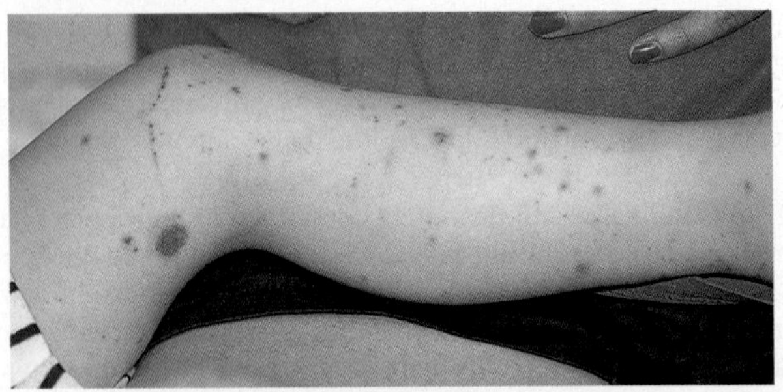

Figure 15-2

(A) Microscopic polyangiitis
(B) Rheumatoid vasculitis
(C) Large vessel vasculitis
(D) Small vessel vasculitis
(E) Urticarial vasculitis

The answer is D: Small vessel vasculitis. The patient in the vignette has Henoch-Schönlein purpura (HSP), which is a small vessel vasculitis. The exact etiology of HSP is unknown; however, the majority of patients have a preceding viral or gastrointestinal infection. HSP is an IgA-mediated autoimmune small vessel vasculitis. IgA forms immune complexes that are then deposited in the small vessels leading to the characteristic rash and other manifestations of the disease. The rash usually begins as blanching maculopapules on the lower trunk, buttocks, and lower extremities and evolves into large non-blanching purpura. Other common signs and symptoms of the disease are arthritis, abdominal pain, vomiting, diarrhea, proteinuria, and hematuria. The diagnosis of HSP is based on palpable purpuric lesions located on the dependent parts of the body. The treatment of HSP is symptomatic with adequate hydration, and use of nonsteroidal anti-inflammatory drugs for joint pain. Urinalysis should be obtained at presentation and followed for 6 months to monitor for signs of chronic renal disease.

(A) Microscopic polyangiitis is a necrotizing small vessel vasculitis. It is mediated by antineutrophil cytoplasmic antibodies rather than by immune complex deposition. **(C)** A large vessel vasculitis would present with involvement of larger vessels, for example, the aorta and its branches as seen in Takayasu arteritis. **(B)** Rheumatoid vasculitis is a small- and medium-sized vessel disease affecting patients with rheumatoid arthritis. **(E)** Urticarial vasculitis is also a leukocytoclastic angiitis like HSP but the appearance of the rash is erythematous wheals that clinically resemble urticaria and are not limited to the dependent surfaces of the body.

7 A 5-year-old boy of Turkish decent has recently transferred care to a new pediatrician. He has a history of recurrent fevers lasting 1 to 4 days with associated abdominal pain and has been hospitalized three times for these episodes. His mother states she was told it was a virus each time. He has a cousin who has experienced similar episodes. On examination, the boy appears healthy with no abnormalities. Confirmatory genetic testing for a periodic fever syndrome is pending.

Of the following, what is the most appropriate treatment for this patient?

(A) nonsteroidal anti-inflammatory drugs (NSAIDs)
(B) Corticosteroids
(C) Etanercept
(D) Chlorambucil
(E) Colchicine

The answer is E: Colchicine. The patient described in the vignette has familial Mediterranean fever (FMF). This is an autosomal recessive disease seen most commonly in patients of Turkish, Armenian, Arabic, and Sephardic Jewish decent. Patients with this disease usually present before 5 years of age with episodes of fever lasting 1 to 4 days. Patients also have at least one of the following: abdominal pain, arthritis/arthralgia, or chest pain. Genetic testing is used to confirm the diagnosis. Attacks of FMF can be prevented by use of colchicine twice daily. Colchicine not only reduces attacks but also decreases the risk for developing amyloidosis. Death from FMF is usually the result of complications due to amyloidosis. **(D)** Chlorambucil has been used in the treatment of amyloidosis but is not used in the treatment of periodic fever syndromes.

Treatment options for other periodic fever syndromes are varied and include **(A)** NSAIDs, **(B)** corticosteroids, and **(C)** etanercept; however, they are not the treatment choice for patients with FMF.

8 A 16-year-old girl is being seen in clinic following an abnormal anti-double-stranded DNA (anti-dsDNA) result and anemia on a recent laboratory workup. She initially presented with complaints of fatigue, joint pain, and swelling, as well as the rash pictured in Figure 15-3. Her vital signs are temperature 37.2°C, heart rate 82 beats/minute, respiratory rate 18 breaths/minute, and blood pressure 145/92 mmHg.

Of the following, which screening test/procedure does the patient require?

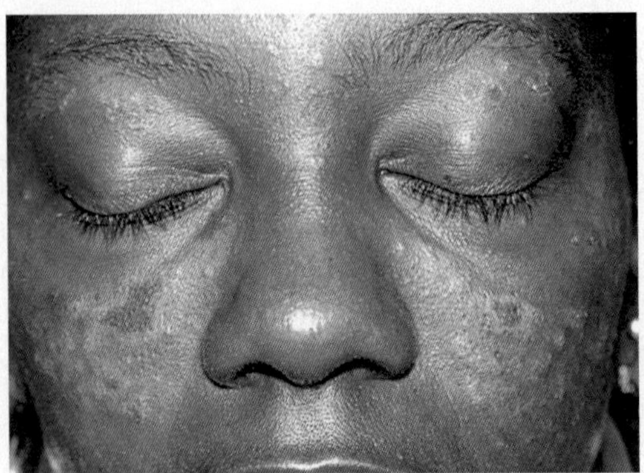

Figure 15-3

(A) Echocardiogram
(B) Chest radiography
(C) Electroencephalogram
(D) Core kidney biopsy
(E) C-reactive protein

The answer is D: Core kidney biopsy. The picture in the vignette is that of a discoid rash. The patient in the vignette has systemic lupus erythematosus (SLE), a chronic inflammatory condition characterized by autoantibodies directed at self-antigen, immune complexes, and immune dysregulation. Kidney disease is one of the most common features in children with SLE and accounts for a significant portion of the morbidity and mortality associated with SLE. Lupus nephritis is present in many patients with SLE and may manifest with hypertension. Therefore, the next best step for the patient in the vignette is to evaluate for renal pathology with a biopsy. Immune complexes are formed from autoantibodies circulating in the body, and then deposited in the glomeruli. Immune complexes are also deposited in the basement membrane by autoantibodies combining with antigens located within the glomeruli themselves. These immune complexes induce an inflammatory response by activating the complement system and attracting lymphocytes, macrophages, and neutrophils.

(A) Echocardiogram is not warranted unless the patient has signs of pericarditis or other cardiac pathology. Although hypertension can be associated with cardiac abnormalities, the more likely etiology for a patient with SLE is renal. **(B)** Chest radiography in patients with SLE is not indicated without respiratory complaints. **(C)** Electroencephalogram would be indicated if the patient had signs of neurologic disease. **(E)** While a C-reactive protein would be expected to be elevated in a patient with SLE, it does not explain her hypertension.

9 The mother of a 17-year-old Lebanese young man is extremely upset because she believes her child has a sexually transmitted disease. She states that she became concerned when she noticed her son limping and he admitted to having sores on his penis. He seemed to be in significant pain and was unable to stand up straight. His confidential HEADDSS history reveals that he is not sexually active. He explains that over the past 12 months he has had recurrent ulcers that appear on his penis for 1 week and are extremely painful. On examination, he has three ulcers located on the glans and shaft of penis. The ulcers are shallow and 4 mm in diameter with surrounding erythema. His buccal mucosa contains several small ulcers and he has edema and decreased range of motion of his left knee.

Of the following, what is the best explanation of this patient's complaints?

(A) Sjogren syndrome
(B) Behçet disease
(C) Herpes simplex virus
(D) Inflammatory bowel disease
(E) Syphilis

The answer is B: Behçet disease. Behçet disease is a waxing and waning condition in which patients have recurrent and painful oral and genital ulcerations. It is most commonly seen in patients of Middle Eastern decent. While the etiology of such conditions is unclear, there is a strong association with HLA-B5 and HLA-B51. This disease process, like many of the connective tissue diseases, is a vasculitis of small- and medium-sized arteries that leads to fibrinoid necrosis and obliteration of the vessel lumens. Patients with Behçet disease have recurrent painful shallow ulcers, 2 to 10 mm in diameter with surrounding erythema that may occur on the buccal mucosa, gingiva, lips, tongue, labia, scrotum, or penis. The ulcers usually persist for 1 to 3 weeks. Patients may also have recurrent asymmetric, polyarticular large joint arthritis. Skin manifestations include erythema nodosum, papulopustular lesions, and acneiform nodules. Ocular manifestations include anterior and posterior uveitis and retinal vasculitis. The central nervous system may also be involved which may lead to meningoencephalitis, cranial nerve palsies, and even psychosis, though this is typically seen late in the disease course.

(A) The patient in the vignette has no complaints of dry mouth or dry eye making Sjogren syndrome unlikely. **(C, E)** Though herpes simplex virus and syphilis should be considered even with a patient denying sexual activity, the triad of arthritis and ulcers in both the mouth and genital area make Behçet disease a more likely diagnosis. **(D)** Patients with inflammatory bowel disease can have recurrent oral ulcers and arthritis years before gastrointestinal symptoms present; however, genital ulcers are not typical.

---

10 An 8-year-old girl presents with a facial and extremity rash as noted in Figures 15-4 and 15-5. Her physical examination is notable for difficulty in lifting her head off the examination table.

Of the following, what laboratory abnormality would best support her findings?

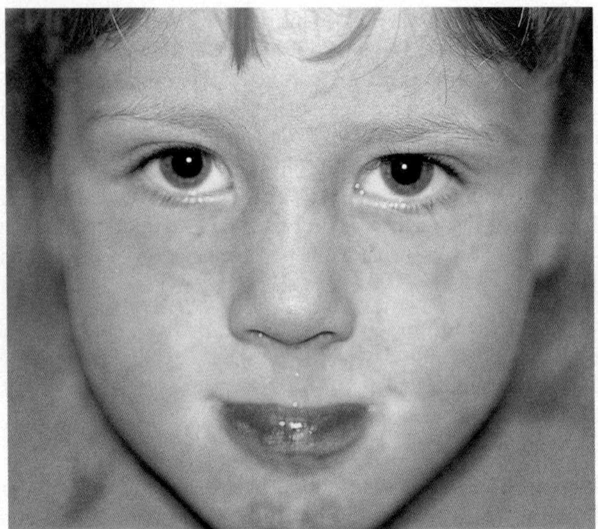

Figure 15-4

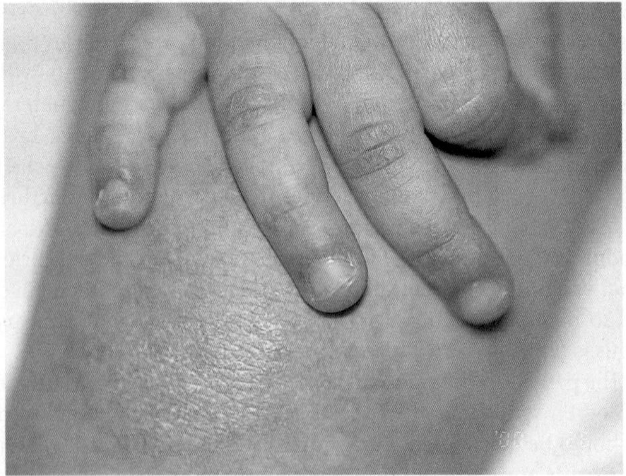

Figure 15-5

(A) Complete blood cell count
(B) Creatine kinase
(C) Prothrombin time
(D) Liver enzymes
(E) Erythrocyte sedimentation rate

The answer is B: Creatine kinase. The patient pictured in the vignette has findings consistent with juvenile dermatomyositis (JDM). JDM is the most common inflammatory pediatric myopathy. The etiology is believed to be a genetic predisposition combined with antigen stimulation and other environmental factors. A history of infection within 3 months of the onset of the disease is usually elicited. The majority of patients present with a characteristic rash on sun-exposed areas. The rash is described as a periorbital violaceous rash that may extend across the nasal bridge in a mask-like distribution. A palpable rash, known as Gottron papules, may be noticed over joints. The metacarpal–phalangeal and intercarpal–phalangeal joints are particularly affected. The rash also may be seen on the joints of the knees, elbows, and medial malleoli. Nailfold telangiectasias, periungual erythema, and hypertrophic, ragged cuticles may be noted. The weakness associated with JDM is proximal in nature making climbing stairs, combing hair, brushing teeth, and getting in or out of a bed, car, or chair difficult. One of the first signs of weakness is neck flexor weakness, which results in the inability to raise one's head from the bed. Diagnosis of JDM is made clinically with the presence of the characteristic rash and symmetric proximal muscle weakness. The diagnosis is supported by elevated muscle enzymes, myopathic changes on electromyography, abnormal muscle biopsy findings, calcinosis, or positive magnetic resonance imaging.

(A, C, D, E) Abnormalities in the complete blood cell count, prothrombin time, liver enzymes, or erythrocyte sedimentation rate are not diagnostic for JDM.

---

11 A previously healthy 16-year-old girl presents to her pediatrician with complaints of right arm tightness and discoloration. She reports a history of the tips of her fingers becoming white followed by redness and paresthesias when she is cold or stressed. Her physical examination is significant for linear thickening of her right forearm. The skin on her right arm appears darker and glossier compared to the other arm.

Of the following, what is her most likely diagnosis?

(A) Reactive arthritis
(B) Henoch-Schönlein purpura (HSP)
(C) Localized burn
(D) Localized scleroderma
(E) Behçet disease

The answer is D: Localized scleroderma. The patient in the vignette has localized scleroderma. Scleroderma is a chronic disease characterized by fibrosis and associated vascular damage and decreased vasculogenesis. It is rare in the pediatric age group and most often affects women in the third to fifth decades of life. Children most commonly have localized scleroderma. In localized scleroderma, the involvement is limited to the skin. Fibrosis can involve the dermis, subcutaneous fat, and muscle and may even involve the bone leading to joint contractures and deformities. Localized scleroderma very rarely evolves into systemic sclerosis. In systemic sclerosis internal organs including the lung, kidney, and gastrointestinal tracts also go through extensive fibrosis.

Evaluation of all patients' with suspected scleroderma should include pulmonary function testing, a contrast upper gastrointestinal study, and an echocardiogram to assess for pulmonary hypertension. Diagnosis of scleroderma is based on diagnostic criteria and requires one major criterion or two minor criteria. The major criterion is sclerodermatous skin changes proximal to the metocarpophalangeal or metatarsophalangeal joints. Minor criteria include sclerodactyly, or skin changes limited to the digits; digital pitting scars resulting from digital ischemia; and bibasilar pulmonary fibrosis not due to primary lung disease. Raynaud phenomenon is commonly seen in patients with scleroderma and the complaints of the finger changes described in the vignette are consistent with Raynaud phenomenon.

(C) Though a localized burn could cause the changes seen in the patient in the vignette there is nothing in the history to suggest such a burn had taken place. Also, an acute burn does not account for the Raynaud phenomenon. **(A)** Reactive arthritis is a postinfectious arthritis that is not associated with Raynaud phenomenon or the additional cutaneous findings described in the vignette. **(E)** Behçet disease involves recurrent oral and genital ulcers. **(B)** HSP is a small vessel vasculitis associated with arthritis, purpura, abdominal pain, and hematuria.

12 A 17-year-old boy presents for a healthcare maintenance visit. He is tall in stature with a long face, high arched palate, and dental crowding. His arm span is noted to be greater than his height, and he has a 3/6 systolic ejection murmur with an associated click on cardiac examination.

Of the following, which abnormality in biosynthesis does he most likely have?

(A) Collagen
(B) Fibrillin-1
(C) Insulin-like growth factor-1 (IGF-1)
(D) Tuberin
(E) Copper transporting protein

The answer is B: Fibrillin-1. The boy in the vignette has characteristics consistent with Marfan syndrome, an autosomal dominant disorder caused by a mutation of FBN1 located on the long arm of chromosome 15 (15q21). This locus encodes for the protein fibrillin-1. Fibrillin-1 is the main constituent of the microfibrils of the extracellular matrix. Diagnostic criteria for Marfan syndrome are mainly clinical and involve the skeletal system (pectus carinatum, pectus excavatum, wrist and thumb hyperlaxity, scoliosis, and high arched palate with dental crowding), ocular system (ectopia lentis, flat cornea, hypoplastic iris, hypoplastic ciliary muscle), cardiovascular system (dilation of aortic root, dissection of the aorta, mitral valve prolapse), pulmonary system (pneumothorax, apical blebs), and skin (striae without weight gain, recurrent hernia).

(A) Collagen defects are associated with many disease processes including Ehler-Danlos and osteogenesis imperfecta. **(C)** IGF-1 abnormalities are associated with gigantism and acromegaly. **(D)** Deficiency in tuberin is associated with tuberous sclerosis. **(E)** Menkes disease is a progressive neurodegenerative condition associated with a mutation in the copper transporting protein.

13 A 14-year-old girl presents to clinic for a sports preparticipation physical examination for track and field. She complains of increased stiffness in her ankles for the past year. The stiffness is worse in the morning and after sitting in school all day. She has tried over-the-counter nonsteroidal medications with some relief of her discomfort. Her past medical history and review of systems are otherwise unremarkable. On physical examination, she has bilateral edema at her ankle joints.

Of the following, what is the most likely cause of her joint stiffness and swelling?

(A) Septic arthritis
(B) Legg-Calvé-Perthes disease
(C) Oligoarticular juvenile idiopathic arthritis (JIA)
(D) Polyarticular JIA
(E) Systemic JIA

The answer is C: Oligoarticular juvenile idiopathic arthritis (JIA). The patient in the vignette has oligoarticular (pauciarticular) JIA. Arthritis is defined as intra-articular swelling and/or limitation of motion with associated pain, warmth, and erythema. The physical findings in JIA are a reflection of the extent of joint involvement. JIA is the most common rheumatologic condition in children and is defined as arthritis occurring for a minimum of 6 weeks' duration in children 16 years or younger. The exact etiology for JIA is unknown; however, there is a strong genetic component.

The three most common subtypes of JIA are as follows:

- Oligoarticular (pauciarticular)
  - Affects ≤4 large joints, for example, knees and ankles
  - Most common—accounting for 50% of the JIA cases
  - Usually seen children aged 2 years and older
  - Female to male ratio is 3:1
- **(D)** Polyarticular
  - Involves ≥5 small joints
  - Accounts for 40% of JIA cases
  - Usually seen in children aged 3 years or older
  - Female to male ratio is 3:1

- **(E) Systemic**
  - o Involves any number of both small and large joints
  - o Accounts for 10% of the JIA cases seen in any age group
  - o Signs and symptoms of systemic involvement
  - o Female to male ratio is 1:1

(A) Septic arthritis is unlikely in this particular patient since she does not have fever and does not have continuous pain. **(B)** Legg-Calvé-Perthes is avascular necrosis of the femoral head that typically presents as hip pain usually presenting in boys aged 3 to 12 years.

CHAPTER

16

Nutrition

TARA ALTEPETER

1 A mother brings her 14-month-old child to the outpatient office. The reason for the visit today is a severe diaper rash that seems to be resistant to all treatments the mother has tried. It has been present for the past 2 months (see *Figure 16-1*). The child is also having a similar red, scaly rash at the corners of her mouth. The mother breastfed the baby for the first year of life, and switched to cow milk around 12 months of age.

Of the following, which deficiency best explains the dermatologic findings in this patient?

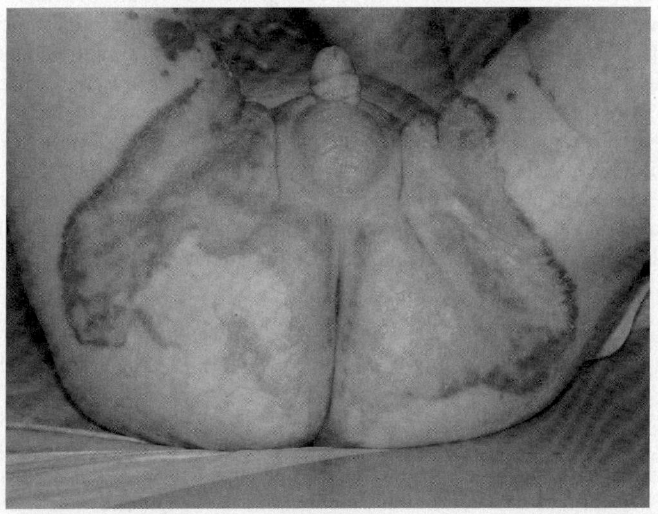

Figure 16-1

(A) Iron
(B) Vitamin B_{12}
(C) Vitamin C
(D) Zinc
(E) Vitamin E

The answer is D: **Zinc.** The patient in the vignette has acrodermatitis enteropathica caused by zinc deficiency. Zinc deficiency can occur from one of two mechanisms: either from inadequate dietary zinc intake, which is more common in developing nations or from an inherited autosomal recessive condition called acrodermatitis enteropathica. Children with acrodermatitis enteropathica have a dramatically reduced ability to absorb zinc from the diet. These patients commonly present shortly after being weaned from breast milk to cow milk. Breast milk contains a ligand, which enhances zinc absorption. Children with acrodermatitis enteropathica typically have a severe, scaly red rash in the diaper and perioral distributions. If left untreated, these patients can go on to develop failure to thrive, diarrhea, alopecia, and nail dystrophy, as well as demonstrate behavioral and neurologic changes. Treatment is with large doses of oral zinc supplementation, which can overcome the significantly reduced absorption that patients with acrodermatitis enteropathica demonstrate.

(A, B, C, E) Deficiencies of iron, vitamin B12, vitamin C, and vitamin E are generally not associated with dermatologic findings. Iron serves as part of the structure of hemoglobin and myoglobin. Deficiency results in a microcytic, hypochromic anemia. Vitamin B12 is absorbed in the ileum and deficiency results in a pernicious, macrocytic anemia. Vitamin C is an antioxidant that aids in iron absorption and collagen stability. Deficiencies present with scurvy, poor wound healing, bleeding gums, and infection. Vitamin E (α-tocopherol) is a potent antioxidant. Premature infants are at particular risk for developing vitamin E deficiency, as vitamin E stores are transferred during the third trimester. Vitamin E deficiency may present with hemolysis, thrombocytosis, and anemia. Vitamin E is a fat-soluble vitamin, and older children with fat malabsorption may also be at risk for becoming deficient.

---

2 A mother brings her 14-month-old child to clinic after 9 months without a visit. The child was born preterm at 28 weeks' gestation and was seen regularly until about 6 months of life. At that time, the family moved away but has returned to the area. The mother reports that the child seems irritable and is having trouble learning to walk. His diet consists mostly of junk food. He does not like milk and drinks only water and apple juice. On examination, his height and weight are less than the 5th percentile, and his lower extremity radiograph is pictured in *Figure 16-2*.

Of the following, which laboratory test would best aid in confirming this patient's diagnosis?

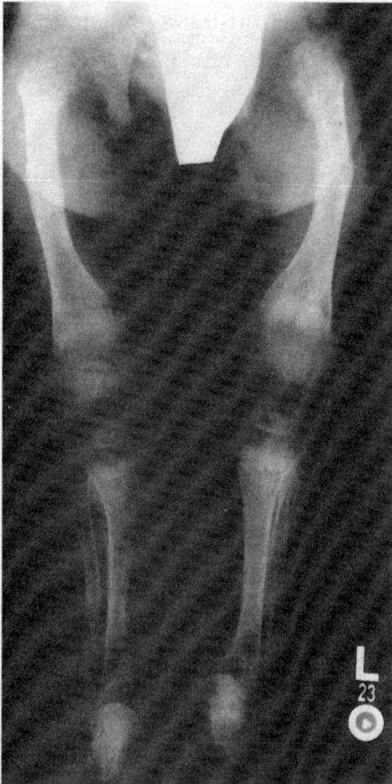

Figure 16-2

(A) 1,25-Hydroxyvitamin D
(B) 25-Hydroxyvitamin D
(C) Alkaline phosphatase
(D) Parathyroid hormone (PTH)
(E) Vitamin A level

The answer is B: 25-Hydroxyvitamin D. The radiography and clinical presentation for the patient in the vignette are consistent for the diagnosis of rickets. The child in the vignette has multiple risk factors for vitamin D deficiency including prematurity and poor milk intake. The recommended daily intake of vitamin D is at least 400 International Units. Vitamin D–deficient rickets and nutritional deficiency are characterized by decreased levels of 25-hydroxyvitamin D. (**C**) Alkaline phosphatase is elevated in patients with rickets, but is not specific for making the diagnosis.

(**D**) PTH levels are also elevated in vitamin D–deficient rickets but are not specific to the disorder. PTH is a counterregulatory hormone that is upregulated in response to low serum calcium. Treatment for vitamin D–deficient rickets is repletion of vitamin D stores. Children with vitamin D deficiency should also receive adequate calcium and phosphorus supplements.

(**A**) Low levels of 1,25-hydroxyvitamin D are seen primarily in children with chronic renal disease due to a failure of the 1-α-hydroxylase enzyme in the kidney. (**E**) Vitamin A levels would not be helpful in the evaluation of the patient in the vignette with findings consistent with vitamin D–deficient rickets. Patients with vitamin A deficiency present with night-blindness, failure to thrive, and poor bone formation.

3 The mother of a premature 7-week-old infant born at 32 weeks' gestation presents to clinic for a checkup after being discharged from the neonatal intensive care unit following a 6-week stay. During her hospitalization, she was intubated for 3 weeks and required nasogastric tube (NG) feedings. The patient was discharged home to continue NG feeds, but her mother reports she is scared of the NG tube and does not understand why her baby feeds poorly by mouth. On examination, she is alert, is in no acute distress, can focus on her mother's face, and has an NG in place.

Of the following, which is the most likely explanation for this patient's symptoms?

(A) Prematurity
(B) Intracranial bleed
(C) Gastroesophageal reflux
(D) Oral aversion
(E) Bronchopulmonary dysplasia

The answer is D: Oral aversion. Oral aversion is a common problem in neonates who have been hospitalized, intubated, and subjected to oral instrumentation. Frequent suctioning and other necessary medical procedures can lead to oral aversion, during which an infant refuses anything placed in his mouth. Preterm infants, patients who have undergone surgery in the neonatal period, and patients with extended periods of intubation are more likely to have an oral aversion. **(A)** Although the infant in the vignette is premature, not all premature infants develop an oral aversion. In a neurologically normal child, oral aversion should improve with time, and children benefit from feeding and speech therapy. Other treatment options include alternate nipple designs, devices to assist breastfeeding, and techniques to decrease oral sensitivity. An NG tube can provide an essential bridge allowing provision of adequate nutrition until the child's feeding skills improve.

(B, E) The patient in the vignette is well appearing on examination, thus making intracranial hemorrhage and bronchopulmonary dysplasia less likely etiologies of her feeding difficulty. **(C)** Although rarely patients with gastroesophageal reflux disease (GERD) develop oral aversion, this would be a later finding and unlikely in the newborn period.

4 A mother has been reading about the differences between breast milk and formula to make the best feeding decision for her baby. She has read that the proteins in breast milk are different than those in the formula and is inquiring which protein is superior.

Of the following, which statement is accurate regarding breast milk and formula composition?

(A) The predominant protein in breast milk is whey protein
(B) The formula contains higher concentrations of fatty acids helpful for brain and eye development
(C) The formula has a higher iron bioavailability
(D) Breast milk and formula contain the same amount of important nutrients
(E) Breast milk does not provide immunoprotection for the newborn

The answer is A: **The predominant protein in breast milk is whey protein.** Parents frequently have questions about the best nutrition for a newborn baby. Breast milk is the best source of nutrition for most healthy, term infants. **(E)** One difference between breast milk and formula is the protein composition. Breast milk is composed of 80% whey protein and 20% casein. The formula is casein predominant. **(B)** Breast milk contains docosahexaenoic acid and arachidonic acid, fatty acids thought to be important for brain and eye development. These compounds are found in some commercially prepared formulas. **(C)** It is true that there is more iron in the formula compared with breast milk; however, the iron in breast milk has much greater bioavailability and is generally sufficient for term infants up to 4 months of life. Breast milk is a complete source of nutrition for healthy term infants. **(E)** In addition to macronutrients, it provides many important substances to boost the infant's immune system such as maternal antibodies, which cannot be included in the formula. When possible, pediatricians should encourage and support mothers in the process of breastfeeding a newborn.

The parents of a 5-week-old infant bring the baby to the clinic with complaints of diarrhea that has been present for 3 days. Today, they note small streaks of blood in the stool. The baby has been fussy, less interested in feeding, and less active. On physical examination, the infant's abdomen is soft with no palpable masses, and there is no evidence of an anal fissure.

Of the following, what is the next best step in the management of this patient?

(A) Switch to a soy-based formula
(B) Switch to an amino acid–based formula
(C) Switch to a hydrolyzed formula
(D) Initiate ranitidine therapy
(E) Initiate loperamide therapy

The answer is C: **Switch to a hydrolyzed formula.** The symptoms described in the vignette are suggestive of milk protein allergy (MPA). The most effective treatment is removal of the offending agent. The first-line treatment is to replace the patient's formula with one whose protein is hydrolyzed. **(A)** A soy protein formula is not appropriate given the significant number of patients with MPA who have a similar reaction to soy protein. A hydrolyzed formula is sufficient to relieve symptoms in the majority of cases. **(B)** Patients who continue to have symptoms while taking a hydrolyzed formula may require an amino acid–based formula.

(D) Ranitidine therapy would be indicated in patients with gastroesophageal reflux disease (GERD). Symptoms of GERD include arching, turning red or crying with feeds, and excessive painful spit-ups. **(E)** Loperamide is an antidiarrheal medication. Treatment with antidiarrheal medications is generally not recommended in pediatric patients, and is never appropriate for an infant of this age.

6 On a medical care mission trip to Asia, many children appear similar to the child in *Figure 16-3*.

Of the following, what is the most likely mechanism responsible for the appearance of his abdomen?

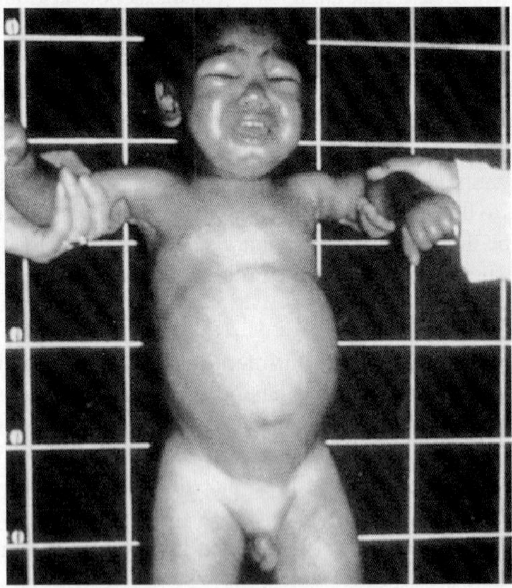

Figure 16-3

(A) Insufficient caloric intake
(B) Insufficient protein intake
(C) Insufficient fat intake
(D) Insufficient milk intake
(E) Insufficient carbohydrate intake

The answer is B: Insufficient protein intake. Severe malnutrition can present with one of two phenotypes. The very thin, emaciated child with loose skin, minimal subcutaneous fat, and a flat abdomen is described as having marasmus, or nonedematous severe malnutrition (see *Figure 16-4*). Alternatively,

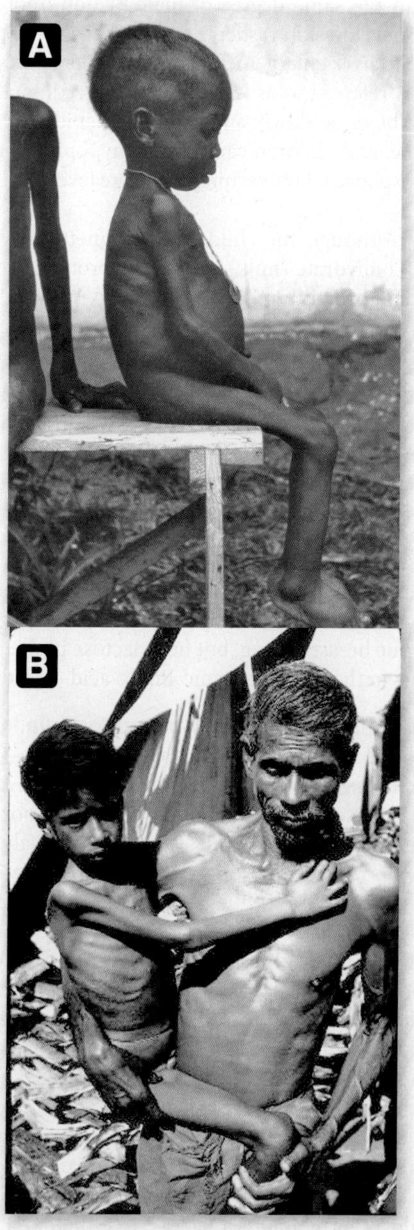

Figure 16-4

some children with the same degree of malnutrition, more specifically protein malnutrition, develop skin rashes, thinning hair, and a protuberant abdomen, which is due to liver enlargement as well as edema secondary to hypoalbuminemia. This is referred to as kwashiorkor. Refeeding a child with severe malnutrition must be done slowly and carefully. Rapid refeeding can result in refeeding syndrome, and children can develop hypophosphatemia due to cellular uptake of phosphorus. Low serum phosphate levels can result in fatal cardiac arrhythmias.

(A, C, D, E) Although the child in the vignette may have insufficient caloric, fat, and carbohydrate (milk) intake, the protuberant abdomen is secondary to insufficient protein.

7 A patient's newborn screening test is positive for galactosemia. The family is contacted to find out how the child is doing. They report that the baby seems well, is breastfeeding every 2 to 3 hours, and they have no concerns.

In explaining the results of the newborn screening test, of the following, which recommendation is likely to be included?

(A) Bring the child to the emergency department
(B) The child will need confirmatory testing in 1 week
(C) Change to a soy-based formula
(D) Continue breastfeeding, but limit lactose in the mother's diet
(E) Change to the hypoallergenic amino acid–based formula

The answer is C: Change to the soy-based formula. Galactosemia is an inherited condition secondary to a deficiency of galactose-1-phosphate uridyl transferase, the enzyme responsible for breaking down galactose. Clinical manifestations of galactosemia can include jaundice, poor feeding, lethargy, hepatomegaly, cataracts, hypoglycemia, and splenomegaly. More frequently, secondary to newborn screening programs, children are identified prior to developing symptoms. Children with galactosemia are at increased risk of bacterial sepsis from *Escherichia coli*. Galactosemia can be rapidly fatal if undiagnosed. Many of the complications can be delayed if not completely avoided by the early removal of all galactose from the diet. Galactose is one of the breakdown products of lactose, a carbohydrate found in breast milk– and cow milk–based formula. **(C)** If the diagnosis of galactosemia is being considered, the first step in the management of the patient is to place the child on a lactose-free formula, such as a soy formula in which the predominant carbohydrate is sucrose rather than lactose. The positive newborn screening test should be confirmed with an enzyme level to make a definitive diagnosis. However, the results generally take some time to return; thus, in the meantime, the safest thing for the child is to maintain a lactose-free diet. **(D)** Galactosemia is a true contraindication to breastfeeding, as breast milk always contains some level of lactose despite dietary restriction. **(E)** Hypoallergenic formulas may still contain some small amounts of lactose. **(A)** The patient in the vignette does not demonstrate any signs of distress on history; thus, there is not an indication to visit the emergency department at this time. **(B)** Waiting 1 week to obtain testing is too long; the confirmatory testing should be obtained as soon as possible.

8 A mother brings her 2-month-old infant to the office for a well-child visit. She has been exclusively breastfeeding and is now interested in starting to introduce other foods into her baby's diet.

Of the following complications, which is most highly associated with early initiation of supplemental foods?

(A) Atopy
(B) Autism
(C) Constipation
(D) Colic
(E) Sudden infant death syndrome

The answer is A: Atopy. Exclusive breastfeeding is recommended until 6 months of age and supplemental foods should generally not be introduced until 4 to 6 months of age in healthy infants. When the child is ready for introduction of solid foods, it is recommended to introduce one food at a time, every 3 to 4 days. This will allow careful assessment to observe if the child is allergic to any of the foods. Typically, it is recommended to start with iron-rich cereals, followed by vegetables and fruits, and finally, meats and mixed meals. **(A)** Increased incidence of atopy and allergy has been reported with the early introduction of supplemental foods.

(B, C, D, E) Increased risk of developing autism, constipation, colic, and sudden infant death syndrome have not been associated with early food introduction.

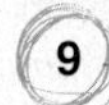

9 A 3-year-old girl has short gut syndrome. She had malrotation with volvulus as an infant and as a result lost 80% of her small bowel, sparing her duodenum. She has been successfully transitioned off total parenteral nutrition and tolerates enteral feedings.

Of the following, which vitamin deficiency is she at risk for developing?

(A) Vitamin A
(B) Vitamin B12
(C) Vitamin K
(D) Vitamin D
(E) Iron

The answer is B: Vitamin B12. Children with short gut syndrome are at risk for many nutrient deficiencies. Children with small bowel resection, particularly of the ileal segment, such as the patient in the vignette, are at greatest risk of developing vitamin B12 deficiency, as B12 absorption occurs in the terminal ileum.

(A, C, D) Vitamins A, D, E, and K are fat-soluble vitamins. Children with fat malabsorption problems, such as cystic fibrosis, pancreatic insufficiency, and chronic cholestasis are at greatest risk of becoming deficient in these vitamins. **(E)** Iron is absorbed in the duodenum; thus, children with duodenal resections are at greater risk of developing this complication.

---

10 A 14-year-old boy presents to the outpatient clinic for a school physical. He has no significant past medical history. His vital signs are as follows: temperature 36.9°C, heart rate 78 beats/min, respiratory rate 14 breaths/min, and blood pressure 140/90 mmHg. His body mass index is 28 kg/m^2. The remainder of his examination is unremarkable except for a large abdominal pannus.

Of the following, which additional finding supports the diagnosis of metabolic syndrome in this patient?

(A) Elevated high-density lipoprotein level
(B) Low high-density lipoprotein level
(C) Elevated low-density lipoprotein level
(D) Low low-density lipoprotein level
(E) Elevated liver function enzymes

The answer is B: Low high-density lipoprotein level. Metabolic syndrome is characterized as at least three of the following: central obesity, hypertriglyceridemia, hypertension, **(A, B)** low high-density lipoprotein (HDL), and elevated fasting glucose levels. This combination is known to put patients at risk for developing diabetes and heart disease. The same condition is now being identified in pediatric patients, who have increasing rates of obesity and related complications.

These risk factors can be associated with the development of nonalcoholic fatty liver disease (NAFLD), which occurs when there is abnormal deposition of fat in the liver. **(E)** NAFLD is often asymptomatic and is picked up when elevated liver enzymes are noted on screening blood work. **(C, D)** Although obese patients may have an elevated low-density lipoprotein level, this is not part of the diagnostic criteria of metabolic syndrome.

---

11 A term infant is brought to the office for a 1-week checkup. The mother seems very anxious and states that breastfeeding is not going well. She describes that she spends hours trying to get her daughter to latch on, but the child will only suck for a few moments. The infant appears thin and jaundiced with dry mucous membranes. The mother reports that the baby made one wet diaper in the past 24 hours. Her birth weight was 4 kg and today she weighs 3.2 kg. When the mother sees the weight, she begins crying and says that she feels like a failure.

Of the following, what is the best next step for this patient?

(A) Supplementation with formula
(B) Admission to the hospital for appropriate hydration
(C) Provide expressed breast milk
(D) Consult a lactation specialist
(E) Start phototherapy

The answer is B: **Admission to the hospital for appropriate hydration.** A loss of more than 10% of birth weight is considered excessive. The initial loss of weight shortly after birth is secondary to diuresis of excess fluid. Within 2 weeks, a thriving child should start to gain weight at a rate of approximately 25 to 30 g/day. Warning signs that a child is not receiving adequate nutrition include a failure to regain birth weight by 10 to 14 days, or a drop from birth weight at any time of greater than 10%. Reasons to consider admission to the hospital for the patient in the vignette include excessive weight loss, dehydration, and further evaluation of the jaundice, which may require phototherapy. **(A, C, D)** Although pumping and providing expressed milk, supplementing breastfeeding with formula, and lactation consultation are all reasonable solutions, appropriate hydration needs to be addressed first. **(E)** Phototherapy may be indicated; however, a serum bilirubin must first be obtained, to assess the extent of hyperbilirubinemia.

12 A 2-year-old boy with a history of repaired biliary atresia presents to the emergency department with profuse epistaxis. After 20 minutes of applied pressure, the bleeding appears to have stopped. Coagulation studies demonstrate a prothrombin time of 18 s, and an international normalized ratio (INR) of 2.4. His hemoglobin is stable.

Of the following, which is the most appropriate next step in the management of this patient?

(A) Cryoprecipitate infusion
(B) Fresh frozen plasma infusion
(C) Vitamin K administration
(D) Vitamin E administration
(E) Nasal packing

The answer is C: **Vitamin K administration.** The patient in the vignette has a coagulopathy likely secondary to vitamin K deficiency. Patients with any type of fat malabsorption are at risk for vitamin K deficiency as it is a fat-soluble vitamin. Children with biliary atresia have diminished transfer of bile, which is important for absorption of fat-soluble vitamins. These patients are typically maintained on fat-soluble vitamin supplements. Given the history for the patient in the vignette, he should receive vitamin K immediately.

(D) Vitamin E deficiency may present as a hemolytic anemia, but is not a cause of active bleeding. **(A, B)** Cryoprecipitate or fresh frozen plasma is more useful in situations in which the bleeding is related to hypofibrinogenemia, such as disseminated intravascular coagulation. **(E)** Nasal packing is appropriate for epistaxis in an otherwise healthy child with normal coagulation studies. It will not address the underlying concern for the patient in the vignette.

A mother has just delivered her newborn infant in Chicago, IL. She has a history of chronic hepatitis C infection. She is interested in breastfeeding her infant and inquires about its safety.

Of the following, which is a contraindication for breastfeeding for this mother?

(A) History of herpes simplex virus
(B) Acute hepatitis B infection
(C) Chronic hepatitis C infection
(D) Human T-lymphotropic virus infection
(E) Latent tuberculosis

The answer is D: Human T-lymphotropic virus infection. The American Academy of Pediatrics recommends exclusive breastfeeding through 6 months of age, whenever safe. In the United States, contraindications to breastfeeding include maternal human T-lymphotropic virus infection, human immunodeficiency virus (HIV) infection, herpes simplex virus infection with open lesions, untreated miliary tuberculosis, and mothers using drugs, chemotherapy agents, or radioactive treatments that preclude breastfeeding. **(A, B, C, E)** Infection with hepatitis B or C, nonactive herpes simplex virus, and latent tuberculosis are not contraindications to breastfeeding. The mother in the vignette should be encouraged to breastfeed her infant.

Although HIV infection is considered a contraindication to breastfeeding in the United States, it should be noted that this is not the case worldwide. In developing nations, where clean water to prepare and provide a safe infant formula is not available, the risk of formula feeding may outweigh the risk of transmission of HIV through breastfeeding.

CHAPTER 17

Surgical Subspecialties

STEPHANIE JENNINGS, HARIT K. BHATT, AND RAMA D. JAGER

1 A mother brings her 6-month-old infant in for evaluation of a lump she noticed on his leg while changing his diaper. She states she left the baby with a babysitter for the past 2 days when she was away on a business trip. The baby has been more fussy than usual and she is having a hard time consoling him. On examination, his right leg appears shorter than his left and there is an obvious deformity and swelling of his right thigh.

Of the following, what is the most likely radiographic finding consistent with this patient's presentation?

(A) Spiral fracture
(B) Buckle fracture
(C) Greenstick fracture
(D) Toddler fracture
(E) Torus fracture

The answer is A: Spiral fracture. The baby in the vignette is non–weight-bearing, and thus is unable to produce the forces on his own necessary to result in this injury. Therefore, abuse is the likely cause. Spiral fractures in non–weight-bearing children are pathognomonic for abuse. Spiral fractures of long bones require a twisting force as the mechanism of action.

(C) A greenstick fracture usually involves the diaphysis of a long bone and is the result of an angulated force. Radiography demonstrates a fracture in only one side of the cortex; appearance on radiography resembles that of a fresh stick in spring that splinters mid-shaft when bent rather than breaking cleanly. **(B, E)** A buckle fracture, also known as a torus fracture, is caused by compression of the distal metaphysis and is seen in young children after falling on an outstretched arm. Often there is not a visible fracture line seen on radiography; however, there is disruption of at least one side of the cortex. **(D)** A toddler fracture is a spiral fracture of the tibia that is often not seen on radiographic films, unless a lateral oblique film is taken. This fracture occurs in children aged 1 to 4 years. The mechanism of a toddler fracture involves a sudden twisting force on the lower extremities that occurs with falling while running. Patients present with a refusal to bear weight on the affected leg.

2 A 5-day-old newborn is seen in the newborn follow-up clinic for his first visit. His mother is very happy and excited to have the baby home with her. He breastfeeds 10 minutes on each breast every 2 hours and sleeps up to 3 hours at a time. On examination, he is able to lift his head while prone. He cries during the abdominal examination but is easily consolable. His testes are descended in the scrotum bilaterally, he is uncircumcised, and his foreskin does not retract.

Of the following, what best describes these findings?

(A) Paraphimosis
(B) Balanitis
(C) Phimosis
(D) Hypospadias
(E) Cryptorchidism

The answer is C: Phimosis. Phimosis describes a tight foreskin that prevents full retraction. Phimosis is present in nearly all full-term newborn males and the majority resolves by 3 months of age. **(A)** Paraphimosis is an emergency and occurs when the foreskin is retracted beyond the coronal sulcus and results in venous stasis, pain, and an inability to reduce the foreskin. **(B)** Balanitis is inflammation of the glans penis and foreskin. **(D)** Hypospadias is the result of incomplete development of the distal urethral meatus with the urethral meatus located anywhere from the glans to the scrotal area. **(E)** Cryptorchidism is the term used to describe undescended testicles.

3 A 3-year-old girl presents to the clinic with a 3-day history of limping. Her mother states she has been a healthy active child besides a flu-like illness she suffered 3 weeks prior to presentation. Her vital signs are heart rate 110 beats/min, respiratory rate 18 breaths/min, blood pressure 98/64 mmHg, and body temperature 37.6°C. Her physical examination notes a well-appearing child sitting on her mother's lap. Cardiac and pulmonary examinations are unremarkable and her extremity examination is pertinent for a left lower extremity that is externally rotated and flexed. She complains of pain with internal rotation and extension of her left lower extremity. There is no erythema, edema, or warmth appreciated on examination. Preliminary laboratory workup reveals an erythrocyte sedimentation rate of 10 mm/hour, C-reactive protein of <1, and a white blood cell count of $9.5 \times 10^3/\mu L$.

Of the following, what is the best explanation of her presentation?

(A) Septic arthritis
(B) Transient synovitis
(C) Osteomyelitis
(D) Child abuse
(E) Osteochondroma

The answer is B: Transient synovitis. The patient described in the vignette has symptoms, examination, and laboratory workup findings consistent with transient synovitis. Transient synovitis is a benign, self-resolving illness often confused with septic arthritis or osteomyelitis and is a diagnosis of exclusion. Children between the ages of 2 and 6 years are most often affected and frequently reveal a history of recent viral syndrome. The treatment is supportive.

It is crucial to rule out a septic arthritis, as this is a medical emergency requiring immediate care to avoid lifelong joint immobility. **(B)** Patients with septic arthritis have elevated white blood cell counts with a left shift as well as elevated acute phase reactants. Outside of the neonatal period, the most common organisms causing septic arthritis are *Staphylococcus aureus, Streptococcus pneumoniae,* and *Kingella* sp. In neonates, group B streptococcus and *Escherichia coli* are common pathogens. When suspecting septic arthritis, a joint aspiration for cell count and gram stain should be obtained and intravenous antibiotic therapy initiated immediately. **(C)** Patients with osteomyelitis present with fever as well as elevated acute phase reactants and point tenderness as well as a limp on physical examination. **(E)** Osteochondroma is a benign tumor consisting of cartilage and bone and often seen at the end of the growth plates in long bones. **(D)** Although it is important to consider child abuse in all pediatric patients, the patient in the vignette has no reported bruising or concerns for neglect to make this the best answer choice.

A 1-month-old infant presents to her pediatrician for her routine health maintenance visit. On examination, she is alert and has positive Moro, Babinski, and grasp reflexes. Her pulmonary and cardiac examinations are within normal limits. Her abdomen is soft with no appreciated masses and her genitalia is sexual maturity rating 1 with mild labial hypertrophy and scant vaginal discharge. Her left leg appears shorter that the right and a clunk is noted during Ortolani examination.

Of the following, what is most likely associated with this condition?

(A) Male gender
(B) Vacuum delivery
(C) Twin gestation
(D) Face presentation
(E) Breech presentation

The answer is E: Breech presentation. The baby described in the vignette has developmental dysplasia of the hip (DDH). DDH describes an abnormal placement of the head of the femur into the hip socket. On examination, gluteal fold asymmetry or leg length discrepancy may be appreciated. The best physical examination tests to assess for DDH are the Barlow and Ortolani maneuvers. The examination is performed while the baby is supine by placing one finger on the head of the trochanter of the femur and applying gentle pressure downward into the examination table. Laxity is felt as the head of the femur dislocates from the hip socket. This is referred to as the Barlow maneuver. The Ortolani maneuver is when the head of the femur relocates with a clunk during abduction. Risks for DDH include **(B)** female gender, breech presentation, and cesarean section especially if it is secondary to breech presentation, and a family history. **(C, D, E)** Face presentation, twin gestation, and vacuum-assisted delivery are not associated with an increased risk of DDH.

5 During a routine male newborn's examination, his left testicle is unable to be palpated.

Of the following, what is the next best step in management?

(A) Refer to surgery
(B) Reassure the family the testicle will descend with time
(C) Order an abdominal ultrasound
(D) Recommend circumcision
(E) Send chromosomal studies

The answer is C: Order an abdominal ultrasound. The boy described in the vignette has an undescended testicle, also known as cryptorchidism. Cryptorchidism is diagnosed via inguinal or abdominal ultrasound to determine the location of the testicle. **(A)** Once the location is properly identified, the patient can be referred to surgery for an orchiopexy. Orchiopexy is the procedure in which the testicle is brought down and tacked to the scrotal sac. If the testicle is left undescended, infertility risk is increased. There remains an increased risk for testicular cancer above the general population even if cryptorchidism is repaired. **(B)** Although many testicles are high riding and will descend with time, if the testicle truly is not palpated in the canal and unable to be gently guided down, an ultrasound is indicated to identify its location. **(E)** There is no reason to suspect the otherwise abnormal genitalia for the boy in the vignette, and therefore chromosomal studies are not indicated. **(D)** There is no reason to suggest circumcision for the boy in the vignette. Circumcision is often recommended for patients with recurrent balanitis or if a paraphimosis occurs.

6 What is the youngest age that the frontal sinuses would be expected to have developed?

(A) Birth
(B) 2 weeks
(C) 4 years
(D) 8 years
(E) 15 years

The answer is D: 8 years. Frontal sinuses develop around 8 to 10 years of age. **(A)** Ethmoid and maxillary sinuses are present at birth. **(B, C)** Sphenoid sinuses develop during the toddler period (around 2 to 5 years of age). **(E)** Given frontal sinuses are the last to develop, all sinuses should be present prior to 15 years of age.

7 A 15-month-old boy presents to clinic with reported fever for 2 days. His mother states that he has been crying, fussy, and taking less oral intake than usual. She says he is tugging on his ears and puts everything into his mouth. She has been giving him ibuprofen every 6 hours with minimal relief. He does not have any known allergies or medical conditions. On examination, his temperature is 38°C, heart rate 120 beats/min, respiratory rate 22 breaths/minute, and oxygen saturation 99% on room air. He is crying with tears but consolable. His right tympanic membrane is erythematous, bulging, and does not appear to have a light reflex. Attempts at pneumatic otoscopy are unsuccessful. His left tympanic membrane appears within normal limits. He has no known allergies.

Of the following, what is the next best step in therapy?

(A) Amoxicillin 80 to 90 mg/kg/day for 7 to 10 days
(B) Azithromycin 10 mg/kg for 1 day, then 5 mg/kg for 4 days
(C) Amoxicillin/clavulanate 90 mg/kg/day for 7 days
(D) Ceftriaxone 100 mg/kg/day for 5 days
(E) Ciprofloxacin/dexamethasone otic drops three times per day for 5 days

The answer is A: Amoxicillin 80 to 90 mg/kg/day for 7 to 10 days. The child described in the vignette has acute otitis media. The first-line therapy for a child with otitis media is high-dose amoxicillin. **(C)** If he were to fail initial therapy, high-dose amoxicillin/clavulanate would be the next appropriate therapeutic step. Ceftriaxone at 50 mg/kg/day can be used in those who do not tolerate oral therapy or are refractory to initial treatment and would be given as a onetime dose that may be repeated up to three times. **(D)** Ceftriaxone at 100 mg/kg/day would not be indicated for otitis media as this is meningitic dosing. **(E)** Otic antibiotic drops are used for otitis externa; however, the patient in the vignette has otitis media. **(B)** Azithromycin may be indicated in children with a true penicillin allergy.

8 The same child returns to clinic 1 week later. His mother states he continues to have fever and is increasingly fussy. His vital signs are temperature 38.5°C, heart rate 142 beats/min, and respiratory rate 26 breaths/min. On examination, his left tympanic membrane remains erythematous, retracted, and nonmobile with insufflation. In addition, the area posterior to his left ear is pictured in Figure 17-1.

Of the following, what is his most likely diagnosis?

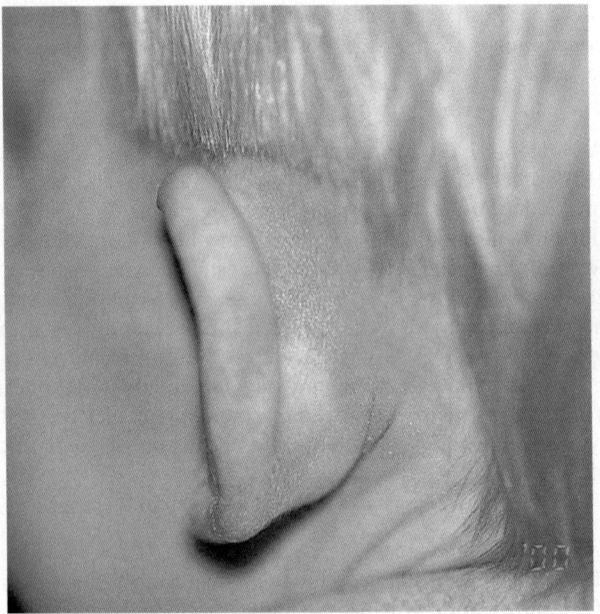

Figure 17-1

(A) Mastoiditis
(B) Otitis externa
(C) Parotitis
(D) Cholesteatoma
(E) Suppurative otitis media

The answer is A: **Mastoiditis.** The boy described in the vignette has mastoiditis. Mastoiditis is a bacterial infection of the mastoid bone and air cells and is a complication of acute otitis media. *Streptococcus pneumoniae* is the most common bacterial pathogen. Treatment should include otorhinolaryngology (ENT) referral for possible mastoidotomy and intravenous antibiotic therapy. Mastoiditis presents similarly to that pictured in the vignette with an erythematous, warm, tender, edematous mastoid region and displacement of the pinna lateral and anteriorly.

(B) Otitis externa is an inflammation in the ear canal often caused by *Pseudomonas aeruginosa*, *Staphylococcus aureus*, *Proteus*, or *Klebsiella*. Otitis externa presents with pain on movement of the pinna, edema, and otorrhea of the ear canal. **(C)** Parotitis is an inflammation in the parotid gland and is most likely secondary to a viral infection. Parotitis would present with swelling anterior to the ear and over the parotid gland. **(D)** Cholesteatoma is often the result of chronic suppurative otitis media and results with keratinized squamous epithelium that grows and invades inwardly. **(E)** Suppurative otitis media is a chronic inflammation of the middle ear and often presents with otorrhea.

9 A 39-week gestational male infant born to a G3P1 woman is examined shortly after delivery. His urethral meatus is found to be located on the ventral surface of the penile shaft.

Of the following, what is his most likely diagnosis?

(A) Clitoromegaly
(B) Hypospadias
(C) Normal genitalia
(D) Epispadias
(E) Congenital adrenal hypoplasia

The answer is B: Hypospadias. The boy in the vignette has hypospadias. Hypospadias is the most common congenital abnormality of the penis. Hypospadias is the result of incomplete development of the distal urethral meatus. There are varying degrees of hypospadias: in first-degree, the meatus is located on the glans; in second-degree, the meatus is on the penile shaft; and in third-degree, it is located in the penoscrotal to scrotal area. Circumcision is contraindicated as the foreskin is often used during surgical correction. **(D)** Epispadias is characterized by an open dorsal urethra.

(E) Congenital adrenal hyperplasia (CAH) is an enzymatic abnormality in the pathway of steroidogenesis and may result in abnormal genitalia. Although the genitalia can appear abnormal in CAH secondary to virilization, this does not often present as hypospadias. **(A)** Clitoromegaly can have a similar appearance as a penis, however, without a urethral opening.

10 A 6-year-old boy presents to the emergency department with complaints of right eye pain and swelling. His mother states that he is an otherwise healthy boy, and only visits his pediatrician for routine health visits. He had his yearly dental examination 1 month prior. He has no surgical history. There is no history of trauma. His vital signs are temperature of 38.2°C, heart rate 98 beats/min, respiratory rate 18 breaths/min, and blood pressure 89/62 mmHg. His examination notes a well-appearing man in no acute distress. His right eye is edematous and erythematous (see *Figure 17-2*). Further examination is limited as he refuses to open his eye and complains of pain with eye movement. A computed tomography of his orbits is included in Figure 17-3.

Of the following, what is the most likely mechanism of his infection?

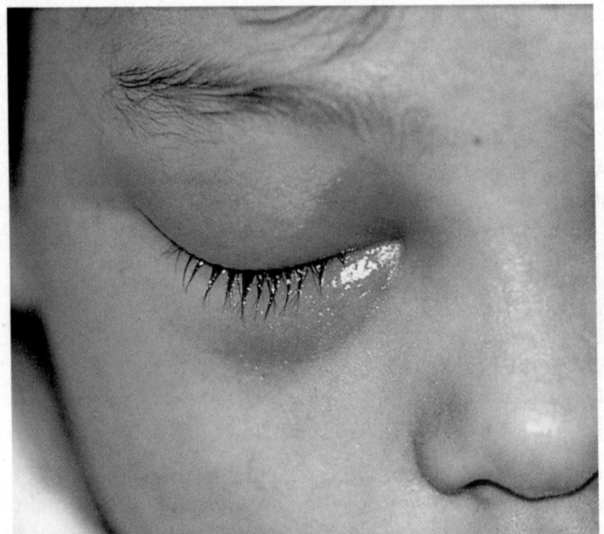

Figure 17-2

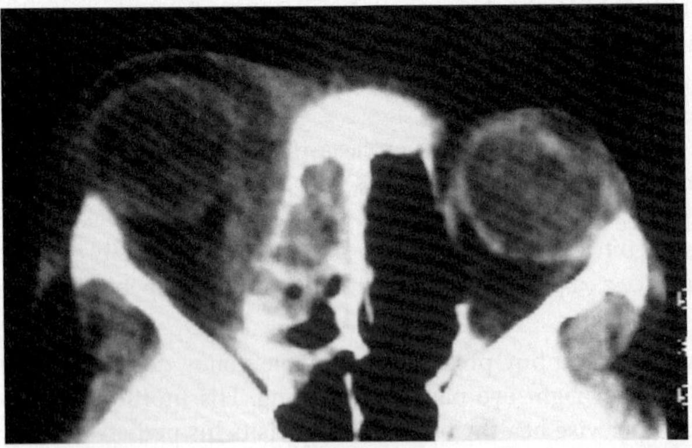

Figure 17-3

(A) Local trauma
(B) Allergy
(C) Direct spread from sinusitis
(D) Insect bite
(E) Foreign body

The answer is C: **Direct spread from sinusitis.** The boy described in the vignette has orbital cellulitis. Orbital cellulitis is an infection and inflammation contained within the orbital rim. Often described as postseptal cellulitis, it is an ophthalmologic emergency, and if left untreated, patients may develop loss of vision, meningitis, and direct intracranial extension with abscess formation. Orbital cellulitis is spread either hematogenously as the veins within the orbits do not contain valves and thus allow bidirectional flow, or through direct spread. Spread occurs from sinusitis (most often of the ethmoid sinus) or dental abscess. The organisms associated with orbital cellulitis are *Streptococcus pneumoniae*, *Staphylococcus aureus* (MRSA), *Haemophilus influenzae* type b, or anaerobes.

(A, D) Periorbital (also known as preseptal) cellulitis is an infection and inflammation anterior to the orbital septum and more often results from local trauma, such as from a scratch or insect bite, maxillary sinusitis, or hematogenous spread. The organisms most often associated with periorbital cellulitis are *Staphylococcus aureus, Streptococcus pyogenes*, or *Streptococcus pneumoniae*. **(B)** Although allergic reactions may cause periorbital edema, the edema is usually bilateral and extraocular muscle activity is unlikely to be impaired. **(E)** There is no history of trauma or surgery, which may indicate a retained foreign body.

11 A 7-year-old boy presents to the acute care clinic with right-sided flank pain radiating toward his testicle. He has had several episodes of vomiting on the day of presentation without diarrhea. He describes the pain as intermittent and intense. He has never had this type of pain before although his mother states she had recently experienced similar symptoms. A urinalysis is positive for red blood cells, no white blood cells, and nitrite and leukocyte esterase negative.

Of the following, what is the most likely test to help identify the etiology of his symptoms?

(A) Basic metabolic panel
(B) Complete blood count
(C) C-reactive protein
(D) Urine creatinine
(E) Thyroid function tests

The answer is A: Basic metabolic panel. The boy described in the vignette has renal stones, also referred to as urolithiasis, based on his history of colicky pain in his abdomen radiating to his groin, hematuria on urinalysis, and a family history. Urolithiasis is twice as common in males as well as in children with metabolic abnormalities. The workup upon initial presentation in patients with urolithiasis should include serum parathyroid hormone, basic metabolic panel, ionized calcium level, uric acid, phosphorus, and urine electrolytes. The basic metabolic panel is important to assess renal function with the blood urea nitrogen and creatinine levels as well as to monitor for hypercalcemia. Most stones are made of calcium, struvite, uric acid, or cystine. **(B, C, D, E)** A complete blood cell count, C-reactive protein, urine creatinine, and thyroid function tests would be nondiagnostic and most likely normal in a patient with urolithiasis.

---

12 A 14-year-old boy presents for his routine school physical. His review of systems is positive for complaints of right-sided leg pain, usually after dinner and sometimes in the middle of the night. The pain is relieved with over-the-counter analgesics. This pain has been occurring for a few months and he reports an intentional weight loss of 5 lb. His HEADDSS history reveals that he has a girlfriend with whom he has recently been sexually active; he smokes marijuana once in a while and has been drunk once at a holiday party. His physical examination notes a normal gait and point tenderness near the right femoral head. A lower extremity radiograph reveals a round lucency with some elevation in bone density surrounding it (see *Figure 17-4*).

Of the following, what is the most likely cause of his pain?

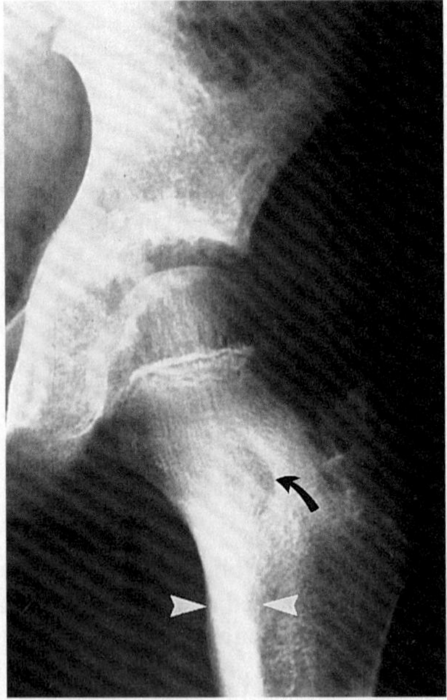

Figure 17-4

(A) Osteomyelitis
(B) Ewing sarcoma
(C) Osteosarcoma
(D) Osteoid osteoma
(E) Chondroma

The answer is D: Osteoid osteoma. The boy described in the vignette has physical and radiographic examinations consistent with osteoid osteoma, a benign bone tumor typically of the long bones although it can arise anywhere. Pain typically is present at night and improves with nonsteroidal anti-inflammatory drug (NSAID) use. Definitive treatment involves surgical removal of the entire nidus.

(A) Osteomyelitis is an infection occurring in bone and usually presents with fever, pain, elevated acute phase reactants, point tenderness, and possibly erythema, edema, and warmth. *Staphylococcus aureus* is the predominant inciting organism for osteomyelitis for all age groups followed by *Streptococcus pneumoniae.* **(B)** Ewing sarcoma is a sarcoma arising from bone, thought to be from neural crest cells of the parasympathetic nervous system and is more common in male adolescents. Radiographic findings typically describe an onion skin appearance surrounding a lytic lesion. Onion skin describes the layers of calcified periosteal elevation (see *Figure 17-5*). **(C)** Osteosarcoma is a malignant tumor of bone, typically arising from the periosteum or the medullary cavity of long bones. It is most often seen in areas of maximum growth such as the proximal tibia, proximal humerus, or distal femur. Radiographic findings describe a sunburst appearance, which is a lytic lesion with periosteal reaction (see *Figure 17-6*). Treatment for osteosarcoma involves chemotherapy, radiation, and surgical resection. **(E)** A chondroma is a benign cartilaginous tumor typically found in bones of the hands or feet (see *Figure 17-7*).

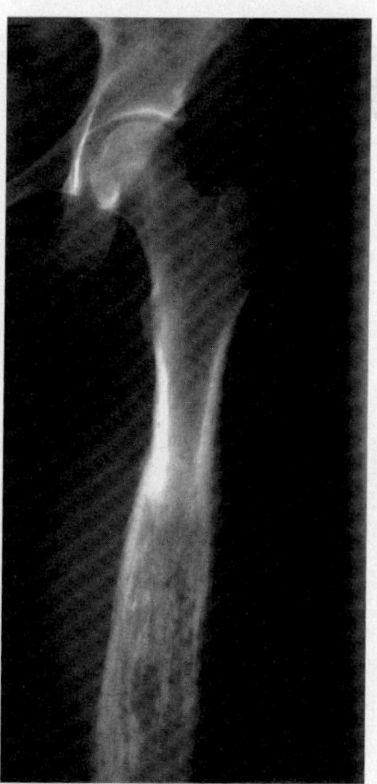

Figure 17-5

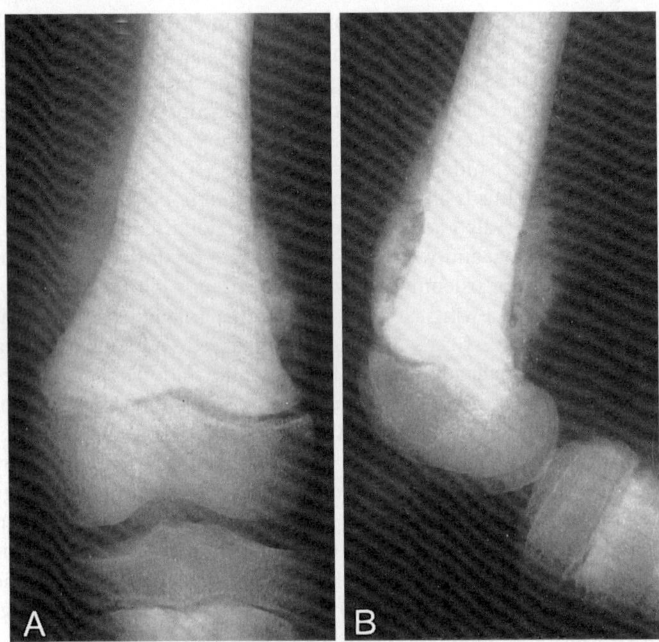

Figure 17-6

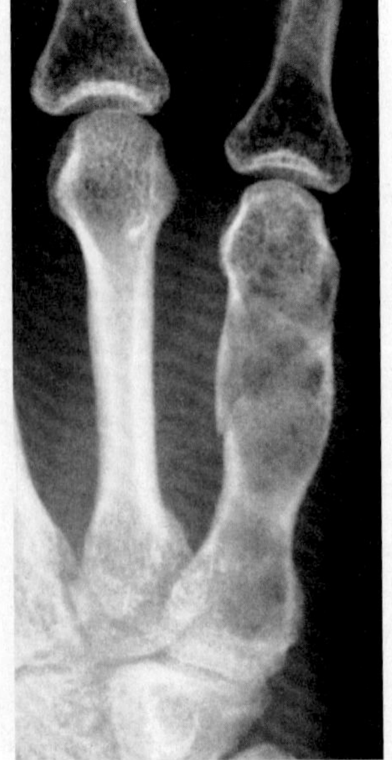

Figure 17-7

13 A 15-month-old girl presents to the walk-in clinic with a 2-day history of worsening drainage from her right eye noted to be spreading toward her left. Her mother states that she started daycare 2 weeks ago and since then has had a cough and runny nose. On examination, her bilateral conjunctivae are injected and inflamed, with copious, thick, mucopurulent drainage and crusting around her lashes.

Of the following, what is her most likely diagnosis?

(A) Bacterial conjunctivitis
(B) Allergic conjunctivitis
(C) Herpes simplex virus (HSV) keratitis
(D) Viral conjunctivitis
(E) Scleritis

The answer is A: Bacterial conjunctivitis. The girl described in the vignette has bacterial conjunctivitis. **(D)** Although viral conjunctivitis is more common, given the copious, thick, mucopurulent drainage, bacterial conjunctivitis is a more likely diagnosis. Viral conjunctivitis is often associated with upper respiratory tract infections along with preauricular lymphadenopathy. Adenovirus is the most common cause of viral conjunctivitis. Bacterial pathogens include nontypeable *Haemophilus influenzae*, *Streptococcus pneumoniae*, and *Staphylococcus aureus.* **(B)** Allergic conjunctivitis presents with watery irritated eyes with edema and itching, without mucopurulent drainage. **(C)** HSV keratitis is a complication of HSV infection and can result in corneal scarring and blindness. **(E)** Scleritis is inflammation of the sclera and often associated with autoimmune disease.

14 A 12-year-old boy presents to the emergency department with an acute onset of abdominal pain and emesis. He is lying extremely still on the stretcher. He is an avid football and basketball player. His HEADDSS history notes two sexual partners with whom he states he uses condoms most of the time. Vital signs are temperature 37.8°C, heart rate 108 beats/minute, blood pressure 137/78 mmHg, and respiratory rate 22 breaths/minute. Physical examination reveals positive abdominal bowel sounds and his abdomen is soft but diffusely tender. He is sexual maturity rating 4 and his left testicle is tender, firm, and in a transverse lie with an absent cremasteric reflex on the left side.

Of the following, what is the most important next step in his management?

(A) Renal ultrasound
(B) Nucleic acid amplification tests for *Neisseria gonorrhea* and *Chlamydia trachomatis*
(C) Abdominal computed tomography with contrast
(D) Urinary catheterization
(E) Doppler testicular ultrasound

The answer is E: Doppler testicular ultrasound. The boy described in the vignette has a testicular torsion. Testicular torsion is a urologic emergency and if left untreated upon 6 hours after presentation the patient has high risk of loss of testicular viability. There are two peaks in age for testicular torsion: neonatal and early adolescence. Physical examination may note a horizontal lie of the testicle, absence of the ipsilateral cremasteric reflex, and failure to relieve pain with the elevation of the testicle. Relief of pain with elevation (Prehn sign) is characteristic in a patient with epididymitis. Immediate testicular ultrasound with Doppler flow and urologic consultation for surgical detorsion are essential in diagnosing and treating testicular torsion.

(B) The patient in the vignette is sexually active and he should be tested for *N. gonorrhea* and *C. trachomatis*; however, epididymitis is not the likely etiology of his current presentation and pursuing this workup is not the next best step in management. **(C)** Abdominal computed tomography with contrast could be useful to evaluate for appendicitis. Appendicitis presents with fever, abdominal pain in the right lower quadrant, as well as guarding and rebound; however, the testicular examination is expected to be within normal limits in patients with acute appendicitis. **(A, D)** Urinary catheterization and renal ultrasound would be useful in the evaluation of a urinary tract infection; however, the patient in the vignette lacks symptoms including dysuria, fever, or urinary frequency.

15 Of the following, what is the most common cause of end-stage renal disease (ESRD) in a 3-year-old boy?

(A) Nephrolithiasis
(B) Posterior urethral valves (PUVs)
(C) Ureteral trauma
(D) Neomycin ingestion
(E) Renal tubular acidosis (RTA)

The answer is B: Posterior urethral valves (PUVs). PUV is the most common cause of ESRD in boys. PUV are often detected on prenatal ultrasound by visualizing hydronephrosis and/or bladder distention. PUVs only occur in males and are the result of abnormal embryologic formation resulting in obstruction within the posterior urethra.

(A) Nephrolithiasis, or kidney stones, infrequently cause ESRD; however, stones may lead to obstruction and/or urinary tract infections. **(C)** Ureteral trauma, if left unrepaired, could lead to ESRD although this would be very unlikely. **(D)** Neomycin is an aminoglycoside and can be nephrotoxic; however, given no reported history of neomycin ingestion, this answer choice is less likely than PUV. **(E)** RTA does not result in ESRD; however, patients with RTA may present with failure to thrive and electrolyte abnormalities including chronic acidosis, hypokalemia, hypercalcemia, kidney stones, and rickets.

16 A 12-year-old boy with sickle cell disease is admitted to the pediatric ward for fever and pain. His vital signs are temperature 37.2°C, heart rate 102 beats/min, respiratory rate 22 breaths/min, and blood pressure 125/78 mmHg. His examination is significant for abdominal pain, and a tender, erect penis.

Of the following, what best describes the mechanism for his pain?

(A) Idiopathic
(B) Increased arterial flow to the cavernosa
(C) Vaso-occlusive crisis in the symphysis pubis
(D) Sildenafil ingestion
(E) Venous obstruction in the corpus cavernosa

The answer is E: **Venous obstruction in the corpus cavernosa.** The boy described in the vignette has priapism. **(A)** Priapism is a sustained erection as a result of either altered arterial flow or obstruction of venous blood. **(B)** The most likely pathophysiology in males with sickle cell is the latter. Venous obstruction of outflow occurs following venous status, hypoxia, and acidosis, which results in sickling of erythrocytes and causes venous occlusion of outflow.

(D) Sildenafil ingestion can result in priapism but would be less likely to have occurred with this boy while admitted to the hospital, without a known ingestion. **(C)** Vaso-occlusive crisis in the symphysis pubis would cause pain; however, it would not cause priapism.

17 A 2-year-old girl is brought to clinic with complaints of fever for 1 day and right ear pain. On examination, her right tympanic membrane is erythematous, retracted, and immobile with insufflation.

Of the following, what is the most likely inciting organism?

(A) *Streptococcus pneumoniae*
(B) *Staphylococcus aureus*
(C) *Streptococcus pyogenes*
(D) *Pseudomonas aeruginosa*
(E) *Moraxella catarrhalis*

The answer is A: *Streptococcus pneumoniae.* The girl described in the vignette has an acute otitis media. Otitis media is inflammation in the middle ear. The most common bacterial causes in the order of prevalence are *Streptococcus pneumoniae*, *Haemophilus influenzae*, and **(E)** *M. catarrhalis*. **(B)** Other less common pathogens include *Mycoplasma* and *Staphylococcus aureus.* **(D)** *P. aeruginosa* is a common pathogen associated with otitis externa, which is characterized by foul-smelling discharge and fluid collection with narrowing of the ear canal. Complications of otitis media include tympanic membrane perforation, hearing loss, mastoiditis, cholesteatoma, paralysis of the facial nerve, as well as labyrinthitis, meningitis, and brain abscess formation. **(C)** *Streptococcus pyogenes* is associated most often with bacterial pharyngitis and is not a pathogen found in acute otitis media.

18 A 15-year-old boy presents with a 1-week history of increasing left lower quadrant abdominal pain as well as testicular pain. Examination is significant for mild erythema of his scrotum, tenderness to palpation of the superior pole of the testicle, and a positive cremasteric reflex. Laboratory workup reveals pyuria on urinalysis.

Of the following, what is the best treatment for him?

(A) Sitz baths
(B) Emergent surgical correction
(C) Acyclovir
(D) Ceftriaxone and doxycycline
(E) Cryotherapy

The answer is D: Ceftriaxone and doxycycline. The boy described in the vignette has epididymitis characterized by inflammation of the epididymis. Epididymitis is often associated with scrotal swelling and tenderness on examination as well as pyuria on urinalysis. The pathogens most often associated with epididymitis are *Chlamydia trachomatis* and *Neisseria gonorrhea.* Treatment should include coverage for both of these pathogens and therefore ceftriaxone along with doxycycline (or azithromycin) is first-line therapy.

(B) Surgical correction is required for testicular torsion and should be done emergently. A torted testicle has about a 6-hour lifespan. The examination of the patient in the vignette is not consistent with testicular torsion as he has been having pain for over a week and the cremasteric reflex remains intact. The cremasteric reflex is elicited with a gentle stroke of the inner thigh leading to ipsilateral rise of the testicle. This reflex is absent in patients with testicular torsion. **(C)** Acyclovir should be used with herpes simplex virus (HSV) infections. There are no vesicular lesions described in the vignette, making HSV infection unlikely. **(E)** Cryotherapy could be used for genital warts. Genital warts are often caused by human papillomavirus (HPV) and have the appearance of cauliflower-like lesions. There were no warts described on the patient in the vignette.

19 A 15-year-old boy presents to the emergency department with complaints of bilateral knee pain that has been present for the past 3 months. He reports increased pain in his right knee although both knees bother him and his parents state that he has started to walk with a limp. He is active in sports at school and he recently started football after completing his wrestling season. He is uncertain if he has sustained any trauma. His body mass index (BMI) is 28 kg/m^2 and he has a past medical history of asthma. On examination, he has limited range of motion with passive flexion and internal rotation of his right hip and some mild limited range of motion on the left. His radiographic imaging is shown in Figure 17-8.

Of the following, what is his most likely diagnosis?

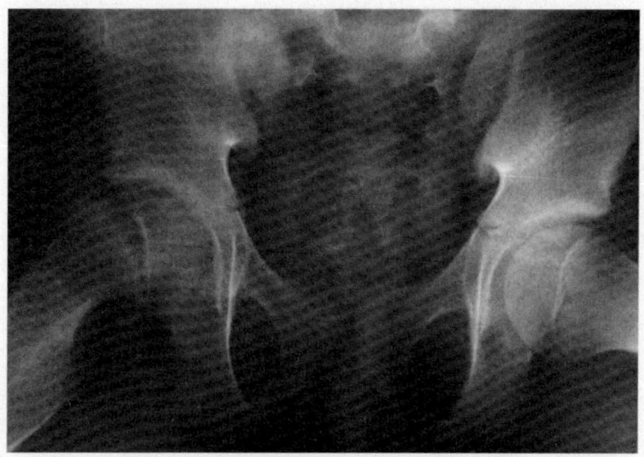

Figure 17-8

(A) Legg-Calvé Perthes disease
(B) Osgood-Schlatter disease
(C) Osteoid osteoma
(D) Baker cyst
(E) Slipped capital femoral epiphysis (SCFE)

The answer is E: **Slipped capital femoral epiphysis (SCFE).** The boy described in the vignette has a SCFE. SCFE often presents as gradual, progressive pain in the knee or hip associated with a limp. More common in obese preteen/teenagers, SCFE is a separation of the head of the femur at the growth plate with the head slipping off the neck of the femur and rotating inferiorly. Up to a quarter of cases are bilateral and therefore both hips should be examined and imaged. On examination, there is limited internal rotation of the hip, and patients often walk with a limp. The diagnostic test of choice is a frog-leg view radiograph.

(A) Legg-Calvé Perthes is a disease characterized by avascular necrosis of the femoral head. It is more commonly seen in boys than in girls and typically presents in the early school-age years. Children present with a painless limp and the physical examination demonstrates limited range of motion with internal rotation, flexion, and abduction at the hip. **(B)** Osgood-Schlatter disease presents with complaints of pain worse with activities such as running, jumping, and squatting, and improves with rest. It is an overuse injury and physical examination reveals swelling and tenderness over the tibial tuberosity (see *Figure 17-9*). Radiographs of the lower extremity may demonstrate irregularity of the tubercle ossification center with some surrounding soft tissue edema. Osgood-Schlatter is often seen in growing preadolescents or adolescents. **(C)** Osteoid osteoma is a benign bone tumor of the long bones although it can arise anywhere. Pain is present at night and improves with nonsteroidal anti-inflammatory drug (NSAID) use. **(D)** Baker cyst, also known as a popliteal cyst, is a benign swelling in the posterior aspect of the knee. Usually Baker cysts require no intervention and resolve spontaneously; however, if it continues to grow or cause pain, surgical excision is often indicated.

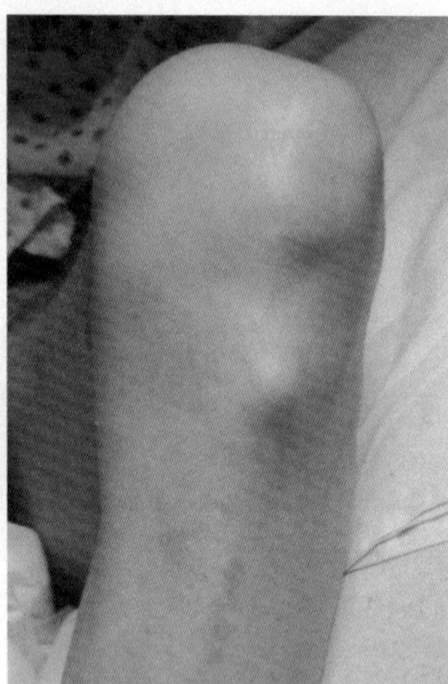

Figure 17-9

20 A 2-year-old boy presents to the emergency department for complaints of fever, neck pain, decreased oral intake, and drooling. A lateral neck radiograph is ordered and shown in Figure 17-10. The film demonstrates edema in the prevertebral area.

Of the following, what best describes his diagnosis?

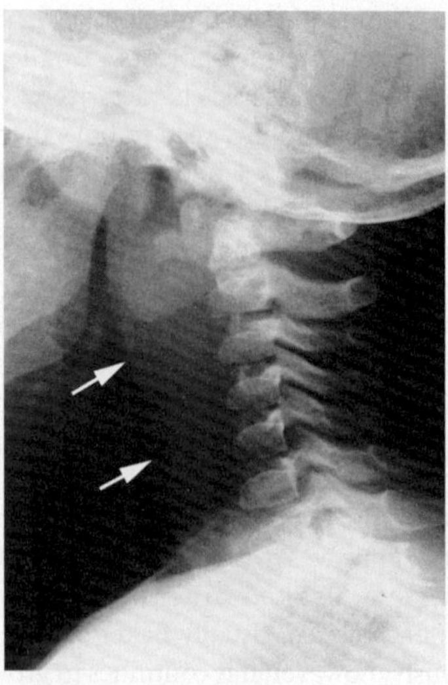

Figure 17-10

(A) Peritonsillar abscess
(B) Pharyngitis
(C) Retropharyngeal abscess
(D) Diphtheria
(E) Adenoiditis

The answer is C: Retropharyngeal abscess. The imaging in the vignette is consistent with a retropharyngeal abscess. A retropharyngeal abscess is an abscess in the potential space between the posterior pharyngeal wall and the prevertebral fascia. Retropharyngeal abscesses are more common in preschool age or younger children and often caused from an infection with *Staphylococcus aureus* or *Streptococcus pyogenes*. The diagnosis is confirmed with lateral neck radiograph demonstrating edema in the prevertebral area that is greater than half the width of the cervical vertebrae and the treatment includes intravenous antibiotic therapy as well as surgical drainage.

(A) A peritonsillar abscess is a bacterial infection within the tonsil and its capsule. Patients usually present with complaints of a sore throat and trismus (difficulty opening their mouths) as well as unilateral tonsillar enlargement. Treatment includes incision and drainage along with antibiotic therapy. **(B)** Pharyngitis is often caused by viral infections, and patients present with sore throat and difficulty swallowing. A lateral neck radiograph would not be diagnostic. **(D)** Diphtheria causes respiratory distress and a gray pseudomembrane covering of the posterior pharynx. Again, a lateral neck radiograph would be noncontributory for this option. **(E)** Adenoiditis is inflammation of the adenoid tissue and may be identified on radiologic imaging; however, the imaging would reveal adenoid hypertrophy rather than the imaging shown in the vignette.

A voiding cystourethrogram is completed to evaluate for vesicoureteral reflux (VUR) and reveals a dilated left ureter with blunting of the renal calyces.

Of the following, which grade of reflux is most consistent with this diagnosis?

(A) Grade I
(B) Grade II
(C) Grade III
(D) Grade IV
(E) Grade V

The answer is C: Grade III. VUR describes retrograde flow of urine from the bladder up to the ureter and renal pelvis. See Figure 17-11 and for an illustration of the VUR grades. **(A)** VUR grade I describes reflux to a nondilated ureter and requires no intervention, only monitoring. **(B)** Grade II describes reflux into the upper collecting system without dilation of the ureter. **(C)** Grade III as described in the vignette is reflux into a dilated ureter with blunting of the renal calyces. **(D)** Grade IV is reflux into a grossly dilated ureter. **(E)** Grade V is significant reflux with ureteral dilation and abnormal renal texture with

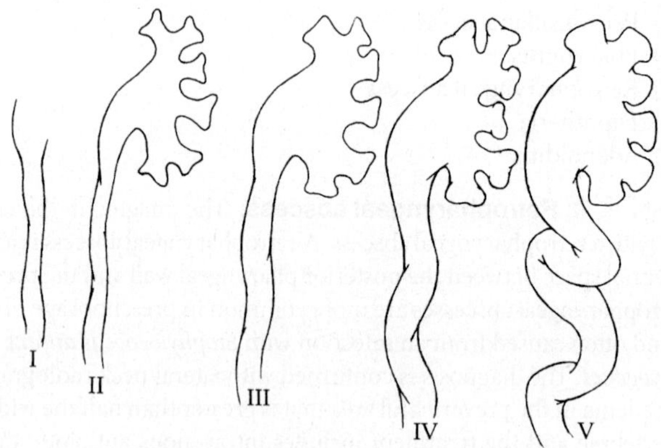

Figure 17-11

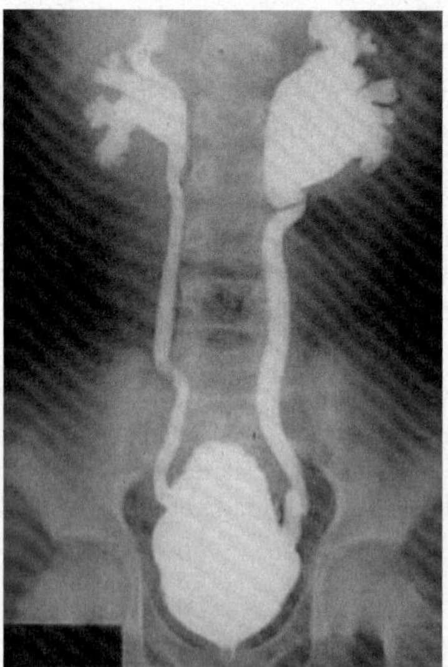

Figure 17-12

loss of renal structure (see *Figure 17-12*). Grades III–V require antibiotic prophylaxis, frequent monitoring, and possibly surgical intervention.

---

22 A 6-year-old boy presents to clinic for a routine physical. His physical examination is significant for a small granuloma formation at his right lower lid (see *Figure 17-13*). He states it is not painful and has been present for several weeks.

Of the following, what is his most likely diagnosis?

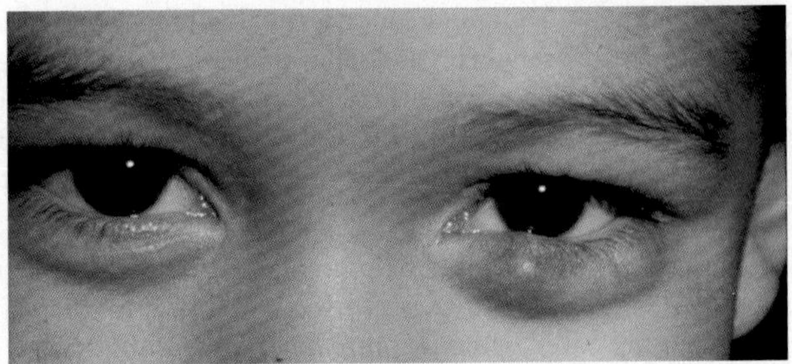

Figure 17-13

(A) Hordeolum
(B) Chalazion
(C) Orbital cellulitis
(D) Dacryostenosis
(E) Ptosis

The answer is B: Chalazion. The boy in the vignette has a chalazion. A chalazion is a subacute or chronic granulomatous formation of the meibomian glands. It presents as a firm nodule that is nontender at the eyelid. Therapy includes warm compresses and possible excision if there is no resolution following several months of supportive care.

(A) Hordeolum (stye) is a bacterial infection of the sebaceous gland (gland of Zeis) or sweat gland (gland of Moll). Hordeola are often self-limited with therapy centered on warm compresses; however, topical antibiotics may be indicated especially for internal hordeola. Hordeola can become inflamed and subsequently painful (see *Figure 17-14*). **(C)** Orbital cellulitis is an infection and inflammation contained within the orbital rim. Often described as postseptal

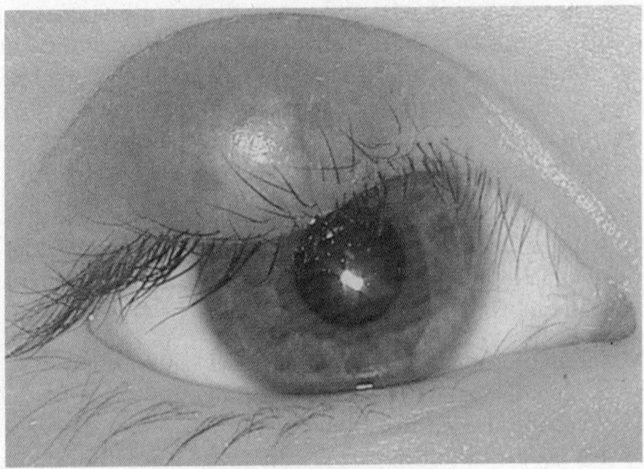

Figure 17-14

cellulitis, it is an ophthalmologic emergency. Orbital cellulitis presents with erythema and edema of the orbital rim as well as pain with eye movements. **(D)** Dacryostenosis is a congenital nasolacrimal duct obstruction and is most often seen in infants. This diagnosis would be unlikely for a 6-year-old boy. **(E)** Ptosis refers to upper eyelid droop, which is not seen in the case in the vignette.

23 A previously well 2-year-old boy presents to a new pediatrician's office for routine care. His mother states she had a healthy pregnancy and her son has been well without complaints. He recently started daycare, is in the process of being toilet trained, and eats what she reports is a balanced diet. She breastfed him until he was 9 months of age and they recently returned from a family reunion in Wisconsin. His physical examination notes a well-appearing active boy. His red reflex is present bilaterally and his right eye deviates medially during the cover–uncover test. His corneal light reflex is off-center.

Of the following, which condition is this patient most likely to develop in the absence of proper therapy?

(A) Strabismus
(B) Glaucoma
(C) Cataracts
(D) Amblyopia
(E) Nystagmus

The answer is D: Amblyopia. The boy described in the vignette has strabismus. **(A)** Strabismus is defined as misalignments of the eyes since the visual axis of each eye is not focused on the same point. **(D)** Amblyopia is a loss or decrease in visual acuity secondary to failure of the visual cortex to properly develop. Amblyopia often results from strabismus, ocular obstruction (hemangioma, cataracts, or severe ptosis), or from refractive errors. The treatment is to either remove the visual obstruction, correct the refractive errors, and/or to patch the unaffected eye in order to strengthen the affected eye. **(B)** Glaucoma may present with corneal clouding, tearing, and increased ocular size. Misalignment is not expected. **(C)** Cataracts present as an abnormal pupil and/or leukocoria. **(E)** Nystagmus is involuntary rhythmic oscillations of the eye, often present bilaterally.

24 Of the following, what is the best advice to give to an 8-year-old boy who complains of epistaxis lasting less than 5 minutes, occurring more frequently in winter, and happening once or twice per month?

(A) See an otorhinolaryngologist for nasal cauterization
(B) Frequently blow nose during the winter months
(C) Prescribe oral antihistamines
(D) Tilt head back and apply pressure to the nares during a bleed
(E) Avoid nose picking

The answer is E: Avoid nose picking. Epistaxis (nose bleed) is a common occurrence in children. The most common etiology in children aged 2 to 10 years is secondary to trauma, for example with nose picking. Other etiologies include foreign bodies within the nares and dry air. **(A)** For frequent or prolonged nose bleeds, otorhinolaryngology referral might be indicated for nasal cauterization. **(B)** Frequent nose blowing could cause an increased risk of epistaxis; however, direct trauma is a more common etiology. **(C)** Oral antihistamines would be indicated for children with seasonal allergies and are not necessarily indicated for children with frequent nosebleeds. Nasal corticosteroid or nasal vasoconstrictor therapy may improve symptoms of epistaxis. **(D)** During an episode the head should be held slightly forward (not back) and pressure applied to the nasal bridge.

---

25 A 14-year-old boy presents with pain in his right leg after playing touch football with his brothers. He has been otherwise well and has a history of a right humerus fracture when he fell off the trampoline 2 years prior. A radiograph of his right leg is shown in Figure 17-15 and is reported to note a fracture through the physis and epiphysis of the distal end of the femur.

Of the following, what is the most accurate description of his fracture?

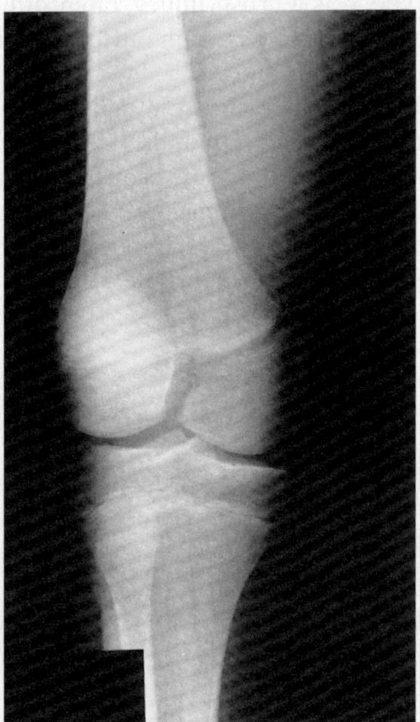

Figure 17-15

(A) Complete fracture
(B) Salter-Harris type II
(C) Salter-Harris type III
(D) Stress fracture
(E) Greenstick fracture

The answer is C: Salter-Harris type III. Salter-Harris classifications of fractures are used to describe fractures that occur through the open growth plate, or physis. Categorization is based on a numbering system of one through five and as the number increases the involvement of the growth plate and risk of permanent damage also increase. This classification system only applies to children with open growth plates. See Figure 17-16 for an illustration of the Salter-Harris classification system. Type I describes a fracture through the physis, the radiographic image is often normal and treatment is supportive with rest, wraps, or a walking boot. **(B)** Type II describes a fracture through the physis and metaphysis. This is the most common type of Salter-Harris fracture and has a very good prognosis. Type II Salter-Harris fractures are often casted or splinted. **(C)** Type III is a fracture involving the physis and epiphysis and often requires open reduction with internal fixation. Type IV is a complete growth plate fracture involving the epiphysis, physis, and metaphysis and requires open reduction with internal fixation. This fracture type has a high risk for abnormal growth in the affected bone. Type V is a crush injury, often difficult to see on plain radiographic imaging, and has a very high rate of permanent growth abnormalities.

(C) A complete fracture is a fracture through the entire cortex of the bone and can be described as displaced or nondisplaced. **(D)** A stress fracture is a fracture that follows repetitive motion and is often seen in athletes or military recruits and not typically visible on imaging. **(E)** A greenstick fracture usually involves the diaphysis of a long bone and occurs with an angulated force. Radiographs of the affected bone demonstrate a break in only one side of the cortex (see *Figure 17-17*).

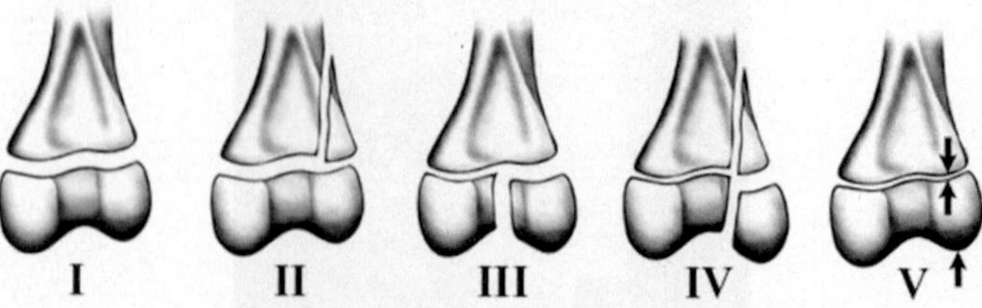

Figure 17-16

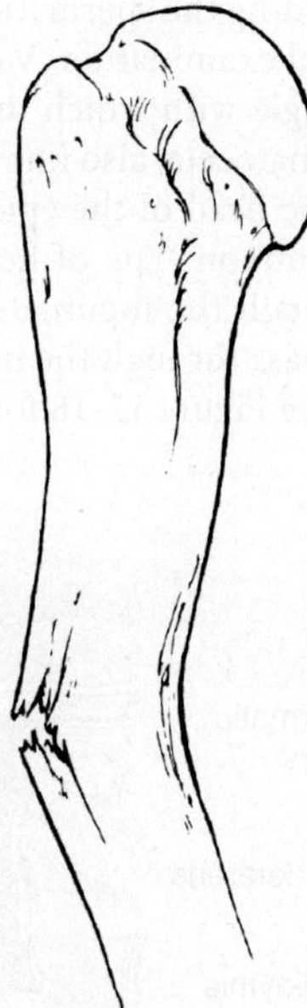

Figure 17-17

26 During a routine physical examination of a 5-month-old infant, transillumination of his left scrotum reveals increased fluid on the left when compared to the right. The mechanism of his scrotal edema is secondary to the failure of the processus vaginalis to close fully.

Of the following, what best describes his diagnosis?

(A) Inguinal hernia
(B) Varicocele
(C) Spermatocele
(D) Communicating hydrocele
(E) Noncommunicating hydrocele

The answer is D: Communicating hydrocele. Hydrocele is a collection of fluid between the visceral and parietal layers of the tunica vaginalis. Communicating hydrocele occurs as the result of the failure of the processus vaginalis to fully close. **(E)** Noncommunicating hydrocele fluid comes from the mesothelial layers of the tunica vaginalis. Hydroceles are common in neonates and often resolve by the time infants begin to walk, around their first birthday. **(B)** A varicocele is a collection of dilated veins in the pampiniform plexus surrounding the spermatic cord and is often described as a bag of worms on physical examination. Varicoceles are more common on the left because of the angle with which the left spermatic vein drains into the renal vein. **(C)** Spermatocele, also known as epididymal cyst, is the result of cyst formation at the head of the epididymis. **(A)** Indirect inguinal hernias are the most common type of hernia seen in children when intestinal contents pass through the inguinal canal, lateral to the vessels, while direct hernias do not pass through the inguinal canal and are medial and inferior to the vessels. See Figure 17-18 for an illustration of the above disorders.

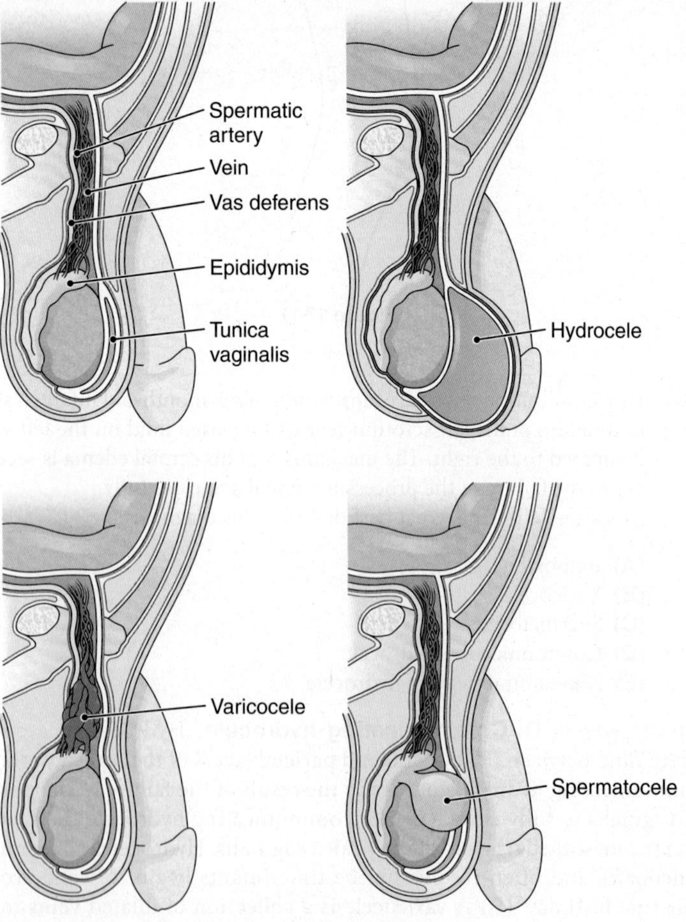

Figure 17-18

27 A 1-day-old neonate born to a 22-year-old woman with poor prenatal care is being evaluated in the newborn nursery. On examination, he is sleeping but easily arousable. His primitive reflexes are intact. His cardiac examination reveals a 1/6 systolic ejection murmur and his lungs are clear. Ophthalmologic examination notes bilateral leukocoria.

Of the following, what is his most likely diagnosis?

(A) Glaucoma
(B) Retinoblastoma
(C) Chlamydia
(D) Papilledema
(E) Congenital cataracts

The answer is E: Congenital cataracts. Leukocoria, or a white pupillary reflex, is an abnormal finding on examination. The most common cause of leukocoria is cataracts. Cataracts are opacities found in the lens. In the neonatal period a quarter of cases are familial while a third are secondary to prenatal infections such as rubella, cytomegalovirus, human immunodeficiency virus, or toxoplasmosis. Galactosemia, an inborn error of metabolism, has a high association with cataracts.

(A) Congenital glaucoma is a rare finding in neonates and presents with corneal clouding or an increase in corneal diameter as well as leukocoria. **(B)** Retinoblastoma is a malignant intraocular tumor that typically presents within the first year of life with leukocoria and strabismus. Although retinoblastoma more often presents unilaterally, familial forms are more often bilateral. Given the age and bilateral nature of the patient in the vignette, congenital cataracts would be more likely than retinoblastoma. **(C)** Chlamydia conjunctivitis is seen in the neonatal period around days 5 to 14 of life with conjunctival injection and drainage but does not present with leukocoria. **(D)** Papilledema is a sign of increased intracranial pressure found on ophthalmoscopic examination with bulging of the optic disks and arterial-venous pulsations. Papilledema does not present with leukocoria.

28 The mother of an 18-month-old girl presents frantically to her pediatrician's office. She reports she grabbed her daughter's arm firmly to prevent her from falling down the stairs approximately 1 hour prior to presentation. She states that since the episode, her daughter has refused to move her arm fully and she is holding her arm partially flexed with her palm facing her abdomen.

Of the following, what is the most likely mechanism occurring in the patient's arm?

(A) Subluxation of the radial head
(B) Spiral fracture of the humerus
(C) Supracondylar fracture
(D) Ulnar nerve injury
(E) Torus fracture

The answer is A: **Subluxation of the radial head.** The description of the child in the vignette is consistent with a common injury in childhood called a nursemaid's elbow. It is a subluxation of the radial head that occurs by way of a pulling force on the child's arm. This injury is not a true dislocation, as a radiograph of the affected area would appear normal. Examination notes the arm to be partially flexed with the palm facing backward as well as refusal to use the affected arm. Reduction is accomplished by one of two methods: flexing and supinating the affected arm, or extending and pronating the affected side. Oftentimes a click is appreciated upon successful reduction and the child returns to normal activity shortly thereafter.

(C) The physical examination can be differentiated from a supracondylar fracture in that the child with a nursemaid's elbow has no obvious deformity, swelling, or tenderness. A supracondylar fracture is a common fracture of the elbow and the history is usually of a child less than 10 years of age who falls on an outstretched arm. Supracondylar fractures require urgent orthopedic consultation as children are at risk for compartment syndrome and neurovascular injury. **(D)** There is no indication for the child in the vignette to have an ulnar nerve injury, as there does not appear to be an obvious fracture. Ulnar nerve injuries present with symptoms of hand weakness. **(B)** Spiral fracture of the humerus would present with a visual deformity of the arm. **(E)** Torus fracture, also known as buckle fracture, is a compression fracture of the distal metaphysis. Diagnosis is made with radiography, and the history would be more consistent with a compression injury rather than a pulling history as was the case described in the vignette.

---

29 A 5-year-old girl with a past medical history significant for sickle cell disease presents to the emergency department with complaints of a 1-week history of fever, progressive pain in her right leg, and refusal to walk. Her baseline hemoglobin is 8 g/dL, and she has never had acute chest syndrome nor required a packed red blood cell transfusion. She was hospitalized twice for pain in her bilateral upper extremities, which she reports as her typical pain crisis. She has never had pain like this before. A complete blood count reveals a white cell count of $25 \times 10^3/\mu L$, hemoglobin 8 g/dL, and platelets $330 \times 10^3/\mu L$. Erythrocyte sedimentation rate and C-reactive protein are 102 mm/h and 10 mg/dL, respectively. A radiograph of her leg is within normal limits.

Of the following, what is the most like organism to cause her infection?

(A) *Pseudomonas aeruginosa*
(B) *Neisseria gonorrhea*
(C) *Staphylococcus aureus*
(D) *Salmonella enteritidis*
(E) *Streptococcus pneumoniae*

The answer is C: *Staphylococcus aureus*. The patient described in the vignette has symptoms and laboratory findings consistent with osteomyelitis. Osteomyelitis is an infection occurring in bone and usually presents with fever, pain, elevated white blood cell count, elevation of inflammatory markers such as erythrocyte sedimentation rate and C-reactive protein, point tenderness, and possibly overlying erythema, edema, and warmth. Radiography may be normal early on, and magnetic resonance imaging is the best test to help identify an osteomyelitis. **(C)** *Staphylococcus aureus* is the predominant inciting organism for osteomyelitis for all age groups followed by *Streptococcus pneumoniae.* **(D)** *Salmonella* sp. is a pathogen that frequently causes osteomyelitis in patients with sickle cell disease; however, *Staphylococcus aureus* remains the most common organism.

Neonates are particularly susceptible to infections with group B streptococcus and *Escherichia coli.* **(B)** Sexually active teenagers are at risk for infections caused by *N. gonorrhea.* **(A)** Puncture wounds through sneakers or other rubber-soled shoes place patients at risk for osteomyelitis caused by *P. aeruginosa.*

30 A newborn baby in the nursery has a short neck, has a low hairline, and is unable to move his head fully from side to side.

Of the following, what is the next best study to order for this patient?

(A) Magnetic resonance imaging of the brain and spinal cord
(B) Echocardiogram
(C) Complete metabolic panel
(D) Ophthalmology examination
(E) Renal ultrasound

The answer is E: Renal ultrasound. The baby described in the vignette has a congenital syndrome called Klippel-Feil syndrome. It is characterized by fusion of the cervical spinal vertebrae. The classic triad of Klippel-Feil syndrome is a short neck with limited range of motion and a low hairline. Associated anomalies for this syndrome include renal anomalies, spina bifida, scoliosis, and hearing loss. A radiograph of the cervical spine would show evidence of vertebral fusion (see *Figure 17-19*). Of the studies provided, only the renal ultrasound is indicated to evaluate for the various renal anomalies associated with Klippel-Feil syndrome.

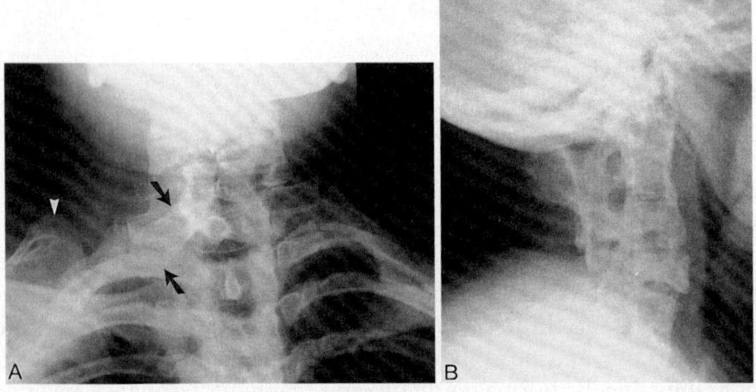

Figure 17-19

(A) Magnetic resonance imaging of the brain and spinal cord would demonstrate vertebral fusion; however, it is not the recommended first-line evaluation for this anomaly. **(B, C, D)** There are no expected abnormalities associated with Klippel-Feil syndrome that would indicate screening with an echocardiogram, ophthalmologic examination, or complete metabolic panel.

---

31 A 16-year-old boy is being seen in adolescent clinic for his school physical. He mentions a lesion he has had on his penis for 2 weeks (see *Figure 17-20*). He states the lesion has not caused him any pain. In addition, he has painless shotty inguinal lymphadenopathy.

Of the following, what is the best diagnostic study to identify the etiology of his lesion?

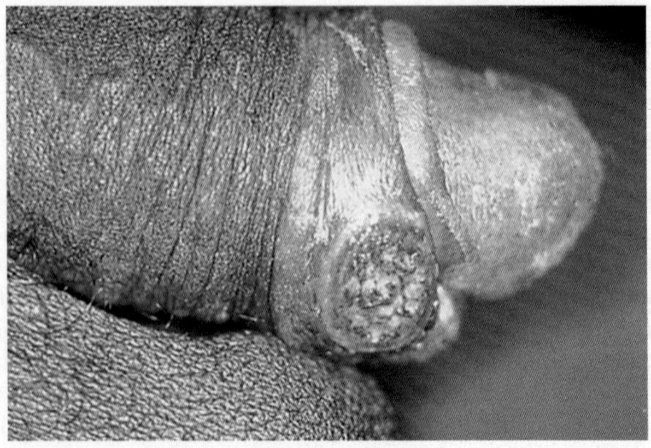
Figure 17-20

(A) Herpes simplex virus (HSV) PCR
(B) Biopsy
(C) Human papillomavirus (HPV) testing
(D) Human immunodeficiency virus titers
(E) Rapid plasma reagin (RPR)

The answer is E: **Rapid plasma reagin (RPR).** The lesion pictured in the vignette is a chancre, the lesion of primary syphilis. A chancre usually develops 2 to 12 weeks following exposure to syphilis and lasts for approximately 3 to 8 weeks. The lesion is painless and often associated with regional lymphadenopathy. Syphilis is identified by nontreponemal serologic testing with either RPR or the venereal disease research laboratory (VDRL) test. If RPR or VDRL are positive, treponemal serologic testing with fluorescent treponemal antibody-absorption can be used for confirmation as this test has a greater sensitivity.

(A) HSV PCR would be used to identify herpes virus. Herpes virus presents with painful ulcerations often associated with painful lymphadenopathy as well as clusters of smaller vesicular lesions. **(C)** HPV testing is useful to identify genital warts caused by the HPV. HPV types 6 and 11 are responsible for the characteristic cauliflower-like warts, and are generally asymptomatic although can be associated with some pain and pruritus. **(D)** Human immunodeficiency virus can be associated with a rash of Kaposi sarcoma. Kaposi sarcoma is not an ulceration but more of a hyperpigmented rash seen throughout the body and not isolated to the genitals. **(B)** A biopsy is not indicated when there is available serologic testing.

---

32 An 8-year-old girl presents to clinic for her routine school physical. She reports to having an active summer vacation and recently attended sleep away camp for 2 weeks. On her physical examination, she has a small mass at the level of her hyoid bone. On palpation, it is solid, nontender, and mobile. On oropharyngeal examination, the mass appears to move when she protrudes her tongue.

Of the following, what best describes her findings?

(A) Branchial cleft cyst
(B) Thyroglossal duct cyst
(C) Cystic hygroma
(D) Fibromatosis coli
(E) Hemangioma

The answer is B: **Thyroglossal duct cyst.** The girl in the vignette has a thyroglossal duct cyst. A thyroglossal duct cyst is a fibrocystic lesion that persists from the thyroglossal duct. Frequently, thyroglossal duct cysts can become infected and require treatment with antibiotic therapy. In addition they may contain ectopic thyroid tissue. Therefore, patients should have thyroid levels checked and surgical excision if indicated.

(**A**) Branchial cleft cysts are also remnants from embryology and form in the lateral neck, often anterior to the sternocleidomastoid muscle. Branchial cleft cysts are often asymptomatic unless infected. (**C**) Cystic hygromas usually present as an irregular, painless, compressible mass in the lateral neck and are often present at birth. (**D**) Fibromatosis coli, also known as congenital torticollis, can present at 1 to 2 weeks of age as a hard nontender mass within the body of the sternocleidomastoid muscle and with the infant's head tilting to one side. (**E**) Hemangiomas are a benign vascular proliferation present at birth or shortly thereafter. There are no reported vascular changes to indicate concern for a hemangioma as the diagnosis for the patient in the vignette.

33 A 6-year-old boy presents to clinic for his preschool physical. He is happy to report all about his summer spent at his lake house. His review of systems is benign aside from complaints of some ear pain on the left. His mother reports there is a green crusting on his pillow in the morning. On examination he has some discomfort with movement of his pinna to insert the otoscope and there is an erythematous and edematous canal making visualization of the tympanic membrane difficult.

Of the following, what is the next best step in management for this patient?

(A) Amoxicillin oral therapy
(B) Ofloxacin otic drops
(C) Hydrogen peroxide otic drops
(D) Otorhinolaryngology referral
(E) Computed tomography scan of head

The answer is B: Ofloxacin otic drops. The boy described in the vignette has otitis externa, also referred to as swimmer's ear. Otitis externa is often associated with a history of swimming or local trauma to the ear canal, such as a foreign body. It is an inflammatory process in the external auditory canal often caused by either fungal (*Aspergillus*, *Candida*) or bacterial (*Pseudomonas*, *Klebsiella*, *Staphylococcus aureus*, *Enterobacter*) infections. The therapy of choice is a broad-spectrum topical antibiotic with or without topical hydrocortisone to help decrease the edema. Preventative measures include drying the ear canal and the use of acetic acid. If left untreated, patients are at risk for malignant otitis externa which is a more invasive disease leading to hearing loss, vertigo, and facial nerve palsy as well as possible osteomyelitis of the temporal bone and intracranial spread.

(**A**) Amoxicillin therapy is indicated for children with acute otitis media. In addition, amoxicillin therapy would be indicated in a 6-year-old with otitis media only if they were febrile for more than 2 days and had already tried supportive measures for pain. **(C)** Hydrogen peroxide is the therapy for impacted cerumen. **(D, E)** Given the boy in the vignette is well appearing and there is no concern for a more aggressive disease process both otorhinolaryngology referral and computed tomography scan are not indicated.

---

34 The father of a 38-month-old girl brings her to the acute care clinic with complaints of burning on urination and a foul-smelling discharge he has noticed in her underwear. She has been otherwise well, without complaints of fevers or chills. She is active, plays with her Yorkshire terrier puppy, attends preschool, and her diet remains healthy and balanced. Her height and weight continue along the 50th percentile. On examination, she is an active girl who cries with attempts to place her on the examination table. She is calm on her father's lap and her examination is completed with her sitting with him. External genitalia examination is significant for an intact hymen, mild erythema, and some excoriation suprapubically as well as a foul-smelling odor.

Of the following, what is the next best step for her management?

(A) Avoid bubble baths
(B) Recommend scented powders to mask the smell
(C) Apply topical estrogen cream
(D) Fluconazole 150 mg orally and repeat in 1 week
(E) Tell him she must remain in your care as you contact social services

The answer is A: Avoid bubble baths. The girl described in the vignette has vulvovaginitis, a common pediatric problem in girls. In toddlers the most common etiology is secondary to irritation from bubble baths, soaps, detergents, or lotions as well as from poor or improper hygiene. Therefore, the best advice for management of vulvovaginitis is proper hygiene, limit bubble bath use, and use mild nonscented detergents. **(B)** Scented powders may exacerbate the symptoms of vulvovaginitis and should be avoided, not recommended for therapy. **(E)** There is no reason to suspect abuse in the case described in the vignette. **(C)** Topical estrogen cream is used occasionally for children with labial adhesions, which the patient in the vignette does not have. **(D)** Fluconazole is used for candidal infections. Patients with candidiasis present with pruritus as well as a cottage cheese-like vaginal discharge.

35 Of the following, what is the most likely etiology for optic neuritis in children?

(A) Multiple sclerosis
(B) Iron toxicity
(C) Viral infection
(D) Bacterial conjunctivitis
(E) Reiter syndrome

The answer is C: Viral infection. Optic neuritis is inflammation of the optic nerve. Optic neuritis in children is often idiopathic or associated with recent viral infections. Herpes simplex virus (HSV) and varicella are often associated infections. **(A)** Multiple sclerosis is associated with optic neuritis but rarely in children. **(B)** Lead toxicity rather than iron toxicity can be associated with optic neuritis. **(D)** Bacterial conjunctivitis does not cause optic neuritis, although infections such as dental abscess, meningitis, or sinusitis may be correlated. **(E)** Reiter syndrome is associated with uveitis rather than optic neuritis along with urethritis and arthritis.

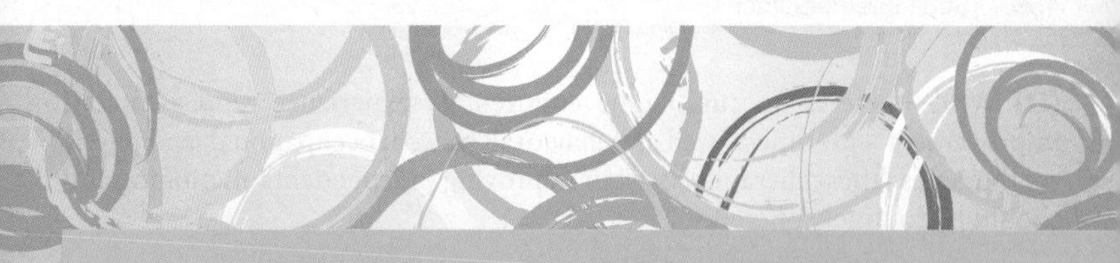

Sample Shelf-Exam

1 A child and his father are visiting for a well-child check necessary for school entry. The child and family have good social, emotional, and therapeutic support services in place. The child displays no verbal communication and little or no eye contact. He also displays intermittent repetitive hand flapping.

Of the following, which is most accurate statement regarding this patient's condition?

(A) It is a group of disorders that includes Rett syndrome
(B) It is caused by a reaction to routine childhood immunizations
(C) It can be detected as early as 9 months old with a validated screening questionnaire
(D) There is no known cure and no therapy has been recommended
(E) It is more common in females

The answer is C: It can be detected as early as 9 months old with a validated screening questionnaire. Autism spectrum disorder is a group of disorders, **(E)** more common in males, which includes classic autism; Asperger syndrome; and pervasive developmental disorder not otherwise specified, also known as atypical autism. Classic autism is marked by verbal and nonverbal communication impairment. Nonverbal communication impairment may include not making eye contact, smiling, or pointing. Social development is also impaired as noted by difficulty sharing emotions and appreciating others' perspectives. Motor development is affected and may be marked by repetitive behaviors like hand flapping. Autism spectrum disorder can be suspected as early as 9 months old through a validated screening questionnaire. It is recommended that all children should be screened for autism spectrum disorder at 9, 18, 24, and 36 months old.

(A) Pervasive developmental disorder is a broader group of disorders and includes the autism spectrum disorders plus childhood disintegrative disorder and Rett syndrome. **(B)** There is no proven link that any routine childhood immunization, in any combination, leads to autism spectrum disorder.

(D) While there is no cure, some children do experience mild symptom improvement with time as well as behavioral, speech, occupational, and physical therapies. These therapies assist in improving independent functioning and should be routinely offered.

An 11-year-old boy presents to the clinic for his sixth-grade school physical. His mother states that she is concerned that he is much smaller than the other children in his class. He has no significant past medical history and he does not take any medications. His mother reports that she had a normal height in school but she did not menstruate until age 16. A wrist radiograph demonstrates a bone age consistent with a 9-year-old boy.

Of the following, what is the most appropriate recommendation for this family at this time?

(A) Refer the patient to endocrinology for initiation of growth hormone therapy
(B) Prescribe testosterone therapy to hasten puberty's onset
(C) Obtain thyroid studies
(D) Advise that the patient see a child psychiatrist to address psychosocial effects of his growth retardation
(E) Reassurance that he will reach his average adult height after his growth cycle is complete

The answer is E: Reassurance that he will reach his average adult height after his growth cycle is complete. Constitutional growth delay occurs when healthy patients have a slower rate of physical development than peers of similar age. Growth rate is normal in early infancy and then declines thereafter. There is usually a history of a parent or family member with a similar history of late-onset puberty, for example, females with delayed menarche and/or males with delayed facial or pubic hair development. Most children with constitutional growth delay eventually reach their expected adult height, although later than their cohort group. Constitutional growth delay is a variant of normal growth, thus medical treatment is not often necessary. Bone age radiographs are used to document delayed bone age in patients with constitutional growth delay as well as primary hypogonadism. Patients with constitutional growth delay have a bone age that is less than the chronological age. Education and reassurance should be given to the parent and the patient.

(A) Growth hormone therapy may be used in various conditions where adolescents are growing slowly secondary to poor growth hormone production from such causes as idiopathic short stature, Turner syndrome, or chronic kidney disease. **(B)** Because there has been controversy surrounding the use of testosterone therapy for boys with constitutional growth delay, reassurance is the best recommendation to give at this time. **(C)** Evaluating thyroid function in a patient with no other complaints and a family history of constitutional growth delay is not indicated. **(D)** Short stature may cause psychosocial issues that may warrant children to be referred for psychotherapy to address issues that may be quite stressful regarding their growth delay; however, the patient in the vignette is not displaying such concerns at this time.

3 A child can pull to a stand and cruise along furniture. When presented cubes, she takes her palm from the table to a pincer grasp and bangs the cubes together. When the cubes are covered with a cloth, she lifts the cloth to find them.

Of the following, what is the youngest age at which these activities are expected?

(A) 4 months old
(B) 6 months old
(C) 9 months old
(D) 12 months old
(E) 18 months old

The answer is C: 9 months old. (A, B, D, E) At 9 months old, infants are developing the motor skills necessary to coordinate multiple actions. Cognitively they have a more developed sense of cause and effect. The combination of these physical and cognitive skills allows for more sequential purposeful actions like standing to then cruise with hands on furniture for balance, or reaching for objects in order to bang them together. Further, object permanence is maturing so infants at 9 months old have developed the critical understanding that even though objects are not immediately visible, the objects are still present, prompting the child to search for them.

4 A 17-year-old girl presents for a health maintenance visit. She reports heavy periods for the last 9 months. Her cycles are 12 days long, and she reports using 10 pads or tampons per day. Her past medical, family, and social histories are negative for any underlying abnormalities or disorders. She has had regular periods since she was 13 years old and is very insistent that she has not been sexually active. On physical examination, her vital signs are temperature 37.6°C, heart rate 95 beats/minute, blood pressure (BP) 100/60 mmHg, and respiratory rate 16 breaths/minute. She is diffusely pale and reports dizziness upon standing. The remainder of her examination is unremarkable. Laboratory evaluation reveals a hemoglobin 8 g/dL with a low mean corpuscular volume (MCV) and a β-human chorionic gonadotropin (β-hCG) level is negative.

Of the following, what is the most likely etiology for this patient's presentation?

(A) Ectopic pregnancy
(B) Hypothyroidism
(C) Dysfunctional uterine bleeding (DUB)
(D) Sexually transmitted infection
(E) Endometriosis

The answer is C: Dysfunctional uterine bleeding (DUB). DUB is a diagnosis that describes abnormal bleeding from the uterus without an organic cause. Etiologies that should be addressed and ruled out when considering this diagnosis include sexually transmitted infections, bleeding disorders such as von Willebrand disease, and pregnancy. Treatment of DUB includes iron therapy and regulating the menstrual cycle with oral contraceptives as DUB is often the result of anovulation. Blood transfusions may be needed to treat symptomatic anemia secondary to prolonged or heavy menstrual periods.

(A) Ectopic pregnancy would be expected to present with more severe abdominal pain and a positive β-hCG level. **(B)** Hypothyroidism can be associated with irregular menses but would be expected to include other findings such as thinning of the hair, dry skin, and bradycardia. **(D)** A sexually transmitted infection is possible but unlikely for the patient in the vignette given the absence of abdominal pain or vaginal discharge. **(E)** Endometriosis as a cause of menorrhagia is less common than DUB in this adolescent.

5 A 4-month-old infant is brought by ambulance to the emergency department. An initial blood gas reveals a pH of 6.9. He is intubated and his initial chest radiograph reveals bilateral pulmonary infiltrates. He is started on a regimen of ceftriaxone and vancomycin. Over the next 24 hours the patient continues to decline and a bronchoalveolar lavage is obtained revealing *Pneumocystis jiroveci.*

Of the following, which is most consistent with a diagnosis of severe combined immunodeficiency (SCID)?

(A) Absolute lymphocyte count >30,000/μL
(B) Elevated levels of IgG and IgM
(C) Positive response to vaccines
(D) Absolute lymphocyte count <2,500/μL
(E) Human immunodeficiency virus (HIV) RNA positivity

The answer is D: Absolute lymphocyte count <2,500/mL. SCID is a group of genetic mutations leading to an absence of innate immunity and natural killer (NK) cell dysfunction. Patients with SCID have an absent or minimal thymus and no circulating thymocytes. X-linked SCID is the most common form of SCID in the United States. Patients with the X-linked form typically have absent T cells, elevated B cells, and absent NK cells. Autosomal recessive SCID disorders include adenosine deaminase (ADA) deficiency which is the most severe, with absolute lymphocyte counts <500/μL and very low numbers of T, B, and NK cells. On physical examination, patients with ADA deficiency have chondro-osseous dysplasia presenting with rib cage abnormalities and multiple skeletal abnormalities at the costochondral junctions.

Patients with SCID typically present within the first several months of life with severe, invasive infections, often with atypical organisms, including *Candida albicans*, *P. jiroveci*, severe adenovirus, cytomegalovirus, and Epstein-Barr virus (EBV). These infections can lead to diarrhea, sepsis, pneumonia, thrush, or failure to thrive. Growth initially appears normal but quickly fades secondary to persistent and recurrent diarrhea.

(A) Laboratory workup demonstrates lymphopenia (<2,500/μL) that is often present at birth. **(B)** Due to the poor function or absence of T cells, serum immunoglobulin levels are low due to the lack of activation and signaling of B cells. **(C)** Similarly, response to vaccine administration is minimal as antibody formation is hindered. Treatment for SCID is a stem cell transplant.

(E) HIV also causes T-cell suppression and can predispose infected individuals to atypical infections such as *P. jiroveci* due to low CD4+ cell counts. Opportunistic infections frequently increase as CD4+ counts decrease below 400/μL. While HIV infection is a consideration for the patient in the vignette, HIV-positive serology is not indicative of also having SCID.

---

6 A 4-year-old girl is a new patient seen in clinic for a preschool checkup. She is of stocky build with her height at the 25th percentile and her weight at the 75th percentile for her age. On examination, she has a round face. Her fourth and fifth digits are shorter than the rest, and the corresponding knuckles are replaced by dimples. She has no palpable thyroid, no murmur, and no abdominal masses or striae. Her laboratory findings are as follows:

Serum calcium	7.2 mg/dL
Serum phosphorus	6.3 mg/dL
Serum intact parathyroid hormone (PTH)	301 pg/mL
Serum 25-hydroxyvitamin D	57 ng/mL

Of the following, which best explains this patient's findings?

(A) Pseudohypoparathyroidism
(B) Hypoparathyroidism
(C) Vitamin D deficiency rickets
(D) Multiple endocrine neoplasia, type 1 (MEN 1)
(E) Multiple endocrine neoplasia, type 2B (MEN 2B)

The answer is A: Pseudohypoparathyroidism. The facial dysmorphism and skeletal anomalies described for this patient in combination with electrolyte changes consistent with hypoparathyroidism (low calcium and high phosphorus) despite elevated PTH levels suggest pseudohypoparathyroidism. This genetic disorder results from decreased PTH receptor responsiveness and may be associated with skeletal changes. Patients may present with tetany, seizures, or other signs of hypocalcemia, which do not typically manifest until 4 to 6 years of age.

(B) In contrast, a patient with hypoparathyroidism is expected to have low levels of PTH causing hypocalcemia and hyperphosphatemia since PTH is responsible for increasing calcium absorption from the gut, releasing calcium from bone, and increasing renal excretion of phosphorus.

(C) Patients with vitamin D deficiency rickets have low levels of vitamin D along with low calcium and low phosphorus levels. This occurs because insufficient vitamin D levels lead to decreased calcium absorption from the gut. The body then responds by secreting increased PTH (secondary hyperparathyroidism) in an attempt to increase the availability of calcium which also increases phosphorus excretion from the kidney. Bony changes can be seen because of poor mineralization such as bowing of the long bones, rachitic changes of the ribs, and cupping of the distal epiphyses leading to widened wrists and ankles. The bony changes described for the patient in this case are not consistent with rickets.

(D, E) MEN syndromes are autosomal dominant collections of a variety of neuroendocrine dyscrasias and tumors. In type 1, patients can develop hyperparathyroidism, pancreatic tumors, and pituitary tumors. In type 2A, also known as Sipple syndrome, patients experience hyperparathyroidism, medullary thyroid carcinoma, and pheochromocytoma. Patients with type 2B typically have medullary thyroid carcinoma and pheochromocytoma but these findings are accompanied by a marfanoid habitus with dermatologic and intestinal neuromas. All patients with MEN 2B have mucosal neuromas of the lips and tongue. Given the autosomal dominant transmission of these diseases as well as their association with malignancy, relatives of affected individuals should have a genetic evaluation as well as a prophylactic thyroidectomy as indicated if MEN 2A or MEN 2B is positive.

At a health maintenance visit, an infant's mother takes a toy her 12-month-old child is chewing on and hands it to an older sibling. The sibling then places the toy in a diaper bag. After initially being upset, the infant is easily soothed and the examination continues. After completing the examination, the infant is assisted off the examination table and goes straight to the diaper bag searching for the toy.

Of the following, which statement best describes the activity observed in this infant?

(A) Object permanence is a developmental milestone signifying the beginning of cause-and-effect reasoning
(B) Self-soothing is a skill not developed until 24 months old
(C) Taking turns is a personal/social developmental milestone attained at 12 months old
(D) Stranger anxiety generally resolves by 6 months old
(E) Exploring objects with one's mouth is a normal developmental process resolved by 9 months old

The answer is A: Object permanence is a developmental milestone signifying the beginning of cause-and-effect reasoning. Object permanence is an important developmental process necessary for cause-and-effect reasoning. While object permanence generally begins when an infant is 9 months old, the process matures by 12 months old and allows recognition that the no-longer-visible object still exists. **(B)** Self-soothing is a critical task achieved by most infants by 2 to 4 months old by placing a fist in their mouth to stimulate non-nutritive sucking. **(C)** Taking turns is often not developed until 36 months old. **(D)** Stranger anxiety and separation anxiety peak near 9 months old and **(E)** exploring objects with one's mouth can last beyond 2 years old.

8 A 5-day-old newborn presents to clinic for his hospital follow-up appointment. He was born full-term via a forceps-assisted vaginal delivery. His birth weight was 4.8 kg. The pregnancy was complicated by a chlamydial infection during the first trimester that was adequately treated and repeat cultures were negative. His mother is currently breastfeeding but states the baby prefers to only feed from her left breast and does not latch well to the right breast. On examination, when placed prone he is able to lift his head toward the right but is unable to turn toward the left. His Moro reflex is intact and he has upgoing Babinski reflex.

Of the following, what is the best next step in management for this infant?

(A) Physical therapy referral
(B) Neurology referral and electromyography testing
(C) Neck ultrasound
(D) Magnetic resonance imaging (MRI) of the head/neck
(E) Lactation consultation

The answer is A: Physical therapy referral. The baby described in the vignette has torticollis, congenital twisting of the neck, likely secondary to fibromatosis colli. Given his presentation occurred in the newborn period it is most likely secondary to birth trauma to the sternocleidomastoid muscle. The treatment for torticollis is physical therapy, exercises, stretching, and massage. **(B)** The baby in the vignette has a symmetric Moro reflex as well as a normal Babinski and therefore is not showing signs or concerns for muscle or nerve damage making neurology referral or electromyography testing unnecessary.

Fibromatosis colli is associated with congenital torticollis and may also involve a mass on the sternocleidomastoid muscle. **(C, D)** This mass may be confused with other cystic or neoplastic causes, but does not require evaluation by ultrasound or MRI. **(E)** His lack of breastfeeding on one side is secondary to his preferred position of comfort of his head and neck and does not require lactation consultation.

9 The concerned parents of a 3-week-old newborn present to the emergency department for evaluation of vomiting. The parents state that the patient has done well since birth, tolerating 2.5 oz of formula every 3 hours with appropriate weight gain. In the last few days, the patient has vomited and is unable to tolerate any formula, although he does appear to still be hungry after each episode of emesis. The parents deny any fevers or sick contacts. On examination, the patient is moderately dehydrated. An abdominal ultrasound confirms the diagnosis.

Of the following, which set of laboratory results is most consistent with this patient's diagnosis?

(A) Sodium: 140 mEq/L, potassium: 2.8 mEq/L, chloride: 88 mEq/L, bicarbonate: 30 mEq/L
(B) Sodium: 132 mEq/L, potassium: 5.4 mEq/L, chloride: 94 mEq/L, bicarbonate: 14 mEq/L
(C) Sodium: 154 mEq/L, potassium: 2.2 mEq/L, chloride: 99 mEq/L, bicarbonate: 21 mEq/L
(D) Sodium: 140 mEq/L, potassium: 4.2 mEq/L, chloride: 100 mEq/L, bicarbonate: 24 mEq/L
(E) Sodium: 128 mEq/L, potassium: 6.8 mEq/L, chloride: 110 mEq/L, bicarbonate: 8 mEq/L

The answer is A: Sodium: 140 mEq/L, potassium: 2.8 mEq/L, chloride: 88 mEq/L, bicarbonate: 30 mEq/L. The differential diagnosis for emesis in the newborn period is broad. Surgical diagnoses include malrotation, pyloric stenosis, and intestinal atresias. Nonsurgical diagnoses include gastroenteritis, adrenal insufficiency, and inborn errors of metabolism. The patient in the vignette has findings consistent with pyloric stenosis, which results in gastric outlet obstruction secondary to the hypertrophy of the pylorus muscle. The incidence is increased in first-born children and males. Symptoms typically begin in the first month of life. The emesis is described as projectile in nature and does not contain bile, as the obstruction is proximal to the duodenum. The recurrent vomiting of gastric contents leads to loss of hydrochloric acid. With prolonged emesis and loss of extracellular volume, there is a relative increase in the bicarbonate concentration that results in a contraction alkalosis. This alkalosis drives the K+/H+ pump in the kidneys to excrete potassium and retain hydrogen ions. **(B, C, D, E)** Therefore, the typical laboratory finding associated with pyloric stenosis is a hypochloremic hypokalemic metabolic alkalosis.

10 A concerned mother brings her 10-year-old son to the clinic after a note from school is sent home stating there has been an outbreak of "strep throat" in class. She reports the boy had a fever earlier in the day and now has a decreased appetite due to throat pain. His examination reveals a boy in no acute distress, enlarged and tender anterior cervical lymph nodes, and oropharyngeal erythema and petechiae. A rapid swab test obtained in the office is positive for *Streptococcus pyogenes*.

Of the following, which is the next best step in the management of this patient?

(A) Treatment with antibiotics is warranted to prevent acute poststreptococcal glomerulonephritis (APSGN)
(B) Treatment with antibiotics is warranted to prevent rheumatic fever (RF)
(C) Complete blood count, blood culture, and erythrocyte sedimentation rate or C-reactive protein should be obtained
(D) Echocardiogram should be ordered to assess for cardiac function and anatomy
(E) Urinalysis should be obtained to evaluate for hematuria

The answer is B: Treatment with antibiotics is warranted to prevent rheumatic fever (RF). *S. pyogenes* is a gram-positive microorganism that can often cause acute pharyngitis and impetigo. Antibiotics can help treat the active infection, although in most cases, the infection is self-limited without treatment. Infection with *S. pyogenes* can trigger an immune response that can cause systemic illness 2 to 3 weeks after the initial infection, such as acute rheumatic fever (ARF) and APSGN. **(A)** Appropriate antibiotic therapy can prevent RF; however, it will not decrease the risk of developing APSGN.

(C) RF is an inflammatory disorder of the connective tissues of the body, including symptoms of carditis, migratory polyarthritis, subcutaneous nodules, erythema marginatum, and Sydenham chorea. If there were concern for RF in the patient in the vignette, ordering a more detailed workup may be indicated.

Patients with APSGN can develop gross hematuria, edema, hypertension, and renal insufficiency. RF and APSGN occur following an initial *S. pyogenes* infection. **(C, D, E)** The boy in the vignette has an acute infection, and therefore, the next best choice would be to treat the patient with antibiotics to eliminate the risk of developing RF.

11 An 11-year-old girl is found to have a BP reading of 132/90 mmHg at her sixth-grade school physical. She has no significant past medical history. There is a family history of grandparents on both sides with adult-onset hypertension and hypercholesterolemia. The remainder of her history, physical examination, and vital signs, including body mass index, are all within normal limits.

Of the following, what is the next best step in the management of this patient?

(A) Prescribe a thiazide diuretic
(B) Assess for target organ damage by ordering an echocardiogram
(C) Order urinalysis, electrolytes, blood urea nitrogen, and creatinine
(D) Repeat the BP in 1 week
(E) Order fasting glucose, insulin, and lipid panel

The answer is D: Repeat the BP in 1 week. Hypertension in the asymptomatic pediatric patient is defined as BP measurements greater than the 95th percentile for age, gender, and height, on three separate occasions. Most children are asymptomatic, and therefore, routine BP should be checked at every visit starting at the age of 3. After multiple measurements are recorded to confirm hypertension, a complete workup should be obtained to differentiate primary, also known as essential hypertension, from secondary causes. **(B, C, E)** The workup should consist of a urinalysis, basic metabolic panel, lipid panel, insulin levels, echocardiogram, and renal ultrasound. The most common cause of secondary hypertension in children is due to renal pathology. **(A)** Prior to starting any therapy, the BP needs to be rechecked and confirmed, followed by a complete diagnostic evaluation for a potential cause. The treatment for children with asymptomatic hypertension without evidence of end-organ damage is therapeutic lifestyle modification with dietary changes and regular exercise as weight loss is the primary therapy in obesity-related hypertension. Indications for medications include patients with symptoms such as headache or vision changes, secondary hypertension, end-organ damage, diabetes mellitus (DM), or hypertension that does not correct with lifestyle changes.

12 A 1-year-old infant has been diagnosed with multiple pyogenic infections including several staphylococcal and streptococcal infections. He had meningitis at 6 months of age, multiple episodes of acute otitis media and conjunctivitis, as well as a recent hospitalization for streptococcal bacteremia. Following an immune workup, he was found to have X-linked agammaglobulinemia.

Of the following, what is the best first-line therapy for this patient?

(A) Stem cell transplant
(B) Intravenous immunoglobulin (IVIG)
(C) Gene therapy
(D) Strict restriction of environment
(E) No therapy indicated

The answer is B: Intravenous immunoglobulin (IVIG). **(A)** Unlike conditions such as severe combined immunodeficiency that are treated with stem cell transplant, **(E)** X-linked agammaglobulinemia, also known as Bruton agammaglobulinemia, is treated with a threefold approach. Treatment begins with antibody replacement with IVIG. IVIG works by replacing the antibodies the affected patient's own body is unable to produce. The second-line treatment is the prompt or prophylactic use of antibiotics. Lastly, these patients with agammaglobulinemia should avoid all live viral vaccines, including measles, mumps, rubella, and varicella.

(D) Although careful treatment with the above methods can be supplemented with being aware of the patient's environment, affected patients do not need to live an isolated, restricted life. **(C)** Similarly while at this time there is no curative therapy, such as gene therapy, with proper IVIG treatment and aggressive management of infections, patients with X-linked agammaglobulinemia can live active lives.

---

13 A 5-year-old girl presents with recurrent and progressive bone pain for the past year. On physical examination, she is less than the 10th percentile for height and weight and has hepatosplenomegaly. Her mother is of Jewish descent. Further laboratory evaluation reveals anemia and thrombocytopenia.

Of the following, which is her most likely diagnosis and treatment plan?

(A) Gaucher disease; enzyme replacement therapy
(B) Systemic lupus erythematosus (SLE); corticosteroids
(C) Juvenile idiopathic arthritis (JIA); nonsteroidal anti-inflammatory drugs
(D) Sanfilippo syndrome; supportive care
(E) Adrenoleukodystrophy; bone marrow transplant

The answer is A: Gaucher disease; enzyme replacement therapy. The patient in the vignette presents with signs and symptoms characteristic of Gaucher disease, a lysosomal storage disorder, found more commonly in the Ashkenazi Jewish population. Gaucher disease is caused by a deficiency of the enzyme β-glucosidase, leading to accumulation of glucocerebroside. These patients generally have hepatosplenomegaly and storage of glucocerebroside in the bone marrow leading to episodes of bone pain and hematologic changes such as anemia, leukopenia, and thrombocytopenia. Recombinant enzyme replacement therapy is the treatment of choice.

(B) SLE may present with arthritis and hematologic changes; however, the patient in the vignette does not currently have enough criteria to establish a diagnosis of SLE as she is presenting with arthralgias, rather than arthritis. **(C)** JIA may present with recurrent bone pain, but would also be expected to have findings on physical examination consistent with arthritis, rather than arthralgias. **(D)** Sanfilippo syndrome is a type of lysosomal storage disorder in the class of mucopolysaccharidoses, which presents with coarse facies, kyphosis, hepatosplenomegaly, and developmental regression. **(E)** Adrenoleukodystrophy is an X-linked condition that presents with adrenal insufficiency, behavioral changes, clumsiness, and hyperpigmentation.

14 An 18-month-old boy presents for his first visit to clinic. The records have not been transferred yet from his previous physician and his mother is unclear of the boy's perinatal course, but states that he went quickly to the neonatal intensive care unit following delivery. His height, weight, and head circumference are at the 10th percentile. On further examination, he is a small boy who is nonverbal and nonmobile. He occasionally grimaces and is drooling with excitement. His upper extremities are held in flexion at the elbows and wrists. The remainder of his examination is within normal limits and his mother notes that this is consistent with his baseline.

Of the following, which is the most likely comorbidity associated with this child's condition?

(A) Regression of developmental milestones
(B) Worsening proximal muscle weakness
(C) Epilepsy
(D) Meningoencephalitis
(E) Child abuse

The answer is C: Epilepsy. The patient described in the vignette has cerebral palsy (CP) placing him at risk for epilepsy. CP is a static and chronic neurologic disorder. Many causes have been proposed including damage to the prenatal, perinatal, or postnatal developing brain as well as birth asphyxia, congenital infections, metabolic disorders, and genetic syndromes. This disorder presents with chronic but unchanging motor abnormalities as described for the child in the vignette. CP can affect motor and cognitive development to varying degrees. Treatment is multidisciplinary and includes support from physicians as well as occupational, physical, and developmental therapists. Associated seizure disorders are controlled with antiepileptic drugs and close follow-up with a neurologist.

(A) Although patients with CP often have delayed developmental milestones they do not regress, in fact, many improve their development with appropriate therapy. **(B)** Worsening proximal muscle weakness can be found in patients with muscular dystrophy. **(D)** Meningoencephalitis is an inflammation of the meninges and brain parenchyma usually of infectious origin. The patient above is not described to have any fevers, altered mental status, headache, or vomiting. **(E)** This patient does not show any signs of trauma but instead is consistent with a diagnosis of CP. It is important to note, however, that often children with CP have a higher incidence of abuse.

---

15 A frantic mother brings her 3-year-old son to the emergency department. She states that the child was playing on the floor when she witnessed him pick a coin up off the floor and put it into his mouth. By the time she was able to reach him, he had swallowed it. On examination, the patient is a smiling, playful child, who is in no acute distress. There is no stridor or drooling present. Chest radiography demonstrates a round opacity at the lower third of the esophagus.

Of the following, which is the next best step in the management of this patient?

(A) Endoscopic removal within 24 hours
(B) Repeat chest radiography in 12 hours
(C) Emergent endoscopic removal of the object
(D) Reassurance and follow-up in 1 week
(E) Administer syrup of ipecac

The answer is B: Repeat chest radiography in 12 hours. The first step to consider in evaluating a patient with a foreign body ingestion is to obtain radiography to determine location. **(C)** A coin lodged in the upper portion of the esophagus is generally removed urgently. If a patient is asymptomatic, a confirmed or suspected foreign body lodged in the lower portion of the esophagus can be observed for up to 24 hours. Many of these swallowed objects will pass into the stomach without incident. A dose of glucagon may be given to help relax the lower esophageal sphincter and increase the likelihood that the object will pass into the stomach. **(B, D)** A repeat radiography examination in 12 hours may be helpful to further evaluate progression of the foreign body. If the foreign body has passed into the stomach, it will likely pass through the rest of the gastrointestinal tract without incident. Such patients can be conservatively managed at home, with parents straining stools to document passage of the object. **(A)** However, if the foreign body remains lodged in the esophagus, endoscopic removal is indicated in 12 to 24 hours following the ingestion to prevent complications such as esophageal perforation. Some foreign body ingestions, such as button batteries or sharp objects, are considered an emergency secondary to the increased risk of esophageal injury, damage, and perforation. If there is any doubt about the identity of a coin-shaped object, it should be removed urgently.

(E) It is never appropriate to administer syrup of ipecac. Potential complications of induced vomiting include aspiration, caustic damage to the esophagus, and a Mallory-Weiss tear.

---

16 A 12-day-old newborn is born at 31 weeks of gestation by caesarean section secondary to fetal distress. His birth weight is 1,850 g. He was admitted to the neonatal intensive care unit and given continuous positive airway pressure ventilation that has been subsequently weaned to 1 L of room air by nasal cannula. He has been tolerating the full volume of neonatal formula via orogastric tube since day of life 6. Overnight, he vomited three times, became tachypneic with increased oxygen demand, and today his abdomen is distended and tympanitic. He had a stool with mixed blood and mucus and subsequently required intubation with mechanical respiratory support.

Of the following, which finding is most consistent with this baby's most likely diagnosis?

(A) Growth on blood culture with group B *Streptococcus*
(B) Plain chest radiograph demonstrating diffuse ground-glass appearance
(C) Plain abdominal radiograph demonstrating paucity of air in the colon and a tissue mass in the right upper quadrant
(D) Plain abdominal radiograph demonstrating a large mass with calcifications that crosses the midline
(E) Plain abdominal radiograph demonstrating gas within the intestinal walls

The answer is E: Plain abdominal radiograph demonstrating gas within the intestinal walls. The neonate in the vignette has developed necrotizing enterocolitis (NEC), a life-threatening disease of infants that is characterized by intestinal necrosis of varying degrees. Risk for NEC is inversely proportional to decreasing gestational age and birthweight. The specific etiology is unknown, but includes infectious and hemodynamic factors. Diagnosis can be suggested by abdominal radiographs showing signs of pneumatosis intestinalis, or gas accumulation within the intestinal submucosa (see *Figure 1*). This can progress to intestinal perforation, peritonitis, sepsis, and death. While NEC is not considered solely an infectious process, it has been associated with bacteremia with gram-negative organisms such as *Escherichia coli, Klebsiella pneumoniae,* or *Clostridium perfringens,* as well as the gram-positive organism *Staphylococcus epidermidis.*

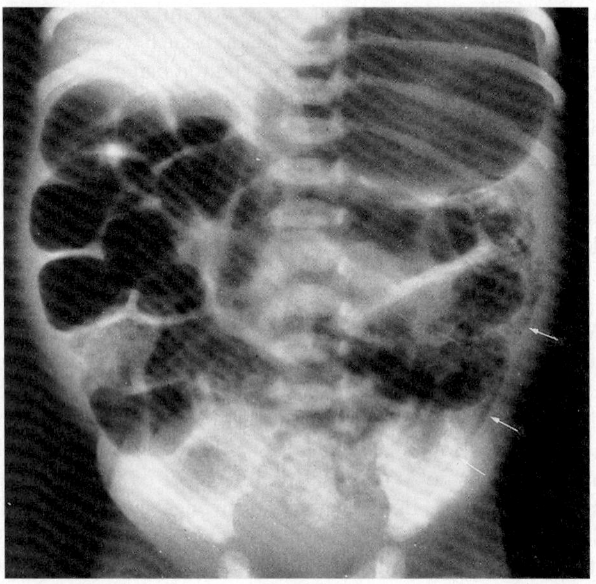

Figure 1

(A) Patients with group B streptococcal infection may present with sepsis but are less likely to have the abdominal findings described in the vignette. **(B)** Respiratory distress syndrome is associated with a ground-glass appearance on chest radiography and is most common in premature infants; however, this etiology is not consistent with the description of NEC in the vignette. **(C)** Abdominal radiographic findings of decreased colonic air and a round tissue mass in the right upper quadrant describes intussusception and is consistent with both abdominal distention and bloody stools, but intussusception is uncommon in the neonatal period. **(D)** A large abdominal mass with calcifications on abdominal radiography is consistent with neuroblastoma; however, this diagnosis does not explain the sudden clinical change or bloody stools as described in the vignette.

---

17 A 12-year-old boy comes to the office for a health maintenance visit. He has no complaints except he wants to know if he is overweight. His body mass index is at the 90th percentile. He eats fruits and vegetables three to four times per week, typically drinks juice and carbonated beverages, and enjoys eating hot dogs. He plays basketball with his friends once a week but otherwise spends his free time playing video games. He is in seventh grade and gets mostly Bs. His vital signs are temperature of 36.7°C, heart rate of 80 beats/minute, respiratory rate of 16 breaths/minute, and BP of 100/70 mmHg. On examination, he is well appearing although overweight. His head and neck are unremarkable and he has no palpable thyroid. His lungs are clear and his heart sounds are within normal limits with no murmur. There are no abdominal masses. His skin is shown in *Figure 2*. On screening laboratory evaluation, his hemoglobin A_1C is 9.6%, fasting glucose is 187 mg/dL, and fasting triglycerides are 145 mg/dL. A urinalysis reveals trace protein and 2+ glucose with no ketones.

Of the following, which best explains this patient's underlying pathology?

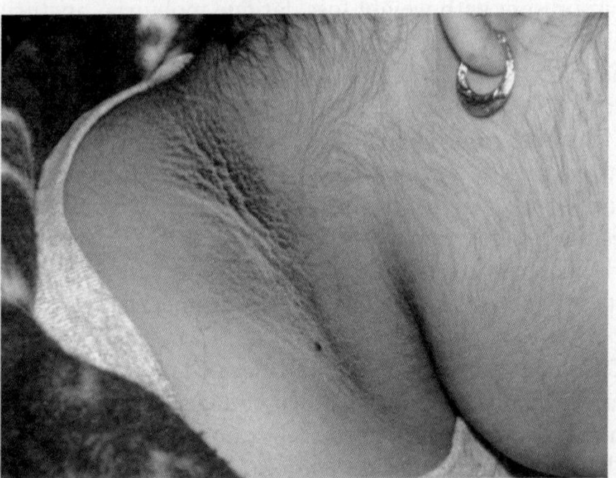

Figure 2

(A) Type 1 diabetes mellitus (DM)
(B) Type 2 DM
(C) Metabolic syndrome
(D) Cushing syndrome
(E) Addison disease

The answer is B: Type 2 diabetes mellitus (DM). DM is a disease characterized by hyperglycemia, whether as a result of decreased insulin levels as in type 1 DM or of diminished insulin function in the face of chronic hyperglycemia as in type 2 DM. As levels of glucose rise, the kidney begins to excrete the surplus resulting in glycosuria. The body is unable to metabolize the glucose properly which makes the body function as if it were in starvation mode; thus, ketone bodies are formed, the byproducts of which can also be seen in the urine. Diabetes may be diagnosed in one of the following ways:

1) Nonfasting blood glucose level >200 mg/dL, and typical symptoms
2) Fasting plasma glucose level >126 mg/dL
3) Two-hour glucose tolerance test value >200 mg/dL after giving a 75 g glucose load

Patients with type 2 DM typically have a large body habitus, a poor diet that is high in simple sugars and starches, and acanthosis nigricans, or dark pigmentation of the axillary, nuchal, and flexural areas. The presentation of type 2 DM is often insidious. Patients may complain of fatigue, abdominal pain, and headaches; however, others may be asymptomatic. Treatment involves diet and lifestyle modification with possible oral medications. **(A)** Patients with type 1 DM have low or absent levels of endogenous insulin and depend on exogenous insulin to prevent the development of ketoacidosis, an acute life-threatening complication of type 1 DM. Patients can present with weight loss, fatigue, polyuria, nocturia, polydipsia, polyphagia, or, in females, recurrent candidal vulvovaginitis. These patients have evidence of autoantibodies such as anti-insulin or anti-β-islet cell antibodies.

(C) Metabolic syndrome is defined as three or more of the following: fasting plasma glucose of greater than 100 mg/dL, hypertension, enlarged waist circumference, elevated triglycerides, and low high density lipoproteins. It increases the risk of coronary artery disease, diabetes, and stroke. Aggressive lifestyle changes can alter the course of this disease. While the patient in the vignette may be at risk for metabolic syndrome, he does not yet fulfill all diagnostic criteria.

(D) Cushing syndrome results from elevated blood glucocorticoid levels from either exogenous (i.e., iatrogenic) or endogenous (i.e., cortisol-secreting adrenal tumor or adrenocorticotropic hormone-secreting pituitary tumor) sources. The most common cause is prolonged administration of glucocorticoid hormones. Patients exhibit hyperglycemia, hypertension, weight gain, linear growth retardation, osteoporosis, moon facies, a buffalo hump, and purplish abdominal striae. **(E)** Patients with Addison disease experience hypoglycemia as opposed to hyperglycemia.

18 An 18-year-old high school senior comes to the office for a routine sports physical. She is on the cross-country team and has received a scholarship to college. Physical examination reveals a thin female. On reviewing her chart, a 5-kg weight loss over the last year is noted. Upon questioning the patient regarding her weight, she states she has to stay thin and would like to lose more weight to stay competitive. She skips breakfast and usually has salad for lunch and dinner. She has not had a menstrual period in the last 6 months.

Of the following, which additional finding is most likely to be found in this patient?

(A) Diarrhea
(B) Hirsutism
(C) Erosion of dental enamel
(D) Bradycardia
(E) Tachypnea

The answer is D: Bradycardia. The patient in the vignette has anorexia nervosa, evidenced by her intense fear of gaining weight, feeling overweight even though she is thin, and having amenorrhea. Death occurs in patients with anorexia from complications of starvation, most likely from cardiac insult secondary to electrolyte abnormalities. **(D)** Bradycardia is a common finding as well as a prolonged QT segment on electrocardiogram. **(B)** Lanugo, or fine, downy hair, is generally found in anorexic patients, as opposed to hirsutism, seen in patients with polycystic ovary syndrome. **(A, C)** Diarrhea and erosion of dental enamel would be more likely to be found in a patient with bulimia nervosa. **(E)** Tachypnea may be a sign of respiratory compensation based on metabolic acidosis; however, this is not a frequent or diagnostic sign seen in patients with anorexia nervosa.

A 15-year-old boy presents with cough and hemoptysis over the past 3 days. He also reports that he has lost 10 lb since last month. He recently emigrated from Mexico. A tuberculin purified protein derivative (PPD) test is placed to be read in 48 to 72 hours.

Of the following, which condition shares the same type of immune-mediated reaction as described in this patient?

(A) Anaphylactic penicillin reaction
(B) Autoimmune hemolytic anemia
(C) Poison ivy contact dermatitis
(D) Serum sickness
(E) Rh incompatibility

The answer is C: Poison ivy contact dermatitis. The Gell and Coombs classification is a way to stratify immunologically mediated adverse reactions. There are four types: immediate hypersensitivity (type I), cytotoxic antibody reactions (type II), immune complex reactions (type III), and delayed hypersensitivity reactions (type IV).

(A) Type I reactions occur when an allergen encounters preformed IgE-mediated antibodies. These antibodies, bound on the surface of mast cells and basophils, cross-link with the antigen causing release of histamines and leukotrienes. The clinical manifestation of immediate hypersensitivity reactions results in urticaria, bronchospasm, and anaphylaxis, as seen with exposure in severe peanut allergy or anaphylactic penicillin reaction.

(B, E) Type II reactions occur when IgG or IgM antibodies recognize an antigen bound to a cell membrane. The antibodies then coat the offending agent's cell and the cell is destroyed through the monocyte/macrophage system and cleared through complement mediators. Neutrophils are recruited to these cells and they autolyze releasing hydrolytic enzymes and anaphylatoxin leading to the destruction of the antigenic cells. Classic examples of cytotoxic antibody reactions include Goodpasture syndrome, Rh incompatibility, and autoimmune hemolytic anemia.

(D) Type III reactions are immune-complex–mediated reactions during which an IgG or IgM antibody binds to a soluble antigen forming a single complex. The immune complex is then deposited in blood vessel walls, within the glomerulus, or within other organs. Diseases such as systemic lupus erythematosus, serum sickness, Jarisch-Herxheimer reaction, or hypersensitivity pneumonitis occur when immune complex deposition causes activation of the complement cascade.

(C) Type IV reactions are mediated by T cells and are referred to as delayed hypersensitivity reactions. CD4 and CD8 cells recognize specific antigens involving the major histocompatibility complex on cells. A reaction occurs 2 to 7 days after exposure. Examples include the PPD, or Mantoux skin test and allergic contact dermatitis.

---

20 A 3-year-old girl presents to the emergency department with pallor, irritability, and edema. Her parents state she has been healthy outside from a recent bloody diarrheal illness. On examination, her vital signs are significant for a heart rate of 130 beats/minute and a blood pressure (BP) of 130/85 mmHg. She appears fatigued and pale and is found to have pinpoint, non-blanching lesions throughout her extremities (see *Figure 3*). Her initial complete blood cell count is significant for hemoglobin of $8.2 \times 10^3/\mu L$ and platelet count of $90 \times 10^3/\mu L$ with the peripheral smear containing schistocytes. Her blood urea nitrogen is 28 mg/dL and her creatinine is 2.0 mg/dL.

Of the following, which is the most likely mechanism for her disease?

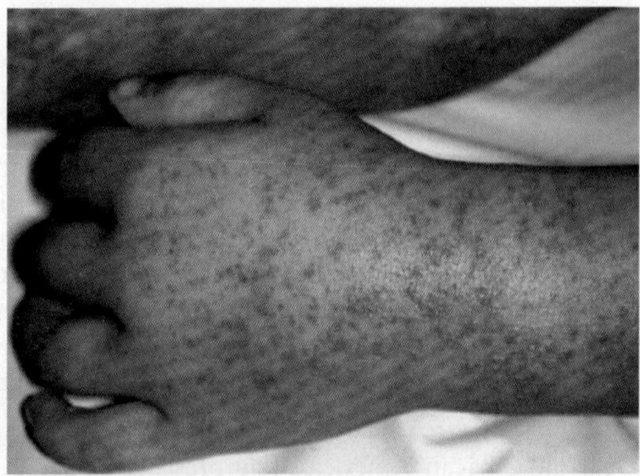

Figure 3

(A) Significant dehydration from diarrhea
(B) Bacteremia causing septic shock
(C) Toxin-mediated injury to endothelial cells
(D) Autoimmune response attacking platelets
(E) Bone marrow infiltration

The answer is C: Toxin-mediated injury to endothelial cells. The patient described in the vignette has symptoms consistent with hemolytic-uremic syndrome (HUS). Typically, HUS is described as the triad of microangiopathic hemolytic anemia, thrombocytopenia, and renal injury. It is commonly associated with a prodromal diarrheal illness, usually due to the verotoxin-producing *Escherichia coli* O157:H7. The toxins bind to specific receptors on endothelial cells causing injury. Shearing of red blood cells through damaged vasculature causes the anemia. These damaged cells appear as schistocytes on the peripheral smear (see *Figure 4*). Platelet aggregation and peripheral destruction cause

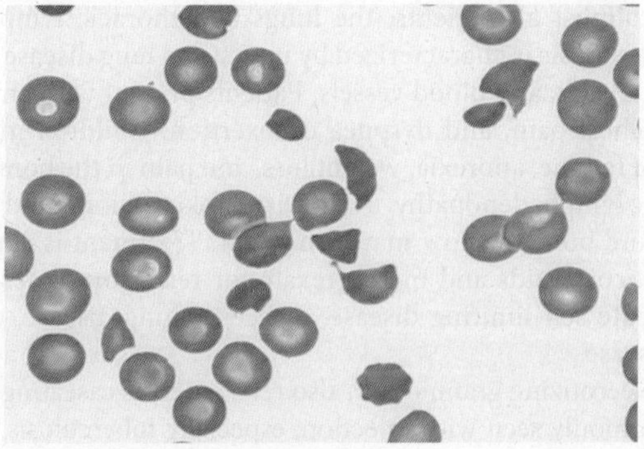

Figure 4

thrombocytopenia, which can present on the skin as petechiae, or pinpoint non-blanching erythematous lesions. Decreased glomerular flow causes compromised renal function that can manifest as edema, hypertension, or acute renal failure.

(A, B) Dehydration and sepsis can cause tachycardia; however, this would be expected to lead to hypotension rather than hypertension. **(D)** An autoimmune response attacking the platelets, such as that seen in idiopathic thrombocytopenic purpura would not be expected to cause a concurrent anemia and renal disease. **(E)** Bone marrow infiltration, as seen in leukemia, can cause anemia and thrombocytopenia; however, it is unlikely to cause renal insufficiency, schistocytes on the peripheral smear, or to follow a diarrheal illness.

21 A 14-year-old African American boy presents to clinic for chronic cough, chest pain, and shortness of breath when he exerts himself. His chest radiograph demonstrates disseminated peribronchial infiltrates and small nodular densities as well as hilar lymphadenopathy. A transbronchial lung biopsy is completed to confirm his diagnosis.

Of the following, what is most likely to be found from the biopsy?

(A) Necrotizing granulomas
(B) Non-caseating, epithelioid granulomas
(C) Caseating granulomas
(D) Langerhans cell histiocytosis
(E) *Pneumocystis jiroveci* pneumonia

The answer is B: Non-caseating, epithelioid granulomas. The patient in the vignette has findings consistent with sarcoidosis which is a chronic multiorgan granulomatous disease with unknown etiology occurring more commonly in the African American population. Definitive diagnosis of the disease requires a biopsy showing the characteristic findings of non-caseating epithelioid granulomas. These granulomas may occur anywhere in the body; however, in almost all patients, the lungs and thoracic lymph nodes are involved. Sarcoidosis is characterized by interstitial lung disease affecting the bronchioles, alveoli, and blood vessels. Patients present with chronic cough, retrosternal chest pain, and dyspnea on exertion. Children may also have complaints of fatigue, anorexia, weight loss, and pain in the bones and joints. Extrathoracic lymphadenopathy, uveitis, iritis, skin lesions, and involvement of the liver and bone marrow may also occur. Treatment is supportive and includes corticosteroids and methotrexate for refractory cases. Sarcoidosis can be an acute self-limiting disease, a chronic lung disease, or relapsing-remitting disease.

(A, C) Necrotizing granulomas, also referred to as caseating granulomas, are most commonly seen with infection, especially tuberculosis. **(D)** Langerhans cell histiocytosis is a histiocytotic disorder where the body accumulates histiocytes leading to organ damage. **(E)** Unlike patients with human immunodeficiency virus (HIV), patients with sarcoidosis are not at increased risk for *P. jiroveci* pneumonia and therefore would be unlikely to be cultured during biopsy.

A 12-year-old girl is being treated for a urinary tract infection caused by *Escherichia coli*. Two days after beginning treatment she breaks out in round, erythematous, pruritic papules on her torso and proximal extremities.

Of the following, which is the most likely etiology of this rash?

(A) Viral exanthem
(B) Drug reaction
(C) Exposure to poison ivy
(D) Cold urticaria
(E) Anaphylaxis

The answer is B: Drug reaction. Drug reactions are an important consideration in a pediatric patient with a new-onset rash. The patient in the vignette likely recently started an antibiotic to treat her urinary tract infection. The majority of drug reactions are actually side effects and only a small percentage are allergic in nature. Drug reactions can range from an urticarial rash to full anaphylaxis. The most common medications to cause allergic reactions are penicillins and semisynthetic penicillins, including amoxicillin, cephalosporins, and trimethoprim–sulfamethoxazole. A drug reaction can occur at any time during the course of treatment or following any number of prior antibiotic courses.

(A) Viral exanthems are common pediatric infections that are associated with the development of a rash. However, these infections rarely present with the rash as the presenting complaint. The cause of the rash of patient in the vignette is more likely secondary to treatment of her recently confirmed bacterial infection rather than an unusual presentation of a concurrent viral infection.

(D) Cold urticaria is a specific disease characterized by the development of hives, localized pruritus, and erythema when exposed to cold temperature. This can be particularly dangerous in patients after full body exposure to cold, such as in swimming, as this can lead to massive vasodilation and hypotension.

(E) Anaphylaxis is a specific type of allergic reaction. It is mediated by IgE stimulation of mast cells leading to involvement of multiple organ systems. While a rash is present in the majority of cases, these patients also often have respiratory symptoms, gastrointestinal tract involvement, and cardiovascular effects including hypotension. The patient in the vignette only has a cutaneous manifestation without involvement of other organ systems and thus is not experiencing anaphylaxis.

(C) While poison ivy does cause a type IV allergic reaction known as a delayed-type hypersensitivity, the patient in the vignette has not reported exposure to poison ivy nor is her rash typical for poison ivy exposure.

23 A 15-year-old Hispanic boy presents to clinic with altered mental status. The family recently relocated from Mexico four months prior. They describe a change in their son's behavior over the last few weeks. He has been more sleepy than normal and his actions are erratic. They note that his grades in school have recently dropped. His parents state he has always helped earn money for the family by working on farms. He recently found a job nearby, and they are concerned he will lose his job if his behavior continues. He frequently complains of a headache, and on examination he is noted to have a brief episode of staring to the right with left-sided tonic–clonic activity.

Of the following, which study is most likely to reveal the etiology of his symptoms?

(A) Computed tomography (CT) scan of the orbits
(B) Chest radiograph
(C) Magnetic resonance imaging (MRI) of the brain
(D) Funduscopic examination
(E) Electroencephalogram (EEG)

The answer is C: **Magnetic resonance imaging (MRI) of the brain.** *Taenia solium*, otherwise known as the pork tapeworm, causes neurocysticercosis and is the reason for the odd behavior, headache, and seizure of the patient in the vignette. This parasite is acquired by ingesting food or water infested with *T. solium* ova. The employment history and immigrant status of the patient in the vignette are risk factors for exposure to this parasite. MRI and CT of the brain are appropriate diagnostic modalities to determine whether the patient has brain cysts and surrounding brain inflammation consistent with a diagnosis of neurocysticercosis. Seizures and focal neurologic signs often correlate with the location of intraparenchymal cysts. Treatment is aimed at prevention of seizures with antiepileptic drugs and decreasing inflammation of the brain parenchyma with steroids. Often the cysts resolve spontaneously; however, if multiple cysts are present, antiparasitic drugs such as albendazole may be prescribed.

(A) A CT scan of the orbits is not indicated for the patient in the vignette as his symptoms appear to be located within the brain parenchyma. **(B)** Chest radiography would be expected to be unchanged in a patient with neurocysticercosis. **(D)** Funduscopic examination may reveal papilledema but this would not be diagnostic. **(E)** While an EEG may demonstrate signs of seizures in this patient, it does not diagnose the etiology of his seizures.

24 A 2-year-old boy presents with facial features as depicted in *Figure 5*, hepatosplenomegaly, profound mental retardation, and corneal clouding.

Of the following, which mode of inheritance is consistent with this patient's presentation?

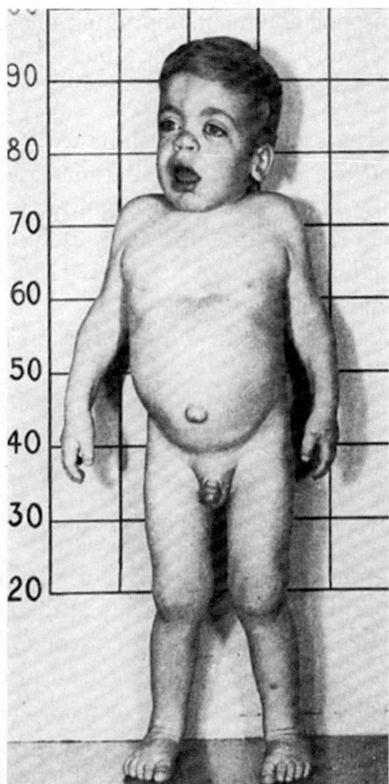

Figure 5

(A) Autosomal recessive
(B) Autosomal dominant
(C) X-linked
(D) Imprinting
(E) Mitochondrial

The answer is A: Autosomal recessive. The patient in the vignette has characteristic features of Hurler syndrome, a mucopolysaccharidosis. Hurler syndrome is a type of lysosomal storage disorder in which deficiencies of certain enzymes result in storage of the precursors in various parts of the body and lead to hepatosplenomegaly, gradual coarsening of facial features, bony problems, profound mental retardation, and cardiopulmonary complications. Patients with these disorders often succumb by the age of 10 years. Corneal clouding in particular is seen in Hurler syndrome, secondary to a deficiency of α-l-iduronidase. **(A)** Hurler syndrome is inherited in an autosomal recessive fashion. **(C)** Another similar mucopolysaccharidosis, Hunter syndrome, is generally differentiated by the lack of corneal clouding and is inherited in an X-linked fashion. **(B, D, E)** Autosomal dominant, imprinting, and mitochondrial inheritance patterns have not been reported for the group of mucopolysaccharidoses.

25 An 8-year-old girl presents to the clinic with concern for red urine since last night. She denies dysuria or increased urinary frequency. She was recently sent home from school for fever, abdominal pain, and sore throat. Those symptoms have resolved. She has not begun menstruating. On examination, her BP is 128/82 mmHg. The rest of her examination is benign.

Of the following what is the most likely cause of her symptoms?

(A) Urinary tract infection
(B) Renal abscess
(C) Nephritic syndrome
(D) Renal calculus
(E) Ureteropelvic junction (UPJ) obstruction

The answer is C: Nephritic syndrome. Nephritic syndrome is the clinical manifestation of glomerular injury, specifically at the endothelial cells. This type of injury leads to hematuria (gross or microscopic), possibly proteinuria, hypertension, and renal insufficiency. Diseases that cause nephritic syndrome include postinfectious glomerulonephritis such as acute poststreptococcal glomerulonephritis (APSGN), IgA nephropathy, membranoproliferative glomerulonephritis, Henoch-Schönlein purpura (HSP), lupus nephritis, Wegener granulomatosis, Goodpasture syndrome, and hemolytic-uremic syndrome. The patient in the vignette likely has nephritic syndrome due to APSGN.

(A, B) Without complaints of fever or dysuria, it would be unlikely for the patient to have an active infection, such as a urinary tract infection or renal abscess. **(D)** The patient does not describe colicky pain similar to that of a kidney stone. **(E)** UPJ obstruction is a congenital condition with obstruction of the ureter at the renal pelvis. Symptoms depend on the amount of obstruction and can manifest as flank pain, hematuria, or recurrent pyelonephritis. With the patient in the vignette's recent illness, hypertension, and sudden onset of hematuria, APSGN is the likely diagnosis.

26 A 7-year-old girl presents to the emergency department with a chief complaint of sudden onset of jaundice, dark urine, fever, and fatigue. She has scleral icterus and an enlarged spleen on examination. Her mother reports that her daughter had jaundice and required a prolonged hospitalization for phototherapy at birth. She also mentions that she has since had two more episodes of jaundice during febrile illnesses. Laboratory testing reveals a hemoglobin concentration of 4 g/dL with a mean corpuscular volume (MCV) of 80 fL and a mean corpuscular hemoglobin concentration (MCHC) of 40 pg/cell.

Of the following, which is this patient's most likely diagnosis?

(A) Glucose-6-phosphate dehydrogenase (G6PD) deficiency
(B) Hereditary elliptocytosis
(C) Hereditary spherocytosis (HS)
(D) Pyruvate kinase deficiency
(E) Phosphofructokinase deficiency

The answer is C: Hereditary spherocytosis (HS). HS is a disorder of the erythrocyte cytoskeleton and is most often transmitted in an autosomal dominant fashion; however, some cases show an autosomal recessive pattern. The disorder is due to a molecular defect in spectrin or ankyrin, which results in red blood cell membrane instability. Spectrin and ankyrin are parts of the cytoskeleton and contribute to the normal biconcave shape of red blood cells. Patients with HS have spherically shaped red blood cell which result from a loss of cell membrane surface area while maintaining intracellular volume. This leads to an increase in the MCHC. The upper limit of normal for MCHC is 36 to 38 g/dL.

Diagnosis of HS can be suggested by the presence of spherocytosis on peripheral smear as shown in *Figure 6* and confirmed with the osmotic fragility test. This test involves incubating a patient's red blood cells in progressively more dilute hypotonic solutions. Spherocytes are more likely to swell or burst than normal biconcave erythrocytes in hypotonic solutions.

Patients can present clinically with severe hemolysis at birth that may require phototherapy or exchange transfusion. The frequency and severity of hemolysis episodes can vary from child to child; however, most children will experience some degree of hemolysis during febrile illnesses. Splenectomy can eliminate most episodes of hemolysis as the spleen is responsible for the breakdown of these abnormally shaped cells. Splenectomy should be reserved

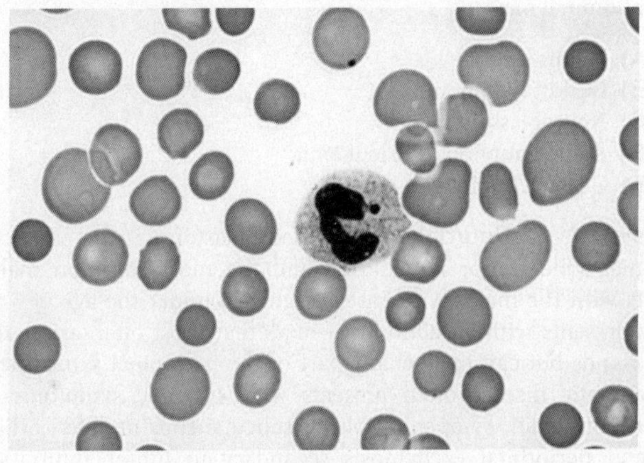

Figure 6

for those patients who experience significant hemolysis since removal of the spleen increases the risk of immunologic issues.

(A) G6PD deficiency also causes hemolysis but is not associated with an elevated MCHC. It is an X-linked disorder; thus, it is most commonly found in male patients. Most patients are asymptomatic except during illnesses or with exposure to certain medications or foods. Some well-known substances to cause hemolysis are sulfonamides, dapsone, trimethoprim–sulfamethoxazole, naphthalene (moth balls), and Fava beans.

(B) Hereditary elliptocytosis is a rare cause of hemolysis in which the red blood cells are elliptical in shape and subject to breakdown in the spleen. Clinical symptoms vary from asymptomatic to severe hemolysis.

(D) Deficiency of pyruvate kinase is an autosomal recessive disorder that can also result in hemolysis. Clinical symptoms vary from minimal to severe. Neonates with this disorder can have severe jaundice resulting in kernicterus. Hemolysis in older children is common during febrile illnesses. MCHC is normal in this disorder.

(E) Phosphofructokinase deficiency is a rare disorder that occurs primarily in patients of Ashkenazi descent. These patients present with hemolysis associated with glycogen storage disease type VII manifesting as muscle weakness, cramps, hemolysis, and possibly myoglobinuria. MCHC is normal in this disorder.

27 A 16-month-old boy presents to the emergency department after his father felt an abdominal fullness while bathing his son. The father also reports that the boy has had low-grade fevers and watery diarrhea over the past 4 days. The boy is in daycare and has an older sibling who recently had a viral illness. On examination, there is a 15-cm firm mass palpated at the right flank as well as bilateral periorbital bruising.

Of the following, which is the most likely cause for this patient's abdominal mass?

(A) Wilms tumor
(B) Burkitt lymphoma
(C) Neuroblastoma
(D) Acute lymphoblastic leukemia
(E) Germ cell tumor

The answer is C: Neuroblastoma. Neuroblastoma is the most common extracranial solid tumor in children and the most common malignancy in infants with the majority of cases diagnosed under the age of 5 years. It typically presents with an abdominal mass that most often arises from the adrenal glands but can involve any part of the paraspinal sympathetic ganglia. Metastatic disease often presents with systemic symptoms, including fever, bony pain, cytopenias, bluish subcutaneous nodules, orbital proptosis, and periorbital ecchymosis secondary to tumor infiltration. The release of catecholamines from the tumor can cause hypertension and the release of vasoactive intestinal peptides can cause secretory diarrhea. Urine vanillylmandelic acid and homovanillic acid are often elevated.

(A) Wilms tumor typically presents as an asymptomatic abdominal mass in older children aged 2 to 5 years. Diarrhea and bruising are not common, but it can be associated with hypertension and hematuria. **(B)** Burkitt lymphoma can present as an abdominal mass but usually in children older than 5 years. This disease commonly involves the bone marrow, which leads to anemia and thrombocytopenia at presentation. Periorbital ecchymosis and diarrhea are not common presenting signs. **(D)** Acute lymphoblastic leukemia does not present as an abdominal mass but can have fevers and bruising. **(E)** Germ cell tumors can arise in the abdomen but generally are not associated with the systemic symptoms described in the vignette.

28 A 15-year-old girl presents to the office with a complaint of right-sided abdominal pain for the last 6 hours. She describes the pain as sharp and crampy in nature. She has no fever, nausea, or vomiting and her appetite is unchanged. Her last menstrual period was 2 weeks ago. She denies sexual activity or alcohol use. She has experienced similar pain about a month prior to presentation; however, the pain was localized to the left side at that time. Her vital signs are temperature 37.2°C, heart rate 88 beats/minute, respiratory rate 19 breaths/minute, and BP 110/80 mmHg. Her physical examination including a pelvic examination is unremarkable, aside from mild diffuse abdominal tenderness.

Of the following, which is the most likely cause of this patient's pain?

(A) Ectopic pregnancy
(B) Acute appendicitis
(C) Intrauterine pregnancy
(D) Ovarian torsion
(E) *Mittelschmerz*

The answer is E: *Mittelschmerz.* The patient in the vignette is most likely experiencing the pain associated with *mittelschmerz* given her benign physical examination and history of menses 2 weeks prior. *Mittelschmerz* is the pain associated with ovulation and occurs mid-cycle. The pain is usually unilateral in the pelvic region. No treatment or intervention is required, although supportive care with over-the-counter analgesics as needed can provide relief.

(A, C) Although ectopic or intrauterine pregnancy is a valid concern in a reproductive-aged woman with unilateral pelvic pain, it is unlikely given the patient's last menstrual cycle began 2 weeks prior to presentation. **(B)** Acute appendicitis presents with right-sided lower abdominal pain, fever, nausea, and vomiting. In addition, her past history of similar mid-cycle pain on the left side is highly suggestive of *mittelschmerz* rather than appendicitis.

(D) Ovarian torsion can present with unilateral pelvic pain; however, she would be expected to have a more suggestive abdominal examination with localized pain as well as pain on pelvic examination.

29 A previously healthy 5-year-old boy is brought to the office due to complaints of diarrhea and stool soiling. The parents report he was previously toilet trained, but over the past week he has been having stool incontinence along with one to two episodes of diarrhea per day.

Of the following, which is the next best step in the evaluation of this patient?

(A) Plain radiograph of the abdomen
(B) Digital rectal examination
(C) Stool cultures
(D) Blood tests for inflammatory markers
(E) Reassurance

The answer is B: Digital rectal examination. The history in the vignette suggests diagnoses of possible infectious diarrhea versus encopresis and stool impaction. The best method to clarify which diagnosis is the cause of the incontinence of the patient in the vignette is to perform a digital rectal examination. The presence of hard formed stool in the rectum would suggest fecal impaction and subsequent stool leakage. The treatment for stool impaction and encopresis involves manual disimpaction, stool softener, and/or laxative use. The treatment for infectious diarrhea is supportive with proper hydration. Antidiarrheal medications are not recommended.

(A) Plain abdominal radiography can be helpful in suspected constipation to assess stool burden, but should not replace a complete physical examination. **(C)** Stool cultures may be indicated if the digital rectal exam does not demonstrate constipation, and bacterial enterocolitis is suspected. **(D)** Blood tests for inflammatory markers should be considered with a possible diagnosis of inflammatory bowel disease. This would not be the first step in a child with 1 week of symptoms, lack of abdominal pain, and lack of blood in the stool. **(E)** Reassurance alone is not appropriate until a complete physical examination is completed.

30 A 4-year-old boy presents with bilateral periorbital edema. He has a history of seasonal allergies, but his mother reports the symptoms appear worse and have not responded to antihistamine therapy. On examination, his vital signs are as follows: temperature of 36.9°C, heart rate of 95 beats/minute, respiratory rate of 15 breaths/minute, and BP of 135/90 mmHg. He is noted to have significant swelling to the upper and lower eyelids of both eyes and bilateral hands. His sclera, conjunctiva, and pupils are normal. A laboratory evaluation is in process.

Of the following, which condition is likely responsible for this patient's symptoms?

(A) Orbital cellulitis
(B) Nephrotic syndrome
(C) Food allergy
(D) Henoch-Schonlein purpura (HSP)
(E) Orthostatic proteinuria

The answer is B: Nephrotic syndrome. With the findings of bilateral, periorbital edema, and hypertension, the patient in the vignette is presenting with signs consistent with renal disease, with the most likely diagnosis being nephrotic syndrome. Nephrotic syndrome is a clinical condition caused by massive loss of protein in the urine due to glomerular pathology, specifically injury at the epithelial cells and basement membrane. The findings include substantial proteinuria, edema (due to decreased oncotic pressure), hypoalbuminemia, and hyperlipidemia. The loss of protein leads the liver to attempt to rapidly replace albumin, which also stimulates lipoprotein synthesis. This manifests as elevated serum lipids. The most common cause for nephrotic syndrome in children is minimal change disease.

(A) Orbital cellulitis is more commonly unilateral and presents with other symptoms, such as fever, eye pain, and erythema. **(C)** Food allergies manifest more commonly as a skin rash (urticaria) than periorbital edema and would not be expected to produce hypertension. **(D)** HSP is a systemic vasculitis that causes a purpuric rash, arthritis, glomerulonephritis, and abdominal pain. **(E)** Patients with orthostatic proteinuria lose small amounts of protein while standing that is not significant enough to cause nephrotic syndrome.

31 During a prenatal visit, prospective parents mention their concern for cystic fibrosis (CF). The mother's brother has CF and they want information about their baby's possibility of having the disease.

Of the following, which is the most accurate statement regarding CF?

(A) One in 50 people of European descent carries the gene
(B) The most common mutation is ΔF508
(C) One in 1,000 newborns in the United States is affected with CF
(D) The newborn screening test detects all cases of CF
(E) The inheritance pattern is X-linked recessive

The answer is B: The most common mutation is ΔF508. CF is an **(E)** autosomal recessive disorder, most common in the Caucasian population. In the United States, **(C)** about 1 in 3,000 Caucasian newborns is born with CF and **(A)** 1 in 25 people of European descent are carriers of the gene. Any patient with a family history of CF should be tested for carrier status.

(B) The most common mutation is ΔF508, which indicates a deletion of phenylalanine at position 508 in the CF transmembrane regulator gene on chromosome 7.

Newborn screening in most states is a two-step process. The first step is measurement of the immunoreactive trypsinogen level, which is elevated in patients with CF. The second step is a genetic mutation study that detects only the most common mutations responsible for the disease; however, there have been hundreds of mutations identified that lead to the disorder; **(D)** therefore, the newborn screening test does not detect all cases of CF.

32 A 16-year-old girl complains of worsening shortness of breath and fatigue with mild activity. Over the past several months she has noticed difficulty walking long distances and climbing stairs. She was diagnosed with acute myeloid leukemia at the age of 5 and underwent chemotherapy with adriamycin and doxorubicin, and she has been in remission for the past 9 years.

Of the following, which will most likely be found during the evaluation for her current symptoms?

(A) Arrhythmogenic right ventricular dysplasia
(B) Pulmonary hypertension
(C) Hypertrophic cardiomyopathy
(D) Restrictive cardiomyopathy
(E) Dilated cardiomyopathy

The answer is E: Dilated cardiomyopathy. Anthracyclines are a class of chemotherapeutic agents with known cardiotoxic effects. Late effects of anthracyclines include dilated cardiomyopathy that manifests with signs and symptoms of congestive heart failure (CHF). Patients often complain of decreased exercise capacity or becoming easily fatigued, and they may have dyspnea and edema.

(C) Hypertrophic cardiomyopathy is a genetic disease popularized as a cause of sudden death among athletes. Certainly, patients with hypertrophic cardiomyopathy may present with symptoms of heart failure; however, there is no association with anthracycline treatment. **(A)** Arrhythmogenic right ventricular dysplasia is also a genetic cardiomyopathy involving fatty infiltration of the myocardium of the right ventricle. It manifests as ventricular arrhythmias. **(B)** Pulmonary hypertension may be a result of pulmonary fibrosis after chemotherapy. Agents such as bleomycin and mitomycin are known to cause pulmonary fibrosis. Radiation therapy to the chest may also be a cause. **(D)** Restrictive cardiomyopathy is the least common form of cardiomyopathy and has no association with anthracyclines.

33 A 16-year-old sexually active girl presents with dysuria and vulvar discomfort for 5 days. Her physical examination reveals vulvar erythema and a thin discharge. Her vaginal pH is 4.5 and a wet mount preparation shows flagellated organisms among numerous white blood cells. She has no abdominal or cervical motion tenderness. She is given the appropriate medication for her condition.

Of the following, what is the best advice to give this patient while taking the medication?

(A) Take the medicine with fatty foods
(B) Take the medicine without food
(C) Her tears may turn orange
(D) Avoid sunlight
(E) Avoid alcohol

The answer is E: Avoid alcohol. The patient in the vignette has *Trichomonas*. The recommended treatment for *Trichomonas* is 2 g of metronidazole orally in a single dose. When taking metronidazole, a disulfiram-like reaction can occur with the ingestion of ethanol and is associated with nausea, vomiting, flushing, and tachycardia.

(A) The antifungal medication, griseofulvin, used to treat tinea capitis should be given with fatty foods to improve absorption. **(D)** Doxycycline has many uses, however, in a sexually active woman it is most often used to treat *Chlamydia trachomatis* infection. Doxycycline causes increased photosensitivity. **(C)** Rifampin, used in the treatment of tuberculosis, produces orange tears and secretions. **(B)** Levothyroxine, a thyroid medication, should be taken without food.

34 A 16-year-old girl presents to the emergency department with complaints of fever, nausea, vomiting, and right upper quadrant abdominal pain. Her initial evaluation included a white blood cell count of $19 \times 10^3/\mu L$ and an unremarkable ultrasound of the gallbladder. On further history, the patient reports she is sexually active and occasionally uses condoms. On physical examination, she is in mild distress and has active bowel sounds with diffuse abdominal tenderness that is greatest in the right upper quadrant. Her abdomen is not distended. A rapid urine pregnancy test is negative.

Of the following options, which is the most appropriate next step to establish a diagnosis?

(A) Liver ultrasound
(B) CT scan of the appendix
(C) Pelvic ultrasound with Doppler study
(D) Plain abdominal radiography
(E) Pelvic examination

The answer is E: Pelvic examination. The adolescent patient in the vignette requires a pelvic examination to exclude pelvic inflammatory disease. Right upper quadrant pain in a sexually active adolescent girl should raise the suspicion for Fitz-Hugh-Curtis syndrome, or perihepatitis most often secondary to infection with *Neisseria gonorrhoeae* or *Chlamydia trachomatis*. Perihepatitis occurs in some cases of pelvic inflammatory disease, in which the bacteria seed the liver capsule. Testing is typically completed by obtaining cultures of endocervical secretions or a urine specimen. Definitive diagnosis is made with an exploratory laparotomy with direct visualization of the liver capsule. **(A)** Involvement of the liver may not be seen with an ultrasound.

(B) Appendicitis generally presents with periumbilical pain followed by right lower quadrant pain and fever and can be diagnosed with ultrasound or CT of the abdomen. **(C)** Pelvic ultrasound with Doppler studies is used to assess for ovarian torsion. Ovarian torsion presents with an acute onset of severe lower quadrant abdominal pain, not often associated with fevers. **(D)** The patient in the vignette does not have signs of obstruction on physical examination, and therefore, a plain abdominal radiograph would not be diagnostic.

35 A new mother brings her 2-week-old infant in for a checkup. She is exclusively breastfeeding, but wants to know if her child would benefit from supplementation with formula. The infant has surpassed his birth weight and appears well.

Of the following, which recommendation is most appropriate for this mother?

(A) Her baby requires supplementation with cow milk formula
(B) Her baby requires supplementation with iron
(C) Her baby requires supplementation with vitamin D
(D) Her baby requires supplementation with a multivitamin
(E) Her baby requires a change to a soy-based formula

The answer is C: Her baby requires supplementation with vitamin D. The American Academy of Pediatrics recommends exclusive breastfeeding for the first 6 months of life. Breast milk provides all the macronutrients needed by term infants. The only supplement that is recommended for exclusively breastfed infants early on is vitamin D. All infants should receive at least 400 IU of vitamin D daily, to prevent complications such as vitamin D–deficient rickets. Breast milk contains a low concentration of vitamin D. Further, many women are vitamin D–deficient themselves, thus, having even lower levels in their breast milk.

(A) An extremely preterm infant may have nutritional needs not fully met by breast milk. For these patients, fortification of breast milk with formula is sometimes needed to allow maximal growth. **(B)** Iron stores in a full-term infant are typically adequate up to 4 months of age. At that point, additional iron is required, and can be provided as iron liquid drops. **(D)** A multivitamin is not required for a full-term, breast-fed infant who is otherwise healthy. **(E)** There is no indication to change to a soy-based formula in this patient.

36 A 7-year-old boy presents with a 3-day history of productive cough, increased respiratory rate, and temperatures reported at home to 103°F. His pediatrician prescribes cefdinir for pneumonia. His mother decided not to fill the cefdinir prescription and instead gives him her left over cefaclor. Within 24 hours of starting the cefaclor he is afebrile and feeling better. On day 7 of his antibiotic course he suddenly develops high spiking fevers, elbow and knee pain, generalized urticaria, and erythema of his hands and feet. His mother calls 911 and he is evaluated in the emergency department. His initial urinalysis reveals red cell casts.

Of the following, what is the most appropriate therapy for his condition?

(A) Intramuscular administration of 1:1,000 epinephrine
(B) Change antibiotic to penicillin
(C) Change antibiotic to clindamycin
(D) Supportive care and symptomatic relief
(E) Cyclophosphamide infusion for his renal disease

The answer is D: **Supportive care and symptomatic relief.** The patient in the vignette has developed serum sickness secondary to the antibiotic he was given for his pneumonia. A type III hypersensitivity reaction, serum sickness, is a self-limited process where a patient's own immune system identifies a medication or anti-venom as an antigen and produces antibodies against it. The antibodies then form antigen–antibody complexes and become deposited within the patient's organs and vessels causing a medium-sized vessel vasculitis. Common inciting agent includes non-human serums (horse serum for diphtheria), anti-venoms, and antibiotics including penicillins, cefaclor specifically, sulfa medications, and minocycline. Laboratory studies demonstrate an elevated erythrocyte sedimentation rate, depressed levels of complement, and hematuria or proteinuria.

Treatment for serum sickness is symptomatic relief with aggressive supportive care. Symptoms typically resolve within 7 to 14 days once the offending agent is identified and removed. Treatment includes antihistamines for pruritus, nonsteroidal anti-inflammatory drugs for fever and arthralgias, and corticosteroids for severe reactions.

(A) Intramuscular administration of 1:1,000 epinephrine is used in the treatment of anaphylaxis and not useful in the initial management of serum sickness. **(E)** Cyclophosphamide is a chemotherapeutic agent used for cancers as well as in autoimmune conditions affecting the kidneys such as in systemic lupus erythematosus or Wegner granulomatosis and would not be indicated in the treatment of serum sickness.

(B, C) Changing of the antibiotic to clindamycin or penicillin is not clinically relevant to the patient because although a partially treated pneumonia developing an empyema is possible, the patient's clinical symptoms fit clearly with serum sickness as his diagnosis.

37 A 2-month-old infant of a mother who received no prenatal care is noted to have microcephaly, and the physical examinations findings and CT findings are depicted in *Figure 7*.

Of the following, which is the most likely TORCH infection affecting this infant?

A

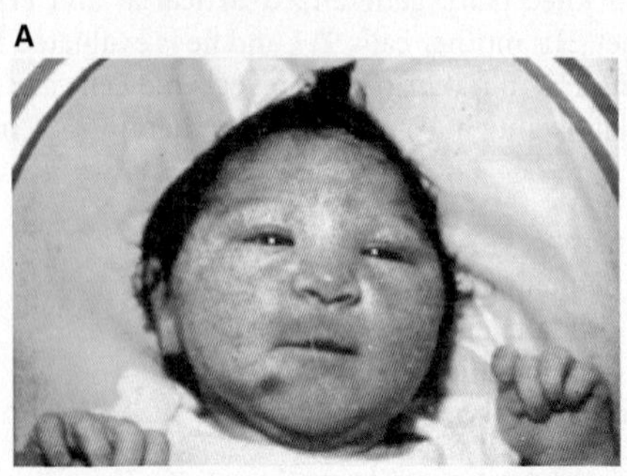

B

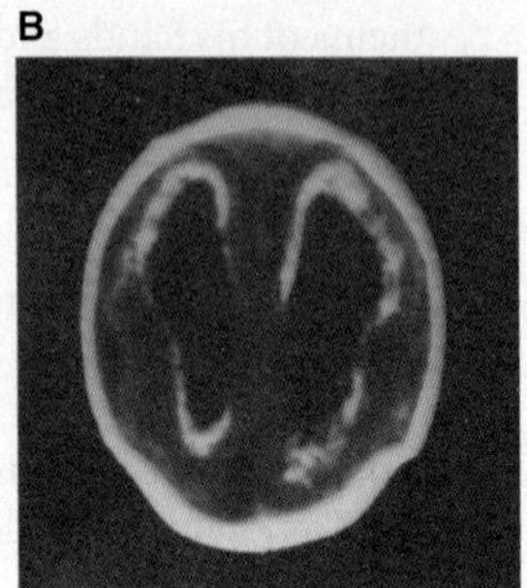

Figure 7

(A) Toxoplasmosis
(B) Cytomegalovirus (CMV)
(C) Herpes simplex virus
(D) Rubella
(E) Syphilis

The answer is B: Cytomegalovirus (CMV). TORCH infections are vertically transmitted from the mother to the infant in utero and screened for in the mother during routine prenatal care. Symptoms and severity of infection vary with not only the cause of infection but also the time of gestation during which the infection was transmitted. Congenital CMV is the most common TORCH infection. Congenital CMV infection results in a spectrum of disease from infants remaining asymptomatic to infants with CMV inclusion disease. CMV inclusion disease results in microcephaly as noted in this infant, periventricular intracranial calcifications, intrauterine growth retardation (IUGR), chorioretinitis, hepatosplenomegaly, jaundice, petechial or purpuric rash, and sensorineural hearing loss.

Many of the above symptoms are nonspecific and present with other TORCH infections as well. **(A)** Some notable characteristics of congenital toxoplasmosis are diffuse intracranial calcifications, IUGR, and possible prenatal exposure to kittens. **(C)** Congenital herpes simplex virus infection is characterized by either a disseminated form presenting like sepsis or localized vesicular disease to the skin, eyes, and mucus membranes. **(D)** Congenital rubella is commonly associated with "blueberry muffin" rash (see *Figure 8*), cataracts, and congenital heart disease such as pulmonary artery stenosis or patent ductus arteriosus. **(E)** Congenital syphilis is associated with a palm and sole rash (see *Figure 9*), keratitis of the eyes, osteochondritis, and "snuffles," or profuse rhinorrhea.

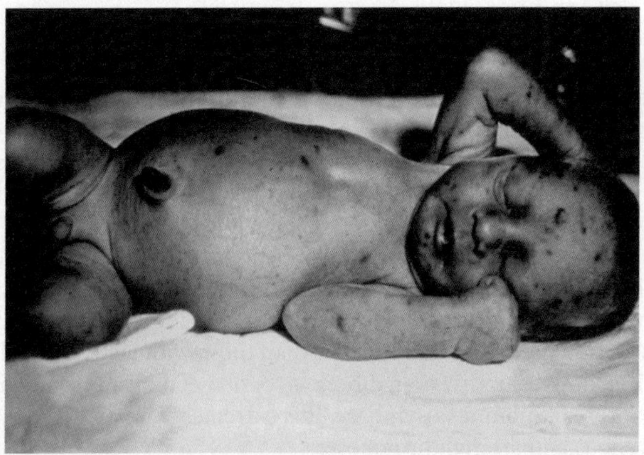

Figure 8

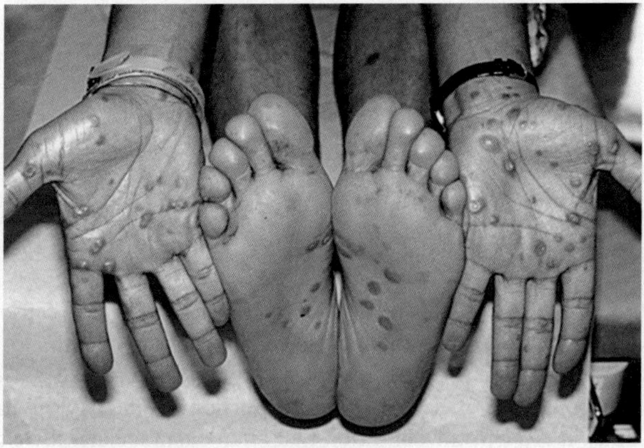

Figure 9

38 A 13-year-old girl presents to the emergency department with a complaint of acute-onset right lower extremity swelling and pain. On examination, her right lower extremity is swollen and erythematous and she reports calf pain with dorsiflexion of her foot.

Of the following inherited conditions, which is the most likely to cause this patient's symptoms?

(A) Factor V Leiden mutation
(B) Protein C deficiency
(C) Protein S deficiency
(D) Antithrombin deficiency
(E) Homocystinuria

The answer is A: **Factor V Leiden mutation.** This patient's history and physical examination are consistent with a deep venous thrombosis of the right lower extremity. Factor V Leiden mutation is the most common inherited thrombotic disorder. The mutation causes factor Va to become resistant to inactivation by activated protein C which leads to thrombosis. The risk is increased in females with this mutation who take oral contraceptives.

(B, C, D) Deficiencies of protein C, protein S, and antithrombin are all less common than factor V Leiden mutation, but individuals with these disorders have a higher risk of thrombosis than those with factor V Leiden.

(E) Homocystinuria is an inborn error of metabolism secondary to a deficiency of cystathionine β-synthase. It is extremely rare and is associated with both venous and arterial thromboses.

39 A 4-year-old girl has just been diagnosed with oligoarticular, previously known as pauciarticular, juvenile idiopathic arthritis (JIA) by her primary pediatrician.

Of the following, an appointment with which subspecialist is most critical within the next 4 weeks?

(A) Ophthalmology
(B) Gastroenterology
(C) Orthopedic surgery
(D) Rheumatology
(E) General office follow-up

The answer is A: **Ophthalmology.** JIA is the most common cause of chronic childhood arthritis. Although JIA is associated with inflammation of other organs, JIA-associated uveitis is the most commonly identified cause of uveitis in childhood. Uveitis affects the anterior portion of the eye, the iris, and the ciliary body. It is a chronic condition that often occurs bilaterally either simultaneously or within a few months of each other. The highest risk of developing uveitis is during the first 2 years of diagnosis, although it can occur at any time. The risk of uveitis decreases considerably 8 years after the onset of disease.

Symptoms of uveitis include pain, light sensitivity, and blurry vision. **(A)** Screening for uveitis is recommended within the first 4 weeks of diagnosis of JIA because the impact on visual acuity may be initially subtle and younger children are less likely to report abnormalities. Untreated uveitis may lead to complications, including cataracts, band keratopathy, and glaucoma. It is important to note that the degree of uveitis is not related to the severity of arthritis.

(D, E) While the patient in the vignette will require follow-up appointments with both her primary care physician and a rheumatologist, they are not as time-sensitive as the ophthalmology appointment. **(B, C)** Evaluation by either a gastroenterologist or orthopedic surgeon is not routinely required with a new diagnosis of JIA.

40 A 14-year-old girl is brought to the outpatient clinic by her mother. The girl reports that she is feeling tired all the time. She used to enjoy playing soccer, but is having difficulty keeping up during practice. The mother reports that she is worried about her daughter's diet. The patient decided to be become a vegetarian this past year and her diet is very limited. Her typical dinner choices include plain pasta with red sauce, rice, and junk food such as chips, soda, and fries. A complete blood count demonstrates a hemoglobin of 9.8 g/dL and a mean corpuscular volume of 70 fL.

Of the following, which nutrient in the patient's diet is most likely deficient?

(A) Folate
(B) Vitamin B_{12}
(C) Iron
(D) Vitamin D
(E) Ascorbic acid

The answer is C: Iron. The complete blood cell count described in the vignette is suggestive of a microcytic anemia. Among the dietary causes of microcytic anemia, iron deficiency is the most common. Foods high in iron content include green leafy vegetable products and red meats. **(A, B)** Deficiencies in vitamin B_{12} and folate are associated with macrocytic anemia. Patients following a strict vegan diet are particularly at risk for developing vitamin B_{12} deficiency.

(E) Deficiency of ascorbic acid, or vitamin C, causes scurvy, a condition seen rarely in the United States. Symptoms can include irritability, tachypnea, fever, tenderness in the lower extremities, and gingival and bony changes. **(D)** Vitamin D insufficiency and deficiency are becoming increasingly identified in the United States. Most children and teenagers with vitamin D deficiency are asymptomatic, although in severe cases children can develop rickets, with multiple bony deformities including craniotabes, rachitic rosary, and bowing of the limbs. Vitamin D deficiency is not associated with microcytic anemia.

A 3-year-old girl is admitted to the hospital for difficulty walking. Her parents report her symptoms have progressed over the past 2 days. She has been a healthy child except for hand-foot-mouth disease 1 month ago that has since resolved. On examination, she has difficulty walking without support. She is unable to complete heel-to-toe or tip-toe walking and appears unsteady while sitting on the examination table. Her patellar deep tendon reflexes are equal and 2+ and she has 5/5 strength throughout. Finger-to-nose testing is clumsy. The remainder of her examination is unremarkable.

Of the following, what is the most likely explanation of this patient's presentation?

(A) Friedreich ataxia
(B) Ataxia-telangiectasia
(C) Rheumatic fever (RF)
(D) Post-viral cerebellitis
(E) Brain tumor

The answer is D: Post-viral cerebellitis. Ataxia is an inability to perform smooth and coordinated movements and is often related to cerebellar dysfunction or injury. The patient in the vignette is suffering from post-viral cerebellitis, otherwise known as acute cerebellar ataxia. This condition most commonly affects young children following a viral infection. Common infections that predispose patients are varicella zoster virus, Coxsackie virus, or echovirus. The prognosis for this condition is excellent and most patients recover fully over days to weeks.

(A) Friedreich ataxia is an autosomal recessive disorder often presenting in school-age children. Patients present with an unsteady gait, dysarthria, and nystagmus. The ataxia is progressive and patients have marked weakness of the lower extremities with decreased or absent reflexes.

(B) Ataxia-telangiectasia is an autosomal recessive neurocutaneous disorder presenting in patients within the first 2 years of life and symptoms often become apparent when infants are learning to ambulate. Patients also have characteristic telangiectasias most commonly on the conjunctiva and the cheeks. Patients with this condition frequently have immune system abnormalities and may have recurrent sinopulmonary infections. **(C)** RF is a postinfectious process that occurs after infection with *Streptococcus pyogenes*, or group A Streptococcus. Diagnosis is based on specific major and minor criteria. Major criteria include Sydenham chorea, which may be mistaken for ataxia but presents as irregular, twisting, dancelike movements rather than the unsteadiness described in the vignette. **(E)** Brain tumor is always a consideration with patients presenting with ataxia. Magnetic resonance imaging of the brain is indicated to obtain the most complete view of the posterior fossa and evaluate the cerebellum. The patient in the vignette is more likely to have postinfectious cerebellitis than a brain tumor.

42 A 2-week-old infant girl born at term presents to the office for her well-child visit. Her birth weight was 8 lb, 11 oz. Her current weight is 10 lb and she is at the 25th percentile for length on the growth curve.

Of the following, at what age would this infant be expected to double her birth weight?

(A) 4 months
(B) 6 months
(C) 9 months
(D) 12 months
(E) 2 years

The answer is A: 4 months. Full-term newborns may lose up to 10% of their birth weight in the first few days of life and regain it by 10 to 14 days. The average newborn gains approximately 30 g/day, or 1 oz/day, during the first 3 months of life. The pattern of weight gain in infancy varies based on nutrition source. Breastfed infants gain more rapidly during the first 3 to 4 months of life compared with formula-fed infants. Weight gain continues at 20 g/day, or 0.67 oz/day, between 3 and 6 months of life and then slows to 10 g/day between 6 and 12 months. **(B, C, D, E)** Infants are expected to double their birth weight by 4 months of age and triple their birth weight by 1 year. Children then gain approximately 2 kg/year, or 4.4 lb year, between age 2 and puberty.

43 A 6-year-old girl is evaluated in clinic for concerns of poor school performance and poor attention. She has had difficulty following along with the rest of her class and her teacher notes she frequently daydreams. In addition to asking both the mother and the teacher to fill out surveys to evaluate for attention-deficit hyperactivity disorder (ADHD), the pediatrician also orders an electroencephalogram (EEG).

Of the following, which EEG finding is most consistent with this patient's presentation?

(A) Spike discharges from the left temporal lobe
(B) 3/second spike and wave discharge
(C) Hypsarrhythmia
(D) 6/second spike and wave discharge with photic stimulation
(E) Normal EEG activity

The answer is B: 3/second spike and wave discharge. The child in the vignette is having absence seizures. This type of childhood epilepsy is characterized by an abrupt pause in activity without loss of tone that lasts for several seconds and resolves as abruptly as it began with resumption of pre-seizure activities. Some children display automatisms during the seizure such as rapid eye-blinking or lip-smacking. There is no post-ictal state.

(B, E) Because absence seizures may occur with a high frequency throughout the day, children often present with concerns for poor attention, but an EEG showing generalized 3/second spike and wave pattern is diagnostic for absence seizures. Ethosuximide is the antiepileptic treatment of choice for absence seizures.

The remaining EEG findings are classic for other types of childhood epilepsy syndromes. Complex partial seizures may be characterized by a brief alteration of mental status with automatisms and could be confused with absence seizures. These seizures typically occur with less frequency than absence seizures and the disorder is less common among the pediatric population. **(A)** EEG findings of spike discharges in the temporal lobe are consistent with complex partial seizures. **(C)** Hypsarrhythmia, or a chaotic pattern of high-voltage, bilaterally asynchronous, slow-wave activity, is the EEG finding associated with infantile spasms. This type of epilepsy usually presents between 4 and 8 months of age and prognosis depends on the presence or absence of associated neurologic symptoms. **(D)** Juvenile myoclonic epilepsy is a seizure disorder that presents during the early teenage years and is associated with significant myoclonic jerks especially during the morning and shows 4 to 6/second spike and wave discharge with photic stimulation. This type of epilepsy requires lifelong treatment.

44 A 4-month-old infant presents for a well-child evaluation. She was diagnosed with congenital heart disease after a harsh murmur was heard at 12 hours of life. Echocardiography showed tetralogy of Fallot with a mild degree of pulmonary stenosis, and the infant was discharged. She has had regular outpatient follow-up appointments with her pediatric cardiologist, and she has not yet required surgical repair. Her examination reveals a 3/6 harsh ejection murmur at the upper left sternal border during systole. During the examination, the infant becomes restless and increasingly irritable. She begins crying and is difficult to console. She has a dusky appearance of her lips and gasping respirations as she continues to cry.

Of the following, which is most accurate regarding the paroxysmal hypercyanotic attacks associated with tetralogy of Fallot?

(A) Decreased systemic vascular resistance (SVR) causes increased right-to-left shunting across the ventricular septal defect (VSD)
(B) The intensity of the murmur increases because the velocity of flow across the right ventricular outflow tract increases
(C) Supplemental oxygen is the definitive treatment as it lowers pulmonary vascular resistance (PVR) without affecting SVR
(D) Milrinone is an effective treatment because it lowers SVR and improves systemic perfusion
(E) Phenylephrine is used in severe spells to increase right-to-left shunting across the VSD and decrease the symptoms

The answer is A: Decreased systemic vascular resistance (SVR) causes increased right-to-left shunting across the ventricular septal defect (VSD). Hypercyanotic attacks (also known as "hypoxic spells" or "tet spells") are caused by an increase in shunting of deoxygenated blood from the right ventricle through the VSD into the left ventricle and into the systemic circulation. This occurs when the SVR is decreased and/or there is increased resistance within the right ventricular outflow tract. In either and both of these situations, the resistance to flow out of the right heart is higher than out of the left heart. The accompanying cyanosis secondary to the right-to-left shunt increases the respiratory drive, which, in turn, increases systemic venous return. This increased return to the right heart reinforces the right-to-left shunt and the cycle is established. Treatments of a hypercyanotic spell are aimed at improving pulmonary blood flow.

The intensity of the murmur corresponds with the amount of pulmonary blood flow. **(B)** Because there is increased resistance across the right ventricular outflow tract during a hypoxic spell, the murmur decreases in intensity. With treatment, the murmur should become louder, owing to increased flow to the lungs. **(C)** While supplemental oxygen is often provided, it is not a definitive treatment during a hypoxic spell because it does little to disrupt the cycle. Oxygen is a pulmonary vasodilator, but does not affect the resistance within the right ventricular outflow tract and, as such, does not substantially improve pulmonary blood flow. **(D)** Milrinone is a phosphodiesterase inhibitor that can lower both systemic and PVR. Typically, it exerts a greater effect on SVR and so would be a poor choice for an infant having a hypercyanotic spell because it would further increase the right-to-left shunt and worsen the cyanosis. **(E)** Phenylephrine is a systemic vasoconstrictor. It can be used during severe hypercyanotic spells to increase SVR and promote flow out of the right ventricular outflow tract and into the lungs. Increasing SVR would improve symptoms by decreasing the right-to-left VSD shunt.

45 A 2-year-old boy presents to clinic for the first time with a known diagnosis of infection with human immunodeficiency virus (HIV).

Which of the following is true regarding prevention of opportunistic infection in children with this infection?

(A) Infants born to HIV-infected mothers should receive prophylaxis against *Pneumocystis jiroveci* until they are determined to be HIV-negative

(B) If an HIV-positive child is exposed to varicella, the varicella vaccine should be given within 24 hours of exposure

(C) Prophylaxis against *Mycobacterium tuberculosis* should be initiated only if the tuberculin skin test produces a reaction greater than 10 mm

(D) Infants should be immunized with the 23-valent pneumococcal polysaccharide vaccine instead of the 13-valent pneumococcal conjugate vaccine

(E) HIV-positive children should not receive the measles, mumps, and rubella (MMR) vaccine

The answer is A: **Infants born to HIV-infected mothers should receive prophylaxis against *Pneumocystis jiroveci* until they are determined to be HIV-negative.** Though the incidence of children with HIV has decreased, patients who are infected with opportunistic infections have the poorest prognosis. In addition to highly active antiretroviral therapy, adequate protection against opportunistic infections is extremely important. Routine immunizations are recommended for all children with HIV with some modifications. **(D)** All children with HIV should receive the 13-valent pneumococcal vaccine at 2, 4, 6, and 12 to 15 months, and they should also receive the 23-valent pneumococcal vaccine at ages 2 and 7 years old. **(E)** The MMR vaccine and varicella zoster vaccine are also recommended for HIV-infected children who are not severely immunocompromised. **(B)** If HIV-infected children are exposed to varicella, they should receive varicella zoster immune globulin.

(A) Routine prophylaxis against *P. jiroveci* is recommended in HIV-infected patients. Though guidelines for prophylaxis depend on CD4 counts, all infants born to HIV-infected mothers should begin prophylaxis for *P. jiroveci* with trimethoprim–sulfamethoxazole at 4 to 6 weeks of age and should be continued until 12 months of age or until they are determined to be HIV-negative. **(C)** Prophylaxis for *M. tuberculosis* is indicated for patients who have a tuberculin skin test reaction greater than or equal to 5 mm, or for patients who have had close contact with an individual with active tuberculosis, regardless of skin test results.

46 A mother comes into the clinic with her 2-month-old infant. Upon entering the room, the smell of tobacco smoke is apparent.

Of the following statements, which is true regarding smoking?

(A) Women who smoke during pregnancy have an increased risk of low birthweight babies
(B) A correlation between maternal smoking and behavioral issues does not exist
(C) Smoking in adolescents is unrelated to risk-taking behaviors
(D) The risk of sudden infant death syndrome (SIDS) is independent of secondhand smoke exposure
(E) Smoking outside is an effective means of preventing exposure to the toxic effects of cigarettes in children

The answer is A: **Women who smoke during pregnancy have an increased risk of low birthweight babies.** Women who smoke during pregnancy have a higher incidence of premature and low birthweight babies. Smoking causes placental damage contributing to low birthweight and prematurity. **(B)** In turn, low birthweight infants are at increased risk for learning disabilities and premature death. **(D)** Smoking during pregnancy and after delivery has been shown to be the biggest risk factor for SIDS. Heavy paternal smoking has also been associated with low birthweight infants. **(C)** Adolescents who smoke generally partake in other high-risk behaviors. **(E)** Smoking cessation is always optimal for the patient and family; however, should a parent continue to smoke once the baby is born, he/she should smoke only outside, away from the baby, with external clothing that can be left outside. Additionally, parents should wash their hands and faces after smoking to prevent toxins from coming into contact with the baby.

47 An 8-year-old girl presents with a 2-day history of fever, abdominal pain, and sore throat. Her oropharynx is erythematous, and a rapid antigen test confirms the diagnosis of group A β-hemolytic streptococcal pharyngitis. A 10-day course of penicillin V is prescribed.

Of the following, what is the primary benefit of antibiotic treatment for streptococcal pharyngitis?

(A) Shorten the clinical course of the illness
(B) Prevention of acute glomerulonephritis
(C) Symptomatic relief
(D) Reduce transmission to others
(E) Prevention of mitral and aortic valvular disease

The answer is E: Prevention of mitral and aortic valvular disease. **(A, C, D)** Antibiotic therapy will shorten the clinical course of streptococcal pharyngitis by only 1 day and may cause some mild symptomatic relief as well as prevent the transmission of the disease; however, this is not the primary reason to treat. The primary benefit to treatment for streptococcal pharyngitis is the prevention of acute rheumatic fever (ARF). The most severe sequela of ARF is rheumatic heart disease, which manifests in most patients as either isolated mitral valve disease or combined mitral and aortic valve disease. Involvement of the right-sided valves is less common. **(B)** Antibiotic therapy does not prevent or decrease the risk of acute glomerulonephritis.

48 An 18-year-old competitive swimmer abruptly loses consciousness during practice. She is not breathing, and cardiopulmonary resuscitation (CPR) is started immediately. Emergency medical personnel take over CPR and attach a cardiac monitor. Her rhythm is displayed in *Figure 10*.

Of the following, which best describes her cardiac rhythm?

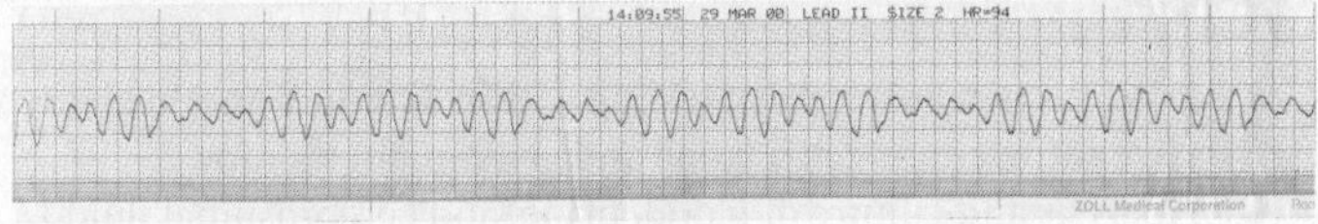

Figure 10

(A) Atrial flutter
(B) Supraventricular tachycardia (SVT)
(C) Ventricular tachycardia
(D) Ectopic atrial tachycardia (EAT)
(E) Ventricular fibrillation

The answer is E: Ventricular fibrillation. The disorganized and irregular appearance of the wide QRS complexes shown in the vignette is most consistent with ventricular fibrillation. **(A)** Atrial flutter appears as rapid atrial signals (F-waves) with QRS complexes that occur at a slower rate (see *Figure 11*). **(B, D)** SVT and EAT are both narrow QRS complex rhythms. In SVT, P-waves are often absent. In EAT, P-waves may be seen, but they are of an abnormal morphology. **(C)** Ventricular tachycardia appears as wide, regular QRS complexes (see *Figure 12*).

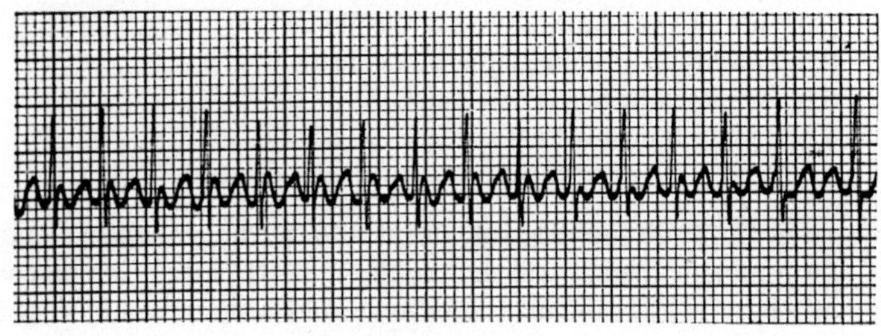

Figure 11

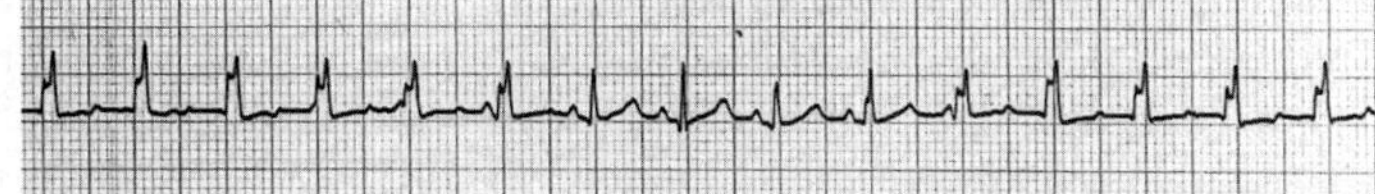

Figure 12

---

49 A 28-year-old woman presents to the emergency department in active labor. She has received no prenatal care and reports that her last menstrual period was approximately 35 weeks prior. A healthy-appearing 3,100 g infant girl is delivered with Apgar scores of 7 and 9 at 1 and 5 minutes, respectively. She is transferred to the nursery for observation.

Of the following, which intervention is most appropriate for this neonate?

(A) Send for newborn screen testing within 12 hours after delivery
(B) Give intravenous ceftriaxone and gentamicin therapy
(C) Analysis and culture of blood, urine, and cerebrospinal fluid
(D) Administration of hepatitis B vaccine
(E) Admit to the neonatal intensive care unit

The answer is D: Administration of hepatitis B vaccine. The mother in the vignette has received no prenatal care and her immunization status is unknown. Despite the lack of prenatal care, the neonate appears healthy and shows no signs of sepsis or other infection. There is a high rate of progression to chronic hepatitis B virus (HBV) infection among exposed infants, thus HBV vaccine is recommended for all infants within the first 2 months of life. Many birthing institutions routinely vaccinate all newborns against HBV before discharge from the nursery. In the event that a mother's prenatal HBV screening results show evidence of HBV infection, hepatitis B immunoglobulin (HBIG) is administered along with routine vaccination to decrease the risk of chronic infection. In the event that the mother's status is unknown, titers should be obtained and the HBIG given within 7 days of birth if she is positive.

(A) Newborn screening is a state-specific, but universal, program designed for early identification of rare but treatable metabolic, endocrinologic, and hematologic diseases. The test involves mass spectroscopy of filter paper saturated with capillary blood that is drawn between 24 and 48 hours of life. **(B, C)** Analysis and culture of blood, urine, and cerebrospinal fluids with intravenous empiric antibiotic therapy is not indicated in the patient in the vignette because there are no signs of infection or distress. **(E)** There is no indication at this point to admit to the neonatal intensive care unit.

50 A 7-year-old previously healthy girl is brought to the emergency department with 3 days of fever, vomiting, diarrhea, and abdominal pain. Today her parents report that she is unable to tolerate any liquids. Her diarrhea has been watery and now has visible bright red blood in it. Laboratory tests note a white blood cell count of $14 \times 10^3/\mu L$. She appears moderately dehydrated. On examination, she is most tender in the right lower quadrant and has voluntary guarding. A CT scan of the abdomen visualizes a normal, non-distended appendix, but is notable for the appearance of multiple mesenteric lymph nodes.

Of the following, which is the next best step in the evaluation of this patient?

(A) Obtain blood cultures and start empiric antibiotics
(B) Start intravenous corticosteroid therapy
(C) Obtain stool cultures for bacterial pathogens
(D) Send stool studies for ova and parasites
(E) Start symptomatic treatment with loperamide

The answer is C: Obtain stool cultures for bacterial pathogens. The clinical presentation of the patient in the vignette is consistent with acute infectious colitis. Bacterial enterocolitis is common in young children. Organisms that specifically cause fever and bloody diarrhea include *Salmonella enteritidis*, *Shigella sonnei*, *Escherichia coli*, *Yersinia pestis*, *Clostridium difficile*, and *Campylobacter jejuni*. *Y. pestis* and *C. jejuni* infections, in particular, can cause a mesenteric adenitis that closely mimics symptoms of appendicitis. Most episodes of bacterial enterocolitis are self-limiting and do not require antibiotic therapy. Stool cultures should be obtained prior to starting antibiotic therapy to rule out *E. coli* O157:H7 infection secondary to the risk of increasing toxin release that may lead to hemolytic-uremic syndrome (HUS).

(A) Blood cultures can be considered for a toxic-appearing patient with infectious colitis, but starting empiric antibiotic therapy is not recommended. **(D)** Ova and parasite studies may be considered in the workup for acute diarrhea after more likely bacterial pathogens have been ruled out, especially for prolonged diarrheal cases. **(E)** Diarrhea is a protective mechanism of the body to remove an offending agent, thus antimotility agents such as loperamide are not recommended to treat patients with infectious etiologies. **(B)** Steroids are not indicated in the treatment of acute infectious diarrhea, but are part of the treatment for inflammatory bowel disease. The history of the patient in the vignette is more consistent with an acute, rather than chronic process.

51 A newborn boy has prolonged bleeding following his circumcision. His family history is significant for a brother who was born with an intracranial bleed and a sister with asthma.

Of the following, which test will most likely reveal the cause of the newborn's prolonged bleeding?

(A) Prothrombin time (PT)
(B) Partial thromboplastin time (PTT)
(C) Factor VIII level
(D) Factor IX level
(E) von Willebrand antigen level

The answer is C: Factor VIII level. The combination of bleeding after circumcision and a family history of intracranial bleeding in a newborn is suggestive of a severe bleeding disorder such as hemophilia. **(D)** Hemophilia A, deficiency of factor VIII, is more common than hemophilia B, deficiency of factor IX. Hemophilia A and B are X-linked disorders. Disease severity is measured as percentage of factor activity (either VIII or IX).

Neither factor VIII nor factor IX crosses the placenta so patients can present with symptoms at birth; however, it is rare to present with intracranial hemorrhage at birth. More commonly, patients present with prolonged bleeding after circumcision. Joint hemorrhage is characteristic of hemophilia but typically does not occur until children begin to bear weight on their extremities. The ankle is the most commonly involved joint. Suspected major bleeding should be treated with an infusion of the missing factor as early as possible to avoid joint degeneration or progression of intracranial bleeds.

(B) PTT is prolonged in patients with hemophilia but it is not diagnostic for the disease. **(A)** PT is normal in these patients. **(E)** von Willebrand disease is characterized by mild bleeding such as easy bruising or epistaxis and is not associated with severe bleeding episodes such as those described in the vignette.

52 An 8-year-old boy presents to clinic for his yearly school physical. He had a great summer vacation and enjoyed swimming, bicycling, and playing basketball and soccer. He is counseled on wearing a helmet while riding his bicycle.

Of the following, what percentage of fatal head injuries could have been avoided by kids if they correctly wore a helmet?

(A) 15%
(B) 38%
(C) 50%
(D) 80%
(E) 99%

The answer is D: **80%.** **(A, B, C, D, E)** Numerous studies have shown that the use of bicycle helmets reduces the risk of death and/or life-threatening head injuries in 60% to 88% of children less than 19 years of age. Most states have instituted bicycle helmet laws and this has begun to help increase the use of helmets among teenagers. Unfortunately, recent studies have shown less than 4% of teenagers report to always wearing a helmet when they ride. Therefore, counseling on proper and safe helmet use is essential during all health maintenance visits.

53 A 17-year-old boy is brought to the emergency department confused and incontinent of urine and stool. His friends report he did not attend basketball practice today so they went to his home. He lives on a grain farm and has been working most of the day. On examination, his heart rate is 44 beats/minute and respiratory rate is 9 breaths/minute. His pupils are constricted.

After initial stabilization, which of the following is the next best step in the management of this patient?

(A) Administer activated charcoal
(B) Administer pralidoxime and atropine
(C) Administer phenobarbital
(D) Provide gastric lavage
(E) Psychiatry consultation

The answer is B: **Administer pralidoxime and atropine.** The patient is presenting with signs and symptoms concerning for toxic ingestion. Given his history of working on a farm, organophosphate poisoning is the most likely exposure. Organophosphates bind with acetylcholinesterase with resulting increased amounts of acetylcholine at nerve synapses. This causes widespread symptoms, including muscarinic effects, nicotinic effects, and central nervous system effects. Symptoms include diarrhea, urination, miosis, bradycardia, bronchospasm, emesis, lacrimation, and salivation. Severe symptoms include seizures, cardiac arrhythmias, shock, coma, and respiratory failure. **(B)** Atropine is useful in treating the muscarinic effects of organophosphate poisoning, while pralidoxime reactivates the acetylcholinesterase, releasing the organophosphate compound, and therefore facilitating its clearance from the body. If pralidoxime is not administered in a timely manner, the chemical bond between the organophosphate compound and acetylcholinesterase becomes permanent, in which case symptoms may persist for weeks awaiting regeneration of the acetylcholinesterase enzyme. Organophosphate compounds are highly lipid soluble and rapidly absorbed.

(A, D) Gastric lavage and activated charcoal administration are unhelpful in the case of organophosphate ingestion. **(C)** While seizures can be part of the presentation in severe organophosphate poisoning, the priority should be to attempt to reverse the underlying chemical problem. **(E)** Toxic ingestion in a teenager should prompt eventual psychiatric evaluation and treatment, but these interventions are best left until after the patient has been medically stabilized.

54 A term infant is born after a prolonged labor complicated by late decelerations in the fetal heart rate indicative of fetal distress. Meconium is noted in the amniotic fluid. The infant is rapidly intubated, and meconium-stained fluid is suctioned from below the vocal cords. In spite of warming and tactile stimulation, she remains minimally responsive. She is cyanotic, tachypneic, and has retractions and nasal flaring. She makes a soft grunting sound with each breath as well.

Of the following, what is the pathophysiology of her condition?

(A) Rapid decline of postnatal PVR
(B) Reversal of right-to-left shunt to a left-to-right shunt at the atrial level
(C) Increase in arterial partial pressure of O_2 following delivery
(D) Persistence of the right-to-left shunt through the ductus arteriosus
(E) Decrease in the arterial partial pressure of CO_2 following delivery

The answer is D: Persistence of the right-to-left shunt through the ductus arteriosus. The patient in the vignette has pulmonary hypertension. Persistent pulmonary hypertension of the newborn (PPHN) is more common in neonates with certain conditions. Birth asphyxia, hyaline membrane disease, pulmonary hypoplasia, and pneumonia due to aspiration of meconium are all predisposing factors for PPHN. The pathophysiology involves persistence of the pattern of fetal circulation, including the right-to-left shunt through the patent ductus arteriosus. The other choices are physiologic changes that occur in the normal infant during transition to extrauterine life. In utero the lungs are fluid-filled, and the fetal

PVR is quite high. This results in shunting of blood from the main pulmonary artery into the aorta (right-to-left). **(A)** After delivery, the PVR rapidly declines **(C)** due to dilation of the pulmonary vasculature as the lungs fill with air and PaO_2 increases **(E)** and $PaCO_2$ decreases. **(B)** The shunting of blood across the foramen ovale reverses and becomes left-to-right as the right-sided pressures fall.

---

55 A boy can briefly stand alone and walk slowly with his mother holding his hand. He can also place blocks in a cup.

Of the following language milestones, which has this boy also likely achieved?

(A) Uses two to six words
(B) Half of his speech is intelligible to strangers
(C) Points to three body parts
(D) Follows a one-step command assisted by gestures
(E) Uses pronouns, though not always correctly

The answer is D: Follows a one-step command assisted by gestures. This patient demonstrates the gross and fine motor skills of a 12-month-old child. The language skills of a 12-month-old child transition from nonspecific attempts to imitate speech to distinct attempts at communication. A 12-month-old child can use "mama" and "dada" specifically, can use one additional word specifically, and follow a one-step command accompanied by a gesture, like retrieving a toy or book accompanied by pointing in the direction of that toy or book. **(A)** The use of two to six words comes at 15 months old, while **(C)** identifying and pointing to three body parts is consistent with the language skills of an 18-month-old child. **(B)** In general, only one-quarter of speech is intelligible by strangers at 12 months old, while **(E)** half of speech will be intelligible at 2 years old, including pronouns that are often incorrectly applied.

Of the following, what is essential to monitor while a patient is taking gentamicin?

(A) Vision
(B) Liver function test
(C) Hearing
(D) White blood cell count
(E) Urinalysis

The answer is C: Hearing. Gentamicin is an aminoglycoside. Aminoglycosides are ototoxic and therefore it is essential to closely monitor hearing for all patients during and after therapy. Other ototoxic medications include furosemide, quinolones, minocycline, cisplatin, vinblastine, quinine, and mefloquine, as well as aspirin. **(A, B, D)** Aminoglycosides do not affect vision, the liver, or white blood cell counts. **(E)** Although aminoglycosides can be nephrotoxic, screening urinalysis is only indicated if symptoms arise.

57 Of the following, what best describes the function of the foramen ovale during fetal life?

(A) It allows deoxygenated blood to reach the lungs by shunting from the left atrium to the right atrium
(B) It allows deoxygenated blood to bypass the lungs by shunting from the right atrium to the left atrium
(C) It allows oxygenated blood to bypass the lungs by shunting from the right atrium to the left atrium
(D) It allows oxygenated blood to bypass the lungs by shunting from the left atrium to the right atrium
(E) It allows oxygenated blood to reach the lungs by shunting from the right atrium to the left atrium

The answer is C: **It allows oxygenated blood to bypass the lungs by shunting from the right atrium to the left atrium.** In the fetus, the organ of respiration and gas exchange is the placenta, not the lungs. Oxygenated blood flows through the umbilical vein and bypasses the liver through the ductus venosus, returning to the heart through the inferior vena cava (IVC). The anatomy of the IVC is such that oxygenated blood flowing into the heart is directed at the atrial septum and through the foramen ovale into the left heart where it exits into the systemic circulation. When the newborn takes a breath and the lungs fill with air, the pulmonary pressures decrease. Left atrial pressure is then higher than right atrial pressure and any atrial-level shunt would be left-to-right. Before delivery, the atrial-level shunt is right-to-left.

58 A girl can draw a cross and square. She recently began speaking in complete compound sentences and her words are essentially completely intelligible to a stranger.

Of the following, what is the youngest age at which these activities are expected?

(A) 2 years old
(B) 4 years old
(C) 5 years old
(D) 6 years old
(E) 12 years old

The answer is B: **4 years old.** The fine motor and language skills displayed by this girl are consistent with a 4-year-old. **(A, C, D, E)** After 2 years old, cognitive development in children allows for progressively more preparation prior to action. However, motor and language skills take time to develop. Thus, actions requiring planning prior to execution, such as intersecting two lines to form a cross or connecting the equal sides of a square, and combining words into sentences with multiple ideas are more readily completed by 4-year-olds, who possess the cognitive, fine motor, and language skills to complete these tasks.

59 The parents of a 6-year-old boy bring him to clinic with concerns about nighttime awakening. His parents describe that he often awakens at night, 2 hours after going to bed, and is crying, sweating, and distressed. He does not respond to his name, is not aware of his surroundings, and is unable to be consoled. He does not recall the events when asked about them the following morning.

Of the following, what is the best explanation of these events?

(A) Nightmare
(B) Night terror
(C) Sleepwalking
(D) Sleeptalking
(E) Seizure

The answer is B: Night terror. Night terrors are common sleep disturbances in school-aged children that are characterized by agitation, confusion, and difficult arousal during the event. Night terrors occur during the first third of the night and may last between 10 and 20 minutes. Children often appear afraid, scream, jump, or act as if they are running away from something frightening. They are not able to be consoled during the episode, and later, when awake, there is no recall of the event. During these episodes, children may also be diaphoretic, tachypneic, tachycardic, and have dilated pupils. Night terrors occur more commonly in boys and often with an associated family history.

(A) Nightmares are frightening, distressing, and often wake a child from sleep. Nightmares occur in the second half of the night. After a nightmare, children have trouble going back to sleep and they are able to recall the nightmare when awake. Recurrent nightmares may be an indicator of a stressor in the child's life. **(C, D)** Sleepwalking and sleeptalking are sleep disturbances that occur when children walk and talk while asleep. These disturbances also occur during the first half of sleep and are associated with amnesia for the event. **(E)** The description of the patient in the vignette is not consistent with a seizure. In addition, the lack of a post-ictal state makes seizure activity less likely.

60 A mother brings her 4-year-old daughter to clinic for enlarged tonsils because she is concerned her daughter will be unable to breathe. She does not have a history of snoring or sleep disturbances, but does have a history of one episode of streptococcal tonsillitis 1 year prior. Her examination is significant for enlarged, but otherwise normal-appearing tonsils with no erythema or exudates.

Of the following what is the next best step in management of this patient?

(A) Refer her to an otolaryngologist
(B) Prescribe a 10-day course of amoxicillin
(C) Refer her for a sleep study
(D) Obtain radiographic studies of the nasopharynx
(E) Reassurance

The answer is E: **Reassurance.** While tonsillar enlargement is often normal, and only requires reassurance, it is important to ensure that the patient does not have any symptoms associated with the enlarged tonsils. A detailed history and physical examination is typically all that is needed to rule out more serious consequences of tonsillar enlargement. Tonsils often reach their maximum size around 4 years of age and then begin to involute.

Tonsils can become large enough to cause airway obstruction. Signs of severe airway obstruction include retractions, cyanosis, and nasal flaring. Airway obstruction can also lead to obstructive sleep apnea (OSA), which presents with snoring and distress during sleep, associated with episodes of gasping and respiratory pauses.

Another etiology of tonsillar enlargement includes infection. Most tonsillitis is due to viral infections such as adenovirus, Epstein-Barr virus (EBV), enterovirus, influenza, and parainfluenza; however, pharyngitis secondary to infection with *Streptococcus pyogenes* is common among school-aged children. Absolute indications for tonsillectomy include suspected malignancy, OSA, or recurrent hemorrhage. **(A)** Because the patient in the vignette does not meet any criteria for tonsillectomy, a referral to an otolaryngologist is not indicated. **(B)** She does not demonstrate any signs of current infection, and therefore does not require antibiotics. **(C, D)** Radiographic studies are completed to evaluate the extent of tonsillar and adenoidal hypertrophy in patients with symptoms of OSA, and thus are not indicated in the patient in the vignette.

61 A previously healthy 13-year-old girl was brought to the emergency department after a syncopal episode. She reports feeling weak for the preceding 1 to 2 days, and was sitting and resting when she collapsed. She had no tonic–clonic movements and was not incontinent. She was unresponsive for less than a minute. She has no significant past medical history. Upon examination she is awake, alert, and communicative. She is afebrile with a BP of 122/72 mmHg, respiratory rate of 16 breaths/minute, pulse of 58 beats/minute, and oxygen saturation 100% on room air. Her neurologic examination is unremarkable. Breath sounds are clear, and the cardiac examination reveals no murmur. Her abdomen is unremarkable and her extremities are warm and well perfused with 2+ pulses. There are no skin rashes or lesions. Complete blood count, basic metabolic panel, urine toxicology, and β-human chorionic gonadotropin (β-hCG) are negative. A head CT scan is also normal. Electrocardiogram is included in *Figure 13*.

Of the following, what additional study will most likely reveal the etiology of this patient's symptoms?

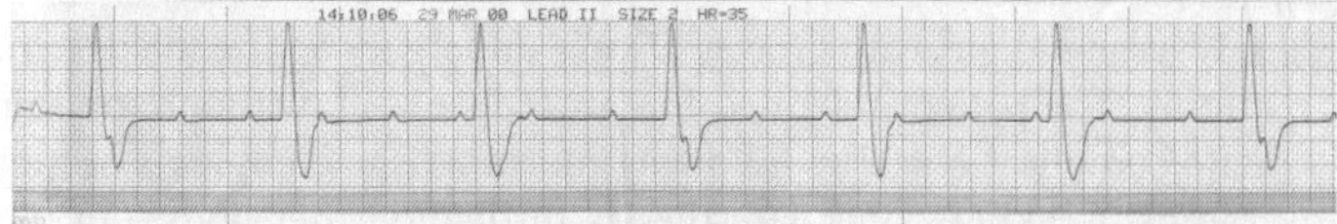

Figure 13

(A) Antibodies against SSA (Ro) and SSB (La)
(B) Antibodies against *Borrelia burgdorferi*
(C) Antistreptolysin O titer
(D) Antiganglioside antibodies (anti-GM1 and anti-GD1)
(E) Antibodies against *Corynebacterium diphtheriae*

The answer is B: **Antibodies against *Borrelia burgdorferi.*** Lyme disease, infection with the spirochete *B. burgdorferi*, may occur through the bite of a tick of the *Ixodes* species. Second- and third-degree atrioventricular (AV) block has been known to occur with Lyme disease. The first sign of the early localized form of the disease is the classically described annular rash, or target lesion, called erythema migrans that occurs around the site of the tick bite. Heart block may occur in patients with early disseminated disease along with neurologic and ophthalmologic signs and symptoms. Late manifestations of Lyme disease may include arthritis, polyneuritis, and encephalitis. Many patients do not remember an insect or tick bite. As such, Lyme disease must not be eliminated from the differential based on the absence of this element from a patient's history.

(A) AV block can occur in the fetus and newborn from damage to the conduction system from maternal IgG antibodies such as SSA and SSB present in systemic lupus erythematosus (SLE). The patient described in the vignette is not an infant, but a previously healthy adolescent. Syncope due to AV block would be an uncommon presentation of SLE. **(C)** A high antistreptolysin O titer demonstrates evidence of a recent or concurrent infection with *Streptococcus pyogenes*. Streptococcal infection is a necessary criterion for the diagnosis of rheumatic fever (RF). While a prolonged PR interval (first-degree AV block) is a minor Jones' criterion, this patient presented with third-degree AV block and has no evidence of rheumatic heart disease. **(D)** The diagnosis of Guillain-Barré syndrome depends upon studies of cerebrospinal fluid; however, antibodies against GM1 and GD1 are occasionally elevated in such patients. The patient described in the vignette has no other presenting symptoms, and Guillain-Barré syndrome is unlikely. **(E)** Diphtheria may produce a toxic cardiomyopathy in up to a quarter of infected patients. Cardiac involvement typically manifests in the second or third week of illness with tachycardia disproportionate to a patient's fever. Prolongation of the PR interval is common, and second- and third-degree AV block may occur as well. The adolescent described in the vignette has no signs or symptoms of respiratory or cutaneous diphtheriae, and laboratory detection of *C. diphtheriae* is made by culture on special media.

62 A 17-year-old girl with Graves disease undergoes a scheduled thyroidectomy. The patient tolerated the procedure well, without any immediate complications. The following morning, she complains of muscle cramps, weakness, and paresthesias throughout her body. On physical examination, when tapping on her face in front of her ear, a facial spasm occurs on the ipsilateral side of her face.

Of the following, which combination of electrolyte abnormality and diagnostic sign is this patient's presentation most consistent with?

(A) Hypocalcemia; Chvostek sign
(B) Hypocalcemia; Trousseau sign
(C) Hypocalcemia; Cullen sign
(D) Hypercalcemia; Trousseau sign
(E) Hypercalcemia; Chvostek sign

The answer is A: **Hypocalcemia; Chvostek sign.** Primary hypoparathyroidism causes significant hypocalcemia. The main causes of primary hypoparathyroidism are congenital malformations, DiGeorge syndrome, surgical procedures secondary to removal of parathyroid glands, or autoimmune diseases. Parathyroid hormone (PTH) responds to low ionized calcium levels in the body. PTH acts to correct the hypocalcemia by mobilizing calcium from the bone and by increasing reabsorption of calcium from the kidney while excreting phosphate. PTH also stimulates vitamin D activation, which in turn also helps to increase serum calcium by enhancing absorption from the gastrointestinal tract. **(A, B, C)** Clinical manifestations of hypocalcemia include those seen in the patient in the vignette, such as muscle cramps, weakness, and paresthesias, along with tetany, seizure-like activity, and laryngospasm. **(A, E)** Tetany can be detected by Chvostek sign (lightly tapping over the facial nerve in front of the ear resulting in facial spasm) or **(B, D)**Trousseau sign (occluding the brachial artery by inflating a BP cuff for 3 to 5 minutes resulting in spasm of the muscles of the hand and forearm). **(E)** Cullen sign is bluish discoloration around the umbilicus associated with intraperitoneal hemorrhage, commonly seen with ruptured ectopic pregnancy or acute hemorrhagic pancreatitis.

63 A child in clinic is able to pedal a tricycle and copy a circle.

Of the following, what is the highest percentage of this child's speech would be expected to be intelligible to strangers?

(A) 10%
(B) 25%
(C) 50%
(D) 75%
(E) 100%

The answer is D: **75%.** This child's gross and fine motor skills, pedaling a tricycle and copying a circle, respectively, are consistent with the skills of a

3-year-old. The language skills of a 3-year-old include a vocabulary of over 250 words, and compiling five- to eight-word sentences using simple adjectives, pronouns, and plurals correctly. Roughly 75% of these words should be intelligible by a stranger. **(A, B)** Generally, 25% of a child's words are intelligible by a stranger at 1 year old, **(C)** 50% by 2 years old, 75% by 3 years old, and **(E)** essentially 100% intelligible by a stranger by 4 years old.

64 A 6-month-old boy presents to the clinic with an extensive erythematous rash on his face, scalp, and chest (see *Figure 14*). His mother states that the rash does not seem to bother the baby and that it has worsened over the past 2 months. The boy has been eating and growing well with no other complaints. On examination, the boy is well appearing and has an erythematous, greasy, scaly, papular rash on his chest and face. There is thick yellowish scaling on the scalp and eyebrows.

Of the following, which intervention is likely to be most effective in treating this patient's overall condition?

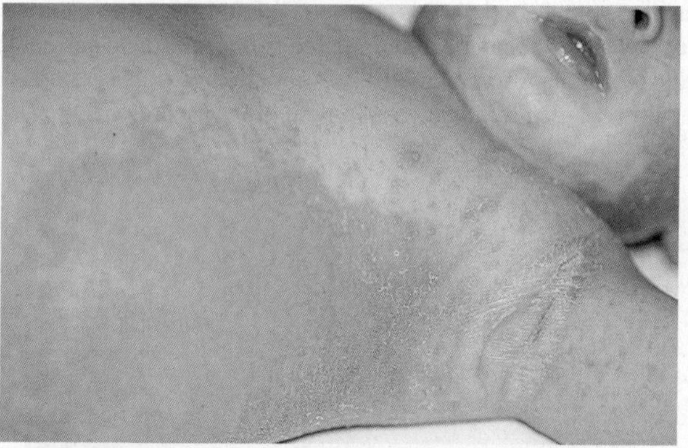

Figure 14

(A) Change to a laundry detergent without dyes or scents
(B) Apply a daily emollient following bathing
(C) Head-to-toe coverage with permethrin 5% cream
(D) Oral griseofulvin therapy
(E) Hydrocortisone ointment and selenium sulfide shampoo

The answer is E: **Hydrocortisone ointment and selenium sulfide shampoo.** The patient in the vignette has seborrheic dermatitis as evidenced by the greasy scale and erythema limited to the scalp, face, and chest. Seborrheic dermatitis may also affect the perineum. It mainly affects two age groups: infants and adolescents. The mechanism is unknown but seborrheic dermatitis has been attributed to overproduction of sebum on the skin surface with an inflammatory response secondary to overgrowth of *Pityrosporum obicularis*.

Treatment is with topical low-potency corticosteroid ointments and antifungal or keratolytic shampoos. Care should be taken to avoid contact with the eyes as the shampoos can cause irritation.

Seborrheic dermatitis may be confused with other common neonatal dermatitides, including atopic dermatitis, contact dermatitis, and scabies. Extensive tinea capitis may be confused with seborrheic dermatitis that is confined to the scalp. **(B)** Atopic dermatitis can be differentiated from seborrheic dermatitis based on distribution. Atopic dermatitis typically involves scaling and erythema of the extremities rather than limited only to the scalp, face, and chest as seen in seborrheic dermatitis. Initial treatment of atopic dermatitis includes daily application of emollients following bathing. **(A)** Similarly, contact dermatitis is expected to only affect those areas that come in contact with the offending substance. For example, a contact dermatitis from a laundry detergent would be expected on the skin of the body and extremities that is covered by clothing. **(C)** Scabies (see *Figure 15*) can be extensive and diffuse in the infant age group and can be distinguished from seborrheic dermatitis with the identification of mites on microscopic examination of scrapings. Scabies is treated with head-to-toe coverage of permethrin 5% cream. **(D)** Extensive tinea capitis caused by *Trichophyton tonsurans* can be differentiated from seborrheic dermatitis limited to the scalp with potassium hydroxide examination of scalp scrapings as well as a fungal culture. Tinea capitis is treated with oral griseofulvin.

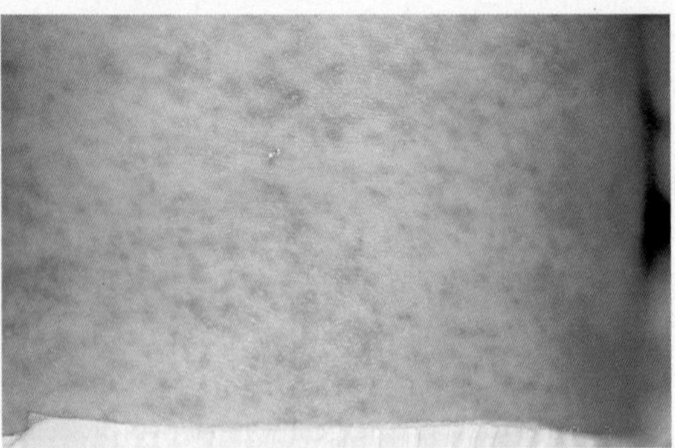

Figure 15

65 A mother brings her 13-year-old daughter to her pediatrician's office because she is concerned her daughter is going bald. She reports that she has noticed her hair is thin and there is a bald spot on the left side of her head. The girl is a straight-A student and has recently started high school. She has had no fevers or any recent illnesses. The examination of her head is shown in *Figure 16*.

Of the following, what is the most likely cause of her examination findings?

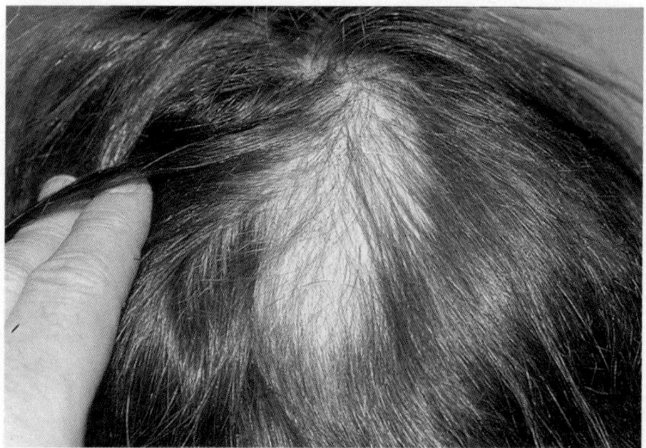

Figure 16

(A) Telogen effluvium
(B) Alopecia areata
(C) Trichotillomania
(D) Tinea capitis
(E) Traction alopecia

The answer is C: Trichotillomania. The patient in the vignette has hair loss secondary to trichotillomania, or a disorder of impulse control that leads to chronic hair pulling. This condition often affects the hair on the frontotemporal or frontoparietal areas, but may also affect eyelashes or eyebrows. Hair loss from pulling results in circumscribed areas with irregular borders and contain several lengths of broken hairs. Hair pulling is more common in females and may be associated with acute stress or other psychiatric conditions.

(A) Telogen effluvium is an acquired diffuse alopecia that often follows a traumatic or stressful event and results in rapid conversion of hairs from an active growing state to a resting state. These hairs are shed over the following several months and may lead to significant thinning. **(B)** Alopecia areata is an autoimmune-mediated process that is described as a well-circumscribed area of complete hair loss involving the scalp hair, body hair, sexual hair, eyelashes, and eyebrows. It is associated with a good prognosis for hair regrowth. **(E)** Traction alopecia (see *Figure 17*) is hair loss secondary to increased tension from various popular hairstyles. **(D)** Tinea capitis is a fungal infection of the scalp and hair that presents as a circumscribed area of hair loss and may be associated with scaling.

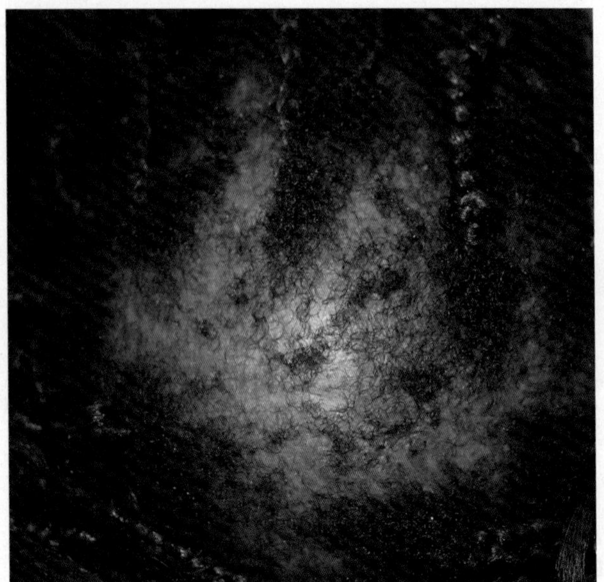

Figure 17

66 What is the typical caloric requirement for a newborn?

(A) 60 kcal/kg/day
(B) 70 kcal/kg/day
(C) 100 kcal/kg/day
(D) 140 kcal/kg/day
(E) 150 kcal/kg/day

The answer is C: 100 kcal/kg/day. A healthy term newborn typically requires between 80 and 120 kcal/kg/day to support growth and development. Children with underlying chronic conditions and increased metabolic demands such as congenital heart disease or chronic respiratory disease may have significantly increased needs. **(D, E)** These patients may require 120 to 140 kcal/kg/day in order to meet increased metabolic demands, which may be accomplished by using a more concentrated formula. **(A, B)** After the newborn period of rapid growth has past, caloric requirements decrease to between 40 and 70 kcal/kg/day for older children and adults.

67 An 18-year-old boy who recently immigrated to the United States presents with a wound he sustained from a nail gun yesterday. His immunization history is unknown. On examination, there is a deep puncture wound on his forearm with surrounding erythema, warmth,

and tenderness. The wound also expresses dark, purulent, and foul-smelling drainage. The wound is cleaned and irrigated.

Of the following, what additional treatment regimen is most appropriate for this patient?

(A) Tetanus immunization, tetanus immunoglobulin, and antibiotics
(B) Tetanus immunization and antibiotics
(C) Tetanus immunoglobulin and antibiotics
(D) Antibiotics and surgical consult for debridement and repair
(E) Antibiotics only

The answer is A: Tetanus immunization, tetanus immunoglobulin, and antibiotics. The decision whether to vaccinate patients against tetanus and administer tetanus immunoglobulin depends on the status of the wound and the patient's vaccination history. The patient in the vignette presents with a dirty wound as it is a penetrating injury that occurred more than 4 hours ago and currently appears infected.

For guidelines regarding tetanus vaccine and immunoglobulin administration, please refer to the below table.

Vaccination History	Clean Wounds	Dirty Wounds
<3 tetanus vaccines or unknown	Tetanus vaccine	Tetanus vaccine + immunoglobulin
>3 tetanus vaccines	*>10 y since last vaccine*: give tetanus vaccine	*>5 y since last vaccine*: give tetanus vaccine + immunoglobulin
	<10 y since last vaccine: nothing needed	*<5 y since last vaccine*: give tetanus vaccine

The dirty wound of the patient in the vignette appears infected and his immunization status is unknown; therefore, he should be given tetanus immunization, tetanus immunoglobulin, and antibiotics.

Tetanus disease is toxin-mediated and is caused by *Clostridium tetani*. It is marked by spastic paralysis. The toxin produced binds to the neuromuscular junction and prevents neurotransmitter release. This results in uninhibited muscle contractions seen locally around the wound or more systemically in generalized disease.

68 An infant with dilated cardiomyopathy presents with difficulty feeding and respiratory distress. His physical examination is significant for tachycardia, tachypnea with accessory muscle use, and a gallop rhythm. The liver edge is palpable 3 cm below the costal margin. Chest

radiography demonstrates cardiomegaly with increased pulmonary vascular markings.

Of the following, which treatment for heart failure is correctly paired with its mechanism of action?

(A) Furosemide causes diuresis by promoting sodium reabsorption
(B) Captopril reduces afterload to the left ventricle by inhibiting production of angiotensin I
(C) Digoxin causes increased contractility by increasing intracellular calcium
(D) Carvedilol may reduce mortality by selectively blocking β_1-adrenergic receptors
(E) Milrinone exerts its inotropic effect by inhibiting phosphodiesterase type 5

The answer is C: Digoxin causes increased contractility by increasing intracellular calcium. The infant described in the vignette has congestive heart failure (CHF). Treatment of CHF depends on identifying its cause. The goal of medical management is not only relief of symptoms, but to prepare the patient for surgical intervention if necessary and support the heart during the postoperative recovery period. Digoxin is a cardiac glycoside that inhibits the function of the Na^+/K^+ ATPase, increasing the concentration of intracellular sodium. This, in turn, affects the membrane Na^+/Ca^{2+} exchanger that relies on Na^+ inflow to pump out Ca^{2+}. The increased concentration of intracellular calcium leads to an increase in contractility.

(A) Furosemide acts to inhibit sodium reabsorption thereby promoting the excretion of water. **(B)** Angiotensin-converting enzyme inhibitors such as captopril prevent the conversion of angiotensin I to angiotensin II, a powerful vasoconstrictor. Angiotensin I is produced by the action of renin on angiotensinogen. **(D)** Carvedilol has both α- and β-blocking action. Metoprolol, which is less frequently used, is a selective β_1-adrenergic receptor antagonist. **(E)** Milrinone is both an inotrope and an afterload reducer by acting as a peripheral vasodilator. It inhibits phosphodiesterase type 3. Sildenafil is an agent sometimes used in the treatment of pulmonary hypertension and inhibits phosphodiesterase type 5.

---

69 A 21-month-old girl presents to the emergency department with a severe cough. Her parents note the cough began yesterday and has progressively worsened. On presentation, the patient is in visible distress and has a loud, harsh cough. Her physical examination is significant for a respiratory rate of 40 breaths/minute, use of accessory muscles, and high-pitched sounds heard on inspiration.

Of the following, which organism is responsible for her disease process?

(A) Respiratory syncytial virus
(B) Human metapneumovirus
(C) Rhinovirus
(D) Parainfluenza virus
(E) Adenovirus

The answer is D: Parainfluenza virus. The symptoms of the child in the vignette are consistent with croup, or laryngotracheobronchitis. Croup is characterized by a loud, bark-like cough, stridor, hoarseness, and varying degrees of respiratory distress. It is most commonly caused by parainfluenza virus. The clinical symptoms of croup are the result of edema of the airways, including the large bronchi, larynx, and trachea. The narrowing of the airway from the edema produces respiratory distress and stridor. Croup is a clinical diagnosis, though a neck or chest radiograph may demonstrate the steeple sign, indicating narrowing of the trachea (see *Figure 18*). Treatment of croup includes keeping the patient calm, corticosteroids, and inhaled racemic epinephrine as needed.

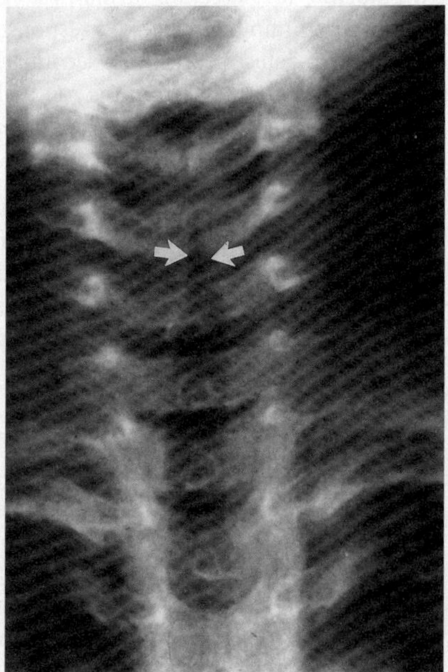

Figure 18

(A, B, C, E) Though the other answer choices can produce a croup-like illness; parainfluenza virus is responsible for the majority of cases of viral croup.

70 Which of the following is essential to include during a 3-year-old's health maintenance visit?

(A) Visual acuity
(B) Fasting lipid panel
(C) Urinalysis
(D) Auditory brain stem response
(E) Complete blood count

The answer is A: Visual acuity. Vision screening is essential during all health maintenance visits. Newborns should be assessed with corneal light and red reflex. From 6 months to 3 years of age, assessment should include red reflex, corneal light reflex, fixation, and cover/uncover test. Starting at age 3 years, visual acuity should be done yearly. By age 6 years children should have 20/20 to 20/40 vision and by 8 years vision should be 20/20 in both eyes.

(B) Fasting lipid panels should be done in obese patients who have abnormal lipid screens or those with a family history of hyperlipidemia. **(A)** There is no standard guideline for screening urinalysis. **(D)** Auditory brain stem response, also known as brain stem–evoked response audiometry, is a neonatal hearing screen used to detect hearing loss secondary to auditory neuropathy. **(E)** Screening complete blood cell count is routinely drawn at 1 year and 2 years of age and then as indicated.

71 A 14-year-old boy presents with 10 days of bloody diarrhea. He is admitted to the hospital for intravenous hydration and further evaluation. He ultimately undergoes a colonoscopy, which demonstrates pancolitis, consistent with a diagnosis of ulcerative colitis.

Of the following, which is the best initial treatment for this child?

(A) 6-Mercaptopurine
(B) Complete bowel rest
(C) Nasogastric tube feedings
(D) Systemic corticosteroids
(E) Supportive care

The answer is D: Systemic corticosteroids. Ulcerative colitis is a chronic inflammatory disorder of the gastrointestinal tract. Typical manifestations include frankly bloody diarrhea, abdominal pain, weight loss, and poor growth. The definitive diagnosis is made by colonoscopy and histologic examination of tissue samples. The pattern of involvement in ulcerative colitis is continuous throughout the colon. If there are patchy areas of involvement then further consideration must be given to the diagnosis of Crohn disease. First-line treatment for ulcerative colitis typically involves the use of 5-aminosalicylate medications. Oral or intravenous steroids are also often necessary at the time of diagnosis, or during an acute flare of the disease, depending on the severity of the presentation. The patient in the vignette presents with a protracted course of bloody diarrhea and will benefit from the immediate anti-inflammatory effects of steroid therapy.

(A) Immune modulators, such as 6-mercaptopurine, are often used to maintain remission. However, these medications take 6 or more weeks to show a clinical effect; thus, immune modulators would not be the first choice for therapy in inflammatory bowel disease. **(B)** Bowel rest is no longer universally recommended during the initial treatment of inflammatory colitis. Some enteral nutrition is important for healing; thus, complete bowel rest is reserved only for situations in which colonic inflammation is severe enough to preclude oral feeding. **(C)** Based on the description of the patient in the vignette, he is able to take feeds by mouth and would not require nasogastric feeds. **(D)** Supportive care is required; however, corticosteroids are the next best step in management for this patient.

72 A 6-month-old boy presents to clinic with cough, rhinorrhea, and fever for 1 day. His vital signs are within normal limits and the infant is well appearing on examination. The parents are instructed how to appropriately suction and to monitor for signs of acute respiratory distress.

Of the following, which sign is most concerning for acute respiratory distress?

(A) Nasal flaring
(B) Post-tussive emesis
(C) Productive cough
(D) Temperature >39°C
(E) Respiratory rate of 40 breaths/minute

The answer is A: Nasal flaring. Infants often present to the outpatient setting with cough and cold-like symptoms. Most of these illnesses are self-limited and do not progress to severe disease. However, it is important that parents be aware of the signs of acute respiratory distress so that patients can be adequately evaluated and treated. These signs include tachypnea, intercostal retractions, abdominal breathing, nasal flaring, and grunting. Intercostal retractions and abdominal breathing are caused by an intrathoracic pressure that is more negative than usual, as is the case in airway obstruction or decreased pulmonary compliance. Dyspnea can manifest as nasal flaring. Grunting is a product of forced expiration against a partially closed glottis and suggests hypoxia, pulmonary edema, atelectasis, or pneumonia. A respiratory rate of 40 breaths/minute is considered within normal limits for a 6-month-old patient.

(B) Post-tussive emesis is a relatively common finding in infants and younger children with a cough; however, by itself, it is not considered a sign of acute respiratory distress. **(C)** Whether a cough is wet- or dry-sounding yields little information about respiratory status. **(D, E)** Children with a fever can be tachycardic and tachypneic, but the fever itself is not a sign of acute respiratory distress.

A 17-year-old boy presents to the emergency department with fevers, purulent nasal discharge, and headaches. Upon review of systems, he admits to several episodes of sinusitis in the past and a 2-month history of diarrhea. He has been diagnosed with three episodes of sinusitis in the past 2 years as well as required hospitalization in the intensive care unit for a pneumonia. Three weeks prior to presentation he was diagnosed with idiopathic thrombocytopenic purpura. His mother reports when younger he was an otherwise healthy child with few infections and no hospitalizations.

Of the following, which diagnostic laboratory testing result is most likely to reveal his underlying disorder?

(A) Pancytopenia
(B) Elevated levels of IgE with normal levels of IgG, IgA, and IgM
(C) Low IgA with otherwise normal levels of IgG, IgM, and IgE
(D) Low C3 and C4 levels
(E) Low IgG, IgM, IgA, and IgE

The answer is E: Low IgG, IgM, IgA, and IgE. The patient in the vignette has common variable immunodeficiency (CVID). CVID is a disorder with variable presentation demonstrated by hypogammaglobulinemia of all immunoglobulin isotypes. Patients with CVID initially have normal immune function and then develop hypogammaglobulinemia in their teens or young adulthood. Patients demonstrate minimal to no B-cell response to antigens, characterized by lack of positive immunity to vaccinations, although the actual number of B cells may be normal. Additionally, patients with CVID have variable T-cell function.

Secondary to the hypogammaglobulinemia, patients are predisposed to mucosal infections such as sinusitis, pneumonias, bronchiectasis, and chronic diarrhea. Physical examination often reveals large tonsils, lymphadenopathy, and splenomegaly. Patients with CVID are at an increased risk for autoimmune hemolytic anemia, thrombocytopenia, and systemic lupus erythematosus (SLE).

Patients with CVID have an increased risk for developing lymphoma and must be monitored routinely. There is also a high predisposition of developing CVID in families with selective IgA deficiency. Treatment includes regular infusions of intravenous immunoglobulin (IVIG) for immunity.

(C) Patients with isolated low IgA levels have selective IgA deficiency. These patients are often asymptomatic; however, they can be predisposed to recurrent sinopulmonary infections, increased food and environmental allergies, and celiac disease. **(B)** Patients with isolated elevated IgE levels have hyper-IgE syndrome, or Job syndrome. Patients with Job syndrome have skin and pulmonary infections, eczema, and predisposition for abscesses especially with fungal organisms. **(D)** Low complement levels are seen in many diseases, including SLE, cryoglobulinemia, liver failure, and pancreatitis. While the patient in the vignette may be at risk for developing a condition that is characterized by low complement, as his symptoms are currently described, he has no indications his complement levels are low.

(A) Although the patient in the vignette could have pancytopenia, this would not be diagnostic of his underlying immunodeficiency.

74 A 24-month-old girl is seen in clinic because her mother states that she is more pale than usual. A complete blood count reveals a hemoglobin concentration of 6.5 g/dL. The white blood cell and platelet counts are both normal. The mean corpuscular volume (MCV) is 78 fL. On examination, her vital signs are as follows: temperature 37.6°C, heart rate 125 beats/minute, respiratory rate 18 breaths/minute, and BP 88/45 mmHg. The child appears well but slightly pale and the remainder of her physical examination is unremarkable.

Of the following, which diagnosis and treatment pair is most appropriate for this patient?

	Diagnosis	Treatment
(A)	Transient erythroblastopenia of childhood (TEC)	Transfusion of red blood cells
(B)	TEC	Observation
(C)	Iron deficiency anemia	Oral iron supplementation
(D)	Diamond-Blackfan syndrome	Corticosteroids
(E)	Diamond-Blackfan syndrome	Bone marrow transplant

The answer is B: TEC: treatment is observation. TEC is the most common acquired red cell aplasia in children and typically occurs between 6 months and 3 years of age. The anemia commonly develops slowly and many children are asymptomatic or experience only mild symptoms. White blood cells and platelets remain unaffected. The anemia is characteristically normocytic. Recovery is spontaneous and occurs over 1 to 2 months. **(A)** Transfusions are generally not needed unless the patient is symptomatic, for example, experiences tachycardia, hypoxia, and shock. The vital signs of the patient in the vignette are normal for a 24-month-old girl.

(D, E) Diamond-Blackfan syndrome is an inherited red cell aplasia that is less common than TEC. This disorder typically has a macrocytic anemia at diagnosis and is associated with physical anomalies such as dysmorphic facies and upper limb defects. The treatment for Diamond-Blackfan syndrome is corticosteroids and the diagnosis is usually made prior to 1 year of age. Bone marrow transplant is an option in refractory cases.

(C) Iron deficiency is a common cause of anemia in the toddler age group and is associated with microcytosis. The mean corpuscular volume (MCV) in the vignette is normocytic, making the diagnosis of iron deficiency unlikely. Iron supplementation is the treatment of choice for iron deficiency anemia.

75 A 10-year-old boy presents to clinic with the chief complaint of headache. His mother also states that he has been more emotional lately. Upon examination, his height is below the 3rd percentile and his visual acuity is 20/50. His sexual maturity rating is 1.

Of the following, which malignancy is most likely to cause this patient's clinical picture?

(A) Brain stem glioma
(B) Medulloblastoma
(C) Cerebellar astrocytoma
(D) Histiocytosis
(E) Craniopharyngioma

The answer is E: Craniopharyngioma. Primary central nervous system tumors are the second most common malignancy in childhood. The most common clinical presentation of a brain tumor generally involves signs of increased intracranial pressure such as headache, nausea, vomiting, and papilledema. However, other symptoms may be present based on the location of the tumor. Craniopharyngiomas often present with endocrinologic abnormalities including short stature and delayed puberty. They can be associated with decreases in visual acuity or visual field defects as well as neurobehavioral abnormalities. The peak age of presentation is 8 to 10 years and the primary treatment is surgical removal.

(A) Brain stem gliomas do not present with endocrine issues, but rather, they can present with double vision, unsteady gait, weakness, swallowing difficulties, or other cranial nerve defects. **(B)** Medulloblastoma is a posterior fossa tumor and presents with headaches, vomiting, and truncal ataxia. Peak incidence is between 5 and 7 years old. **(C)** Cerebellar astrocytomas often present similarly to a medulloblastoma but with a several month history of ataxia, vomiting, and headaches. **(D)** Histiocytosis can present with pituitary dysfunction and classically patients develop diabetes insipidus. Patients with this diagnosis often have other clinical manifestations such as bony pain or swelling; rash involving the scalp, diaper area, axilla, or posterior auricular region; lymphadenopathy; hepatosplenomegaly; or exophthalmos.

Of the following, which form of atrioventricular (AV) block is correctly paired?

(A)	First-degree AV block	There is progressive prolongation of the PR interval until the impulse is not conducted to the ventricle
(B)	Type I second-degree AV block	P-waves occur at regular intervals, but are dissociated from the QRS complexes, which occur at a slower rate
(C)	Type II second-degree AV block	The PR interval is normal and consistent. Impulses are either normally conducted or completely blocked
(D)	Third-degree AV block	The PR interval is prolonged above the upper limit of normal for age. Conduction to the ventricles is normal
(E)	Complete AV block	The PR interval and conduction into the ventricles is normal, but the heart rate varies with respiration

The answer is C: Type II second-degree AV block—the PR interval is normal and consistent. Impulses are either normally conducted or completely blocked. (**A**) First-degree AV block occurs when the PR interval is longer than the upper limit of normal for age and heart rate. It is typically a benign phenomenon and can be seen in healthy children and adolescents.

(**B**) Second-degree AV block occurs in two forms, based on where the block occurs within the conduction system. Type I (Mobitz type I) second-degree AV block is also called Wenckebach AV block. The block is at the level of the AV node. It appears on the ECG as progressively lengthening of the PR interval until the electrical impulse is not propagated into the ventricle. Typically, it is also benign. It can occur in patients with increased vagal tone, such as highly conditioned athletes, but can also be seen in some pathologic conditions. Type II (Mobitz type II) second-degree AV block is more worrisome than type I second-degree AV block. It occurs below the AV node, at the bundle of His. There is often a normal PR interval; however, conduction to the ventricle may be blocked abruptly. This appears as a P-wave without a QRS complex. It is important to distinguish this from type I in which the PR intervals of the preceding beats progressively lengthen.

(**D, E**) Third-degree AV block and complete AV block are synonymous. P-waves (atrial impulses) and QRS complexes (ventricular impulses) are entirely dissociated, or independent of one another. This is a particularly concerning rhythm as the ventricular rate is usually much slower than the normal sinus rate. The ventricular rate may be insufficient to provide appropriate cardiac output and patients may experience presyncope, syncope, or even sudden death.

See *Figure 19* for a diagram of the various types of heart block.

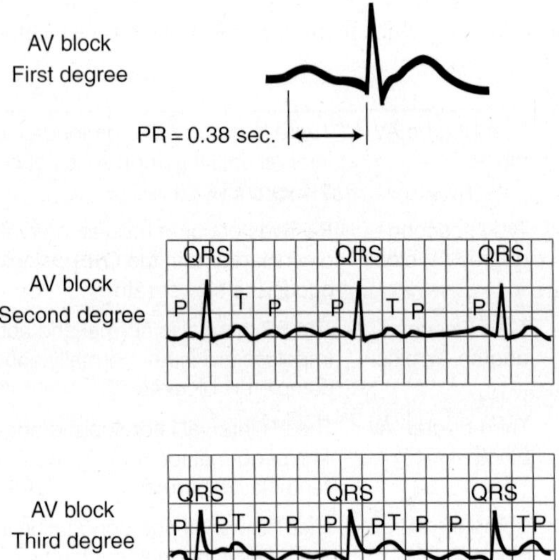

Figure 19

---

77 A full-term baby boy at day of life 2 is admitted to the neonatal intensive care unit because of a seizure. An echocardiogram demonstrates a ventricular septal defect (VSD) and a chest radiograph demonstrates the absence of a thymic shadow. Laboratory results after the seizure revealed the following:

Sodium	141 mEq/L
Potassium	4.1 mEq/L
Chloride	103 mEq/L
CO_2	19 mEq/L
Urea nitrogen	9 mg/dL
Creatinine	0.6 mg/dL
Glucose	89 mg/dL
Calcium	6.5 mg/dL
WBC	8.1×10^3 cells/μL
Hemoglobin	15.4 gm/dL
Hematocrit	46.3%
Platelets	227×10^3 cells/μL

Of the following, which best explains the underlying mechanism of this patient's disease?

(A) Perinatal hypoxic insult
(B) Chromosomal nondisjunction
(C) Congenital thyroid deficiency
(D) Chromosomal microdeletion
(E) Intrauterine cocaine exposure

The answer is D: Chromosomal microdeletion. The most significant finding on the laboratory results of the patient in the vignette is severe hypocalcemia and may explain the seizure he experienced. Also important to recognize is this patient's athymia on imaging. These two findings in combination with a cardiac defect strongly suggest DiGeorge syndrome as the patient's underlying diagnosis. DiGeorge syndrome results from abnormal development of the third and fourth pharyngeal pouches secondary to a microdeletion on chromosome 22q11.2, which can cause a wide variety of features, the most classic of which are hypocalcemia from parathyroid hypoplasia, immunodeficiency secondary to thymic hypoplasia, and cardiac defects. Other findings include palatal defects, facial dysmorphism, and intellectual disabilities.

(A) Neonatal seizures can occur in full-term infants for a variety of reasons. Perinatal asphyxia is a common cause and may result in hypoxic–ischemic encephalopathy. Seizures, oxidative stress, and inflammation are thought to be triggered by a reperfusion injury after an initial anoxic period. Infants at risk are those who experience preterm birth, abnormal heart rate patterns, or thick meconium in the amniotic fluid.

(B) The most common cause of a trisomy is nondisjunction, which is the failure of chromosomes to separate normally during meiosis. The most common trisomy resulting in a viable infant is trisomy 21. These infants may have a wide variety of findings including congenital heart defects, intestinal defects, typical facies, and intellectual disability. These patients are not typically affected by hypoparathyroidism or immunodeficiency although they do have an increased risk of autoimmune diseases and leukemia.

(C) Patients with congenital hypothyroidism present with symptoms including hypotonia, constipation, poor feeding, prolonged jaundice, and large anterior fontanelle. This presentation is the result of some form of thyroid dysgenesis resulting in a lack of sufficient thyroid hormone, but it does present with immunodeficiency or hypocalcemia.

(E) Fetal cocaine exposure can result in preterm birth and increases the risk of spontaneous abortion, low birth weight, placental abruption, maternal and fetal vitamin deficiencies, postnatal respiratory distress syndrome, and infarction of the bowels. However, these babies generally do not develop hypocalcemic seizure or lack a thymus.

78 A first-time mother brings her 2-month-old baby girl to the emergency department for concerns of decreased activity. The mother states that her baby was thriving the first month of life while she was breastfeeding. Since she switched the baby to formula, the patient appears to be more irritable and weak. She states the patient is still drinking an adequate amount of formula and making slightly fewer wet diapers. On examination, the child has a high-pitched cry, dry mucous membranes, and a doughy feel to her pinched abdominal skin. Laboratory results reveal the baby's serum sodium is 164 mEq/L.

Of the following, which is most likely responsible for this patient's condition?

(A) Water intoxication
(B) Syndrome of inappropriate antidiuretic hormone (SIADH)
(C) Nephrogenic diabetes insipidus
(D) Non-accidental trauma
(E) Improperly mixed formula

The answer is E: Improperly mixed formula. The patient in the vignette presents with hypernatremic dehydration. Children with hypernatremia can present with signs of dehydration, or more specifically irritability, lethargy, high-pitched cry, fever, and doughy feeling skin due to loss of intracellular water. Hypernatremia is caused by increased sodium intake (iatrogenic administration of sodium bicarbonate), increased water loss (diabetes insipidus), or increased water and sodium loss (diarrhea). For the patient in the vignette, the symptoms appear to have started soon after the mother switched the baby to formula; thus, the most likely explanation involves formula. **(E)** This first-time mother is at risk for improper mixing of formula, with a higher-than-recommended amount of formula powder to water concentration, leading to hypernatremic dehydration.

(C) Without an increase in urine output, nephrogenic diabetes insipidus is unlikely. **(A, B)** Water intoxication and the SIADH both lead to hyponatremic disturbances. **(D)** Non-accidental trauma can be considered in an infant brought to medical attention for decreased activity, but this would explain neither the electrolyte abnormality nor the symptoms of dehydration for the patient in the vignette.

79 A 2-month-old infant is seen for a routine health maintenance visit. He is growing well and he will receive the appropriate immunizations at this visit.

In addition to age-appropriate anticipatory guidance, which of the following recommendations are best to give at this visit?

(A) Infants should sleep in their own crib until they consistently sleep more than 6 hours per night, then they may co-sleep
(B) Water heaters should be set to 49°C (120°F) to minimize the risk of accidental scald burns
(C) Two-month-old infants should be given one to two teaspoons of rice cereal added to their bottles at feeds
(D) Car seats should be rear-facing until 6 months of age, then face forward until age 2
(E) Introduction of free water is needed at 2 months to guarantee adequate hydration and regular stools

The answer is B: Water heaters should be set to 49°C (120°F) to minimize the risk of accidental scald burns. Injuries represent one of the most important causes of preventable pediatric morbidity and mortality and account for the most common cause of death in childhood and adolescence. Age-specific anticipatory guidance aids in the efforts to control and prevent nonfatal and fatal injuries. Water heaters should be set to no higher than 49°C (120°F) to minimize the risk of accidental scald burns in children. Water temperatures at 150°F produce a full-thickness burn after only about 2 seconds of exposure.

(A) Infants should sleep in their own cribs starting at birth. They should be placed on their backs to sleep and avoid soft surfaces and/or bedding accessories in the crib. Bed sharing (co-sleeping) is a risk factor for sudden infant death syndrome (SIDS) and should be avoided. **(D)** Children should use rear-facing car seats until age 2 years. **(C, E)** Solids and free water are not recommended for infants before age 6 months.

---

80 A 6-year-old patient is brought to the emergency department after ingestion of lamp oil. The parents note the ingestion occurred 1 hour ago, at which point the patient was gagging and coughing. Since then, the patient has not had any symptoms. Physical examination is unremarkable.

Of the following, which complication is he at highest risk for developing?

(A) Liquefaction necrosis of the esophagus
(B) Tachycardia and hypertension
(C) Convulsions and delirium
(D) Chemical pneumonitis
(E) Respiratory depression and coma

The answer is D: Chemical pneumonitis. Toxic ingestions are a frequent occurrence in pediatrics and cause a myriad of symptoms including those mentioned in the above answer choices. The specific toxidrome depends on the specific substance ingested. The patient in the vignette ingested lamp oil, a hydrocarbon. Volatile hydrocarbons typically have minimal systemic effects after reaching the stomach but can be extremely hazardous when aspirated into the lungs. When volatile hydrocarbons are ingested, emesis should never be induced and gastric lavage should never be performed. Examples of volatile hydrocarbons include furniture polish, turpentine, gasoline, kerosene, charcoal lighter fluid, and lamp oil. **(D)** When aspirated, these substances produce a chemical pneumonitis and patients present with cough and respiratory distress, usually about 30 minutes after ingestion though onset of symptoms may occur hours later. Radiographic changes of a chemical pneumonitis may not be apparent immediately following an aspiration, but these findings can include bibasilar infiltrates, fine perihilar opacities, and atelectasis. Treatment for volatile hydrocarbon aspiration is supportive and may require intubation and mechanical ventilation if pneumonitis is present.

(A) Liquefaction necrosis of the esophagus is caused by ingestion of alkali agents such as drain cleaner. **(B)** Tachycardia and hypertension are associated with sympathomimetic overdose. **(C)** Convulsions and delirium may be associated with ethanol withdrawal. **(E)** Isopropyl alcohol, or rubbing alcohol, ingestion can lead to respiratory depression and coma.

81 A mother presents at 38 weeks of gestation in active labor. Her examination is significant for oligohydramnios. Upon delivery, the baby's abdomen is unusually soft, even while crying and the overlying skin appears wrinkled. His testicles are difficult to palpate and do not appear to be in the scrotum.

Of the following conditions, which is this baby most likely to develop?

(A) Pneumonia
(B) Recurrent urinary tract infections
(C) Necrotizing enterocolitis (NEC)
(D) Meningitis
(E) Congenital heart disease

The answer is B: Recurrent urinary tract infections. The patient in the vignette has characteristics consistent with prune-belly syndrome, or Eagle-Barrett syndrome, with the classic finding of deficient abdominal wall musculature. These patients typically have undescended testicles and significant urinary tract abnormalities, specifically urethral obstruction leading to dilated ureters. The in utero result of urinary obstruction leads to oligohydramnios, and subsequently, can cause pulmonary hypoplasia. **(A, C, D)** Patients with Eagle-Barrett syndrome are not at increased risk for pneumonia, meningitis, or NEC. **(E)** Although cardiac anomalies can be seen in these patients, it is a much more rare association in Eagle-Barrett syndrome than urinary tract infections. The most common complication in this patient population is recurrent urinary tract infections secondary to defective emptying of the bladder and a dilated urinary collecting system. Both can lead to urinary stasis and allow for recurrent infections that can be difficult to clear.

82 A 5-year-old girl presents to the clinic for evaluation of developmental delay. Her mother reports her daughter to have global delay as assessed by her therapists, has no speech, and walks awkwardly. On evaluation, she laughs throughout the examination, and has fair hair and pigmentation.

Of the following, which is the most likely inheritance pattern for the condition described in this patient?

(A) Autosomal recessive
(B) Autosomal dominant
(C) Translocation
(D) Uniparental disomy
(E) Triplet repeat

The answer is D: Uniparental disomy. The patient in the vignette has Angelman syndrome, a condition in which patients present with severe mental retardation, impaired or absent speech, inappropriate laughter, and an ataxic gait. These patients may go on to develop seizures as well. Angelman syndrome can be inherited in one of two ways, either as a microdeletion on the maternal chromosome 15 (imprinting), or as uniparental disomy in which the patient has two normal copies derived paternally. In either situation, the syndrome arises as a result of a lack of a maternal copy of chromosome 15. Testing to diagnose this condition entails either a microarray to look for microdeletions or methylation testing to look for uniparental disomy. **(A, B, C, E)** Translocation, triplet repeat, autosomal recessive, and autosomal dominant disease are not the modes whereby Angelman syndrome is inherited.

83 A 3-week-old infant is brought to the office by his mother. She reports that over the past week his stools have become watery and frequent. He is stooling eight times per day and today she noticed small streaks of bright red blood in his diaper. He has been feeding 2 oz of regular infant formula every 2 hours. He has been a little more fussy than normal and spits up with several feedings each day. However, he is still eating well. On examination, the infant is well hydrated and nontoxic appearing. The remainder of his examination is benign, including a careful examination of the rectal area, which does not demonstrate any evidence of a fissure.

Of the following options, which is the likely cause of this patient's bloody stool?

(A) Enterocolitis
(B) Midgut volvulus
(C) Intussusception
(D) Meckel diverticulum
(E) Rotavirus infection

The answer is A: Enterocolitis. The patient in the vignette has a presentation consistent with milk protein allergy. Milk protein–induced enterocolitis is a condition that results from non-IgE-mediated allergy to milk. In infants, the offending agent is most commonly cow milk protein. Symptoms can range from mild diarrhea or constipation and fussiness, to severe vomiting, diarrhea, hypotension, and shock. Milk protein enterocolitis typically presents between 1 week and 3 months of age. Treatment is avoidance of the offending agent.

In formula-fed infants, the initial course of action is to change to a hypoallergenic formula, in which the cow milk proteins are hydrolyzed. Soy formula should be avoided in this condition because of cross-reactivity between soy proteins and milk proteins. In a breastfed infant, the mother can opt to remove all milk and soy products from her diet. This is challenging, but may be an option for those who wish to continue breastfeeding.

(B) Midgut volvulus presents with bilious emesis and signs of shock. **(C)** Intussusception is a condition in which a portion of the bowel telescopes into itself. It commonly presents with episodic colicky abdominal pain and can progress to frankly bloody stools when intestinal necrosis occurs. This necrosis is often described as looking like currant jelly. Intussusception would be a rare finding in a 3-week-old infant. **(D)** A Meckel diverticulum typically causes a large amount of painless frank rectal bleeding rather than diarrhea as described in the vignette. **(E)** Rotavirus infection is common in infants and causes large amounts of watery, non-bloody diarrhea.

84 Shortly after evaluating a child in the emergency department who was brought in following a motor vehicle accident, the patient's oxygen saturation begins to drop. Examination of the patient reveals deviated trachea to the right, expanded chest, distended neck veins, hypotension, and absent breath sounds on the left.

Of the following, what is the next best step in her management?

(A) Cardiopulmonary resuscitation (CPR)
(B) Administer intravenous fluids
(C) Chest radiography
(D) Placement of a chest tube
(E) Needle thoracostomy

The answer is E: Needle thoracostomy. The patient in the vignette is presenting with signs of a left-sided tension pneumothorax. Lung perforation may occur secondary to trauma and may result in an air leak into the pleural space. As the pleural space expands, it collapses the ipsilateral lung and pushes the thoracic contents, including the trachea contralaterally. Tension pneumothorax is a medical emergency that can quickly lead to respiratory failure and death if the pressure is not relieved. **(E)** The next best step in management for the patient in the vignette is immediate decompression via needle thoracostomy **(D)** followed by chest tube placement. **(C)** Chest radiography (see *Figure 20*) will only delay decompression, and **(A)** CPR is not warranted in a conscious patient. **(B)** Hypotension in patients with tension pneumothorax is secondary to decreased venous return from the increased intrathoracic pressure; therefore, intravenous fluids will not solve the problem and is not the recommended next step.

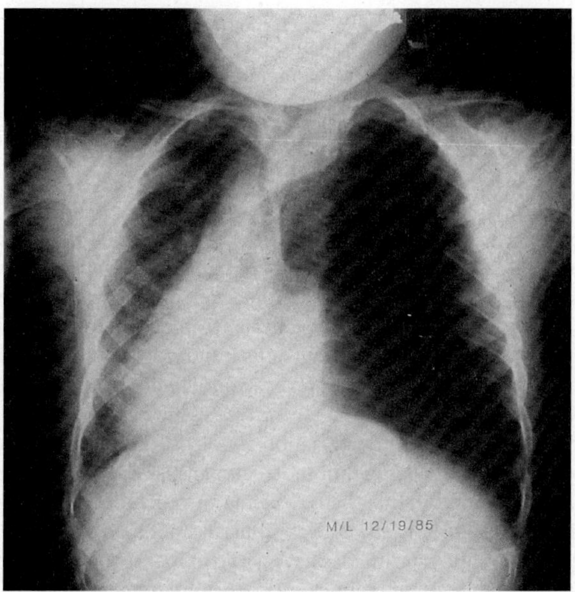

Figure 20

85 A 3-year-old boy is seen by his pediatrician for fever, irritability, and worsening conjunctivitis. His mother states that he has not been eating much since his fever began a week ago, and she is concerned that he is dehydrated. His lips and tongue are erythematous and dry, and he has a swollen lymph node on the left side of his neck. His lungs are clear, and there is no heart murmur. His extremities have full range of motion without joint swelling or erythema, but his hands and feet are somewhat edematous and erythematous. There is also a fine erythematous rash on his chest and back.

Of the following, which is a correct initial treatment for this patient's illness?

(A) Aspirin 80 to 100 mg/kg/day PO
(B) Nafcillin 200 mg/kg/day IV
(C) Penicillin VK 250 mg PO
(D) Ibuprofen 10 mg/kg/dose PO
(E) Prednisone 2 mg/kg/day

The answer is A: Aspirin 80 to 100 mg/kg/day PO. The patient in the vignette has physical examination findings consistent with Kawasaki disease (KD). KD is an inflammatory vasculitis that occurs predominantly in children younger than 4 to 5 years of age. It is a clinical diagnosis that is characterized by at least 5 days of high fever along with four of the five following findings on examination:

- Bilateral non-exudative conjunctivitis
- Unilateral cervical lymphadenopathy
- Changes of the hands and feet that include edema and erythema of the palms and soles
- Changes of the oral mucosa including drying and cracking of the lips and tongue
- A diffuse rash often occurring over the trunk

KD can be associated with dilation of the coronary arteries, particularly in children who remain untreated. Management during the acute phase includes aspirin. Aspirin is used for both its antiplatelet properties, to help prevent coronary artery aneurysms and may offer anti-inflammatory effects as well. Another mainstay of therapy is intravenous immunoglobulin (IVIG). Almost all patients experience relief of their fever within 48 hours of receiving IVIG.

(B) Nafcillin is a correct choice for the treatment of streptococcal endocarditis. Endocarditis may present with a more indolent course, and classic features include splinter hemorrhages within the fingernails, Janeway lesions (painless), and Osler nodes (painful) rather than erythema and edema of the hands and feet. **(D)** Penicillin (or erythromycin) is an appropriate antibiotic treatment for rheumatic fever (RF). While aspirin does have a role in the treatment of the arthritis and/or carditis in acute RF, antibiotics are not helpful in the management of KD. **(D)** Ibuprofen is an effective anti-inflammatory medication; however, it does not have the same antiplatelet activity that is needed for the initial treatment of KD. **(E)** Steroids are used for patients with carditis secondary to RF and may be used as an adjunctive medication for patients with KD whose fever persists in spite of IVIG. It is not, however, included in the initial treatment of KD.

86 A father brings his 3-year-old daughter in to clinic because of complaints of an intermittent wobbly walk. Her gait is off balance intermittently throughout her examination. She is interactive and follows commands without difficulty. She has noticeable nystagmus and states she feels better if she lies down and closes her eyes.

Of the following, what best describes her diagnosis?

(A) Tinnitus
(B) Benign paroxysmal vertigo (BPV)
(C) Pseudotumor cerebri
(D) Encephalitis
(E) Guillain-Barré syndrome

The answer is B: Benign paroxysmal vertigo (BPV). The patient in the vignette has BPV, the most common form of vertigo. Patients often complain of intermittent bouts of dizziness as if the room is spinning around them. Toddlers are unable to articulate the sensation and therefore often present with an ataxic gait. It is more common in females and the typical age range is 2 to

12 years. The differential diagnosis of BPV includes migraine headache, labyrinthitis, intracranial tumors, trauma, and Ménière disease (abnormal fluid balance in the inner ear with associated vertigo, tinnitus, and hearing loss). BPV is a diagnosis of exclusion and often resolves without treatment.

(A) Tinnitus is ringing in the ear. Tinnitus is often associated with middle ear disease or in children with hearing loss or aspirin toxicity. **(C)** Pseudotumor cerebri is more common in overweight adolescents and presents with headache, vomiting, and papilledema. The gait in patients with pseudotumor cerebri is normal and their symptoms are not intermittent. **(D)** Encephalitis could present with ataxia; however, the patient in the vignette would be expected to have more severe constant symptoms, including lethargy, vomiting, and fever. **(E)** Guillain-Barré syndrome is an ascending motor nerve paralysis starting typically in the lower extremities. The gait abnormalities would be different from those seen in the vignette as it is secondary to a muscle weakness that would not be intermittent.

87 An infant is born at 30 weeks of gestation and is small for gestational age due to placental insufficiency. At 1 week of life, his vital signs are heart rate 190 beats/minute, respiratory rate 52 breaths/minute, and a BP of 85/30 mmHg. Physical examination reveals bounding pulses and a continuous, harsh murmur across the chest that can also be heard on the infant's back. A patent ductus arteriosus is suspected. Intravenous indomethacin is ordered to attempt medical closure of the ductus arteriosus.

Of the following, what is the mechanism of action of indomethacin?

(A) Inhibits conversion of arachidonic acid to leukotriene A_4
(B) Inhibits conversion of arachidonic acid to prostaglandin H_2(PGH_2)
(C) Inhibits conversion of PGH_2 to thromboxane A_2(TXA_2)
(D) Inhibits conversion of PGH_2 to prostaglandin E_2(PGE_2)
(E) Inhibits conversion of PGH_2 to prostacyclin I_2(PGI_2)

The answer is B: Inhibits conversion of arachidonic acid to prostaglandin H_2 (PGH_2). Indomethacin is a nonselective inhibitor of cyclooxygenase (COX) enzymes. Both COX-1 and COX-2 synthesize PGH_2 from arachidonic acid. PGH_2 may be acted on by prostacyclin synthase or thromboxane synthase to form PGI_2 or TXA_2, respectively. PGE_2 can also be synthesized from PGH_2 by PGE synthase. Leukotrienes are formed along a separate pathway, starting at arachidonic acid, and using 5-lipooxygenase rather than cyclooxygenase. **(A, C, D, E)** Although PGE_2 is a major vasodilator and the cause of smooth muscle relaxation that is responsible for maintaining patency of the ductus arteriosus, indomethacin exerts its effect a step earlier in the eicosanoid synthesis pathway by inhibiting conversion of arachidonic acid to PGH_2.

88 Laboratory results from a 9-year-old female patient that had presented with mild weight loss and episodes of fast heart rate reveal a thyroid-stimulating hormone (TSH) level of 0.2 μU/mL and free thyroxine (fT4) of 17 ng/dL. Her examination demonstrates a heart rate of 121 beats/minute and a mild resting tremor.

Of the following, which is the best first-line treatment option for this condition?

(A) Methimazole oral therapy
(B) Subtotal thyroidectomy
(C) Propylthiouracil (PTU) oral therapy
(D) Radioactive iodine ablation
(E) Propranolol oral therapy alone

The answer is A: Methimazole oral therapy. The laboratory results of the patient in the vignette suggest a hyperthyroid state. The elevated fT4 with an expected low TSH is due to the negative feedback loop on the pituitary. The history and physical examination in the vignette are consistent with a hyperthyroid state, revealing weight loss, tachycardia, and tremor. **(E)** All of the above-listed options are possible treatments for hyperthyroidism except for the use of propranolol therapy alone, although it can be used as adjunctive therapy for symptomatic relief. **(A, C)** Antithyroid medications such as methimazole and PTU can be effective although require daily administration, have side-effect profiles, and rates of remission are low. Methimazole is 10 times more potent, has a longer half-life than PTU, and can be taken once instead of three times a day. PTU does not cross the placenta or enter breast milk; thus, it is preferred during pregnancy and lactation, but it carries a risk of severe liver disease and, as a result, methimazole is the drug of choice in young, nonpregnant children. **(D)** Radioactive iodine ablation has the putative risk of increasing the chance of future malignancy; therefore, it is not used in children less than 10 years of age. **(B)** A surgical approach may be favorable in cases where medication adherence is poor and ablation is not an option, although total thyroidectomies are superior to subtotal thyroidectomies when performed by experienced surgeons. There remain the risks of anesthesia and any surgical interventions. Thus, many pediatric endocrinologists choose antithyroid medications as first-line therapy for hyperthyroidism.

89 A mother brings her healthy 1-month-old boy for his health maintenance visit. She states that she would like to set up a home apnea monitor for her son because her niece died of sudden infant death syndrome (SIDS) and she is worried the same will happen to her baby.

Of the following, which is the best advice regarding home apnea monitors?

(A) Home apnea monitoring is indicated with a positive family history of SIDS
(B) Her anxiety will be greatly eased with a home apnea monitor
(C) There is no indication for home apnea monitoring of healthy infants
(D) Her baby needs a sleep study prior to prescription for a home apnea monitor
(E) Home apnea monitoring is indicated if the baby were to have an apparent life-threatening event (ALTE)

The answer is C: There is no indication for home apnea monitoring of healthy infants. SIDS is defined as the sudden death of an infant without findings in the history, examination of the home, or postmortem examination indicating a cause of death. Important risk factors for SIDS include sleeping in the prone position, maternal smoking, low birthweight, low socioeconomic status, young maternal age, single motherhood, and multiparity. It is important to discuss these risk factors with families and advise them on safe sleeping habits for infants. Studies have failed to indicate a familial correlation with SIDS.

An ALTE is defined as an episode that involves apnea, change in tone, color change, choking, or gagging, which is frightening to an observer. The differential diagnosis for an ALTE is very broad and ranges from apnea, congenital heart disease, infections, seizures and other neurologic diseases, cardiac dysrhythmias, gastroesophageal reflux, airway anomalies, and non-accidental trauma. It is important to note that most SIDS victims do not have a history of an ALTE.

(A, E) Home apnea monitoring has not been shown to prevent SIDS or prevent the recurrence of future ALTEs. **(C)** While home apnea monitoring may be indicated in some clinical scenarios, it is not indicated in a healthy child. It is also not routinely indicated in a child who has had an ALTE. **(B)** Home apnea monitors do not reduce parental anxiety; in fact, parental anxiety may be worsened due to alerts in an otherwise healthy child. **(D)** Sleep studies are not indicated for identifying infants at risk for ALTEs or SIDS.

---

90 A 5-year-old boy presents with a 9-day history of fevers. His parents report he has been cranky and not interested in playing or eating his favorite foods. They deny any sick contacts, cough, rhinorrhea, diarrhea, or vomiting. On examination, his temperature is 40°C, heart rate 115 beats/minute, BP 98/65 mmHg, and respiratory rate 22 breaths/minute. His conjunctivae are injected and he has dried, cracked lips. His cardiopulmonary examination notes a 2/6 systolic ejection murmur and his lungs are clear. His abdomen is soft with no appreciated masses. Cutaneous examination notes a rash in his groin region as well as peeling of his fingers.

Of the following, what is the most important diagnostic test to perform?

(A) Echocardiogram
(B) Throat culture
(C) Blood culture
(D) Complete metabolic panel
(E) Immunoglobulin levels

The answer is A: Echocardiogram. The patient in the vignette has findings consistent with Kawasaki disease (KD), an acute vasculitis that affects mostly medium-sized arteries with a predilection for the coronary arteries. It is a disease that is predominately seen in young children with the majority of cases occurring in children younger than 5 years of age. Clinical manifestations of KD must include a fever for at least 5 days without a known source. In addition to fever, diagnostic criteria require at least four characteristic findings that include the following: bilateral bulbar nonpurulent conjunctival injection; erythema of the oral and pharyngeal mucosa with strawberry tongue and dry, cracked, fissured lips; edema and erythema of the hands and feet; maculopapular rash with possible accentuation in the groin area; unilateral cervical lymphadenopathy greater than 1 cm; and perineal desquamation. Other symptoms may include irritability, diarrhea, urethritis, sterile pyuria, hydrops of the gallbladder, and arthritis.

The most serious manifestation of KD is cardiac involvement. Coronary aneurysms appear in the second to third week of the illness in roughly a quarter of untreated children.

Of the choices listed, the most appropriate diagnostic test to perform is an echocardiogram. The recommendation is to obtain a baseline echocardiogram at the time of diagnosis, repeat at 2 to 3 weeks and again at 6 to 8 weeks after the onset of illness. If no cardiac abnormality is seen at 8 weeks and the acute phase reactants have returned to normal, follow-up echocardiograms are at the discretion of the treating physician.

(B, C, E) Both a throat culture and blood culture as well as immunoglobulin levels are non-diagnostic in a patient with KD. **(D)** A complete metabolic panel may reveal mildly elevated liver enzymes or bilirubin; however, this is a non-diagnostic finding.

91 A 3-day-old neonate is admitted to the neonatal intensive care unit the day following his circumcision because of a desquamating rash that is pictured in *Figure 21*. On examination, his temperature is 37.2°C, heart rate is 130 beats/minute, and respiratory rate is 34 breaths/minute. His skin is erythematous and tender with several flaccid bullae and large areas of denuded skin. Gentle pressure on the skin causes unroofing of eroded areas. His oral mucous membranes are moist without any lesions.

Of the following, which is the most accurate statement regarding this patient's underlying disorder?

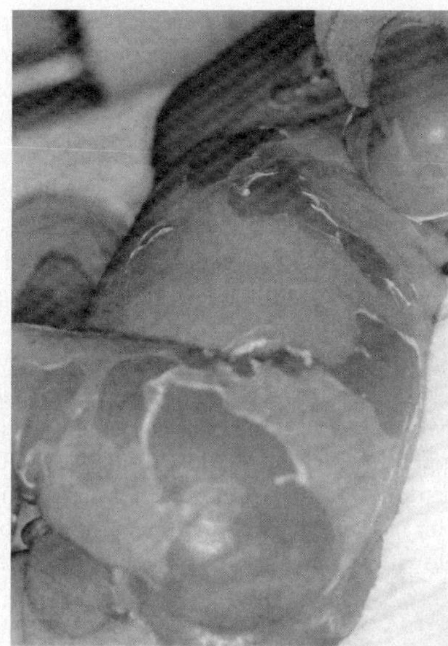

Figure 21

(A) Culture of the fluid from the bullae will likely grow *Staphylococcus aureus*
(B) Culture of the fluid from the bullae will likely grow *Streptococcus pyogenes*
(C) The skin erosions are toxin-mediated
(D) Histologic evaluation of a bulla roof will reveal full-thickness epidermis
(E) This disorder is associated with coronary artery aneurysms

The answer is C: The skin erosions are toxin-mediated. The picture and scenario described in the vignette are consistent with staphylococcal scalded skin syndrome (SSSS). SSSS is a disorder caused by an exfoliative toxin produced by specific types of **(B)** *S. aureus*. While the exfoliation can be quite extensive, it spreads hematogenously from an infection at the primary site. **(A, B)** The flaccid bullae rupture easily and contain sterile fluid. The primary site of infection for the infant in the vignette is likely his circumcision site. Other common sites of infection that can lead to SSSS include conjunctivae, nares, and the perioral region. Diagnosis is made by culture of the primary site of infection as well as histologic evidence of epidermal separation at the granular layer rather than full-thickness epidermis. Treatment with oral antistaphylococcal agents may be adequate in older patients with mild involvement; however, the patient in the vignette and patients who are toxic-appearing require parenteral antibiotics and admission for close observation and support.

Stevens-Johnson syndrome (SJS) is a cutaneous eruption associated with tense bullae and mucous membrane involvement often following recent drug ingestion. **(D)** Histologic evaluation of the blister roof in patients with SJS demonstrates full-thickness epidermis. **(E)** Kawasaki disease (KD) is a vasculitic disease associated with an exfoliative rash especially in the groin and hands and feet and can lead to coronary artery aneurysm. It is unlikely in the neonatal period.

---

92 A 5-week-old infant presents to clinic with parental concern for what they describe as noisy breathing. Per the parents, she makes a "wheezing" noise while breathing, which gets worse when she is upset. Symptoms began 2 weeks ago and have gotten progressively worse. They deny fever, cough, rhinorrhea, or feeding problems. The baby had an uncomplicated delivery and has done well at home with good weight gain. She is well-appearing on examination, though lung auscultation reveals high-pitched sounds on inspiration, with good air entry throughout all lung fields. Her oxygen saturation is 100% on pulse oximetry.

Of the following, what is the most likely cause of this infant's breathing pattern?

(A) Bronchopulmonary dysplasia (BPD)
(B) Tracheomalacia
(C) Pneumonia
(D) Bronchiolitis
(E) Tracheoesophageal fistula

The answer is B: Tracheomalacia. The symptoms described of the baby in the vignette are most consistent with tracheomalacia. Tracheomalacia is the result of a floppy tracheal wall. The extrathoracic component of the trachea collapses during inspiration and produces stridor. This condition is benign and generally resolves with growth. Diagnosis can be made with fluoroscopy of the airway. Tracheomalacia does not require any treatment.

(A) BPD is a consequence of neonatal respiratory distress syndrome and oxygen damage to the lungs. The patient in the vignette does not have a history of oxygen requirement at birth, making BPD unlikely. **(C, D)** Pneumonia and bronchiolitis generally do not produce stridor and the patient in the vignette does not have any symptoms of infection. **(E)** Most tracheoesophageal fistulas present shortly after birth with drooling and respiratory distress along with the inability to fully pass a nasogastric tube.

---

93 A 4-month-old child is seen for a health maintenance visit. On examination, there is flattening of the right posterior skull that causes the anterior right skull to protrude as seen in *Figure 22*. He has been growing normally and appropriately meeting all of his developmental milestones. The remainder of the examination is benign.

Of the following, what is the most likely diagnosis?

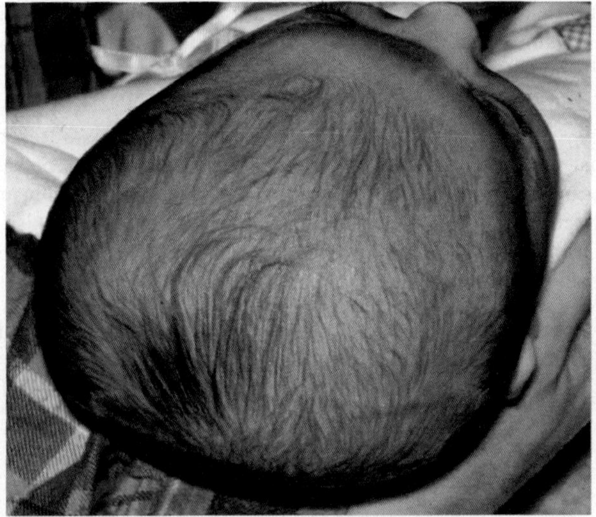

Figure 22

(A) Craniosynostosis
(B) Hydrocephalus
(C) Anencephaly
(D) Positional plagiocephaly
(E) Skull fracture

The answer is D: Positional plagiocephaly. The child in the vignette has plagiocephaly, a physiologic flattening of the head due to positioning. Plagiocephaly and craniosynostosis are easily confused and can be differentiated with a thorough physical examination. Plagiocephaly is a deformation of head shape that often occurs when an infant is left to lie on his back; however, the sutures remain open and unfused. **(A)** Craniosynostosis is defined as premature closure of the cranial sutures with prominent bony ridges at the site of the closure and skull elongation in the axis parallel to the fused suture. When diagnosing positional plagiocephaly, reassurance can be given that this condition usually resolves on its own as the child grows. If the malposition is significant, a helmet may be considered to help encourage proper skull growth. Therapy for most types of craniosynostosis is surgical management to ensure proper brain growth.

(B) Hydrocephalus is an abnormal accumulation of cerebrospinal fluid in the ventricles causing ventriculomegaly. The signs and symptoms of hydrocephalus in an infant include a bulging fontanelle, increased sleepiness, and enlarging head circumference. **(C)** Anencephaly is a malformation of the anterior spinal cord causing defects in brain development. This condition is not compatible with life and patients are born severely disfigured or stillborn. **(E)** A skull fracture usually presents after trauma with bruising and a possible bony depression felt on physical examination.

---

94 A 14-year-old boy comes to the office with complaints of fever, sore throat, and swollen neck glands. On physical examination, he has tonsillar hypertrophy with exudates and a palpable spleen 3 cm below the costal margin.

Of the following, which is most appropriate regarding anticipatory guidance for this patient and family?

(A) Avoid contact sports until symptoms and splenomegaly resolve
(B) Complete bedrest for 12 weeks
(C) Return to school without restriction following treatment for 24 hours
(D) Monitor for hematuria
(E) Amoxicillin for 10 days

The answer is A: **Avoid contact sports until symptoms and splenomegaly resolve.** The combination of symptoms and physical examination findings described in the vignette is consistent with infectious mononucleosis, a viral illness caused by an infection with Epstein-Barr virus (EBV). The typical presentation is that of fever, sore throat, malaise, headache, abdominal pain, and myalgia. Treatment of mononucleosis syndrome is supportive and includes proper hydration and rest; **(B)** however, complete bedrest for extended periods of time is not necessary. The illness typically lasts 2 to 4 weeks, but significant fatigue may last up to 6 weeks in uncomplicated patients. Splenic rupture is the most feared complication, and generally occurs secondary to blunt abdominal trauma in a patient with an enlarged spleen. Accordingly, children with EBV should be kept out of sports for at least 3 to 6 weeks and until the splenomegaly has completely resolved on physical examination.

(E) Antibiotic therapy is not indicated for a viral infection. When administered to patients with EBV infection can cause a diffuse maculopapular eruption. **(C)** Patients with streptococcal pharyngitis may return to school after 24 hours of antibiotic therapy and symptom improvement. Patients with EBV infection may return to school 24 hours after the resolution of fever and with improvement in fatigue. **(D)** Patients with EBV are not at increased risk for developing postinfectious glomerulonephritis.

---

95 A 1-month-old newborn comes to clinic for her first visit. Her mother reports that she was born full term by vaginal delivery and the neonatal period was unremarkable except she needed to stay in the nursery for 5 extra days for phototherapy. Her birth weight was 7 lb 6 oz (3.3 kg).

She reports that the girl has been difficult to rouse for feeds and she only takes 1½ oz of formula every 2 to 3 hours. She also states that the girl breathes noisily and often seems to stop breathing for several seconds at a time. She has a hard, formed stool every 3 to 4 days. On examination, her temperature is 35.5°C, heart rate is 120 beats/minute, and respiratory rate is 32 breaths/minute. Her weight is 3.45 kg. Review of the newborn screen thyroid testing results suggests the diagnosis.

Of the following, what is the most likely mechanism for this infant's clinical findings?

(A) Thyroid dysgenesis
(B) Inborn error in thyroxine synthesis
(C) Maternal thyrotropin-receptor antagonist
(D) Iodine deficiency
(E) Excessive secretion of thyroid hormone

The answer is A: Thyroid dysgenesis. The infant in the vignette has congenital hypothyroidism and exhibits signs and symptoms consistent with decreased levels of thyroid hormone, such as failure to thrive, difficulty feeding, prolonged hyperbilirubinemia, and constipation. If left untreated, this disorder can lead to significant delays in both physical and mental development. Infants with congenital hypothyroidism may be asymptomatic at birth secondary to moderate transplacental transport of maternal thyroxine. The newborn screening program has greatly increased detection and thus decreased the irreversible consequences of long-term congenital hypothyroidism.

(A) Thyroid dysgenesis secondary to aplasia, hypoplasia, or ectopic gland accounts for a large majority of infants born with congenital hypothyroidism. **(B, C)** The remaining causes include inborn errors in thyroxine synthesis and transplacental passage of maternal thyrotropin-receptor antagonists. **(D)** Iodine deficiency is a significant cause of primary hypothyroidism in developing countries; however, this cause is uncommon in congenital hypothyroidism. **(E)** Excessive secretion of thyroid hormone would lead to hyperthyroidism and would not be consistent with the clinical findings described in the vignette.

96 A 12-year-old girl is followed as an outpatient for chronic abdominal pain. Her pain is intermittent multiple times throughout the week. She denies vomiting and has daily stools that are normal in consistency. She has a good appetite, is growing well, and denies any recent weight loss. She has not been able to identify any triggers for her pain and she denies symptoms associated with food. Her parents report that their daughter is an A student, and involved in many activities after school. They describe her as anxious and a perfectionist.

Of the following, what is the next best step to treat this patient's most likely condition?

(A) Acetaminophen with codeine as needed for pain
(B) Ibuprofen as needed for pain
(C) Stress reduction education
(D) Proton pump inhibitor
(E) Antacid therapy

The answer is C: Stress reduction education. Functional abdominal pain is a common finding in pediatric patients and is a diagnosis of exclusion. The physician must screen carefully for any worrisome symptoms that would prompt more aggressive evaluation. Concerning symptoms include weight loss, dysphagia, prolonged diarrhea, hematochezia, hematemesis, anemia, delayed growth, delayed puberty, arthritis, pain that awakens the child from sleep, and unexplained fever or rash. In the absence of any of these more concerning symptoms, a diagnosis of functional abdominal pain can be considered. Functional abdominal pain is a subacute condition that has been present for greater than 3 months. It presents most commonly in children 6 to 14 years old and often occurs in stressed individuals. Functional abdominal pain is not consistent with malingering. Functional abdominal pain is challenging to treat. It is important to educate the family that the child's pain is real, but that there is not an organic, treatable cause within the gastrointestinal tract. Treatment options include supportive counseling and stress reduction techniques.

(A, B, D, E) Acetaminophen, ibuprofen, proton pump therapy, and antacid therapy are unlikely to benefit the patient in the vignette without any symptoms of gastroesophageal reflux, and without an identifiable cause to the pain itself.

97 A 4-month-old girl is seen in clinic. She was born to a G1P0 woman with adequate prenatal care without reported complications. Her mother states the baby's left eye has yellow crusted discharge on occasion and often it seems she is crying from that eye. On examination, she is a healthy 4-month-old infant with mild tear production on the left. She has a symmetric red reflex and her conjunctivae are clear and without injection.

Of the following, what is the best advice to give her mother?

(A) She should massage the nasolacrimal region with a warm cloth
(B) She should use erythromycin ointment for 1 week
(C) She should take the baby emergently to an ophthalmologist
(D) She should place gloves on her daughter's hands so she cannot scratch her face or eye
(E) She should change to a more hydrolyzed formula

The answer is A: She should massage the nasolacrimal region with a warm cloth. The baby described in the vignette has nasolacrimal duct obstruction. The initial management for this is to have parents perform gentle massage of the nasolacrimal region and wipe away any crusted discharge. **(B)** There is a slight risk of infection and if patients develop excessive purulent drainage or conjunctival injection then antibiotic therapy should be initiated.

First-line therapy for bacterial conjunctivitis is erythromycin ointment. **(C)** This is not an ophthalmologic emergency; however, if the duct does not open by 1 year of age, then the child should be referred to ophthalmology for possible surgical dilation of the nasolacrimal duct. **(D)** Mittens are not recommended as infants prefer to soothe themselves by sucking on their hands and the baby in the vignette is not presenting as if she has a corneal abrasion. A corneal abrasion would present with pain, crying, and increased fussiness. **(E)** A more hydrolyzed formula should be used in infants with milk protein allergy which would present with more systemic signs than described in the vignette, including rash, emesis, diarrhea or constipation with blood streaked stools, and failure to thrive.

98 The mother of a healthy 11-year-old boy seeks guidance regarding her son's school performance. His teacher notes that he is easily distracted and has a hard time keeping up and completing homework assignments. At home, he has difficulty paying attention, completing chores, and is constantly on the move. His physical examination is unremarkable.

Of the following, what is the next best step in the management of this patient?

(A) Refer to a developmental specialist
(B) Begin therapy with a tricyclic antidepressant
(C) Order thyroid function testing
(D) Distribute parent and teacher questionnaires
(E) Obtain a diet history

The answer is D: Distribute parent and teacher questionnaires. The patient in the vignette displays behaviors consistent with attention-deficit hyperactivity disorder (ADHD). ADHD is one of the most common chronic health problems affecting school-aged children and is characterized by problems with inattention, impulse control, and motor hyperactivity. The first step in making an appropriate diagnosis of ADHD involves careful history-taking in particular with regard to other complicating conditions or situations that may cloud the clinical picture. An assessment should be made as to whether the child is in under any unusual social stress at school or at home, suffers from a sleep or mood disorder, is involved in some sort of substance abuse, or has a learning disability, such as dyslexia. Questionnaires should be distributed to parents and teachers to confirm that the behaviors are present in separate locations. **(A)** Treatment for ADHD includes both pharmacologic and behavioral medication therapies. First-line pharmacologic treatment agents for ADHD are psychostimulants, including methylphenidates and dextroamphetamines.

(B) While tricyclic antidepressant medication may play a role in pharmacotherapy for ADHD, they are not first-line treatment options and should not be started prior to confirming a diagnosis with questionnaires. **(C)** While symptoms of hyperthyroidism can mimic ADHD, additional associated findings include tachycardia, weight loss, and temperature instability. **(E)** Dietary history, especially excessive caffeine, sugar, or chocolate intake play little if any role in the diagnosis of ADHD.

99 An 18-month-old girl presents to the emergency department after her 5-year-old brother hit her in the arm with a foam football. Upper extremity radiographic findings reveal a radial comminuted fracture. On physical examination, in addition to the deformity of her upper extremity she is noted to have blue sclera. Her mother asks about what the future will hold for her child.

Of the following, what is she at most risk to develop?

(A) Renal failure
(B) Epilepsy
(C) Hearing loss
(D) Blindness
(E) Mental retardation

The answer is C: Hearing loss. The child described in the vignette has osteogenesis imperfecta (OI). OI is commonly divided into four types of inheritable disorders all with variable abnormal synthesis in type 1 collagen and therefore result in brittle bones secondary to poor bone matrix. The autosomal dominant forms (types 1 and 4) are often milder while autosomal recessive forms (types 2 and 3) are more severe and can be fatal. **(A, C, D, E)** Children with OI have normal intelligence and vision and are not at increased risk for seizures nor renal disease. However, secondary to poor bone composition, they are at risk for hearing loss, delayed dental eruption, and weak teeth as well as ligamentous abnormalities.

100 A 15-year-old girl presents to an urgent care center for fatigue on a hot July day. She has been with her father for the past 2 days and at an outdoor water park with her older cousins. She denies fevers, dizziness, vomiting, diarrhea, cough, chest pain, or palpitations. Her vital signs reveal a temperature of 37.5°C, heart rate of 120 beats per minute, and a BP of 100/70 mmHg. Her examination is significant for dry lips, tachycardia, 2+ pulses throughout, and capillary refill less than 2 seconds. On further questioning, she denies taking any drugs or over-the-counter medications.

Of the following, which is the most likely explanation for this patient's tachycardia?

(A) Cocaine
(B) Thyroid hormone dysfunction
(C) Pheochromocytoma
(D) Dehydration
(E) Supraventricular tachycardia (SVT)

The answer is D: Dehydration. The most likely explanation for the patient in the vignette's fatigue, dry lips, and tachycardia is moderate dehydration. Children are at risk for dehydration if their losses are not adequately replaced. Increased insensible water losses occur during the summer months when children are active outdoors without taking the time to properly hydrate. Moderately dehydrated patients will be tachycardic and normotensive. Once the dehydration becomes severe, patients are at risk for hypotension and hypovolemic shock. **(A)** Cocaine, amphetamine, and other sympathomimetics can cause tachycardia; however, patients will typically also have other symptoms such as hypertension, hyperthermia, mydriasis, and diaphoresis. **(B, C)** Endocrinopathies, such as hyperthyroidism and pheochromocytoma, can also cause tachycardia, but are less likely for the patient in the vignette without any other symptomatology. **(E)** Patients with SVT will present with chest pain, palpitations, syncope, and dizziness.

Figure 1-1 Chung EK, Atkinson-McEvoy LR, Boom JA, et al. *Visual Diagnosis and Treatment in Pediatrics*. 2nd ed. Philadelphia, PA: Lippincott Williams & Wilkins; 2010.

Figure 1-2 Fleisher GR, Ludwig W, Baskin MN. *Atlas of Pediatric Emergency Medicine*. Philadelphia, PA: Lippincott Williams & Wilkins; 2004.

Figure 1-3 Fleisher GR, Ludwig W, Baskin MN. *Atlas of Pediatric Emergency Medicine*. Philadelphia, PA: Lippincott Williams & Wilkins; 2004.

Figure 1-4 Modified with permission from Marshall WA, Tanner JM. Variations in patterns of pubertal changes in girls. *Arch Dis Child*. 1969;44:291-303; Root AW. Endocrinology of puberty: 1. Normal sexual maturation. *J Pediatr*. 1973;83:1-19.

Figure 1-5 Fleisher GR, Ludwig S. *Textbook of Pediatric Emergency Medicine*. 6th ed. Philadelphia, PA: Lippincott Williams & Wilkins; 2010.

Figure 1-6 Chung EK, Atkinson-McEvoy LR, Boom JA, et al. *Visual Diagnosis and Treatment in Pediatrics*. 2nd ed. Philadelphia, PA: Lippincott Williams & Wilkins; 2010.

Figure 2-1 MacDonald MG, Seshia MMK, Mullett MD. *Avery's Neonatology Pathophysiology & Management of the Newborn*. 6th ed. Philadelphia, PA: Lippincott Williams & Wilkins; 2005.

Figure 2-2 MacDonald MG, Seshia MMK, Mullett MD. *Avery's Neonatology Pathophysiology & Management of the Newborn*. 6th ed. Philadelphia, PA: Lippincott Williams & Wilkins; 2005.

Figure 2-3 Frymoyer JW, Wiesel SW. *The Adult and Pediatric Spine*. Philadelphia, PA: Lippincott Williams & Wilkins; 2004.

Figure 2-4 Eisenberg RL. *An Atlas of Differential Diagnosis*. 4th ed. Philadelphia, PA: Lippincott Williams & Wilkins; 2003.

Figure 2-5 Chung EK, Atkinson-McEvoy LR, Boom JA, et al. *Visual Diagnosis and Treatment in Pediatrics*. 2nd ed. Philadelphia, PA: Lippincott Williams & Wilkins; 2010.

Figure 2-6 Mulholland MW, Lillemoe KD, Doherty GM, et al. *Greenfield's Surgery Scientific Principles and Practice*. 4th ed. Philadelphia, PA: Lippincott Williams & Wilkins; 2006.

Figure 2-7 Chung EK, Atkinson-McEvoy LR, Boom JA, et al. *Visual Diagnosis and Treatment in Pediatrics*. 2nd ed. Philadelphia, PA: Lippincott Williams & Wilkins; 2010.

Figure 2-8 Avery GB, Fletcher MA, MacDonald MG. *Neonatology: Pathophysiology and Management of the Newborn*. 5th ed. Philadelphia, PA: Lippincott Williams & Wilkins; 1999.

Figure 2-9 Fleisher GR, Ludwig S, Baskin MN. *Atlas of Pediatric Emergency Medicine*. Philadelphia, PA: Lippincott Williams & Wilkins; 2004.

Figure 2-10 Chung EK, Atkinson-McEvoy LR, Boom JA, et al. *Visual Diagnosis and Treatment in Pediatrics*. 2nd ed. Philadelphia, PA: Lippincott Williams & Wilkins; 2010.

Figure 2-11 Fleisher GR, Ludwig S. *Textbook of Pediatric Emergency Medicine*. 6th ed. Philadelphia, PA: Lippincott Williams & Wilkins; 2010.

Figure 2-12 Pillitteri A. *Maternal and Child Nursing*. 4th ed. Philadelphia, PA: Lippincott Williams & Wilkins; 2003.

Figure 3-1 Klossner NJ, Hatfield NT. *Introductory Maternity and Pediatric Nursing*. 2nd ed. Philadelphia, PA: Lippincott Williams & Wilkins; 2009.

Figure 3-2 Cohen BJ, Wood DL. *Memmler's the Human Body in Health and Disease*. 10th ed. Baltimore, MD: Lippincott Williams & Wilkins; 2004.

Figure 4-1 Frymoyer JW, Wiesel SW. *The Adult and Pediatric Spine*. Philadelphia, PA: Lippincott Williams & Wilkins; 2004.

Figure 4-2 Fleisher GR, Ludwig S, Baskin MN. *Atlas of Pediatric Emergency Medicine*. Philadelphia, PA: Lippincott Williams & Wilkins; 2004.

Figure 4-3 Sweet RL, Gibbs RS. *Atlas of Infectious Diseases of the Female Genital Tract*. Philadelphia, PA: Lippincott Williams & Wilkins; 2005.

Figure 5-1 Klossner NJ, Hatfield NT. *Introductory Maternity and Pediatric Nursing*. 2nd ed. Philadelphia, PA: Lippincott Williams & Wilkins; 2009.

Figure 5-2 Chung EK, Atkinson-McEvoy LR, Boom JA, et al. *Visual Diagnosis and Treatment in Pediatrics*. 2nd ed. Philadelphia, PA: Lippincott Williams & Wilkins; 2010.

Figure 5-3 MacDonald MG, Seshia MMK, Mullett MD. *Avery's Neonatology Pathophysiology & Management of the Newborn*. 6th ed. Philadelphia, PA: Lippincott Williams & Wilkins; 2005.

Figure 5-4 McConnell TH. *The Nature of Disease: Pathology for the Health Professions*. Philadelphia, PA: Lippincott Williams & Wilkins; 2007.

Figure 5-5 Chung EK, Atkinson-McEvoy LR, Boom JA, et al. *Visual Diagnosis and Treatment in Pediatrics*. 2nd ed. Philadelphia, PA: Lippincott Williams & Wilkins; 2010.

Figure 6-1 Smeltzer SC, Bare BG, Hinkle JL, et al. *Brunner and Suddarth's Textbook of Medical Surgical Nursing*. 12th ed. Philadelphia, PA: Lippincott Williams & Wilkins; 2009.

Figure 6-2 Harwood-Nuss A, Wolfson AB, Linden CH, et al. *The Clinical Practice of Emergency Medicine*. 3rd ed. Philadelphia, PA: Lippincott Williams & Wilkins; 2001.

Figure 6-3 Smeltzer SC, Bare BG, Hinkle JL, et al. *Brunner and Suddarth's Textbook of Medical Surgical Nursing*. 12th ed. Philadelphia, PA: Lippincott Williams & Wilkins; 2009.

Figure 6-4 Schwartz MW. *The 5-Minute Pediatric Consult*. 6th ed. Philadelphia, PA: Lippincott Williams & Wilkins; 2012.

Figure 6-5 Gold DH, Weingeist TA. *Color Atlas of the Eye in Systemic Disease*. Baltimore, MD: Lippincott Williams & Wilkins; 2001.

Figure 6-6 Tasman W, Jaeger E. *The Wills Eye Hospital Atlas of Clinical Ophthalmology*. 2nd ed. Philadelphia, PA: Lippincott Williams & Wilkins; 2001.

Figure 6-8 Eisenberg RL. *An Atlas of Differential Diagnosis*. 4th ed. Philadelphia, PA: Lippincott Williams & Wilkins; 2003.

Figure 6-10 Berg D, Worzala K. *Atlas of Adult Physical Diagnosis*. Philadelphia, PA: Lippincott Williams & Wilkins; 2006.

Figure 6-11 Berg D, Worzala K. *Atlas of Adult Physical Diagnosis*. Philadelphia, PA: Lippincott Williams & Wilkins; 2006.

Figure 6-13 Baim DS. *Grossman's Cardiac Catheterization, Angiography, and Intervention*. 7th ed. Philadelphia, PA: Lippincott Williams & Wilkins; 2006.

Figure 6-14 Porth CM. *Essentials of Pathophysiology Concepts of Altered Health States*. 2nd ed. Philadelphia, PA: Lippincott Williams & Wilkins; 2007.

Figure 6-15 Sadler T. *Langman's Medical Embryology*. 9th ed. Baltimore, MD: Lippincott Williams & Wilkins; 2003.

Figure 6-16 Harwood-Nuss A, Wolfson AB, Linden CH, et al. *The Clinical Practice of Emergency Medicine*. 3rd ed. Philadelphia, PA: Lippincott Williams & Wilkins; 2001.

Figure 6-17 Fleisher GR, Ludwig S, Baskin MN. *Atlas of Pediatric Emergency Medicine*. 6th ed. Philadelphia, PA: Lippincott Williams & Wilkins; 2010.

Figure 6-19 Nixon JV, Alpert JS, Aurigemma GP, et al. *The AHA Clinical Cardiac Consult*. 3rd ed. Philadelphia, PA: Lippincott Williams & Wilkins; 2011.

Figure 6-20 Harwood-Nuss A, Wolfson AB, Linden CH, et al. *The Clinical Practice of Emergency Medicine*. 3rd ed. Philadelphia, PA: Lippincott Williams & Wilkins; 2001.

Figure 6-21 Menkes JH, Sarnat HB, Maria BL. *Child Neurology*. 7th ed. Philadelphia, PA: Lippincott Williams & Wilkins; 2005.

Figure 7-1 Daffner RH. *Clinical Radiology: The Essentials*. 3rd ed. Philadelphia, PA: Lippincott Williams & Wilkins; 2007.

Figure 7-2 Chung EK, Atkinson-McEvoy LR, Boom JA, et al. *Visual Diagnosis and Treatment in Pediatrics*. 2nd ed. Philadelphia, PA: Lippincott Williams & Wilkins; 2010.

Figure 7-3 Fleisher GR, Ludwig S. *Textbook of Pediatric Emergency Medicine*. 6th ed. Philadelphia, PA: Lippincott Williams & Wilkins; 2010.

Figure 7-4 Chung EK, Atkinson-McEvoy LR, Boom JA, et al. *Visual Diagnosis and Treatment in Pediatrics*. 2nd ed. Philadelphia, PA: Lippincott Williams & Wilkins; 2010.

Figure 7-5 Mulholland MW, Lillemoe KD, Doherty GM, et al. *Greenfield's Surgery: Scientific Principles and Practice*. 4th ed. Philadelphia, PA: Lippincott Williams & Wilkins; 2006.

Figure 7-6 Mulholland MW, Lillemoe KD, Doherty GM, et al. *Greenfield's Surgery: Scientific Principles and Practice*. 4th ed. Philadelphia, PA: Lippincott Williams & Wilkins; 2006.

Figure 7-7 Mulholland MW, Lillemoe KD, Doherty GM, et al. *Greenfield's Surgery: Scientific Principles and Practice*. 4th ed. Philadelphia, PA: Lippincott Williams & Wilkins; 2006.

Figure 7-8 Fleisher GR, Ludwig W, Baskin MN. *Atlas of Pediatric Emergency Medicine*. Philadelphia, PA: Lippincott Williams & Wilkins; 2004.

Figure 7-9 Fleisher GR, Ludwig W, Baskin MN. *Atlas of Pediatric Emergency Medicine*. Philadelphia, PA: Lippincott Williams & Wilkins; 2004.

Figure 7-10 MacDonald MG, Seshia MMK, Mullett MD. *Avery's Neonatology Pathophysiology & Management of the Newborn*. 6th ed. Philadelphia, PA: Lippincott Williams & Wilkins; 2005.

Figure 7-11 Eisenberg RL. *An Atlas of Differential Diagnosis*. 4th ed. Philadelphia, PA: Lippincott Williams & Wilkins; 2003.

Figure 7-12 Goodheart HP. *Goodheart's Photoguide of Common Skin Disorders*. 2nd ed. Philadelphia, PA: Lippincott Williams & Wilkins; 2003.

Figure 7-13 Adapted with permission from Shamberger RC. Chest wall deformities. In: Shields TW, ed. *General Thoracic Surgery*. 4th ed. Baltimore, MD: Williams & Wilkins; 1994:529-557.

Figure 8-1 Sweet RL, Gibbs RS. *Atlas of Infectious Diseases of the Female Genital Tract*. Philadelphia, PA: Lippincott Williams & Wilkins; 2005.

Figure 8-2 Blackbourne LH. *Advanced Surgical Recall*. 2nd ed. Baltimore, MD: Lippincott Williams & Wilkins; 2004.

Figure 8-3 Chung EK, Atkinson-McEvoy LR, Boom JA, et al. *Visual Diagnosis and Treatment in Pediatrics*. 2nd ed. Philadelphia, PA: Lippincott Williams & Wilkins; 2010.

Figure 8-4 McConnell TH. *The Nature of Disease: Pathology for the Health Professions*. Philadelphia, PA: Lippincott Williams & Wilkins; 2007.

Figure 8-5 Goodheart HP. *Goodheart's Photoguide of Common Skin Disorders*. 2nd ed. Philadelphia, PA: Lippincott Williams & Wilkins; 2003.

Figure 9-1 Becker KL, Bilezikian JP, Brenner WJ, et al. *Principles and Practice of Endocrinology and Metabolism*. 3rd ed. Philadelphia, PA: Lippincott Williams & Wilkins; 2001.

Figure 10-1 Developed by the National Center for Health Statistics in Collaboration with the National Center for Chronic Disease Prevention and Health Promotion (2000). http://www.cdc.gov/growthcharts.

Figure 10-2 Campbell WW. *DeJong's The Neurologic Examination*. 6th ed. Philadelphia, PA: Lippincott Williams & Wilkins; 2005.

Figure 10-3 Fleisher GR, Ludwig S. *Textbook of Pediatric Emergency Medicine*. 6th ed. Philadelphia, PA: Lippincott Williams & Wilkins; 2010.

Figure 10-4 Becker KL, Bilezikian JP, Brenner WJ, et al. *Principles and Practice of Endocrinology and Metabolism*. 3rd ed. Philadelphia, PA: Lippincott Williams & Wilkins; 2001.

Figure 10-5 Pillitteri, A. *Maternal and Child Nursing*. 4th ed. Philadelphia, PA: Lippincott, Williams & Wilkins; 2003.

Figure 10-6 Pillitteri, A. *Maternal and Child Nursing*. 4th ed. Philadelphia, PA: Lippincott, Williams & Wilkins; 2003.

Figure 10-7 Becker KL, Bilezikian JP, Brenner WJ, et al. *Principles and Practice of Endocrinology and Metabolism*. 3rd ed. Philadelphia, PA: Lippincott Williams & Wilkins; 2001.

Figure 10-8 Marino BS, Fine KS. *Blueprints Pediatrics*. 5th ed. Philadelphia, PA: Lippincott Williams & Wilkins; 2009.

Figure 10-9 Developed by the National Center for Health Statistics in Collaboration with the National Center for Chronic Disease Prevention and Health Promotion (2000). http://www.cdc.gov/growthcharts.

Figure 10-10: Bickley LS, Szilagyi P. *Bates' Guide to Physical Examination and History Taking*. 8th ed. Philadelphia, PA: Lippincott Williams & Wilkins; 2003.

Figure 10-11 Eisenberg RL. *An Atlas of Differential Diagnosis*. 4th ed. Philadelphia, PA: Lippincott Williams & Wilkins; 2003.

Figure 11-1 Fleisher GR, Ludwig W, Baskin MN. *Atlas of Pediatric Emergency Medicine*. Philadelphia, PA: Lippincott Williams & Wilkins; 2004.

Figure 11-2 Goodheart HP. *Goodheart's Photoguide of Common Skin Disorders*. 2nd ed. Philadelphia, PA: Lippincott Williams & Wilkins; 2003.

Figure 11-3 Goodheart HP. *Goodheart's Photoguide of Common Skin Disorders*. 2nd ed. Philadelphia, PA: Lippincott Williams & Wilkins; 2003.

Figure 11-4 Chung EK, Atkinson-McEvoy LR, Boom JA, et al. *Visual Diagnosis and Treatment in Pediatrics*. 2nd ed. Philadelphia, PA: Lippincott Williams & Wilkins; 2010.

Figure 11-5 Chung EK, Atkinson-McEvoy LR, Boom JA, et al. *Visual Diagnosis and Treatment in Pediatrics*. 2nd ed. Philadelphia, PA: Lippincott Williams & Wilkins; 2010.

Figure 11-6 Chung EK, Atkinson-McEvoy LR, Boom JA, et al. *Visual Diagnosis and Treatment in Pediatrics*. 2nd ed. Philadelphia, PA: Lippincott Williams & Wilkins; 2010.

Figure 11-7 Goodheart HP. *Goodheart's Photoguide of Common Skin Disorders*. 2nd ed. Philadelphia, PA: Lippincott Williams & Wilkins; 2003.

Figure 11-8 Chung EK, Atkinson-McEvoy LR, Boom JA, et al. *Visual Diagnosis and Treatment in Pediatrics*. 2nd ed. Philadelphia, PA: Lippincott Williams & Wilkins; 2010.

Figure 11-9 Sauer GC, Hall JC. *Manual of Skin Diseases*, 7th ed. Philadelphia, PA: Lippincott-Raven; 1996.

Figure 11-10 Goodheart HP. *Goodheart's Photoguide of Common Skin Disorders*. 2nd ed. Philadelphia, PA: Lippincott Williams & Wilkins; 2003.

Figure 11-11 Goodheart HP. *Goodheart's Photoguide of Common Skin Disorders*. 2nd ed. Philadelphia, PA: Lippincott Williams & Wilkins; 2003.

Figure 11-12 Chung EK, Atkinson-McEvoy LR, Boom JA, et al. *Visual Diagnosis and Treatment in Pediatrics*. 2nd ed. Philadelphia, PA: Lippincott Williams & Wilkins; 2010.

Figure 11-13 Sauer GC. *Manual of Skin Diseases*. 5th ed. Philadelphia, PA: JB Lippincott; 1985.

Figure 11-14 Fleisher GR, Ludwig W, Baskin MN. *Atlas of Pediatric Emergency Medicine*. Philadelphia, PA: Lippincott Williams & Wilkins; 2004.

Figure 11-15 *Stedman's Medical Dictionary*. 27th ed. Philadelphia, PA: Lippincott Williams & Wilkins; 2008.

Figure 11-16 Neville B, Damm DD, White DK, et al. *Color Atlas of Clinical Oral Pathology*. Philadelphia, PA: Lea & Febiger; 1991.

Figure 11-17 Chung EK, Atkinson-McEvoy LR, Boom JA, et al. *Visual Diagnosis and Treatment in Pediatrics*. 2nd ed. Philadelphia, PA: Lippincott Williams & Wilkins; 2010.

Figure 11-18 Goodheart HP. *Goodheart's Photoguide of Common Skin Disorders*. 2nd ed. Philadelphia, PA: Lippincott Williams & Wilkins; 2003.

Figure 11-19 Goodheart HP. *Goodheart's Photoguide of Common Skin Disorders*. 2nd ed. Philadelphia, PA: Lippincott Williams & Wilkins; 2003.

Figure 11-20 Fleisher GR, Ludwig W, Baskin MN. *Atlas of Pediatric Emergency Medicine*. Philadelphia, PA: Lippincott Williams & Wilkins; 2004.

Figure 11-21 Goodheart HP. *Goodheart's Photoguide of Common Skin Disorders*. 2nd ed. Philadelphia, PA: Lippincott Williams & Wilkins; 2003.

Figure 12-1 Goodheart HP. *Goodheart's Photoguide of Common Skin Disorders*. 2nd ed. Philadelphia, PA: Lippincott Williams & Wilkins; 2003.

Figure 12-2 Engleberg NC, Dermody T, DiRita V. *Schaecter's Mechanisms of Microbial Disease*. 4th ed. Baltimore, MD: Lippincott Williams & Wilkins; 2007.

Figure 12-3 Eisenberg RL. *An Atlas of Differential Diagnosis*. 4th ed. Philadelphia, PA: Lippincott Williams & Wilkins; 2003.

Figure 13-1 Berg D, Worzala K. *Atlas of Adult Physical Diagnosis*. Philadelphia, PA: Lippincott Williams & Wilkins; 2006.

Figure 13-2 Fleisher GR, Ludwig W, Baskin MN. *Atlas of Pediatric Emergency Medicine*. Philadelphia, PA: Lippincott Williams & Wilkins; 2004.

Figure 13-3 Chung EK, Atkinson-McEvoy LR, Boom JA, et al. *Visual Diagnosis and Treatment in Pediatrics*. 2nd ed. Philadelphia, PA: Lippincott Williams & Wilkins; 2010.

Figure 13-4 Goodheart HP. *A Photoguide of Common Skin Disorders: Diagnosis and Management*. Baltimore, MD: Lippincott Williams & Wilkins; 1999.

Figure 13-5 Goodheart HP. *A Photoguide of Common Skin Disorders: Diagnosis and Management*. Baltimore, MD: Lippincott Williams & Wilkins; 1999.

Figure 13-6 Fleisher GR, Ludwig S. *Textbook of Pediatric Emergency Medicine*. 6th ed. Philadelphia, PA: Lippincott Williams & Wilkins; 2010.

Figure 13-7 Fleisher GR, Ludwig W, Baskin MN. *Atlas of Pediatric Emergency Medicine*. Philadelphia, PA: Lippincott Williams & Wilkins; 2004.

Figure 13-8 Fleisher GR, Ludwig W, Baskin MN. *Atlas of Pediatric Emergency Medicine*. Philadelphia, PA: Lippincott Williams & Wilkins; 2004.

Figure 13-9 Fleisher GR, Ludwig W, Baskin MN. *Atlas of Pediatric Emergency*

Medicine. Philadelphia, PA: Lippincott Williams & Wilkins; 2004.

Figure 13-10 Fleisher GR, Ludwig S. *Textbook of Pediatric Emergency Medicine*. 6th ed. Philadelphia, PA: Lippincott Williams & Wilkins; 2010.

Figure 13-11 Schwartz MW. *The 5-Minute Pediatric Consult*. 6th ed. Philadelphia, PA: Lippincott Williams & Wilkins; 2012.

Figure 13-12 Klossner NJ, Hatfield NT. *Introductory Maternity and Pediatric Nursing*. 2nd ed. Philadelphia, PA: Lippincott Williams & Wilkins; 2009.

Figure 13-13 Tasman W, Jaeger E. *The Wills Eye Hospital Atlas of Clinical Ophthalmology*. 2nd ed. Philadelphia, PA: Lippincott Williams & Wilkins; 2001.

Figure 14-1 Rubin E, Farber JL. *Pathology*. 3rd ed. Philadelphia, PA: Lippincott Williams & Wilkins; 1999.

Figure 14-2 Fleisher GR, Ludwig W, Baskin MN. *Atlas of Pediatric Emergency Medicine*. Philadelphia, PA: Lippincott Williams & Wilkins; 2004.

Figure 14-3 Goodheart HP. *Goodheart's Photoguide of Common Skin Disorders*. 2nd ed. Philadelphia, PA: Lippincott Williams & Wilkins; 2003.

Figure 14-4 Topol EJ, Califf RM, Prystowsky EN, et al. *Textbook of Cardiovascular Medicine*. 3rd ed. Philadelphia, PA: Lippincott Williams & Wilkins; 2006.

Figure 14-5 Chung EK, Atkinson-McEvoy LR, Boom JA, et al. *Visual Diagnosis and Treatment in Pediatrics*. 2nd ed. Philadelphia, PA: Lippincott Williams & Wilkins; 2010.

Figure 14-6 Rubin R, Strayer DS. *Rubin's Pathology: Clinicopathologic Foundations of Medicine*. 5th ed. Philadelphia, PA: Lippincott Williams & Wilkins; 2008.

Figure 14-7 Yochum TR, Rowe LJ. *Yochum and Rowe's Essentials of Skeletal Radiology*, 3rd ed. Philadelphia, PA: Lippincott Williams & Wilkins; 2004.

Figure 14-8 Yochum TR, Rowe LJ. *Yochum and Rowe's Essentials of Skeletal Radiology*. 3rd ed. Philadelphia, PA: Lippincott Williams & Wilkins; 2004.

Figure 14-9 Lee GR, Foerster LG, Lukens J, et al. *Wintrobe's Clinical Hematology*. 10th ed. Philadelphia, PA: Lippincott Williams & Wilkins; 1998.

Figure 15-1 Goodheart HP. *Goodheart's Photoguide of Common Skin Disorders*. 2nd ed. Philadelphia, PA: Lippincott Williams & Wilkins; 2003.

Figure 15-2 Fleisher GR, Ludwig W, Baskin MN. *Atlas of Pediatric Emergency Medicine*. Philadelphia, PA: Lippincott Williams & Wilkins; 2004.

Figure 15-3 Goodheart HP. *Goodheart's Photoguide of Common Skin Disorders*. 2nd ed. Philadelphia, PA: Lippincott Williams & Wilkins; 2003.

Figure 15-4 Fleisher GR, Ludwig W, Baskin MN. *Atlas of Pediatric Emergency Medicine*. Philadelphia, PA: Lippincott Williams & Wilkins; 2004.

Figure 15-5 Fleisher GR, Ludwig W, Baskin MN. *Atlas of Pediatric Emergency Medicine*. Philadelphia, PA: Lippincott Williams & Wilkins; 2004.

Figure 16-1 MacDonald MG, Seshia MMK, Mullett MD. *Avery's Neonatology Pathophysiology & Management of the Newborn*. 6th ed. Philadelphia, PA: Lippincott Williams & Wilkins; 2005.

Figure 16-2 Becker KL, Bilezikian JP, Brenner WJ, et al. *Principles and Practice of Endocrinology and Metabolism*. 3rd ed. Philadelphia, PA: Lippincott Williams & Wilkins; 2001.

Figure 16-3 Klossner NJ, Hatfield NT. *Introductory Maternity and Pediatric Nursing*. 2nd ed. Philadelphia, PA: Lippincott Williams & Wilkins; 2009.

Figure 16-4 Harvey RA, Ferrier DR. *Lippincott's Illustrated Reviews: Biochemistry*.

5th ed. Baltimore, MD: Lippincott Williams & Wilkins; 2011.

Figure 17-1 Fleisher GR, Ludwig W, Baskin MN. *Atlas of Pediatric Emergency Medicine*. Philadelphia, PA: Lippincott Williams & Wilkins; 2004.

Figure 17-2 Fleisher GR, Ludwig W, Baskin MN. *Atlas of Pediatric Emergency Medicine*. Philadelphia, PA: Lippincott Williams & Wilkins; 2004.

Figure 17-3 Fleisher GR, Ludwig W, Baskin MN. *Atlas of Pediatric Emergency Medicine*. Philadelphia, PA: Lippincott Williams & Wilkins; 2004.

Figure 17-4 Yochum TR, Rowe LJ. *Yochum and Rowe's Essentials of Skeletal Radiology*. 3rd ed. Philadelphia, PA: Lippincott Williams & Wilkins; 2004.

Figure 17-5 Rubin R, Strayer DS. *Rubin's Pathology: Clinicopathologic Foundations of Medicine*. 5th ed. Philadelphia, PA: Lippincott Williams & Wilkins; 2008.

Figure 17-6 Yochum TR, Rowe LJ. *Yochum and Rowe's Essentials of Skeletal Radiology*. 3rd ed. Philadelphia, PA: Lippincott Williams & Wilkins; 2004.

Figure 17-7 Bucholz RW, Heckman JD. *Rockwood & Green's Fractures in Adults*. 5th ed. Philadelphia, PA: Lippincott Williams & Wilkins; 2001.

Figure 17-8 Fleisher GR, Ludwig S. *Textbook of Pediatric Emergency Medicine*. 6th ed. Philadelphia, PA: Lippincott Williams & Wilkins; 2010.

Figure 17-9 Berg D, Worzala K. *Atlas of Adult Physical Diagnosis*. Philadelphia, PA: Lippincott Williams & Wilkins; 2006.

Figure 17-10 Yochum TR, Rowe LJ. *Yochum and Rowe's Essentials of Skeletal Radiology*. 3rd ed. Philadelphia, PA: Lippincott Williams & Wilkins; 2004.

Figure 17-11 Blackbourne LH. *Advanced Surgical Recall*. 2nd ed. Baltimore, MD: Lippincott Williams & Wilkins; 2004.

Figure 17-12 Mulholland MW, Lillemoe KD, Doherty GM, et al. *Greenfield's Surgery: Scientific Principles and Practice*. 4th ed. Philadelphia, PA: Lippincott Williams & Wilkins; 2006.

Figure 17-13 Chung EK, Atkinson-McEvoy LR, Boom JA, et al. *Visual Diagnosis and Treatment in Pediatrics*. 2nd ed. Philadelphia, PA: Lippincott Williams & Wilkins; 2010.

Figure 17-14 Berg D, Worzala K. *Atlas of Adult Physical Diagnosis*. Philadelphia, PA: Lippincott Williams & Wilkins; 2006.

Figure 17-15 Mulholland MW, Lillemoe KD, Doherty GM, et al. *Greenfield's Surgery: Scientific Principles and Practice*. 4th ed. Philadelphia, PA: Lippincott Williams & Wilkins; 2006.

Figure 17-16 Strickland JW, Graham TJ. *Master Techniques in Orthopaedic Surgery: The Hand*. 2nd ed. Philadelphia, PA: Lippincott Williams & Wilkins; 2005.

Figure 17-17 Cohen BJ. *Medical Terminology*. 4th ed. Philadelphia, PA: Lippincott Williams & Wilkins; 2003.

Figure 17-18 Cohen BJ. *Medical Terminology*. 4th ed. Philadelphia, PA: Lippincott Williams & Wilkins; 2003.

Figure 17-19 Yochum TR, Rowe LJ. *Yochum and Rowe's Essentials of Skeletal Radiology*. 3rd ed. Philadelphia, PA: Lippincott Williams & Wilkins; 2004.

Figure 17-20 Goodheart HP. *Goodheart's Photoguide of Common Skin Disorders*. 2nd ed. Philadelphia, PA: Lippincott Williams & Wilkins; 2003.

Figure 1 Daffner RH. *Clinical Radiology: The Essentials*. 3rd ed. Philadelphia, PA: Lippincott Williams & Wilkins; 2007.

Figure 2 Goodheart HP. *Goodheart's Photoguide of Common Skin Disorders*. 2nd ed. Philadelphia, PA: Lippincott Williams & Wilkins; 2003.

Figure 3 McConnell TH. *The Nature of Disease Pathology for the Health Professions.* Philadelphia, PA: Lippincott Williams & Wilkins; 2007.

Figure 4 Anderson SC. *Anderson's Atlas of Hematology.* Philadelphia, PA: Lippincott Williams & Wilkins; 2003.

Figure 5 Menkes JH, Sarnat HB, Maria BL. *Child Neurology.* 7th ed. Philadelphia, PA: Lippincott Williams & Wilkins; 2005.

Figure 6 Rubin R, Strayer DS. *Rubin's Pathology: Clinicopathologic Foundations of Medicine.* 5th ed. Philadelphia, PA: Lippincott Williams & Wilkins; 2008.

Figure 7 Engleberg NC, Dermody T, DiRita V. *Schaecter's Mechanisms of Microbial Disease.* 4th ed. Baltimore, MD: Lippincott Williams & Wilkins; 2007.

Figure 8 Sweet RL, Gibbs RS. *Atlas of Infectious Diseases of the Female Genital Tract.* Philadelphia, PA: Lippincott Williams & Wilkins; 2005.

Figure 9 Goodheart HP. *Goodheart's Photoguide of Common Skin Disorders.* 2nd ed. Philadelphia, PA: Lippincott Williams & Wilkins; 2003.

Figure 10 Nixon JV, Alpert JS, Aurigemma GP, et al. *The AHA Clinical Cardiac Consult.* 3rd ed. Philadelphia, PA: Lippincott Williams & Wilkins; 2011.

Figure 11 Fleisher GR, Ludwig S. *Textbook of Pediatric Emergency Medicine.* 6th ed. Philadelphia, PA: Lippincott Williams & Wilkins; 2010.

Figure 12 MacDonald MG, Seshia MMK, Mullett MD. *Avery's Neonatology Pathophysiology & Management of the Newborn.* 6th ed. Philadelphia, PA: Lippincott Williams & Wilkins; 2005.

Figure 13 Nixon JV, Alpert JS, Aurigemma GP, et al. *The AHA Clinical Cardiac Consult.* 3rd ed. Philadelphia, PA: Lippincott Williams & Wilkins; 2011.

Figure 14 Fleisher GR, Ludwig W, Baskin MN. *Atlas of Pediatric Emergency Medicine.* Philadelphia, PA: Lippincott Williams & Wilkins; 2004.

Figure 15 Fleisher GR, Ludwig W, Baskin MN. *Atlas of Pediatric Emergency Medicine.* Philadelphia, PA: Lippincott Williams & Wilkins; 2004.

Figure 16 Goodheart HP. *Goodheart's Photoguide of Common Skin Disorders.* 2nd ed. Philadelphia, PA: Lippincott Williams & Wilkins; 2003.

Figure 17 *Stedman's Medical Dictionary.* 27th ed. Philadelphia, PA: Lippincott Williams & Wilkins; 2008.

Figure 18 Daffner RH. *Clinical Radiology: The Essentials.* 3rd ed. Philadelphia, PA: Lippincott Williams & Wilkins; 2007.

Figure 19 Porth CM. *Pathophysiology Concepts of Altered Health States.* 7th ed. Philadelphia, PA: Lippincott Williams & Wilkins; 2005.

Figure 20 Fleisher GR, Ludwig S. *Textbook of Pediatric Emergency Medicine.* 6th ed. Philadelphia, PA: Lippincott Williams & Wilkins; 2010.

Figure 21 Avery GB, Fletcher MA, MacDonald MG. *Neonatology: Pathophysiology and Management of the Newborn.* 5th ed. Philadelphia, PA: Lippincott Williams & Wilkins; 1999.

Figure 22 Chung EK, Atkinson-McEvoy LR, Boom JA, et al. *Visual Diagnosis and Treatment in Pediatrics.* 2nd ed. Philadelphia, PA: Lippincott Williams & Wilkins; 2010.

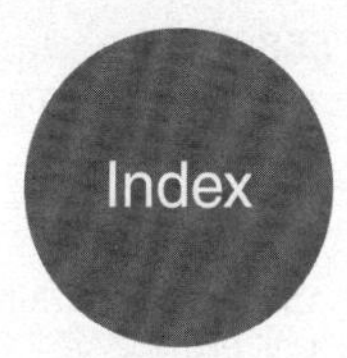

Note: Page numbers followed by *f* indicate figures; those followed by *t* indicate tables.

A

D

E

K

L

M

N

O

Q

R

T

U

V

W